D1548934

HEALTH INFORMATICS

Studies in Health Technology and Informatics

This book series was started in 1990 to promote research conducted under the auspices of the EC programmes' Advanced Informatics in Medicine (AIM) and Biomedical and Health Research (BHR) bioengineering branch. A driving aspect of international health informatics is that telecommunication technology, rehabilitative technology, intelligent home technology and many other components are moving together and form one integrated world of information and communication media. The complete series has been accepted in Medline. Volumes from 2005 onwards are available online.

Series Editors:
Dr. O. Bodenreider, Dr. J.P. Christensen, Prof. G. de Moor, Prof. A. Famili, Dr. U. Fors, Prof. A. Hasman, Prof. E.J.S. Hovenga, Prof. L. Hunter, Dr. I. Iakovidis, Dr. Z. Kolitsi, Mr. O. Le Dour, Dr. A. Lymberis, Prof. J. Mantas, Prof. M.A. Musen, Prof. P.F. Niederer, Prof. A. Pedotti, Prof. O. Rienhoff, Prof. F.H. Roger France, Dr. N. Rossing, Prof. N. Saranummi, Dr. E.R. Siegel and Dr. P. Wilson

Volume 151

Recently published in this series

ISSN 0926-9630

Health Informatics

An Overview

Edited by

Evelyn J.S. Hovenga RN PhD (UNSW) FACHI FACS
Professor and Director, eHealth Education Pty Ltd, Australia

Michael R. Kidd MBBS MD DCCH, DipRACOG, FRACGP, FACHI, FAFPM (Hon), FHKCFP (Hon), FRNZCGP (Hon), MAICD
Executive Dean, Faculty of Health Sciences, Flinders University, Australia

Sebastian Garde Dr. sc. hum., Dipl.-Inform. Med., FACHI
Senior Developer, Ocean Informatics, Düsseldorf, Germany

and

Carola Hullin Lucay Cossio RN, BN (Hons), PhD (Melb. Uni)
Global Health Informatics Consultant, Melbourne, Australia

Amsterdam • Berlin • Tokyo • Washington, DC

ISBN 978-1-60750-092-6 (print)
ISBN 978-1-60750-476-4 (online)
Library of Congress Control Number: 2010920424

Publisher
IOS Press BV
Nieuwe Hemweg 6B
1013 BG Amsterdam
Netherlands
fax: +31 20 687 0019
e-mail: order@iospress.nl

Distributor in the USA and Canada
IOS Press, Inc.
4502 Rachael Manor Drive
Fairfax, VA 22032
USA
fax: +1 703 323 3668
e-mail: iosbooks@iospress.com

Health Informatics
E.J.S. Hovenga et al. (Eds.)
IOS Press, 2010

Foreword

Compared to other fields in biomedicine and in the health sciences, the field of health informatics is still a relatively young one. Health informatics – others may call it also medical informatics – has nevertheless matured considerably. Today, its impact on the quality and efficiency of health care has even become crucial. Because of this development, health care professionals, who are well-educated in health informatics, are urgently needed.

This book, edited by Drs. Evelyn Hovenga, Michael Kidd, Sebastian Garde and Carola Hullin Lucay Cossio, with sections

– setting the scene (introduction),
– basic health informatics concepts,
– supporting clinical practice,
– supporting health care service delivery management,
– supporting clinical and health informatics research, and
– health informatics education

is a broad introduction to the field of health informatics. With contributions of many distinguished authors, it is a valuable resource for health care professionals and health informatics students. In its second edition, new developments in a rapidly changing and expanding field have been considered.

My congratulations go to all, who contributed to this book, in particular to the editors for having composed an attractive overview, and especially to Evelyn Hovenga, the 'spiritus rector', not only for this project.

Prof. Dr. Reinhold HAUX
Peter L. Reichertz Institute for Medical Informatics, Braunschweig and Hannover, Germany
President of IMIA, the International Medical Informatics Association

Preface and Acknowledgements

This text was originally published in Australia in 1996. Since then, the world has changed significantly. The emergence of the Internet and World Wide Web with its enormous possibilities had just begun, standardisation was in its infancy, broadband was unheard of, we had just started thinking about the Y2K bug, supply chain management was more theory than practice, Google wasn't even founded, nor would anybody have had dreams or nightmares about Google Health or Microsoft HealthVault to store your personal health information and make it accessible when needed. To say it with the words of Thomas Friedman [1], since 1996, the world has been flattened in the sense that many people have been empowered significantly and now have a far more equal opportunity to achieve, create, collaborate and compete with each other than used to be the case, in healthcare as well as in any other business.

Thus, this second edition has been extensively reviewed, updated and a number of new topics have been included in order to meet contemporary issues and challenges. The text has a strong focus on health viewed from a computing perspective. It was compiled primarily for health professionals who now require knowledge about how these new technologies of information and communication may be used to enhance their practice. It aims to provide an overview of the health informatics discipline. The contents reflect what we consider are the basics for continuing education purposes and for inclusion into any curriculum which prepares a student for practice in any of the health professional disciplines. It is suitable for use as a basic text in both undergraduate and post graduate curricula. Each chapter can be expanded upon as required. Guidelines for health informatics education are provided in the last few chapters of this text.

This text is not all inclusive or exhaustive; most of the chapters could be expanded individually into a book on its own.

This text deliberately avoids a focus on any one of the health professions. Health care has become more and more integrated between the various sectors ranging from primary care to hospitals, as well as becoming more interdisciplinary between the various health professions. Also there is a trend to empowering the patient to play a more active part in decision making. All this requires clinical information to be available across sectors and across professions and necessitates integrated clinical (computer) systems such as 'professional' or 'clinician' workstations that support the focus on the patient as the centre of care rather than a discipline or departmental focus. Clinical data from multiple sources are integrated and support multiple types of clinical decision making. This also has implications for the language or terminology used and may well influence changes in how individuals practice their profession at the point of care.

The book is divided into six sections, an overview of the discipline, basic health informatics concepts, the application of health informatics supporting clinical practice, health care service delivery management, clinical research and health informatics education. We first present the history of computing in health followed by an overview of the discipline and outline some of the basic principles underlying this health discipline, including the need to balance the technology with our underlying commitment to patient care. In section two we discuss the basic concepts which need to be grasped about computing and explain how these apply to the health professions to best meet the needs as detailed in section 1. The next four sections demonstrate how these new technologies can assist our daily work, in clinical practice, management, education and research enabling us to realize our global e-health vision.

We thank the Spanish language editorial team, Carola Hullin Lucay Cossio, Erika Caballero Muñoz, Lorena Camus, Alejandro Gigoux Múller, Antonio Jose Ibarra Fernandez, and Maria Pilar Marin Villasante who managed the translation process prior to this book's publication by Mediterraneo, Santiago, Chile.

Reference

[1] Friedman T.L. 2006 The world is flat: The globalised world in the twenty-first century. 2nd expanded edition. Penguin Books Ltd., London UK.

Contents

x

Section 5. Supporting Health Informatics and Clinical Research

Section 6. Health Informatics Education

Section 1

Setting the Scene

Health Informatics
E.J.S. Hovenga et al. (Eds.)
IOS Press, 2010
doi:10.3233/978-1-60750-476-4-3

1. History of Health Informatics: A Global Perspective

Branko CESNIK[a] (deceased 2007, edited by Michael R KIDD[1b])
[a]Co-editor of Health Informatics: an overview 1st edition, Past Associate Professor and Director of Medical Informatics, Faculty of Medicine, Monash University, Australia
[b]MBBS, MD, DCCH, DipRACOG, FRACGP, FACHI, FAFPM (Hon), FHKCFP (Hon), FRNZCGP (Hon), MAICD
Executive Dean, Faculty of Health Sciences, Flinders University, Australia

Abstract. In considering a 'history' of Health Informatics it is important to be aware that the discipline encompasses a wide array of activities, products, research and theories. Health Informatics is as much a result of evolution as planned philosophy, having its roots in the histories of information technology and medicine. The process of its growth continues so that today's work is tomorrow's history. A 'historical' discussion of the area is its history to date, a report rather than a summation.

As well as its successes, the history of Health Informatics is populated with visionary promises that have failed to materialise despite the best intentions. For those studying the subject or working in the field, the experiences of others' use of Information Technologies for the betterment of health care can provide a necessary perspective. This chapter starts by noting some of the major events and people that form a technological backdrop to Health Informatics and ends with some thoughts on the future. This chapter gives an educational overview of:

- The history of computing
- The beginnings of the health informatics discipline

Keywords. Medical Informatics, computer systems, history

'Those who cannot remember the past are condemned to repeat it.'
George Santayana (1863-1952), American philosopher, poet

1. History of Computing

While thousands of individuals have been part of the evolution of computing in the last century, some perspective on the history of computing development is useful in understanding the current level of development and sophistication (or lack of it) in today's computing environment.

The desire to represent information in ways that allow real world issues to be more easily managed has been a common pursuit for centuries. As far back as in the 17th century Wilhelm Von Liebnitz was advocating the idea that it might be possible to represent the entire nature of human behaviour in some codified form. This principle

---

[1] Corresponding Author: Michael.Kidd@Flinders.edu.au

still forms the basis on which many software developers, especially in medicine, view coding. That is, if we developed a fine enough coding system, then all things may be classified (not that Herr Liebnitz was in possession of tools that could assist in this desire).

The first example of how such tools might be created and the uses to which they could be put can reliably be ascribed to Charles Babbage in the 19th Century. It is generally agreed that Mr Babbage created the first computer, a mechanical device aimed at solving mathematical problems. The machine never succeeded in functioning as desired and he stumbled from funding source to funding source (Kings, Queens and Heads of State). The issue of whether or not his 'analytical engine' could ever have succeeded is moot, however his machine not only still exists, but has also been recreated in an attempt to settle the argument. It appears that, if accurate enough engineering techniques had been available, his life work could have succeeded.

The above two historical figures highlight the fact that the principles underlying today's use of computers has been around for a very long time. The punch card system devised by Herman Hollerith in the 1890's to manage the United States census data demonstrates the effectiveness of technologies that do not use the microchip capabilities of today.

This system was so successful that it was still being used after World War II. It involved hundreds of workers developing the ability to punch cards and also to pass long needles through trays of such cards to perform data analysis. Even when digital (electronic) computers were developed, punch cards were still used as the major form of data input, as any computer science student of the 50's and 60's can verify. Despite the development of ever increasingly powerful computers over this time, it was not until the end of the 1960's that this technique finally was laid to rest.

2.   The Electronic Computer

The need for information management during World War II spurred the development of electronic computers. The first digital or electronic computer was ENIAC, created in the 1940's. This device occupied a large room and ran on valves with enormous power consumption and remains at the Smithsonian institute as a reminder of the scale of change in this century. Post WWII computers continued to evolve in speed, capacity, sophistication and reliability, they also continued to reduce in size. Due to the specialised environments, space and support needed to run these devices, the concept of mainframe computing evolved.

Mainframe computing implies a central computer which supports users at distance through the provision of 'dumb' terminals. Note that the idea of computing at distance (via a terminal) only occurred in the late 40's and early 50's. This centralised form of computing services supported by an Information Management Service (IMS) remained the norm until the late 60's, early 70's.

In the late 1950's Ledley and Lusted, living in a world of now powerful new computing devices, where among many who recognised the potential of computer-assisted medical decision making. While access, cost, and implementation were seen as limiting the ability to provide such support in a widely available fashion, the belief was evident that increasing computational power could be harnessed to model, assist and enhance health care. While the 'dumb terminal' - mainframe model of computing services was not able to adequately address this desire, the coming years would see the 'personal computer' become a reality, initially as the minicomputer.

The emergence of minicomputers in the late 60's provided what were, in essence, stripped down mainframes with their own storage ability, aimed at supporting a small number of local user and promising a future of 'personal' computing. These were still very expensive but were a major leap forward from the distributed, 'dumb terminal' philosophy of previous decades. So enthusiastic were many of the proponents of minicomputers that advertisements from the 60's and 70's described the desirability for Medical Practitioners to purchase them to improve their office and patient management. The promise that such technologies could so intimately assist health professionals at a personal level remains today. That promise is satisfied more often today than then but disappointment often remains even with current advanced systems.

3.   Microcomputers Arrive

The highly personal availability of computing technologies became more possible with the advent of the microcomputer. The Apple II microcomputer (6502 chip, monochrome display, tape or floppy storage) provided the first real personal computer, Whilst many other microcomputers existed (Tandy, Commodore, Zenith etc) this was the first that encouraged average users to indulge in programming and the production of software on a large scale destined for personal use.

While these machines initially penetrated the home / hobbyist market rather than business, the introduction of the program VISICALC (the first, functional, spreadsheet program) altered the perception of microcomputers and their usefulness. The business world suddenly had a powerful new tool for financial modeling offering a familiar paradigm (an accounting sheet) with the power of microcomputer based technologies behind it. Such applications did not escape the attention of those responsible for the financial management of health care. As for all aspects of society, the personal computer found its way into practice environments, hospital systems, organisations working in epidemiological work and a host of other health related areas.

In 1982 IBM released the IBM PC (640K, cassette or floppy storage, colour display). It appears that IBM did not consider this machine as a serious project and that the explosion of clones, acceptance by business and the massive secondary industry generated by software developers was completely unpredicted. Initial projections were for a few thousand sales. The currently installed base of machines with this architecture is well into the millions.

The release of the Macintosh computer (evolved from the Xerox PARC work and the Apple Lisa) offered a whole new principle in how users could interact with computers. Now called the WIMP interface (Windows, Icons, Mouse and Popdown menus), this was the first practical, commercially available, Graphic User Interface or GUI and its underlying philosophy can be attributed in large part to Douglas Engelbart, the inventor of the mouse as a pointing device.

As these microcomputers became increasingly powerful and popular through the 1980's IMS groups finally started agreeing that these 'toys' should have some access to mainframes, usually if they agreed to behave as dumb terminals. Users also found the need to connect PC's together resulting in the development of Local Area Networks (LANs).

Without an agreed standard for these endeavours we have the current situation with a wide (but reducing) number of ways to link PC's together. LAN structures now communicate with each other forming Wide Area Networks (WAN) with links into mainframe services.

Overall, this progression of increasingly powerful, smaller and faster computing possibilities has resulted in the availability of the 'personal' computer. Ideally, technology should be an additional tool for individuals providing connectivity to resources far greater than personal experience, education or traditional paper based repositories of information could provide.

All of this is possible because of the development of the microchip or integrated circuit, predominantly developed by the companies INTEL and MOTOROLA. These 'chips' are evolving at a rapid pace providing more and more processing power. These 'hardware' advances are not matched by developments in software; processors spend much of their time doing nothing. The widespread adoption of the GUI interface, larger and more sophisticated software creations and the need to enhance the means whereby users interact with the computer means that the hoped for developments of handwriting and speech recognition in a highly interactive graphic environment are now occurring.

4.   Computer Languages - Telling the Computer What To Do

The software programs have evolved along with the hardware base itself, although at differing rates. These languages range from telling the computer what to do at a very low level, such as assembly language, to much more abstracted means of representation provided by Object Orientated Systems, Natural language tools, Artificial Intelligence methodologies and a variety of others. In an inevitable progression, the increased hardware capabilities are used by developers to create more and more sophisticated means of 'communicating' with the computer to manage information in more and more natural ways.

While the above is promising, the actual tools we use on computers today are still in their infancy in many ways. The vast majority of computer human interaction is via the keyboard, itself an unfriendly legacy of the past. The QWERTY keyboard design aims to reduce typing speed so as to decrease the possibility of the letter 'hammers' jamming, despite the fact that such typewriters are now museum pieces.

Health care poses some of the greatest challenges for both the technologies and those seeking to apply them to patient care. Health care often deals with the most abstract of ideas such as 'well', 'pain', 'happy', 'sad'. Health care also generates enormous volumes of information regarding the community and its needs. Thus understanding Health Informatics requires not only familiarity with the technology but, more importantly, insight into the nature in which health care delivery occurs. These questions are not yet answered but Health Informatics lays claim to some of the possible directions and solutions most likely to be of benefit.

5.   Health Informatics - a Discipline

Health Informatics is often described as a new discipline. It has evolved to address the desires to apply and explore the uses of these relatively new tools for the better provision of health care. This is a bold claim with some merit. The successes of the field in living up to the claim have been less than expected and have, at times, disrupted the timely delivery of health care rather than enhanced it. This is not entirely surprising given the accelerating rate of change in technologies and the relatively 'young' nature of a discipline which is now examining itself to clarify its role. Health Informatics began as Medical and Nursing Informatics during the 1970s, a period described by van Bemmel & Shortliffe [1] as undergoing exponential development due to the growing availability of steadily less expensive hardware, more powerful software and the advent of microcomputers.

A gradual change from electronic data processing in health, through the use of informatics in medical care, to health informatics, is discernable from the types of papers presented at the three yearly World Congresses on Medical Informatics (Medinfo), which began in 1974 in Stockholm. The use of computers to support medical decision making, including artificial intelligence, was strong during the 1980s. The linkage of systems emerged in 1989 when multiple disciplines began to work together to develop integrated systems utilising new database technology and the power of networks. This produced synergistic applications where the whole became greater than the sum of its parts. The most popular papers presented at Medinfo'92 in Geneva were those on knowledge based work such as concepts, methodologies, software and other tools, systems and evaluations of systems and experiences [2] These congresses were organised by the International Medical Informatics Association (IMIA), which began as a special interest group of IFIP.

While Health Informatics aims to articulate its place in health care, other health care professionals continue to adopt the technologies into their own areas. For example, the use of computing systems in radiological imaging is extensive. Amongst the lessons to be learned from the history of Health Informatics is that Health Informatics as a discipline must be cognisant of, and involved in, the aims and activities of health care itself. Technologies are becoming ubiquitous in their availability with ever increasingly powerful tools allowing health care workers to readily create systems for their own benefit. Health Informatics should communicate to the health care profession the lessons of its past, just as Health Informatics needs to learn from the work and activities of this same community.

The benefits of the technology as well as the ability to demonstrate such benefits to others are becoming compulsory. The reasons for this include: the effect of computer usage by practitioners on patients themselves; the security of medical information; the need for new skills to be learned; and the price of the technology at a time when rising health care costs are an international concern.

Health Informatics strives to enhance all aspects of health care at all times. If this is kept in mind, the lessons of history to date will be heeded and incorporated into the future of Information Technology in health care, rather than ignored.

Tribute:

Professor Branko Cesnik was an international leader in the discipline of Health Informatics. In the 1990's he established Australia's first academic research and education unit for medical informatics. He was co-editor of the original edition of this publication. This chapter is reproduced as a tribute to Branko and his life's work.

References:

[1]   van Bemmel J.H. and Shortliffe E.H. 1986 Foreword to the Fifth World Congress on Medical Informatics *(Medinfo '86) Proceedings* edited by Salamon R., Blum B., Jorgensen M., North-Holland, Amsterdam p.x.
[2]   Mandil S.H. 1992 From "EDP in Health" to Health Informatics. In: *Proceedings of the Seventh World Congress on Medical Informatics* edited by Lun K.C., Degoulet P., Piemme T.E., Rienhoff O., North-Holland, Amsterdam p.xxxiv

Health Informatics
E.J.S. Hovenga et al. (Eds.)
IOS Press, 2010
© 2010 The authors and IOS Press. All rights reserved.
doi:10.3233/978-1-60750-476-4-9

2. Health Informatics - An Introduction

Evelyn.J.S.HOVENGA[1], RN, PhD (UNSW), FACHI, FACS[a], Michael R KIDD,
MBBS, MD, DCCH, DipRACOG, FRACGP, FACHI, FAFPM (Hon), FHKCFP
(Hon), FRNZCGP (Hon), MAICD[b], Sebastian GARDE Dr. sc. hum., Dipl.-Inform.
Med., FACHI[c], Carola HULLIN LUCAY COSSIO RN, BN, Hons, PhD (Melb.Uni)[d]
*[a]Director, eHealth Education, Consultant, openEHR Foundation, and Honorary
Senior Research Associate, Centre for Health Informatics & Multiprofessional
Education, University College London, Honorary Academic Fellow, Austin Health,
Melbourne, Adjunct Professor, Central Queensland University Rockhampton,
Queensland, and Victoria University, Melbourne, Australia*
[b]Executive Dean, Faculty of Health Sciences, Flinders University, Australia
[c]Senior Developer, Ocean Informatics, Düsseldorf, Germany
[d]Co-Founder eHealth Systems, Santiago, Chile, Melbourne, Australia

Abstract. This chapter gives an educational overview of:
- the scope of the health informatics discipline
- health informatics and e-health definitions
- health informatics professional networks
- potential benefits of applying health informatics technologies

Keywords. Medical Informatics, Information Systems, Health, Computer Systems,
Knowledge

Introduction

Health Informatics is a highly interdisciplinary field that may be defined as "an
evolving scientific discipline that deals with the collection, storage, retrieval,
communication and optimal use of health related data, information and knowledge. The
discipline utilises the methods and technologies of the information sciences for the
purposes of problem solving, decision making and assuring highest quality health care
in all basic and applied areas of the biomedical sciences" [1].

1. eHealth

The term e-health only came into widespread usage a few years ago at the turn of the
century. It was preceded by telemedicine, teleradiology or telehealth. As this became
more common place most people realised that telemedicine or telehealth was simply

---

[1] Corresponding Author: e.hovenga@ehealtheducation.net

about the delivery of health care via the use of telecommunications. With rapid advances and the convergence of these technologies with information technologies these terms became obsolete. There is no agreed definition for e-health, yet this term is widely used by many. Oh et al. [2] undertook a systematic review of 1209 abstracts and 430 citations and found 10 different definitions for the term eHealth, and from a Google search an additional 41 unique definitions were located ranging in length from 3 to 74 words. The most common universal themes were health and technology. In addition 6 less frequently mentioned themes emerged: commerce, stakeholders, outcomes, place and perspectives. The word Internet was mentioned in 27 of the 51 definitions and only one definition included the term *integration*.

The adoption of technologies to better manage health information and communication within a nation's health industry enables significant productivity and efficiency improvements to be achieved. It enables the provision of a more effective and efficient health workforce who are thus enabled to provide higher quality, safer and more accessible care in multiple locations producing better health outcomes. The adoption of health informatics or e-health is simply a requirement of doing business in 21st century healthcare [3]. This requires educational organizations to build the necessary workforce capacity so that these technologies can be developed, implemented and used optimally.

2. Health Informatics Discipline

The discipline of health informatics has arisen from the earlier established science of medical informatics [4] [5] [6]. The field of health informatics is very extensive. For example at the twelfth's world congress on medical informatics held in Brisbane in 2007, Australia close to 300 papers and as many posters were presented and classified into any one of 71 different topics covering all aspects of the technology and many different applications by a vast array of health professionals in all types of health care related settings, including clinical, management, administrative, policy and research based in community and institutional settings. It is noted that the first world congress on medical informatics was held in 1974 in Stockholm, Sweden . Although the two disciplines share many concepts, and the terms are often interchangeable, in this textbook we have chosen to focus on the use of information technology in all areas of health care, rather than just focus on the delivery of medical services by medical practitioners. The term health informatics is all embracing and medical informatics could be viewed as a subset of health informatics along with nursing or dental informatics.

Many countries have established a health informatics group, society or association. Such organizations then choose to become a member of the International Medical Informatics Association (IMIA) and this organization hosts international conferences together with the local national member organization to promote the discipline, enable international networking to take place and to share experiences. IMIA has set about to define the health informatics discipline via its scientific map and the educational recommendations. Both are IMIA endorsed documents available from www.imia.org although they are both in the process of being updated[7]. The current scientific map has seven categories as detailed in Table 1:

Table 1 IMIA Scientific Map Categories

Applied Technology	Information Technology Infrastructure	Applications and Products	Data-Infrastructure Related	Human-Organizational	Education and Knowledge	Clinical Disciplines

These original IMIA Scientific Map categories have been extended to fourteen organizing concepts or categories in the latest draft, these are presented in the Table 2.

Table 2– IMIA's 2008 Draft Organizing Concepts of the Health Informatics Discipline

1. ICT (Computer Science) for Health	8. People in Organisations
2. Health & Social Care processes	9. Politics & Policy
3. Health (Care) Records	10. Technologies for Health
4. Health & Social Care industry	11. Terminology, Classification & Grouping
5. Health Informatics Standards	12. Uses of Clinical Information
6. Knowledge Domains & Knowledge Discovery	13. Using Informatics to Support Clinical
7. Legal & Ethical	14. Computer Systems Applications in Health (Toolkit)

Numerous concepts fit within each category ranging from around 20 to more than 60 indicating the enormous scope of this discipline. This clearly demonstrates not only the scope of the Health Informatics discipline but also the needs from a healthcare system perspective.

The discipline is very broad, has lots of depth and may be classified into computing (incl. all information and communications technologies) or health (incl. healthy living, population health, health service delivery, health policy) problem spaces. This means that no health informatician has the same set of knowledge and skills as another, each tends to focus on their own strengths and areas of interests in either problem space although all need to possess a basic set of competencies. The figures below show the key differences for each problem space [8]. The shaded portion in Figure 1 represents Health Informatics in the problem space of computing. Health Informaticians need knowledge/skills throughout the spectrum in the computing space, from some practical knowledge in Computer Hardware and Architecture to a profound theoretical understanding as well as application skills on the organisational and information systems layer.

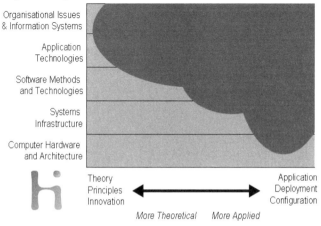

Figure 1: The Overall Place of Health Informatics in the Problem Space of Computing

The Health problem space is complex. For example, sharing electronic health records is a more complex task than sharing financial information or travel bookings. There are lots of different types of information; progress notes, appointments, documents, collections of images, laboratory results, registries etc. The variety of information is obvious in the paper world where there are hundreds or thousands of different forms in just one hospital, putting at risk people receiving healthcare services. Health care is constantly changing in three ways (breadth, depth, complexity): new information, information in finer-grained detail, and new relationships are always being discovered or becoming relevant complicating this space further. Therefore – more than in other computing discipline - in addition to an understanding of content in the computing problem space, an understanding of the health problem space content is fundamental for Health Informaticians. The shaded portion in Figure 2 represents Health Informatics in the health problem space which is essentially the reverse of the depth of skills and knowledge required from the computing space.

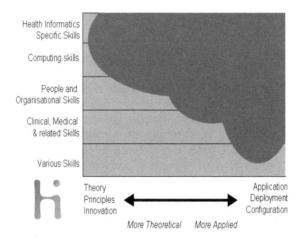

Figure 2 The Overall Place of Health Informatics in the Health Problem Space

Every health informatics project requires a team of people who collectively contribute the necessary set of skills and knowledge to that project, thus teamwork and the ability to work collaboratively with others are skills every health informatician requires. The difference between information systems specialists and health information systems specialists is that the latter place a greater emphasis on the application of the technology/systems in health care. They focus on solving very complex medical or health related problems using the information technology to the fullest extent as the tool to achieve that. This often means the need for a change in work practices.

3. Potential Benefits of Applying ICT in the Health Industry

The application of cutting edge technologies pertaining to the computer, communication and information sciences has much to offer the health sciences. We are of the view that appropriate use of these technologies will result in improved health, lower costs and improved service delivery methods [9]. To achieve this, healthcare professionals need to be aware of the possibilities today and in the future and participate in this discipline's further development.

Close to 40 years ago Martin and Norman [10[p.222]] predicted that in medicine the computer promised revolutionary changes. Today the same may be said about communications and knowledge management technologies. We have witnessed a convergence between communications, computing and television or broadcasting technologies enabling the merging of all types of data into integrated multimedia information, providing rapid interactions between people from any location. The speed by which these changes impact upon health service delivery is determined by and dependent upon how quickly the health professions accept the role of these new technologies in their workplace. It is they who need to identify the potential use of these technologies within the health care industry.

The international network of health informaticians is growing rapidly. There is evidence of an approaching critical number such that the process of change is now self sustaining. This network could be compared with what Marilyn Ferguson describes as an Aquarian conspiracy where conspirators (read health informaticians) collude to change social institutions, modes of problem solving and distribution of power [11[p.20]]. They are characterised by rethinking everything, examining old assumptions, by looking differently at their work, relationships, health, political power, experts, goals and values. They are leading the way towards a paradigm shift; they have a new perspective towards health care. Ferguson [11[p.28]] notes that:

"New paradigms are nearly always received with coolness, even mockery and hostility. Their discoveries are attacked for their heresy. (For historic examples, consider Copernicus, Galileo, Pasteur, Mesmer). The idea may appear bizarre, even fuzzy, at first because the discoverer made an intuitive leap and does not have all the data in place yet."

Many health informatics network members can no doubt identify with these sentiments. This book is dedicated to these pioneers who dared to be out of step with their peers and who have provided the building blocks for this paradigm shift. It has proved difficult for the discipline to gain acceptance from mainstream health professionals and recipients of health care. Also enabling procedures and legislations have been and continue to be slow to emerge. For example the European eHealth action plan developed in 2004 lists a number of activities associated with legal and regulatory issues that need to be completed by 2009 [12]. In 2005 the World Health Organisation's (WHO) world assembly adopted a resolution on e-health [13] recognising that eHealth is the cost-effective and secure use of information and communications technologies in support of health and health-related fields, including health-care services, health surveillance, health literature, and health education, knowledge and research. All member states were urged to develop and implement an e-health strategy.

Health informatics is about data, information and knowledge and what we do with all this as health professionals. From a national perspective these technologies need to be used to support the implementation and performance monitoring of a country's health policies. It is no accident that the advent of low cost easily accessible computer technology has occurred at the same time as the so-called information explosion that has affected all areas of modern life. The problem of managing the ever increasing volume of information and developing methods to help keep abreast of important changes in knowledge is particularly applicable to those of us working in health care.

It is becoming increasingly difficult to practice as a health professional without the use of information technologies to support daily practice. This challenge is going to continue as expectations of increasing quality of health care is demanded by the consumers of our services. Improved information management of health care data became an accepted essential element of the infrastructure of all contemporary health care systems some time ago [14[p.2]].

4. Learning About Health Informatics

Those of you who have had little past experience in the use of computers may be reticent about approaching this text. Information technology can be a daunting challenge for those of us who missed out on being part of the 'computer generation' currently graduating from our high schools and tertiary institutions. Remember that you don't need to be a computer genius to use a computer effectively in your professional life. You just need to understand the basic concepts. It's like driving a car; you don't need to know exactly how the engine works but you do need to learn how to drive the machine, to identify when something is wrong and to understand the road rules so that you minimise the risk of getting into trouble.

If you are already computer literate, you can enjoy applying your acquired skills to the health sciences and learn how to use information technology to support the provision of high quality health care. The computer age poses real challenges for us all. We hope that you find this text useful in assisting you to meet the challenges ahead.

References

[1]   Graham I 1994 *HISA* - informatics enhancing health. Health Informatics Society of Australia, Melbourne
[2]   Oh H, Rizo C, Enkin M, Jadad A. 2005 What Is eHealth (3): A Systematic Review of Published Definitions, *Journal of Medical Internet Research;7(1)*:e1 viewed June 2008 at http://www.jmir.org/2005/1/e1/
[3]   Australian Health Informatics Council (AHIC) 2007 *eHealth Future Directions Briefing Paper* for the Australian Health Ministers Advisory Council (AHMAC) meeting October 2007 - http://www.health.gov.au/internet/main/publishing.nsf/Content/ehealth-futuredirections accessed 5 May 2008.
[4]   Shortliffe E.H., Perreault L.E., Wiederhold G., Fagan L.M. (Eds) 1990 *Medical informatics - computer applications in health care.* Addison Wesley
[5]   Hannan T 1991 Medical informatics - an Australian perspective. *Australian and New Zealand Journal of Medicine 21: 363-378*
[6]   Coiera E 1994 Medical informatics. *Medical Journal of Australia 160: 438-440*
[7]   International Medical Informatics Association (IMIA) – *Scientific Map 2002* http://www.imia.org/2002_scientific_map.html accessed 5 May 2008
[8]   Garde S, Harrison D, Hovenga E 2005 Australian Skill Needs Analysis of Health Informatics Professionals, *Research Report 1,2,3 &4 of the Health Informatics Research Group* Central Queensland University, Rockhampton, Qld
[9]   Chaudrey B, Wang J, Wu S, Maglione M, Mojica W, Roth E, Morton SC, Shelelle PG 2006 Systematic review: impact of health information technology on quality, efficiency, and costs of medical care. *Ann Intern Med 2006 May 16;* 144(10): 742-52 Accessed 7 May 2008 from: http://www.annals.org/cgi/reprint/144/10/742.pdf

[10] Martin J and Norman A R D 1970 *The computerized society: an appraisal of the impact of computers over the next fifteen years.* Prentice Hall, Englewood Cliffs, NJ p.222)
[11] Ferguson M 1980 The Aquarian conspiracy. Paladin Grafton Books, London
[12] European Commission 2004 *"e-Health - making healthcare better for European citizens: An action plan* for a European e-Health Area" [COM(2004) 356 final - not published in the Official Journal] - Communication from the Commission to the Council, the European Parliament, the European Economic and Social Committee and the Committee of the Regions of 30 April 2004 accessed on 7 May 2008 from http://europa.eu/scadplus/leg/en/lvb/l24226f.htm .
[13] World Health Organisation (WHO), *World Health Assembly resolution on eHealth* (WHA58.28, May 2005), viewed June 2008 from http://www.euro.who.int/telemed/20060713_1
[14] Dick R.S. and Steen E.B (Eds) 1991 *The computer based patient record - an essential technology for health care.* National Academy Press, Washington

Review Questions

1. What is your understanding of the Health Informatics discipline?
2. Describe how the adoption of e-Health policy strategies are likely to impact upon:
    a. The population at large
    b. Health care providers (clinicians)
3. Explain how a health workforce with Health Informatics skills and knowledge are able to improve health services.
4. Identify changes required in your work environment to enable optimal use of available technologies.

Health Informatics
E.J.S. Hovenga et al. (Eds.)
IOS Press, 2010
© *2010 The authors and IOS Press. All rights reserved.*
doi:10.3233/978-1-60750-476-4-16

3. Health Care Services, Information Systems & Sustainability

Evelyn J.S. HOVENGA[1], RN, PhD (UNSW), FACHI, FACS

Director, eHealth Education, Consultant, openEHR Foundation, and Honorary Senior Research Associate, Centre for Health Informatics & Multiprofessional Education, University College London, Honorary Academic Fellow, Austin Health, Melbourne, Adjunct Professor, Central Queensland University Rockhampton, Queensland, and Victoria University, Melbourne, Australia

Abstract. This chapter gives an educational overview of:
- many competing characteristics within national health systems
- national primary information and knowledge flows between health care entities.
- the role of information technologies in assisting health organizations become sustainable enterprises.
- the business of maintaining healthy populations for any nation
- desirable e-health strategy objectives

Keywords. Health Care Systems, Health Facilities, Health Services Administration, Health Policy, Public Health Informatics, Sustainability

1. Healthy Populations

Health is a complex concept. The most widely accepted definition of health is that used by the World Health Organisation (WHO) that views health from a holistic perspective and defines it as: a state of complete physical, mental and social well being and not merely the absence of disease and infirmity [1]. The WHO Constitution indicates that the promotion and protection of health is of value to all. It is in this spirit that governments approach health planning and policy development.

In many countries everyone in need of health care gets treated or cared for, although in many instances one's ability to access or pay and the policies of funding organisations do govern what service is provided for whom and under what conditions. A nation's primary health concerns or burden of disease influences health policy development and implementation. For example Australia has identified seven health priorities that altogether contribute 80% to its national burden of disease and injury [2]. These are arthritis and musculoskeletal conditions, asthma, cancer control, cardiovascular health, diabetes mellitus, injury prevention and control, and mental health. These were first identified in response to the World Health Organization's global strategy *Health for All by the year 2000* and its subsequent revision. Monitoring

---

[1] Corresponding Author: e.hovenga@ehealtheducation.net

for trends and progress made in reducing such disease burdens is achieved via the adoption of a series of indicators [3].

WHO collects and manages national statistics from its member States for 50 core indicators on mortality, morbidity, risk factors, service coverage and health systems for all member States (nations) enabling performance comparisons to be made [4]. Individual nations collect and manage their own statistics in addition to those collected for WHO or such information is collected via ad hoc surveys. For example the Australian Institute of Health and Welfare publishes a biennial health report *Australia's Health* 2008 that is made available via their website free of charge in pdf format [5]. Canada and other countries produce similar statistics.

At the first International Conference on Health Promotion in Ottawa, Canada in November 1986, delegates drafted an International Charter for Health Promotion[6]. This Charter, supported by WHO and other international health organisations, built on the progress made since 1978 through the WHO Declaration of Alma Ata on Primary Health Care [7]. When reading this it becomes apparent that there are a number of environmental, socioeconomic and political determinants of health that vary between countries. These also need to be considered when defining the business of health. From a public health perspective we need to focus on prevention such as ensuring food and water are not contaminated or limiting the spread of disease via compulsory infectious and other disease reporting, constant surveillance, vaccination programs, screening programs and numerous health promotion programs all of which have the potential to significantly reduce the demand for health services and prevent major disease outbreaks with potential dire consequences. These days the maintenance of a nation's bio-security is equally as important.

2. Health Industry Business Drivers

The health domain as an industry is extensive. It consumes anywhere between 8 to 14 percent of the gross domestic product (GDP) in most countries and increasing annually but this is significantly less in developing nations. The European Commission reported that "without significant reforms, including the better use of eHealth, health expenditure is expected to increase from 9% of GDP at present to around 16% by 2020 in response to an 'ageing' Europe" [8]. The following general health system characteristics may be viewed in general terms as key business drivers for change in most if not all nations. Priorities, details and significance of drivers will vary between nations.

- An Ageing population increasing the demand for health services
- Changing patterns of disease and medicine
- Increasing incidence of environmental health hazards
- Increasing complexity of treatments and case mix
- Increasing workload for all health professionals
- Shortages in qualified staff
- Increasing patient expectations in terms of access and quality care
- Patient empowerment
- A need to control costs
- A recognised need to improve patient safety and reduce the incidence of error

- Information, knowledge and communication technology advances and society's rate of adoption
- Greater Political commitment

Many entities collectively make up a nation's health system. Viewing a health system's infrastructure from a business perspective requires us to identify the drivers and context of a health system's operations. We have an increasingly mobile population who expect to have seamless access to health care at any location. People living in communities where the provider to population ratio is low, or where there are great distances between the population and various types of health service providers, expect to have access to the same levels of care as people living in communities with high provider to population ratios or living in denser populated areas. The nation's population as a whole expects all health services to be integrated so that their care is facilitated through an exchange of all relevant health related information.

Any nation's health industry business is about improving and maintaining the health of its population. Most commonly it is a nation's government that determines how a national health care system is structured to best meet these business needs. This is influenced by a government's ideological persuasion, various historical events, political influences, resource availability and distribution, workforce characteristics, medical advances, equipment and technology availability, the integration of research and adoption of best or evidence based practice. It is also influenced by activities undertaken for public health purposes in the relevant time period, such as the provision of HIV/AIDS management, or the establishment of infectious diseases facilities when this is a major public health problem. A historical example is the provision of quarantine services during Sydney's early settlement days. In the days when there was a belief that mental illness could only be treated by means of long term institutional care, we witnessed the establishment of facilities to accommodate this perceived need but this need has now changed. Indeed we are now witnessing many changes in healthcare delivery modes, all of which need to be able to be supported by the e-health infrastructure.

Thus it is apparent that not only the incidence of actual ill- health episodes determines a health care system's structure, it is also influenced by health prevention, promotion and the perceived best treatment and care options adopted at the time. Similarly during the 1960s we didn't have dedicated intensive care units but with the many advances in various technologies this became necessary to best treat seriously ill patients. These historical shifts indicate that a health system needs to be flexible to be able to accommodate such changes.

Health care services may be delivered in the community, such as at home, school or work, as a primary health care service mostly provided by general practitioners, community care such as child care services, day surgery provided by specialists, diagnostic services such as organ imaging, pathology, outpatient or private specialist consulting services, bush (remote) nursing centres, or care provided by alternative health care services such as acupuncture or natural pathology. Residential health services include: acute, rehabilitation, residential and aged care. The boundaries of practice, in terms of who provides which type of service, varies considerably between countries, specially in developing countries where some specialties mentioned above do not exist in their own right.

Other factors greatly influencing a country's health care system infrastructure are the available health care workforce, their knowledge and skill competencies, professional regulation, education and other support services such as those industries who manufacture and supply drugs, equipment, surgical supplies and many technologies including computer hardware and software as well as those who provide administrative support services such as insurance companies, funders, those managing health care statistics, quality and safety organisations, patient complaint facilities and more. Thus any health system has many and varied stakeholders who need to work collaboratively. In some healthcare contexts it is not normal practice to share and exchange information. In developing countries this is also dependent upon the energy and water availability as well as other environmental factors that impact upon the manner a health system interoperates between its decision makers.

There are many and varied direct health care delivery services, many support functions and related industries, a mix of private and public or government funded operations and a number of national reporting requirements. All of these variables have an impact upon how well any national health system functions in terms of efficiency, that is achieving the best possible return on investment combined with a good use of available resources, and effectiveness in terms of achieving best patient and population health outcomes.

In summary health systems are complex highly connected social constructs that control: funding, access to services, workforce supply and demand, availability and cost of drugs, supplies, equipment, physical facilities and technologies, research opportunities and adoption of research results. This shapes consumer expectations and ultimately clinical outcomes. All these processes and outputs are constrained by a nation's political, legal, workplace, cultural, financial and business systems [9].

3.   National Government Roles

Governments play a number of vital roles that influence how all business associated with health care is managed. Essentially this is the result of high level health policy directions and complimentary legislation. Examples from Australia and Chile are Medicare [10], a universal health system providing all Australians with access to free or low-cost medical, optometrical and hospital care and the Chilean Government's adoption of listing all conditions for which care provision is provided by a Universal Access and Explicit Guarantees Plan (AUGE) covering health promotion, treatment and rehabilitation [11]. These policy directions then became the primary drivers of how all health related business processes need to operate. In essence Governments tend to determine:

- who is funded together with the funding rules by type of service to be provided and their location such as for example how many funded acute or aged care beds private aged care providers should have access to or who should own and manage buildings and highly specialised equipment.
- available resource allocation and distribution across the many different entities
- health services organization, structure and e-health infrastructure
- legislative and regulatory controls for the health care sector including in some instances contractual arrangements between service providers.
- target populations for specific health programs and policies
- direct health services provided by the Government
- national reporting requirements, information and knowledge management infrastructure

- desired standards of health service delivery
- educational opportunities for the health workforce and at what cost to individuals
- funding of health related research.

The list above is not comprehensive but serves to demonstrate that governments have a far reaching influence on the health of a nation. Governments need to manage a tension between the rights of the individual to health care and the common good of the nation's population as a whole, as well as access to healthcare relative to location and workforce capacity. In other words the tension is between available resources and a demand for service within the context of information flow and overall system functionality.

The role of government regarding the improvements in health extends beyond the health care system and touches most if not all government departments in one way or another. Examples are in trade in terms of approved medications, safety requirements related to all imported equipment and supplies used in the health industry, regulations regarding occupational health and safety, as well as health promotion matters such the use of safety belts or helmets for cyclists and motorbike riders [12] [13] [14] [15].

4.   Sustainable Health System Characteristics

According to the World Business Council for Sustainable Development (WBCSD) 'nearly everyone agrees that the way we manage health today is unsustainable – it costs more than we can afford, and delivers less than we expect'. Yet future health systems will have to treat proportionately more people, with more illness, higher expectations, often using more expensive technologies, and using relatively fewer tax dollars and workers [16]. We need to explicitly design and implement new sustainable systems. What does a sustainable health system look like and how do we set about building it?

The WBCSD has adopted three pillars, economic growth, ecological balance and social progress to guide sustainable activities. Boxer [17] argues that all business leaders need to promote and adopt a sustainable way of operating to achieve organisational survival. He argues that a sustainable way of operation requires paying equal respect to the demands of society, the environment and financial needs. A simple model for visualising whether an organization has a sustainability problem is the 'funnel' diagram, which plots consumption of resources against resource availability (Figure 1). In real systems, a growing gap between resource supply and demand cannot be sustained for long, and corrections must be made to bring supply and demand into balance.

Sustainable organizations have developed strategies that fine tune and maintain this balance in ways that avoid the need for periodic, reactionary, large and usually painful structural adjustments, or even collapse. Creating a sustainable health system therefore requires us to focus on providing the best possible match between demand and supply by reducing technology, quality and demographic driven demands and by maximising resource availability such as workforce capacity and funding. Resources such as workforce expertise should not be lost to the system. We need to avoid accumulating costs to the system by for example an increase in the demand for renal dialysis that may be better dealt with via a prevention strategy. Individuals also have a role to play in reducing demand as we are increasingly witnessing self inflicted ill health due to poor lifestyle choices such as poor nutrition, alcoholism, drug or risk taking. Healthcare is embedded in a wider national system.

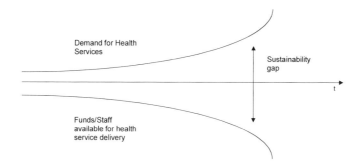

Figure 1: The Sustainability Funnel – when resource availability and utilization diverge we have a sustainability gap [18].

In summary the framework adopted as the base from which to document any national health care system will influence its structure. If the intention is to reduce the cost of health care then this may result in rationing care provision. If the intent is to keep all people alive and fully functioning at any cost then the focus will be on the necessary research and the widespread adoption of the latest technological advances. If the focus is on minimal intervention and promoting the adoption of healthy lifestyles then there is a need to focus on sociological, environmental and psychological perspectives. If the aim is prevention then the focus is on risk management strategies such as the introduction of seatbelts, screening for early detection of disease and strategies to reduce smoking etc.

A national e-health framework needs to focus on the best possible use of information and communication technologies to support the business of health care in accordance with national directions. In other words when a national e-health strategy is being considered one needs to assess these many perspectives in terms of the extent of their adoption and how these are being operationalised.

5. National Health System Entities

Any nation's health care system consists of all the stakeholders who collectively make up a nation's health industry. Many nations have states, provinces or territories that collectively make up a nation. The governing arrangements in terms of jurisdictional control, and the funding and reporting of health services as well as workforce capacity building vary considerably between nations. This in turn influences work and information flows as well as the extent to which additional support services are required and provided.

Health care providers consist of two different types of entities, organizations, facilities or enterprises and individuals. Support services may be provided to both. Such services can have an individual patient or subject of care focus, or a family focus or a community or public health focus. Communities may be described in terms of homogeneous subjects of care, such as people with diabetes requiring the provision of care from multiple different health care providers or communities may be defined based on location such as remote communities. Environmental (e.g., polluted water supply or air) or endemic genetic factors (e.g., sickle cell anaemia) or lifestyle/cultural factors (i.e., high incidence of smokers or alcohol consumption or petrol sniffing), tend to differentiate communities in terms of their specific disease burden and the mix of health services required in any specific location. This in turn influences the support service requirements as well as information flows to support the delivery of health care, for supply chain management (related to e-commerce), and to meet jurisdictional reporting requirements.

Supply chain refers to the process of moving any supply item from the manufacturer to the point of use from raw materials via manufacturer, wholesaler, distributor, transport, purchasing, warehousing, and in-house storage and distribution processes. This concept is presented in more detail from an informatics perspective in Chapter 28. A similar process is adopted for the provision of various services.

Jurisdictional reporting requirements are governed primarily by the way the health system is funded as well as governmental priorities and policy initiatives. A jurisdiction is the highest authority controlling and taking responsibility for the services provided. This defines the scope over which this authority is exercised. These authorities will, for example, determine the legal parameters concerned with the maintenance of privacy and confidentiality of all health related information. Any country may find it useful to develop a national health information model and use this as a guide for the development of the many aspects of its e-health directions. Details about Australia's national health information model may be used as an example [19]. This model has been used to guide the development of the National registry of meta-data (METeOR) available on-line [20].

6. Information Flows

Once you have a diagram reflecting the health system of interest you can begin to think about the possible information flows that information and communication technologies need to be able to support. An analysis of information and work flows is a necessary pre-cursor to the development of system architectures that meet these business needs. You may refer to various possible patient journeys through the health system and associated information flow needs or you may adopt any of the perspectives listed in Box 1 to assist this process.

Box 1 Perspectives for Information Flow Analysis

• Follow the information required to enable the provision of a specific service.
• identify which entities need to be able to share information to enable the provision of aged care services or chronic disease management.
• Follow all patient related information from first contact with a health service provider to discharge or from birth to death.
• Identify and follow the information required to manage a supply chain.
• Identify and follow the information required to allocate resources in-house enabling the service provider to meet service demand.
• Identify and follow the information required by a jurisdiction to monitor trends or to support resource allocation, workforce planning activities or health policy development.
• Identify and follow the information required by health insurers to pay providers of care or to reimburse subjects of care for payments made.
• Identify and follow information needs to enable the monitoring of the quality of care provided.

7. Health Knowledge

The health industry is knowledge intensive. There is a strong need for all health care providers to analyse, create, share and use the most up-to-date and available knowledge to support the delivery of health care services to improve outcomes of care. Knowledge is information in context so that it may be applied to guide actions. Health knowledge is acquired by a variety of means: through experience, engaging in learning processes, research and data mining. Health knowledge is constantly changing as a result of ongoing research activities and various medical and technical advances. Consequently it is difficult for any health care provider to keep up-to-date. To assist this process some organisations are dedicating their efforts to acquiring, evaluating and packaging this knowledge in readily accessible formats such as 'best practice guidelines' or care protocols . Ideally we develop clinical systems that automate new knowledge discovery using practice based evidence. This concept is presented in some detail in Chapter 31.

The knowledge used as a basis for clinical, management and policy decision making to support health care, varies in terms of quality, accuracy and soundness. It is often clouded by values, opinions and other people's views, and consists of or comes from a number of possible sources listed in box 2.

Box 2 Possible Sources of Health Knowledge

- tradition, 'we've always done it this way'
- authority, position power and perceived expertise
- borrowing/transferring knowledge from other disciplines
- what was learned during professional education and from textbooks
- reasoning, trial and error, 'let's try this and see'
- experience, 'this worked for me the last time'
- rules, regulations, procedures and protocols
- a role model or mentor, someone perceived as having expertise
- journal articles, popular press, the Internet, sales representatives
- processed data collected routinely and systematically such as trend data
- research, both qualitative and quantitative and including randomised clinical trials usually conducted by others.

Evidence based practice is about less reliance on most of the above and a greater reliance on the best possible evidence available about what works and what doesn't. This requires an ability to look for, retrieve and assess what is good evidence and what is not. In addition such evidence needs to be made available at the point of care when required.

The Cochrane Collaboration [21] is one of the leading organisations promoting the adoption of evidence based practice (EBP). It is an international organisation that aims to help people make well-informed decisions about health care by preparing, maintaining and promoting the accessibility of systematic reviews of the effects of health care interventions. Its focus is on the conduct of systematic reviews of randomised contol trials (RCTs). This all began in 1972 with a publication by Archie L Cochrane titled, *Effectiveness and efficiency: random reflections on health services*. A coding and classification group was registered with the Cochrane collaboration centre in 1995 and many discipline focused groups are also registered.

However their strategic plan makes no mention of the need for the health industry to adopt controlled terminologies, a reference terminology, or clinical minimum data sets to facilitate the use of clinical information systems to evaluate practice in real world settings. Their systematic reviews are based on the results of randomised controlled trials. Systematic reviews, using meta–analysis are replacing 'expert opinion' reviews as a basis for guidelines and health care decisions. Journals like *Evidence Based Medicine* and *Evidence Based Nursing* are other sources of information to find the good and the clinically useful research. The Australian National Institute of Clinical Studies (NICS) was established to assist clinicians to bridge the gap between what clinicians know and what they do [22].

Most health care decisions are not based on any of these types of evidence. Furthermore once such evidence is obtained, the decision maker needs to first decide if that evidence applies to the situation for which a decision needs to be made. Are the circumstances the same or sufficiently similar? An alternative is the use of knowledge networks which are less research but more practice oriented. Knowledge and information management concepts are presented in detail in chapters 8, 9 and 10, the use of knowledge in decision support systems is dealt with in more detail in Chapters 23 and 24.

8.   New Technologies

Technology may be defined as any new way of doing something. It may be using very expensive or very basic equipment, devices or new processes. New technologies impact the way health care providers can or should be providing health services. Frequently there is an overlap period where both the old and the new technologies continue to be used concurrently thus adding to the costs incurred. For example when echo-cardiography was first introduced cardiac surgeons still needed to do angiograms to enable them to determine their surgical approach. This tends to change over time with widespread acceptance and changes to work practices. Some new technologies are very expensive and the benefits of their use may be illusive when first introduced. For example the Australian Government controlled the introduction of Magnetic Resonance Imaging (MRI) equipment and its use to contain costs. The same is true for new drug therapies and a variety of new medical devices. Consequently, the government has systems in place to evaluate these under controlled conditions prior to them becoming readily available. Similarly health service providers need to conduct an impact analysis from various perspectives prior to introducing a new service or new equipment to support an existing service.

New technologies also impact on ethics and morals. This is particularly evident in the new reproductive technologies, genomics and advances in organ transplants. The latter impacts on how we value human life. In some countries this may lead to the selling of a variety of spare parts with enormous social consequences. There is also a danger that the adoption of new technologies make clinicians 'forget' about other older and inexpensive technologies or practices including physical observations. These issues should alert you to the types of problems policy makers may be facing in the very near future and the impact they may have on health business processes. The Australian Government's therapeutic goods administration (TGA) deals with many of these issues [13]. You can learn all about them by visiting the TGA website.

9.   e-Health Strategies

Today we need to integrate all health care with e-health technologies. Noting the potential impact that advances in information and communication technologies could have on health care and health-related activities. The integration of technologies to improve health service delivery is not new. During the late 1920s and early 1930s, Australia experienced a great example of combining medicine, aviation and radio to bring health care to those people who live, work and travel in remote locations. The Royal Flying Doctor Service continues to provide a unique range of primary health care and emergency services throughout the country [23]. This service is now supported via the adoption of e-health technologies.

Many of the crucial data feeds needed to monitor health system behaviour come from patient records, wherever they are held, or in whatever structure or format, hence the focus on patient-centred health care and record management. Making the best possible use of available technologies to safely deliver quality health services requires every nation to establish some electronic means for storing these patient data. The electronic health record thus becomes the foundation for our sustainability infrastructure. This is discussed in detail in the next chapter.

Coiera and Hovenga [9] noted that in addition a health system's operational effectiveness requires the ability to evaluate performance not only in terms of quality and safety of clinical care but also in terms of overall service quality, cost, dependability, flexibility and speed. Consequently health information systems need to be able to provide significant amounts of data about clinical and administrative processes, describing for example the flows of patients through a system, the status and availability of clinical staff, the availability and utilization of resources such as drugs and beds. With increasing monitoring of process data, we are better able to see the actual dynamic behaviour of organizations, and use that data to first build meaningful models of the ways different processes interact, and then track any changes we make to the system.

All of these information needs are best met via the establishment of a framework to enable health professionals and health information systems to communicate with each other in a timely and reliable manner. Such a framework consists primarily of the adoption of any number of agreed health informatics standards but also on agreed policies and methods of operation. This creates a new national health information environment facilitating all appropriate stakeholders (users) to find, request, retrieve and provide access to relevant patient records, data, information and knowledge rapidly and accurately subject to patient authorisation where relevant. Such an approach takes advantage of significant investments made in the acquisition of telecommunication and information technologies nationally and by many health care providers within the country.

Many now argue that optimum efficiencies can only be achieved with the widespread adoption of *semantically* interoperable information systems i.e. systems capable of transferring, sharing, exchanging and meaningfully using information, in a machine processable format maintaining context, for decision support, regulatory reporting, population surveillance, clinical practice evaluation, outcome analysis and more [24] [25]. In other words, interoperability should enable the reuse (and avoid the 'waste') of data for multiple, often very different purposes [9]. One recent study of information sharing and integration in the public sector [26] supports this view by identifying that the primary integration problems are semantic issues: relationships between information and decision rules, data quality, inter-organisational interactions, collaboration and trust.

A number of countries are increasingly looking towards the establishment of an e-health nation through the adoption and implementation of health information and communication technologies. A European e-Health focus group produced a report on current and future standardization issues in the eHealth domain in 2005 based on the European Council for Employment, Social Policy, Health and Consumer Affairs recognition that: "electronic health cards, electronic health dedicated national and regional networks and the use of other information technology tools can achieve significant improvements in the quality and safety of the health care that is delivered to patients in an environment of increasing pressures in health care systems, while contributing to cost savings in the longer term" [27 p.5]. They listed key strategic aims, critical applications and infrastructure needs for any e-health nation to realize the stated benefits. These are presented in Table 1

Table 1 CEN/ISSS e-Health Focus Group's Strategic Aims, Critical Applications and Infrastructure Needs.

Key Strategic Aims	Critical Applications (p.7)	Infrastructure Needs
• improving access to clinical records • enabling patient mobility and cross-border access to health care • reducing clinical errors and improving safety • improving access to qualify information on health for patients and health care professionals • improving efficiency of health care processes.	• electronic health/patient records including health record and business architectures • electronic transfer of prescriptions • electronic health data messages between hospitals and primary care particularly communication of service requests and reports for laboratory investigations, • discharge summaries and patient referrals • digital imaging and associated service requests and reports • e-prescribing with decision support • core data sets (e.g. for public health and assessing quality of clinical care).	• management of patient identification • protecting personal information • terminological systems for clinical records and medicines • data cards and portals • achieving semantic interoperability.

This work has resulted in the development of the European Commission's mandate (M/403) on standardization in the field of e-health [28]. This mandate (M/403) aims to provide a consistent set of standards to address the needs of this rapidly-evolving field for the benefit of future healthcare provision. In February 2008 CEN, CENELEC, and ETSI, the three European Standards Organizations (ESOs) launched a joint project 'eHEALTH-INTEROP' to address this mandate's requirements [29] [30]. The latest most common general vision statements in the literature are about person-centred health systems improving access, quality and efficiency. eHealth and telehealth concepts are presented in more detail in Chapter 20.

The implementation of national e-health strategies is well advanced in a number of nations but for everyone this remains a work in progress. Given the number of stakeholders and settings, the necessary changes in work practices take some time to become the norm. Achieving sustainable health services supported by e-health requires a significant emphasis on change management and changing organisational processes, as recent explorations into sustainable public health services is demonstrating [31] [32].

This chapter has provided an overview of the many factors influencing national health systems' ability to have a healthy population. Various health industry business drivers influencing health information and knowledge needs as well as communication flows were identified. It is imperative that e-health implementation efforts use the need to achieve a sustainable health system as their guide. E-health strategies are now common around the globe, many examples can be found via web searches and in the literature. A number of the concepts introduced in this chapter will be explained in greater detail in the remainder of this book.

References

[1] World Health Organisation (WHO) *constitution* viewed 8 May 2008 http://www.who.int/governance/
[2] Australian Government. Budget Overview – Ensuring a sustainable health system 2006. http://www.budget.gov.au/2005-06/overview/html/overview_19.htm
[3] Australian Institute of Health and Welfare, (AIHW) and the National Health Priority Areas (NHPA) last updated in 2005 http://www.aihw.gov.au/nhpa/index.cfm viewed June 2008.
[4] WHO *World Health Statistics 2008* http://www.who.int/whosis/whostat/2008/en/index.html viewed June 2008.
[5] Australian Institute of Health and Welfare, (AIHW)., *Australia's Health 2008*, viewed June 2008, http://www.aihw.gov.au/publications/index.cfm/title/10585
[6] Ottawa Charter for Health Promotion, 1986 viewed on 12 May 2008 http://www.euro.who.int/AboutWHO/Policy/20010827_2
[7] WHO 1978 *Declaration of Alma Ata* http://www.who.int/hpr/NPH/docs/declaration_almaata.pdf. viewed June 2008
[8] Commission of the European Communities, Brussels, 21.12.2007 http://eur-lex.europa.eu/LexUriServ/site/en/com/2007/com2007_0860en01.pdf. viewed 12 may 2008.
[9] Coiera E and Hovenga EJS 2007 Building a Sustainable Helath System in: *Yearbook 07 of Medical Informatics:* Biomedical Informatcs for Sustainable Health Systems, Schattauer, Stuttgart, Germany p.11
[10] Medicare Australia http://www.medicareaustralia.gov.au/public/register/index.shtml
[11] Red Salud de Chile (Ministerio de Salud de la Republica de Chile) , *Garantías Explicitas en Salud*, viewed 27th June 2008 http://www.redsalud.gov.cl/gesauge/ges.html
[12] Australian Council for Safety and Quality in Health Care (ACSQHC) 2005, *About us*, viewed 22 May 2006, http://www.safetyandquality.org/index.cfm?page=About
[13] Therapeutic Goods Administration (TGA) http://www.tga.gov.au/
[14] The pharmacy Guild of Australia 2006, *News and updates*, viewed 22 May 2006, http://www.guild.org.au/
[15] Australian Council on Healthcare Standards 2002, *Safety, quality, performance*, viewed 22 May 2006, http://www.achs.org.au/
[16] World Business Council for Sustainable Development (WBCSD), *A Healthy Tomorrow?* Health Systems: Facts & Trends Affecting Business Decisions Today. www.wbcsd.org 2006, viewed 8 January 2007
[17] Boxer LJ. *The Sustainable Way*. Melbourne: Brolga Publishing; 2005.
[18] The Natural Step. The natural step framework guidebook; 2000.
[19] Australian Institute of Health and Welfare (AIHW), 2003 *National Health Information Model* http://www.aihw.gov.au/publications/hwi/nhimv2/index.html viewed June 2008.
[20] Australian Institute of Health and Welfare (AIHW) *METeOR* http://meteor.aihw.gov.au/content/index.phtml/itemId/181162 cited June 2008
[21] Cochrane collaboration http://www.cochrane.org/index.htm
[22] Australian National Institute for Clinical Studies (NICS) 2001, *Strategic plan 2001–2004*, viewed 22 May 2006 http://www.nicsl.com.au
[23] Royal Flying Doctor Service of Australia n.d., History, viewed 22 May 2006, http://flyingdoctor.net/history.htm

[24] Hovenga E.J.S 2008 Importance of Achieving Semantic Interoperability for National Health Information Systems *Text & Context Nursing Journal* Vol.17 No.1 pp.158-167 http://www.textoecontexto.ufsc.br/archive.php.

[25] Hovenga E.J., Garde S, EHRs, Semantic Interoperability and Politics, *eJHI* accepted for publication October 2009 www.ejhi.net

[26] Dawes S, Cresswell A, Pardo T, Tompson F. Modeling, the social and technical processes of interorganisational information integration. *ACM International Conference Proceedings Series Vol.89* - Proceedings of the 2005 national conference on Digital government research 2005:289-90.

[27] European Committee for Standardization/Information Society Standardization System (CEN/ISSS), e-Health Standardization Focus Group 2005, *Current and future standardization issues in the e-health domain: Achieving interoperability.* Executive Summary, viewed 12 May 2008, http://www.cen.eu/CENORM/businessdomains/businessdomains/isss/activity/ehealth_fg.asp

[28] European Commission (EC) *eHealth Mandate M/403* 2007 viewed May 2008 http://ec.europa.eu/enterprise/standards_policy/action_plan/doc/mandate_m403en.pdf

[29] European Standards Organisations (ESOs) Positive Prognosis for e-Health Standardization, *Press Release 7 February 2008* http://www.cen.eu/CENORM/businessdomains/businessdomains/isss/activity/0802ehealthinterop.pdf viewed 12 May 2008

[30] SA/CEN/ENTR/000/2007-20 *eHealth Mandate M/403 – Phase 1 Report* http://www.ehealth-interop.eu viewed 14 November 2009

[31] Brown A, Grootjans J, Ritchie J, Townsend W, Verrinder G. *Sustainabilty and Health – Supporting Global Ecological Integrity in Public Health*: Alan and Unwin; 2005.

[32] Shediac-Rizkallah MC, Bone LR. Planning for the sustainability of community-based health programs: conceptual frameworks and future directions for research, practice and policy *Health Education Research* 1998; 13: 87-108

Further Reading

- Australian Health Information Council 2004, Welcome to Australian health information, cited 22 May 2006, http://www.ahic.org.au/index.html

- Australian Science at Work (ASW) 2006, *Commission for the Future bibliography*, viewed 30 June 2006, http://www.austehc.unimelb.edu.au/asaw/bib_home.htm

- Braa J, Monteiro E, Sahay S 2004 Networks of Action: Sustainable Health Information Systems Across Developing Countries. *MIS Quarterly Vol.28 No.3 pp.337-362*

- Eng T n.d., *The e-health landscape* – a terrain map of emerging information and communication technologies in health and health care, Princeton, NJ, The Robert Wood Johnson Foundation, viewed May 2008 http://www.informatics-review.com/thoughts/rwjf.html

- Health Information Strategy Steering Committee. *Health Information Strategy for New Zealand 2005*. Ministry of Health http://www.moh.govt.nz/moh.nsf/0/1912064EEFEC8EBCCC2570430003DAD1/$File/health-information-strategy.pdf. viewed June 2008

- Oh, H, Rizo, C, Enkin, M & Jadad, A 2005, 'What is ehealth (3): A systematic review of published definitions', *Journal of Medical Internet Research, vol. 7, Issue 1, Article e1*, viewed 22 May 2006, http://www.jmir.org/2005/1/e1/

- Pagliari, C, Sloan, D, Gregor, P, Sullivan, F, Kahan, D, Oortwijn, W & MacGillivray, S 2005, 'What is ehealth: A scoping exercise to map the field', *Journal of Medical Internet Research, vol. 7, Issue 1 Article e9,* viewed 22 May 2006, http://www.jmir.org/2005/1/e9/

- Standards Australia n.d., Health Informatics Brochure e-HEALTH, viewed 22 May 2006, http://www.standards.org.au/

- Therapeutic Guidelines Limited (TGL) n.d., Welcome, viewed 22 May 2006, http://www.tg.com.au/home/index.html.

- Williams, J (ed.) 2001, Australian dictionary of clinical abbreviations, acronyms & symbols, viewed 22 May 2006, http://www.himaa.org.au/bookstore.html.

- WHO (World Health Organization) 2005 eHealth: proposed tools and services EB117/15 http://www.who.int/gb/ebwha/pdf_files/EB117/B117_15-en.pdf

- WHO (World Health Organization), cited 30 June 2006, http://www.who.int/en/

Review Questions

1. Are any of your national health system's characteristics competing with each other in a manner that impedes your country's ability to have a sustainable health system in the future?
2. How does patient information and clinical knowledge flow between healthcare providers who collectively provide services for individual patients?
3. Can you identify and describe national and/or local health system sustainability characteristics?
4. Provide an argument, for or against the view that optimal use of information, knowledge management and communication technologies will enable any healthcare enterprise to be sustainable.
5. What type of e-Health policy strategies would you like to see adopted by your country and/or local healthcare provider organizations?

Health Informatics
E.J.S. Hovenga et al. (Eds.)
IOS Press, 2010
doi:10.3233/978-1-60750-476-4-30

4.   E-Health Records and Future Healthcare

Evelyn J.S. HOVENGA[1], RN, PhD (UNSW), FACHI, FACS[a], Sam HEARD
MBBS, FACHI[b]

[a] *Director, eHealth Education, Consultant, openEHR Foundation, and Honorary
Senior Research Associate, Centre for Health Informatics & Multiprofessional
Education, University College London, Honorary Academic Fellow, Austin
Health, Melbourne, Adjunct Professor, Central Queensland University
Rockhampton, Queensland, and Victoria University, Melbourne, Australia*
[b] *Chief Executive Officer, Ocean Informatics, Director, openEHR Foundation,
Senior Visiting Research Fellow, University College London, England*

Abstract. This chapter gives an educational overview of:
- Data collected, stored in health records and used for multiple purposes
- Electronic health records and how these are likely to influence our future
- Personal health records
- Clinical systems and their relationship to national data collections
- Potential future use of new technologies

Keywords. Medical; record systems – computerized, Forms and records control,
Personal information, Computer communication networks, Internet, Data
collection, Documentation, Telemedicine

Introduction

Information and knowledge about our own health and the health services we receive
during our lifetime are usually documented in records kept by ourselves and the many
different health care service providers we interact with. Now that we have entered the
electronic era we expect these records to be maintained in an electronic form.
Achieving this in a manner that truly is worth the investment and that provides a real
benefit to us requires a paradigm shift in thinking. Adoption and use of the latest
information, communication and knowledge management technologies enable us all to
be globally empowered in what Friedman [1] refers to as the latest version of
globalisation. He identified ten major political events, innovations and companies as
forces that have occurred since 1989 to flatten the world resulting in multiple new ways
for us to do business including the adoption of various tools enabling collaboration.
Key to this change was the world wide web, a platform that enabled convergence of
these forces. Further progress came about as visionaries and early adopters worked
with technology experts changing many business practices such as the introduction of

---

[1] Corresponding Author: e.hovenga@ehealtheducation.net

on-line banking or shopping. This was followed by the integration of various digital communication media such as the convergence of personal computers with TV broadcasts via broadband. Consequently within the health industry we now have to work with *"new players, on a new playing field, developing new processes and habits for horizontal collaboration……… the most important force shaping global economics and politics in the early twenty-first century"* [1[p.212]]. This chapter explores this paradigm shift as it relates to e-(electronic) health records (EHRs) and the delivery of future healthcare services.

1. Information is Key

Health care concerns all of us. It is about maintaining our physical, functional, emotional, mental, and spiritual wellbeing within our environment; within its own physical, social and family contexts. We need to know about preventing ill health or injury and how to best manage any genetic, acquired or environmental limitations or disabilities in a manner that optimises our sense of well being. There is more information about our body and how it functions, more research and more effort optimising its function than any other aspect of life. The business of maintaining health and delivering health care is certainly information and knowledge intensive. This makes the business management aspects of healthcare ideally suited to this new web enabled communication and media-intensive global paradigm.

When a person engages with anyone in the health industry they communicate by providing information that needs to be interpreted by the receiver. Shannon (1948) referred to such communication as a 'mathematical information theory of communications' described by Nelson [2[p.11]] as follows. The sender originates a message, an encoder converts the content into a code such as words, letters, symbols or a computer code that needs to be sent via a channel such as sound waves, telephone lines or paper. Noise such as background sounds may occupy space on the channel but is not part of the message. A decoder converts the message to enable the receiver to understand the message. In other words information is the result of an organization and interpretation of data that results in our ability to understand the message. This has to do with not only the language used but also with the way data (the message) is presented.

Healthcare professionals rely on all types of information presented by the patient. They use all their senses and prior knowledge to interpret such information. For example the taking of a body's temperature produces a reading. The reading itself is data such as 37 that becomes information once we apply the knowledge that this figure represents a body temperature measurement. Further meaning is obtained by applying our knowledge that a reading of 37 degrees Celcius represents a normal body temperature. This provides us with the information that this patient does not have a fever. However in the first instance a touch of a child's forehead may well have provided that same indication in the first instance, the measurement and reading confirms this.

Information is key to successful problem solving and health service delivery. Problem solving includes deciding on an investigative strategy, making a correct diagnosis, assessing care needs, and choosing the most appropriate treatment option. Ideally information is verifiable, free from bias, clearly communicated, appropriate and accurate. Some information may be quantifiable, comprehensive or timely. All necessary information needs to be accessible. These characteristics then are the precursors or requirements of electronic information systems.

People using such systems also have requirements to be effective; they must have 'information literacy'. This can be defined "as an understanding and set of abilities enabling individuals to recognize when information is needed and have the capacity to locate, evaluate and use effectively the needed information" [3]. Information literacy used to be a concept embraced by librarians however the relationship between information literacy concepts and computer or information technology literacy in health care facilities became apparent during the 1990s [4]. Consequently it is argued that health professionals need both traditional literacy skills and this new information literacy.

Optimising the use of information and communication technologies to support the management of health and the delivery of health care services requires the engagement of visionaries, computing experts, innovators, risk takers, movers and shakers and a change of thinking by managers, purchasing decision makers, legislators, policy developers and implementers. It requires an ability to clearly define all health concepts that need to be electronically managed in a standard manner to minimise loss of meaning. This is explained in some detail in chapter 6 on important health information concepts. The focus of this chapter is about information acquisition, communication, documentation and use, some of which requires convergence with knowledge management technologies via electronic health records. One key but yet to be resolved issue is a person's health information governance, ownership, control, access and use. The indications are that we should be more concerned about health information access than ownership in this new paradigm; specifically control of access.

2. Patient Controlled

Generally speaking patients, or their parent or guardian or carer, decide when to make contact with the health system. In cases of injury patients may have a say in where and by whom they wish to be treated but when severe ill health episodes or injuries occur they may lose that control. We have all experienced being in control of aspects of our life and understand how this contributed to our own sense of wellbeing; this undoubtedly extends beyond our activities and behaviours to what others know about us. The transmission of information about ourselves is fundamental to our autonomy. Just as it is known that being engaged, participating and managing one's own work related activities contributes to job satisfaction and improved productivity.

Similarly it is well known that patients who are in control of their own health management enjoy better overall outcomes. This is especially so patients requiring chronic disease management. However this also means that health professionals as well as information systems need to be able to support such patient empowerment and patients themselves need to have the necessary information and skills to access and use this information. Consequently all technologies used for this purpose need to be well designed to suit the average health care consumer. The consequent transparency is a major change for older generations who simply hold the belief that 'doctor knows best' and for many health professionals who still maintain a paternalistic attitude that influences their 'doctor-patient' relationship.

Patient control and empowerment is now in everyone's best interest as it has the capacity to not only improve health outcomes but also reduce the demand for health services; this translates into significant cost savings especially if there is less need for contact with health professionals. Such a change in focus offers some hope in providing for an increasingly ageing society, who are themselves proving adept at using new technology, with an increased need for long term management of chronic diseases when there are major shortages in the health workforce. These facts plus a demand from people now accustomed to managing their lives in an electronic environment, are expected to push new health policies and procedures towards enabling patients to take charge of their own health care management. Good use of available technologies contributes to our ability to create sustainable national health systems.

2.1 Hand Held, Distributed or Centralised

So far we have established that information is key, that patients need to be in control and that all stakeholders need to possess the relevant information and technology literacy to effectively manage our health care. Thus health information needs to be patient centred, recorded and managed in a manner that enables ease of documentation (data/information collection), storage, access, retrieval, timely and multi-purpose use. Our primary focus is therefore the patient information record or container that has traditionally been paper based but now needs to be structured to meet these fundamental electronic requirements. These records have been spread around our community with each provider maintaining their own record. Only the patient knows about all providers who have or had a record about them. Such records are usually not kept forever. Yet ideally our health records contain all the information about our past, present and future planned care. It is very difficult to predict what information is of no use in the future. A minor flu-like illness may indicate the onset of a chronic viral condition some time later, a tick bite gives the clue of Lyme's disease or a gastrectomy many years previously indicates that vitamin B12 deficiency might be the cause of neurological symptoms. Computers are wonderful tools for getting the information that we need at a particular moment.

In President Bush's State of the Union address in January 2004 he outlined a plan to ensure that most Americans have electronic health records within the next 10 years. He stated: "By computerizing health records, we can avoid dangerous medical mistakes, reduce costs, and improve care" [5]. He was of the view that a health care system must put "the needs and the values of the patient first and give[s] patients information they need to make clinical and economic decisions – in consultation with dedicated health care professionals". In August 2009 the Obama administration unveiled $1.2 billion in federal grants for electronic health records systems to create vast records sharing networks as part of its health care reform plan aimed at cutting future health care costs and improving care [6].

Given that people are often mobile, especially throughout a lifetime, they are expected to have encounters with a variety of healthcare providers in numerous different locations. Despite this their health information is ideally kept up to date and complete to ensure continuity of care, to avoid unnecessary investigations and most importantly to ensure the safety of the care provided. In the absence of such access people have been expected to simply remember all significant health events such as allergies, vaccinations, surgical interventions, current drug treatments. With current technologies we can do so much better but we need to decide what controls there are to be for access to our e-health records; the electronic data that is akin to the paper record. There are choices to be made regarding health record storage: should these be on handheld devices such as our mobile phone with a local barrier, in distributed systems at the institutions where we seek health care or in one centralised repository so that it can be accessed simply by ourselves and those providing care?

The reality is inevitably all of the above. Home recording of blood pressures or blood sugars, now known to be highly accurate, necessitates some local capacity even if it is limited to the device itself. Health care providers will be legally bound to record and maintain information they have offered and will require ongoing access to this. Some information, such as severe allergy, may be best made available to all and a wristband is unlikely to be the most appropriate location when more and more transactions take place electronically. The solutions offered should not dictate the storage scheme. The scale of the implementation and differing views on the appropriateness of centralisation of information and access control will force governments to abandon single source systems as a solution in this space.

When e-health records are distributed amongst various healthcare providers they may be linked to enable data sharing. However, this apparently straightforward step requires that each system shares a single logical information model. Therefore a precursor of achieving information sharing is a standardized structure to house the content of e-health records.

3. Standardised Content

Back in the 1960's Professor Larry Weed designed the problem oriented medical record (POMR) that was adopted by many; in fact it became ubiquitous in clinical documentation [7]. It provided a structured framework for the recording of patient information that enabled better medical decisions to be made. What is now needed is an international standard way for holding clinical data electronically to enable reliable and accurate electronic communication of all clinical data between systems and health care providers to achieve further improvements to patient outcomes. There are several fundamental standards requirements whose international or at least national adoption will ensure that these benefits can be realised. They are presented in summary form in Table 1. These concepts are discussed in greater detail in chapter 11 on national standards in health informatics. The standards required for clinical data types, terminology and clinical domain models are also discussed in greater depth in chapter 6 on important health information concepts.

The "Integrated Care Electronic Health Record" (EHR) is defined by the International Organization for Standardization [8] as:

> "...a repository of information regarding the health of a subject of care in computer processable form, stored and transmitted securely, and accessible by multiple authorised users. It has a commonly agreed logical information model which is independent of EHR systems. Its primary purpose is the support of continuing, efficient and quality integrated health care and it contains information which is retrospective, concurrent and prospective."

Table 1 Fundamental Standards Enabling the Realisation of Benefits via the Use of e-Health Records

Standard Required	Explanation
e-Health record structure/ architecture/information model	A structured record facilitates ease and accuracy of data extraction including data types suitable for holding clinical content
Set of clinical content models and terminology	To ensure that all clinical data stored within these records are structured in a standard manner and use standard terminology, thus enabling data/information comparison and aggregation without loss of meaning.
Unique patient identifier	To ensure that data from one provider record can be added to another provider's or patient held record that belongs to the same patient.
Unique individual and organisational provider identifier	To ensure that patient records maintained by an individual provider will be associated with that provider only and no other.

According to Garde, Knaup, et al [9] this means in practical terms that an EHR has the following characteristics:

- The EHR is **patient-centred**: one EHR relates to one subject of care, not to an episode of care at an institution;
- The EHR is **longitudinal**: it is a long-term record of care, possibly birth to death;
- The EHR is **comprehensive**: it includes a record of care events from all types of carers and provider institutions tending to a patient, not just one specialty; in other words there are no important care events of any kind not in the EHR;
- The EHR is **prospective**: not only are previous events recorded, so is decisional and prospective information such as plans, goals, orders and evaluations.

3.1 Personal Health Records (PHRs)

Since Bush's 2004 State of Union address and a parallel push for patient empowerment we are witnessing the promotion and increasing uptake of personal health records (PHRs). The international definition of an e-health record is "Repository of information regarding the health status of a subject of care, in computer processable form " [8] although more than 20 definitions for EHRs and their equivalent are provided in various standards. A PHR is a term used to describe both electronic patient centred records within healthcare organisations (such as primary care in the United Kingdom) as well as records kept by individuals (in most other countries). The differences will be content, who compiles, owns and has access to the record. These are issues yet to be resolved. In any event patient/personal records may be stored on any server with web access or on handheld devices or consist of a module within a large integrated information system that allows patients and their providers to share an online record and use decision support tools.

A personal health record for a child with 'special health care needs' may also be developed specifically for the child's parents/guardian and carers enabling them to help their children receive the best possible care [10p.997]. Personal health records are usually established independently of healthcare providers by people who simply wish to maintain their own health record. Indeed a growing number of companies specialise in providing such web-based opportunities. Alternatively a person can simply use their own PC to maintain such a record and make it available to any provider as required via a memory stick or printed copy. In the simplest form it could consist of a print out listing current medications or allergies carried in one's pocket, briefcase or handbag. Some people carry an alert wrist band that could be classified as a PHR.

Until there is wide agreement on the standardisation of content, the opportunity to hold one's entire health record as a PHR is not possible. Ideally the PHR will conform to the model used in clinical systems to enable people to keep the information they deem important and to allow electronic communication of this information without relying on consent of third parties.

The American Health Information Management Association has launched a website, [www.myphr.com] that explains how the adoption of PHRs assists people to play a more active role in their health care. It also provides instructions on how to best maintain such a record. This topic is covered in greater detail in chapter 16 on consumer health informatics.

3.2 Clinical Systems

Clinical information systems are software applications using clinical data and information to support all clinical activities such as prescribing, medication management, order entry for pathology, clinical records and diagnostic imaging services. Clinical systems usually provide decision support services and access to clinical practice guidelines. Ideally such systems include telehealth and home monitoring data and make use of and contribute to standard e-health records. Clinical systems may be referred to as e-health record systems. Section 3 includes chapters covering various clinical systems and the e-health record relationship in more detail. One Government department's [11] business case for the adoption of clinical systems includes the following anticipated outcomes:

- Reduced medication errors
- Reduced redundant pathology tests by minimising transcription errors
- Reduced clinician administrative tasks, resulting in more time spent with patients
- Improvements in turnaround times for medication orders
- Increased use of less expensive drugs and tests
- Reduced delays in patient discharge from speedy availability of test results
- Reduction in additional bed-days associated with adverse events.

However clinical systems also have the potential to compromise patient safety [12]. Anyone able to program can develop a clinical system and make it available for use by clinicians as there is no control or regulatory mechanism. Clinical outcomes are rarely measured making it difficult to detect errors. Coiera and Westbrook [13] noted that "it takes something like 10 years for a new compound to go from laboratory to clinical trial, and many more before a drug's safety and efficacy are proven" and asked why a similar process does not exist for clinical software? The answer is that it is early days and we do not derive sufficient benefit from clinical systems to warrant such restrictions. Systems are generally adopted on the basis of their coverage of functions required rather than measurable benefits. Improved access to records in hospitals is often sufficient to make the investment worthwhile from a management perspective.

3.3 National Repositories

The World Health Organisation (WHO) collects national statistics for 50 core indicators organized into six major areas: mortality and burden of disease, health service coverage, risk factors, health system inputs, differentials in health outcome and coverage, as well as basic socio-demographic statistics from 193 member nations to monitor trends of global public health. The availability of this data, provided by individual nations, enables the WHO to provide leadership in all matters that are critical to the health of these nations. Many nations collect data additional to that required by the WHO for their own public health purposes. For example, Australia has a minimum data set collection for admitted patient episodes and numerous additional registries, many of which also share their data with international public health organisations such as for example the Centre for Disease Control (CDC) or the International Association of Cancer Registries (IARC).

National repositories are dependent upon the adoption of a standard metadata schema that enable data linkage from multiple data sources. These repositories and registries all require data normally stored in patient health records which most commonly tend to be extracted from those records manually.

Agreement about the standardised representation of clinical content in e-health records not only allows more accurate automated retrieval of data for reporting purposes, it provides a means of establishing a reporting process. For instance, a national collection which is deemed critical may require that a person's weight is recorded in order that other values can be interpreted safely. Having agreed on the representation of body weight in the health record and the other values, it is possible to request that these values are always present in a health record of the target population. Thus, standardisation of clinical content should take the needs of this 'secondary' data collection into account.

3.4 Registries

Registries are used for public health surveillance purposes such as bio-surveillance security, chronic diseases and for diseases with rapid treatment advancement such as the blood cancers. Registries provide valuable epidemiological, demographic and social indicators about the health of a population. Ideally such registries contain information needed for health policy development or analysis to enable the implementation of appropriately planned responses to meet health service demands. The ability to link data repositories enhances their value, but this is dependent upon standardisation and the adoption of a generalised registry infrastructure for each domain. Data to populate these registries come from clinical systems such as pathology or imaging or from paper or e-health records using a variety of data collection methods. To clearly understand the types of knowledge represented in these data collections one needs to analyse the relationships between the data entities. Only then is it possible to develop the system requirements suited to maximizing the usability of the data collected taking advantage of today's technology [14]. Standardisation of clinical content is also relevant in this context.

3.5 Research

The availability of standardised content in PHRs, clinical systems, national repositories and registries enables greater use of such data for research purposes as more and more relationships between clinical and personal information become important in determining the best treatments. People will be able to consent personally for their data to be used in research and be aware of possible benefits to themselves and others. They will be able to add relevant personal health information as part of this process. This is covered in some depth in chapters 31 and 32 on practice based evidence for clinical practice improvement and integration of data for research. To enable outcomes monitoring it becomes necessary to have full e-health record linkage between multiple providers as only then will it be possible to assess each patient journey through the health system based on a clear indication of the many and varied diagnostic/treatment/care processes undertaken by multiple providers as a contribution to the final outcome over any given time period.

4. Clinical Engagement

Given that the business of maintaining health and delivering health care is information intensive, it is critical that clinicians are engaged in determining health record and clinical system requirements, in fact to be the primary drivers of clinical content. The agreed content must support their work flow and they must be motivated in the process of engagement. However the clinicians in turn need to appreciate not only the information needs relevant to their own discipline but also the information needs of other clinicians as well as organisational and national information reporting needs. Clinical business analysts are hard to find as few if any existing educational programs prepare clinicians to competently undertake such tasks. Every clinical discipline has its own information domain although these are small compared to the information shared between specialties and disciplines. This is an area that needs attention as standardised content introduces a need for discipline specific electronic knowledge and information governance. This will become clearer once you have read the other chapters in this book, especially chapter 17 on engaging clinicians.

4.1 Appropriate Quality Controls

As mentioned previously clinical systems can compromise patient safety, hence it is important for clinicians using such systems to be reassured that the content is processed according to the latest available knowledge. This is only possible if proper quality control procedures are put in place.

The United States has established a Certification Commission for Healthcare Information Technology which has the responsibility for certifying all clinical systems maintaining e-health records and their networks. Their mission is to *"accelerate the adoption of health information technology by creating an efficient, credible and sustainable certification program"* [15] [16]. Companies need to make their product available for rigorous testing and evaluation against a long list of criteria based on a carefully scripted product demonstration observed by a jury of three people. These criteria are open for public comment for several weeks every time these are updated.

Several European countries initiated accreditation schemes for e-health systems but there is no international standard set of evaluation criteria. The European Institute for Health Records established in 2002 is now the European authorised certification body [17]. It defines functional and other criteria to support EHRs certification development, testing and assessment. Their certification criteria is freely available via their website. The Australian Medical Association (AMA) [18] supports the development of a regulatory framework to standardise and govern the use of clinical software in medical practice. It is the AMA's view that such an approach will contribute to reducing potential risks and improve quality and safety related to the use of information technology. Their position statement indicates that clinical engagement in this process is essential.

4.2 Builds Clinician Trust

Adoption of the AMA's position regarding the need for a regulatory framework and governance with clinical engagement is a good start to building clinician trust of the functions performed by clinical systems. It is essential for clinician's to be assured that clinical systems purchased and implemented are kept up to date regarding for example the use of clinical guidelines or latest research findings. In addition such systems must be safe. They need to be able to have trust that the system will process all information accurately and consistently.

5. Overcome the Tyranny of Distance

Adoption of a national broadband service and the latest communication technologies does mean that clinicians with specialised knowledge can be available to people and providers in any location at any time. It also has the capacity to promote people with chronic diseases taking greater responsibility for their own care via, for example, home monitoring under supervision. Such scenarios have the potential to greatly reduce the demand for health services and improve patient outcomes. The technologies used include interactive video, data and image transfer using store and forward technologies, multimedia including the Internet, file transfer, web video and data streaming. These technologies are used for patient consultations, to obtain second opinions, diagnostic support, clinical information transfer including real time in support of trauma cases, remote and home patient monitoring, continuing professional education and more. A number of legal issues such as jurisdictional licencing and funding tele-consultations often require legislation. Chapter 20 on e-health, telehealth and remote access covers this topic in some detail.

5.1 Video Consultations Where Required

Australia has been using video conferencing since the mid 1990's mostly for educational purposes. The biggest clinical user is mental health. Its use by health professionals from a number of specialty areas continues to increase with significant benefits reported for Queensland Health for example [19]. Video consultations are now routine in this setting and used on an as required basis. The availability of high quality personal webcams and free internet communications will increase the pressure on healthcare providers to deliver e-health care at the patient's home or other location without attending in person. Preliminary consultations, which are brief and include visual information, have great potential to save huge amounts of time for patients and doctors alike. The added value is greatest when brief access is provided to experienced clinicians most able to deal effectively with the issue at hand.

5.2 Second Opinions from Centres of Excellence

Technologies are now available that enable real time video images to be transmitted enabling clinicians or even patients to obtain second opinions from centres of excellence on an as required basis. This is particularly important to assist clinicians working in remote areas or for community nurses making home visits. In many situations it is only with the aid of visual analysis that second opinions can be given. Use of these technologies can save many hours of patient travel which in some settings can be measured in thousands of dollars. Effective implementation may require changes to existing legislation or funding arrangements.

5.3 Examination Centres

Many devices now have communication channels to allow data to be entered in an e-health record. The combination of video and access to information derived from measurement of physical attributes such as weight, blood pressure, blood sugar etc will transform the ability of clinicians to provide health care at a distance. In small remote townships this may extend to ultrasound data, near patient laboratory testing and Xray data without a clinician being physically present.

More isolated pharmacies and remote health outstations of the future may have examination centres that allow such comprehensive physical examination data to be collected locally and used by the clinician at a distance. The introduction of such facilities is easy to research but have the risk of overestimating the benefits based on the enthusiasm of the initiators of the project; the Hawthorn effect. Sometimes just having the equipment there is reassuring for people living in a very remote setting and maintenance and training can be limited due to the availability of experienced operators via video and remote control.

6. Assists Understanding

E-health records have the possibility to assist understanding by taking standardised content and displaying this in a manner that is appropriate to the viewer. Terminology can be transformed to use more non-professional terms if this is helpful; for example, coronary thrombosis of the left anterior descending coronary artery can be displayed as myocardial infarction if the latter is not understood, or heart attack if that definition is not helpful. Information for specific purposes can be presented to clinicians or patients themselves. A review of medication that presents which medications have indications that are known side-effects of other medications being used is particularly helpful to prevent poly pharmacy. The way this is presented might be very different for different users. Some information might be better presented in a consistent manner. Laboratory results, company logos aside, can be presented consistently in the same environment ensuring users recognise the meaning of the data on the screen.

6.1 E-health Records Influence Our Future

The e-health record provides the foundation data for health care. All knowledge access and computerised assistance, such as automated lookup, decision support and notifications, work much more efficiently and effectively with electronic access to the e-health record but standardised representation of content is a prerequisite. We can all see the future, even the politicians around the world. The reality is that the gap between what is possible and what is available is growing rapidly. Standardisation of the e-health record, not clinical systems, is the missing link. Consistent representation of important clinical concepts will save enormous amounts of time and money by eliminating the clinical configuration now required by hospital systems, often taking many years to complete. A shared international terminology is now a reality. The next decade will see clinical systems finally realising their potential.

The next section provides a good overview of the many basic health informatics concepts, including interoperability, terminologies, clinical knowledge management and more, to enable improved understanding of the many features identified in this introductory section.

References

[1] Friedman T.L. 2006 *The world is flat: The globalised world in the twenty-first century*. 2nd expanded edition. Penguin Books Ltd., London UK
[2] Nelson R. 2002 Major Theories Supporting Health Care Informatics in: Englebardt S P, Nelson R (Eds) *Health Care Informatics: an interdisciplinary approach*. Mosby, St Louis
[3] ALA 1989, *Presidential committee on information literacy*, American Library Association: Chicago. Australian Medical Association (AMA) Position Statement: Safety and Quality of E-Health Systems – 2006 viewed 8 May 2008 from http://www.ama.com.au/web.nsf/doc/WEEN-6VD2PW
[4] Carty, B. and P. Rosenfield, From Computer Technology to Information Technology: Findings from a national study of nursing education. *Computers in Nursing, 1998*. 16(5): p. 259-265.
[5] Bush G 2004 Promoting Innovation and Competitiveness, *President Bush's Technology Agenda* viewed 8 May 2008 from http://www.whitehouse.gov/infocus/technology/economic_policy200404/chap3.htm
[6] O'Harrow R U.S. to Dole Out $1.2 Billion for Health Records Technology. *The Washington Post, Friday, August 21, 2009* http://www.washingtonpost.com/wp-dyn/content/article/2009/08/21 viewed 12 November 2009
[7] Johnson C D, Zeiger R F,Das A K, Goldstein M K, 2006 Task Analysis of Writing Hospital Admission Orders: Evidence of a Problem-Based Approach. *AMIA Annu Symp Proc. 2006; 389–393* viewed 8 May 2008 from http://www.pubmedcentral.nih.gov/articlerender.fcgi?artid=1839659
[8] *ISO TR 20514:2004* Health Informatics - EHR Definition, Scope, & Context.
[9] Garde S, Knaup P, Hovenga E, Heard S (2007): Towards Semantic Interoperability for Electronic Health Records: Domain Knowledge Governance for openEHR Archetypes. *Methods of Information in Medicine. 46(3): 332-343.* http://dx.doi.org/doi:10.1160/ME5001
[10] Rocha R A, Romeo A N, Norlin C. 2007 Core features of a parent-controlled pediatric medical home record. In K.Kuhn et al (Eds) *Medinfo2007*, IOS Press, Amsterdam
[11] *Victorian State Government 2008 HealthSMART Office of Health Information Systems* of the Metropolitan Health and Aged Care Services. Division of the Victorian State Government, Department of Human Services, Australia viewed 8 May 2008 from http://www.health.vic.gov.au/healthsmart/clinsys.htm
[12] Ash JS, Berg M, Coiera E. 2004 Some unintended consequences of information technology in health care: the nature of patient care information system-related errors. *J Am Med Inform Assoc. 2004 Mar-Apr;11(2):121-4.* viewed 8 May 2008 from http://www.pubmedcentral.nih.gov/articlerender.fcgi?tool=pubmed&pubmedid=14633936
[13] Coiera E and Westbrook J 2006 Editorial: Should Clinical software be regulated? *The Medical Journal of Australia 2006;* 184 (12): 600-601 viewed 8 May 2008 http://www.mja.com.au/public/issues/184_12_190606/coi10287_fm.html

[14] Safran, C., Bloomrosen, M., Hammond, W. E., Labkoff, S., Markel-Fox, S., Tang, P. C. & Detmer, D. E. (2007) Toward a National Framework for the Secondary Use of Health Data: an American Medical Informatics Association white paper. *JAMIA,* 14, 1-9
[15] Certification Commission for Healthcare Information Technology *(CCHIT)* viewed 8 May 2008 http://www.cchit.org/about/index.asp
[16] CCHIT *2007 Physician's Guide to Certification for Ambulatory Electronic Health Records.* Accessed 8 May 2008 http://www.cchit.org/files/CCHITPhysiciansGuide2007.pdf
[17] *European Institute for Health Records* http://www.eurorec.org/index.cfm?actief=home
[18] Australian Medical Association (AMA) *Position Statement on Safety and Quality of eHealth Systems -* 2006 viewed 12 November 2009 http://www.ama.com.au/node/2509
[19] Kennedy C, Blignault I, Hornsby D, Yellowlees P. 2001 Videoconferencing in the Queensland health service. *Journal of Telemedicine and Telecare, Volume 7, Number 5,* 1 October 2001, pp. 266-271(6)

Review Questions

1. Make a list of possible uses of clinical data collected at the point of care.
2. Identify and describe issues associated with such secondary data usage and consider how a balance between individual private use and public good is best obtained.
3. How would you like to see better use made of clinical data to improve population benefits.
4. Describe how individuals should be able to make good use of Personal Health Records.

Section 2

Basic Health Informatics Concepts

Health Informatics
E.J.S. Hovenga et al. (Eds.)
IOS Press, 2010
doi:10.3233/978-1-60750-476-4-45

5. Interoperability

Dennis H JARVIS[1a,b], Jacqueline H JARVIS [a,c]

[a] *Central Queensland University, Rockhampton, Australia*
[b] *Associate Professor, School of Computing Sciences*
[c] *Senior Lecturer, School of Management and Information Systems*

Abstract. This chapter gives an educational overview of:

- the roles that ontology and process play in interoperability
- the processes that can be employed to realise interoperability and their supporting technologies
- interoperability solutions employed in the health informatics sector within the conceptual model presented in the chapter
- directions for future research in the area of interoperability for health informatics

Keywords. Information Systems, Health, Computer Communication Networks, Computer Systems, Interoperability, Connectivity, Ontology

Introduction

In this chapter, we present an overview of interoperability from a software engineering perspective. That is, we look at interoperability as a property of distributed systems and examine how it can be realised. In this regard, we clearly distinguish between the **process** that is employed to achieve interoperability and the **content** that is transferred by these processes.

Interoperability is an issue that is becoming increasingly important in the IT industry in general and the Health Informatics field in particular. The IEEE has defined interoperability as *"the ability of two or more systems or components to exchange information and to use the information that has been exchanged"* [1].

This definition identifies two key processes – information exchange and information use – that are required for interoperability of systems. However, it does not specify what constitutes information, exchange or use. We begin by considering information. Information is normally contrasted with data on the one hand and knowledge on the other. In the knowledge management literature, it is the generally accepted view [2] that

- data constitutes simple facts
- information arises from the combination data into meaningful structures, and
- knowledge is information situated in a particular context

For example, a blood pressure reading might constitute a data item. The collection of validated data items in a patient record gives rise to information about a patient and aspects of that information become knowledge when a patient is admitted with chest pains.

---

[1] Corresponding Author: d.jarvis@cqu.edu.au

The goal of interoperability (as defined by IEEE) is not to exchange knowledge, but to exchange information (as defined above) and data. Knowledge transfer is currently outside the scope of mainstream interoperability solutions and is an area of active research, particularly within the multi-agent systems community. The key problem is that knowledge is dynamic - it requires interpretation, via appropriate procedures, of information that is situated within a particular context. For example, a control system for an Unmanned Air Vehicle (UAV) needs to determine (procedures) whether the aircraft it has identified (information) from its on board sensors (data) are hostile (knowledge). In a medical environment, a decision support system (procedure) may need to determine whether the blood pressure reading (information) for a patient is consistent with other patient data and whether it is indicative of a particular problem (knowledge). In general, knowledge generation is an activity that requires sophisticated reasoning, as evidenced by activities such as medical diagnosis, patient planning and in the military domain, battle space awareness. At present, there is no consensus on how knowledge should be generated for particular domains, let alone shared between applications. Various models for sharing knowledge have been implemented, such as joint intentions [3], team beliefs [4] and goal context propagation [5]. However, this research has been grounded in agent based systems and has therefore not impacted on mainstream software development

The relationship between data, information and knowledge within an application is illustrated in Figure 1.

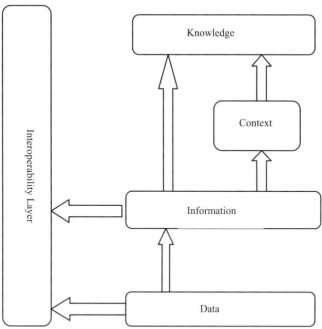

Figure 1. The Relationship Between Data, Information and Knowledge Within an Application. Vertical arrows represent the application of procedural knowledge. Horizontal arrows represent transfer of application content.

Information exchange between computer systems is generally understood in terms of communication protocols, which are rules that specify the types of messages that can be sent, the types of messages that can be received and instructions for message delivery. For example, with the postal system, we can send and receive letters and parcels. If we want the letter or parcel to be delivered, we need to provide the name and address of the recipient. We also provide our name and address in case it cannot be delivered, perhaps because the recipient has changed address. However, the delivery protocol that we use does not specify the contents of our letters. Letters can be bill payments or personal correspondence; they can be written in Japanese or English – it has no effect on the protocol. Note that additional (application specific) protocols can be employed on top of the basic delivery protocol. For example, companies employ specific protocols for overdue bills – initial invoice, 30 day reminder, 90 day reminder, threat of legal action etc.

The concepts of data, information and communication protocols, provide a generic framework for discussing interoperability. However, such a model, as presented in Figure 2, does not address the content (syntax) or the meaning (semantics) of the data and information that is transported between applications.

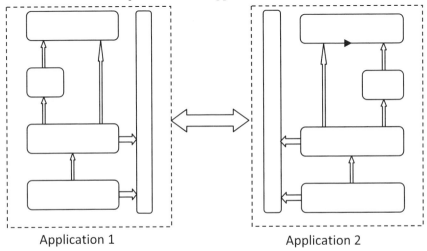

Figure 2. A Conceptual Model for Interoperability. Interaction between application 1 and application 2 is mediated by protocols. The internal structure for an application is as detailed in Figure 1.

Also, the model assumes that the purpose of protocols is to transfer individual data items (data) or aggregate data items (information) between applications. Manipulation of message content (ie conversion of data to information and information to knowledge) is the responsibility of the recipient and is outside the scope of interoperability. However, it is now well accepted that applications should be able to interoperate at the level of services as well as data. This is exemplified in the business sector with the widespread interest in web services. Other approaches, such as distributed objects (as in CORBA) and remote procedure calls (RPCs) are firmly entrenched in general distributed systems development. In the multi-agent systems community, speech acts [6] are widely used, and form the basis of the FIPA standards [7].Typically, on service completion, data will be returned. This data might just be an acknowledgement of the success or failure of the requested service, or it might correspond to the result of the service (for example, an updated patient record or test results).

Service requests can be very specific (e.g. perform a colonoscopy on patient x) or more general in nature (e.g. check patient x for bowel problems). In the latter case, the servicer has autonomy over how the request is realised. What is being requested of the servicer is that it is to achieve a particular goal – it is free to achieve that goal in whatever way it considers appropriate. In the former case, the requester is specifying the service that is to be performed and the servicer has limited flexibility in its behaviour. Note that some services (such as bill generation) may be realised entirely in software, whereas other services (such as performing a colonoscopy) will require human involvement. In the latter case, the software application is concerned with the management of the requested service (logging, scheduling, etc) and not the actual conduct of the service.

The above considerations have led us to classify interoperability approaches in terms of whether interoperability is defined at the level of

1.   message transport,
2.   data,
3.   services or
4.   goals.

In this classification, data refers to both data and information, as defined by Tuomi [2]. Thus the data-oriented approach (level 2) is not restricted to a consideration of individual data items – it encompasses data aggregates as well. We also distinguish between goals and services. A goal defines an objective that is to be achieved or a process that is to be performed (e.g. check for bowel problems), but it does not specify how that objective or process is to be achieved, i.e. the services that are to be employed.

In terms of content, agreed upon vocabularies (ontologies) are mandatory for interoperability to be realised at levels 2-4. With the data-oriented approach, this means that agreement must be reached on the names of data items. That is that we must have a complete, consistent and standardised vocabulary for constructing message content. HL7's Object Identifiers[2] , its vocabulary resources and SNOMED CT are examples of such vocabularies in the health informatics domain. However, as we progress from level 2 through to level 4, the scope of the vocabulary increases as we need to have standardised and consistent terminology and models to describe both services and goals as well as data.

In the case of the service-oriented approach, standardisation is achieved through the employment of a common object model in application development. In the health informatics sector, examples include HL7's RIM (Reference Information Model) [8] and OpenEHR's Archetype models [9]. These efforts still retain a data focus, as services are yet to be the subject of standardisation. However, by adopting an object perspective, they become extensible in that direction. Also, in the case of archetypes, the object perspective allows constraint models for data to be easily specified and reused, meaning that data can be readily and consistently validated. This is infeasible in data-oriented approaches, even those that employ XML technology [10].

As with the service-oriented approach, the applicability of the goal-oriented approach is limited because of the lack of standard terminology – in this case for goals, as well as for services. Adoption of the approach within the health informatics community is a long way off, as there are major research issues to resolve before a standard terminology for goals can be specified. It is included in this chapter for completeness.

---

[2] Registry of OIDs at http://www.hl7.org/oid/index.cfm

In terms of meaning, the approach adopted within the health informatics community has been to define the semantics for each term in a standard vocabulary, such as HL7 or SNOMED CT. These definitions can either be informal (textual descriptions) or formal (e.g. logic based). One then either uses the term directly, or, as in the case of OpenEHR archetypes, one can bind a "local" term to a standard term. In essence, the same approach can be adopted to specify the semantics of services and ultimately, goals.

In the remainder of this chapter, we will discuss the four levels of interoperability that we identified above, in more detail. In particular, we will relate them to the underlying technologies that they employ. We will then conclude with a discussion of where interoperability is headed in the health informatics domain.

1. The Transport-Oriented Approach (Level 1)

In the traditional approach to software development, individual software applications are developed using an appropriate process model, such as the waterfall model, prototyping or evolutionary models [11]. All process models incorporate a requirements specification activity, although its location within the system lifecycle may vary. Requirements are classified as being either functional or non-functional. A functional requirement is a service (such as data validation) that is to be provided by the system under normal operating conditions. On the other hand, a non-functional requirement is an attribute of the system (such as performance or maintainability) that is required for a viable system implementation and that exists over the entire system lifecycle. Examples of non-functional requirements include performance, reliability and maintainability [12]. Interoperability has traditionally been viewed by the software engineering community as a non-functional requirement.

The problem interoperability poses for the system developer is that it is generally impossible to predict in advance what external interfaces will be required over the lifetime of the system, let alone what information will be required. Consequently, lowest common denominator solutions have been traditionally employed with systems being provided with standard interfaces appropriate for the application, such as HTTP for web servers and TCP/IP for general data communication [12].

In the transport-oriented approach, interoperability is seen as essentially a transport issue – what is provided are standardised mechanisms (in the form of communication protocols such as TCP/IP and HTTP) for transferring data. Message content and meaning is outside the scope of this view of interoperability. Analogies include the postal service, discussed previously and the rail system. In the latter case, a standard infrastructure in terms of track with standard gauge and containers of specified dimensions is provided. As with the postal system, the contents of containers are not specified, except in general terms.

In seeking a generic solution, the transport-oriented approach to interoperability provides limited infrastructure to support software development. It becomes the developer's responsibility to pack and unpack messages and to interpret and act upon message content. The remaining approaches seek to provide developers with a richer infrastructure – this is achieved by relaxing the genericity constraint to provide domain-specific infrastructure, as illustrated in Figure 3.

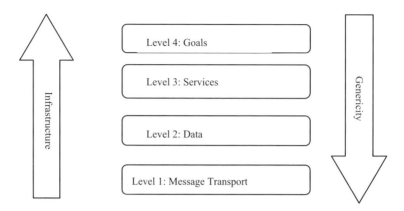

Figure 3. How the Genericity and Functionality of Interoperability Infrastructure Varies with Interoperability Level.

2.   The Data-Oriented Approach (Level 2)

The assumptions underpinning the transport-oriented approach are twofold:
1.   Standardised communication protocols will exhibit long term stability and support
2.   Message content is a data modelling issue and as such is not an interoperability issue.

The first assumption is reasonable if one employs mature standards. However, picking winners can be problematic for standards early in their lifecycle. For example, TCP/IP is a sensible choice for general data communications, but when it was first proposed in 1983 as a realisation of the transport layer in the OSI model [13] there was much debate as to its suitability for general purpose use because of efficiency considerations. In the late 1980's, MAP/TOP [13] looked set to become the dominant protocol in manufacturing enterprises, but it has since lost out to TCP/IP.

Another benefit of maturity is that usage patterns stabilise and pragmatism wins out over rigid adherence to standards. This is exemplified with the OSI model – its session and presentation layers are rarely used [14]. Rather, most applications will deal directly with the transport layer through the raw TCP/IP functionality provided by the networking libraries in Java and .NET. If more sophisticated interaction is required, such as remote procedure calls or distributed object invocation, then the session and presentation layers are replaced with a middle ware layer built on top of a TCP/IP transport layer [14].

The second assumption reflects a past in which applications were developed in isolation and with specific applications in mind. This view is still prevalent in the systems analysis community where the focus is still on the development of data models for particular applications [15]. The assumption is that each application requires its own specific data model which is generated either from application specific data or from other applications that have their own data models.

Particular sectors, such as health, e-business, defence simulation and manufacturing have recognised a need for consistent use of terminology and in response have compiled domain-specific vocabularies for the definition of message content. However, standardisation efforts have in general been limited to the syntactical issues of vocabulary and message structure and the specification of semantic content by and large remains a research issue [16].

The use of XML and its associated protocols (eg SOAP and HTTP) for data transfer [17] has become increasingly popular over the past decade. XML provides a flexible and extensible mechanism for creating domain specific data representation languages, of which document markup languages, such as XHTML [18] can be viewed as a special case. The XML product suite supports service definition through UDDI and WSDL and process definition through WS-BPEL. However, these languages are still data representation languages – they generate (as in XHTML) structured data in which data fields are delimited by tags that give information about that field. A data field may correspond to a method or service, but the details of that method or service is specified elsewhere. The use of XML technology to access and utilise remote web-based services is an area that has attracted much interest in the business sector, but it does not appear to be delivering on its initial promise of providing a new business model for service organisations. Individual organisations are tending to use web services in house rather than making the services available to external organisations [19].

3. The Service-Oriented Approach (Level 3)

A service-oriented approach to interoperability can be realised using either a distributed object model, such as CORBA [20] or a distributed service model, as in remote procedure calls (RPCs) [21]. In this regard, web services can be viewed as providing RPC functionality [17]. The difference between the two models is subtle – in the former case, remote objects are created and services are associated with remote object instances. In the latter case, services are statically associated with a single server process and no objects are created in order to perform a service [20].

An object is a software entity that, in its purest form, is accessed only through a well defined set of services – the underlying data that is used by the services is hidden from users of the object. Furthermore, services can be classified into those that are accessible to the user, and those that, like the underlying data, are hidden. For example, a patient's blood pressure history might be represented as an object, with methods to add and remove readings, display the history and so on. The underlying representation of the history and services for persisting the history might be hidden from the user.

It is now well understood within the software engineering community that object models make a better starting point for the analysis and design of software systems than data models. The reasons for this are twofold:

1. The key objects in a system are less likely to change over time than the data in a system. For example, the concept of blood pressure as a pair of pressure readings is unlikely to change, whereas it is conceivable that the units used may change.
2. An object, by being selective about what services and data are accessible to users of the object, is better able to hide changes in representation from users of the object. For example, if a blood pressure history was persisted to a database, the underlying database could be changed without impacting on users of the object.

In the distributed object approach, the focus of interoperability now becomes the definition of domain specific object models and the requesting of remote applications to perform particular services specified in the object model. Data is still transferred – either as input to the requested service or as the output of a requested service. However, this data can be transferred either as individual data elements or incorporated into an object instance. Object-based messaging differs from TCP/IP messaging in that the messages are persistent – they are typically queued within the middleware layer and a connection between the sender and receiver does not need to be established before transfer can be initiated, as in connection-oriented protocols such as TCP/IP.

Domain specific object models are an example of reference models, and encapsulate the key concepts in a domain and the relationships between those concepts. Reference models are characteristic of a mature domain, as they represent a general consensus within a particular community as to what are the key concepts and relationships in applications characteristic of their domain. For example, in health informatics, the primary concept is the patient record and in agent-based manufacturing, the primary concepts are parts, orders and resources. These concepts are then further refined through processes of classification and aggregation. As an example of classification, the patient record for a day surgery patient might be modelled as a specialisation of that for a long term patient. A patient record contains a collection of different medical reports and data – this is an example of aggregation.

From an interoperability viewpoint, adopting an object-centric approach suffers from the same problems as the data centric approach – there needs to be agreement on the vocabulary that is used. In the case of an object model, this means that agreement needs to be reached on object class names and on the class interfaces – that is, the methods and data of an object that will be publicly accessible.

The RPC approach differs from the distributed object approach in that the local application interacts with a remote application by invoking services that the remote application has made available to external applications. No objects are created in this interaction – only method (procedure) invocation occurs. The RPC approach originated in the work of [22] and was popularised with an implementation for the Sun workstation [21]. In traditional implementations, RPC methods were accessible to an individual application as pre-compiled library functions. However, with web services, a higher level of abstraction is provided. Descriptions of the service are developed by the service provider using WSDL (Web Service Description Language) and these descriptions are then made available in a UDDI (Universal Description, Discovery and Integration) registry. An application then interrogates registries to find suitable service providers and then interacts with the service provider directly using the SOAP protocol [17]. This process is summarised in Figure 4.

As with the distributed object approach, web services (and the RPC approach in general) requires agreement on the services that are to be provided and the vocabulary to be used. WSDL provides a general framework for describing services and how to access them, but the actual vocabulary employed needs to be agreed upon.

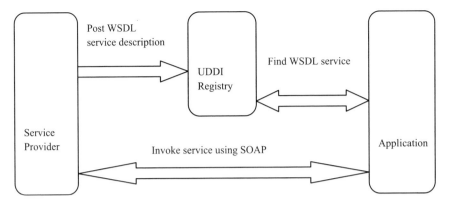

Figure 4. Web Service Invocation.

4.   The Agent-Oriented Approach (Level 4)

Agents extend the notion of encapsulation by encapsulating both data and behaviour. An agent is then able to exhibit a degree of autonomy when it is requested to perform a service, unlike an object. An agent may choose to decline to perform a service; if it accepts, it is free to realise the service in any manner that it chooses, so long as it meets the constraints of the service contract.   The agent-centric approach allows interoperability to be defined at the level of goal exchange.

Adoption of an agent-oriented approach permits a shift in perspective. For example, in the health informatics sector, rather than having applications that exchange health records and perform particular, well-defined functions, one can view the system in terms of patient proxies (represented as agents) that interact with service providers (also represented as agents). The idea is that in a hospitalisation scenario, for example, the patient proxy would drive the treatment process from admission through to release. A similar perspective has been employed in agent-based manufacturing, through the employment of the PROSA reference model [23]. In this approach, orders drive the production process by interacting with resource agents, that provide processing services and part agents, that provide processing plans. Staff agents are available to assist order agents when required. Initial studies (eg [24] [25]) indicate that the adoption of such a viewpoint shows promise in terms of producing simpler and more maintainable systems. Whether its application in the health informatics sector would yield similar benefits is an interesting research question.

As with the other approaches, agreement needs to be reached in terms of terminology and in the agent-centric approach this consensus needs to cover goals as well as objects and data items. Although industrial-strength agent applications have been deployed in niche areas for the past 25 years and commercially supported systems are available, the use of goals to realise interoperability is a recent innovation [5].

5. Current Practice

Traditionally, interoperability has been viewed in terms of information exchange, as demonstrated by the definition presented at the start of this chapter. In this perspective, the focus is on content at the expense of process – different levels of interoperability are distinguished according to the semantic interpretations of the information (data and data aggregates) that is exchanged. This is clearly reflected in the LCIM model proposed in Tolk [26] for defence simulation; the different levels in LCIM relate to information being tied to increasingly more sophisticated semantic interpretations, culminating in its attachment to shared conceptual models. It also gives rise to the common classification of interoperability in terms of syntactic interoperability and semantic interoperability. Again, the focus is on content – process is a secondary consideration.

The Health Informatics community has likewise focused on information exchange – it has been a leader in terms of ontology development as detailed in chapters 9 and 10. However, it is now exploring object models through, for example, HL7's RIM and OpenEHR's archetypes. Interoperability is still at the data level, although archetypes do provide data validation in the form of constraint models. Explicit validation models or services are not provided; rather validation is performed implicitly when an archetype instance is created. It was noted in Bird, Goodchild and Tun [10] that XML technologies such as XSLT are unable to adequately validate archetype constraints and that validation was best specified procedurally within the archetype. However, the option of describing validation (or other functions) as web services using WSDL remains an option. Interoperability at the goal level, while an attractive proposition, remains a research endeavour.

6.   Conclusion

In this chapter, we have presented a conceptual model for interoperability that clearly distinguishes between content and process. Four key processes – message transport, data transfer, service requests and goal exchange – were identified in the model, of which only the first three are widely used. Ontologies and object models, such as the SNOMED CT terminology and OpenEHR's Archetype Models, then provide these processes with the content that is to be exchanged. We noted that the focus of existing interoperability solutions available for health informatics is on data transfer, but they are able to draw upon rich ontological support at both the syntactic and semantic levels.

References

[1]   IEEE, 1990. *IEEE Standard Computer Dictionary: A Compilation of IEEE Standard Computer Glossaries.* IEEE Press, New York.
[2]   Tuomi, I. , 1999. **"D**ata is more than knowledge: implications of the reversed knowledge hierarchy for knowledge management and organizational memory", in HICSS-32. Proceedings of the 32nd Annual Hawaii International Conference on System Sciences.
[3]   Tambe, M., 1997. "Towards Flexible Teamwork", Journal of Artificial Intelligence Research, Vol. 7, pp. 83-124
[4]   Agent Oriented Software Group, 2008. "JACK™ Documentation", http://www.aosgrp.com/index.html cited June 2008
[5]   Rönnquist, R. and Jarvis, D. "Interoperability with Goal-Oriented Teams", In Proceedings of the Agent-based Technologies and Applications for Enterprise Interoperability ATOP 2008 Workshop, 7th International Joint Conference on Autonomous Agents & Multiagent Systems (AAMAS 2008) Estoril, Portugal, May 2008.
[6]   Wooldridge, M., 2002. *An Introduction to MultiAgent Systems*, Wiley.

[7]   IEEE Foundation for Intelligent Physical Agents, 2008. "The Foundation for Intelligent Physical Agents", http://www.fipa.org.
[8]   Health Level Seven Inc., 2008. "HL7", http://www.hl7.org
[9]   openEHR Foundation www.openEHR.org
[10] Bird, L., Goodchild, A. and Tun, Z., 2003. "Experiences with a Two-Level Modelling Approach to Electronic Health Records", Journal of Research and Practice in Information Technology, Vol. 35, No. 2, pp. 121-138
[11] Sommerville, I., 2007. *Software Engineering. 8th Edition*, Addison-Wesley.
[12] O'Brien, F., 2004. *The Engineering of Software Quality*, Pearson Education Australia.
[13] Tanenbaum, A., 1989. *Computer Networks. 2nd Edition.* Prentice-Hall.
[14] Tanenbaum, A. and Van Steen, M., 2007. *Distributed Systems: Principles and paradigms. 2nd Edition.* Prentice-Hall.
[15] Shelly, G.,Cashman, T. and Rosenblatt, H., 2008. *Systems Analysis and Design. 7th Edition.* Thomson Course Technology
[16] Noy, N., Doan, A. and Halevy, A., (2005). "Semantic Integration", AI Magazine, Vol. 20, No. 1, pp. 7-9.
[17] Chatterjee, S. and Webber, J., 2004. *Developing Enterprise Web Services. An Architect's Guide.* Prentice Hall. NY
[18] Musciano, C. and Kennedy, B., 2002. *HTML and XHTML: The Definitive Guide, Fifth Edition.* O'Reilly.
[19] Hart, C., Kauffman, J., Sussman, D. and Ullman, C., 2006. *Beginning ASP.NET 2.0.* Wiley.
[20] Coulouris, G., Dollimore, J. and Kindberg, T., 2005. *Distributed Systems: Concepts and Design. 4th Edition.* Addison Wesley
[21] Brown, C., 1994. *UNIX Distributed programming*, Prentice-Hall. NY
[22] Birrell, A. and Nelson, B., 1984. "Implementing Remote Procedure Calls", ACM Transactions on Computer Systems. Vol. 2, No. 1, pp. 39-59
[23] Van Brussell, H., Wyns, J., Valckenaers, P., Bongaerts, L. and Peeters, P., 1998. "Reference Architecture for Holonic Manufacturing Systems: PROSA". Computers in Industry, Vol. 37, pp. 255-274.
[24] Jarvis, J., Jarvis, D., Rönnquist, R. and Jain, L., 2008. *Holonic Execution: A BDI Approach.* Springer.
[25] Bussman, S., Jennings, N. and Wooldridge, M., 2004. *Multiagent Systems for Manufacturing Control: A Design Methodology.* Springer. NY
[26] Tolk, A., 2003. "The Levels of Conceptual Interoperability Model", in Proceedings of the 2003 Fall Simulation Interoperability Workshop, Orlando, Florida.

Review Questions

1. Explain how ontology and process roles contribute to achieving interoperability.

2. Describe the processes and supporting technologies that can be employed in the Health Informatics sector to realize interoperability.

3. What interoperability solutions are employed in your organization? Describe this relative to the conceptual model presented in this chapter.

4. How would you like to see future research in the area of interoperability progress for the benefit the health industry and the population as a whole?

56

Health Informatics
E.J.S. Hovenga et al. (Eds.)
IOS Press, 2010
© 2010 The authors and IOS Press. All rights reserved.
doi:10.3233/978-1-60750-476-4-56

6. Important Health Information Concepts

Heather GRAIN[1] A.Dip MRA, RMRA, GD DP, MHI, FACHI
Academic Fellow Austin Health, Director E-Health Education and Director Pavillion
Prime Care, Melbourne, Australia

Abstract. This chapter gives an educational overview of:
- The difference between actual patient information and information structure and metadata
- The purpose of defining health information concepts
- How health concepts are defined
- The components used to define health concepts and their relationship to expressing meaning clearly and safely.

Keywords. Information Science, Information Management, Terminology, Data Collection, Metadata, Information Services, Health, Database, Data Management Systems, Systematised Nomenclature of Medicine

1. What is a Health Concept and Why Does It Matter?

In health informatics a concept is the representation of an idea in health care. In a manual environment these ideas are expressed many ways, verbally, in writing, including in the patient's medical record, and in orders and letters of correspondence. Figure 1 indicates the basic components of data in a health care environment.

Example: A simple order for a test to be performed contains many health concepts: The test must identify the person (who is considered a patient), thereby establishing the information that relates to that person, such as their age, name, identifying numbers. This information is constant for the person (for example: the person's age doesn't change just because they are a patient).

A person may become a patient or be a provider of health care, this is called their role. When a provider there are additional information associated with the person such as their qualifications.

The patient has an event (visit to see a provider) that has information associated with it, such as a date and place and there are then the vast complexity of information collected about that event. These healthcare concepts are presented in Figure 1.

2. Concept Representation Components

The general concepts in healthcare include considerable detail to be clear and useful. For example it is not possible to describe a patient's condition when they arrive at the general practitioners or the emergency department without collecting information from the patient about symptoms, situations (falls or other accidents) and their own medical history. The provider then makes observations, such as blood pressure, temperature,

---

[1] Corresponding author: heather+lginformatics.com

pulse and test results. Whether data is collected on a paper based system, or in a computer data is structured. In a paper based system that structure is found through the form design. A traditional health record has forms such as operation reports, pathology reports, progress notes, medication delivery. Each of these forms has headings and special sections to remind the provider to complete information, and to make access to that information quick and simple (it is always in the same place in the record).

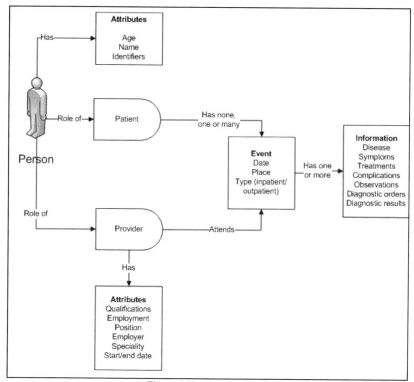

Figure 1 Concepts in Healthcare

The same requirement exists in computer based systems, where there will be screens (equivalent to forms), data elements (equivalent to the heading) and data values (the codes used to record details of the individual in the record). A person may be able to read a statement like 'fell down stairs and # arm' and understand that this statement includes details of the cause of injury (fall down stairs) as well as the diagnosis (fracture of arm). Computers find this type of mixed concept difficult to process. For this reason computer based information tends to be highly compartmentalised. This technical requirement does not mean that information cannot be presented in a user friendly manner. The other difference between the manual and the computer approach is that the manual system, once recorded in a particular place (form and heading) can only be found by looking at that form under that heading (location of information is physically unchanged). Computers offer a totally different approach to data. Once data is recorded in the computer it is possible for the computer to access that data and to display or present it on any other screen or report. It is also possible for a computer to identify the 'fracture of arm' is an injury and thereby to aggregate information for reporting without people having to review and analyse the original content of the data element.

The way we understand data is also impacted by the way the data is presented. Computer systems use colour, size and position on the screen to give impact and in some cases meaning. To achieve this effectively computer systems use a technique to describe each element of data very precisely. This precision supports the ability to consistently define, and therefore consistently use and understand the content of any given data element. This data about data is called Metadata [1].

3.   Metadata – What Is It and Why Is It Important

Metadata is used to describe data for different purposes [1]. It is the '*underlying definition or structured description of the content, quality, condition or other characteristics of data*' [2]. A dictionary is a traditional form of metadata. Information technology have extended and more clearly defined the content and structure needed to support clear metadata definition. Metadata design and use leads to better data and more efficient system development and use, though enabling all people who collect, use or exchange data to share the same understanding of its meaning and representation [3].

Health Information metadata has a wide usage. The specification of details about each element of data you wish to capture assists the developer and users to understand clearly exactly what they wish to collect, the level of detail, the way it is to be collected and how it could be used. Once established it is important that metadata is openly available to all those who collect or use the data, or who have an interest in similar data (as existing metadata can assist others in development of similar information to support data collection in other related areas).

Metadata has a specific structure that has been established through international standards. This structure includes the specification of data elements, value domains. The use of specific data also requires a structure for the record, metadata about record content and use are often represented in information models.

3.1 Metadata Structure

The international standard for metadata registration [4] identifies the following structure to metadata. Figure 2 shows the most common elements of metadata structure.

- The Data Set Specification (a group of data elements collected for a given purpose – e.g.: morbidity data collection, operation report, patient registration). A data set specification 'specifies the standardized output of a data set that has been agreed by stakeholders' [2]. Each data specification uses data elements also specified in the metadata. Different Data Set Specifications may choose to include data elements used by other data sets (e.g. date of birth may be used in data set specification I, and in Data Set Specification II. The data element has two components, what the element is, and how it is represented. For example: The data element 'patient height' can be described as the patient's measured height (without shoes) when standing. This is a specific concept that is described (patient's height). This is the data element concept and it is represented in a specific way, centimetres, and (the value domain). Though each data element is different some may use the same value domain to describe them. For example: height uses a value domain of centimetres, so could a data element that represents the size of a patient's burn injury. The value domain can be re-used as can the data element.

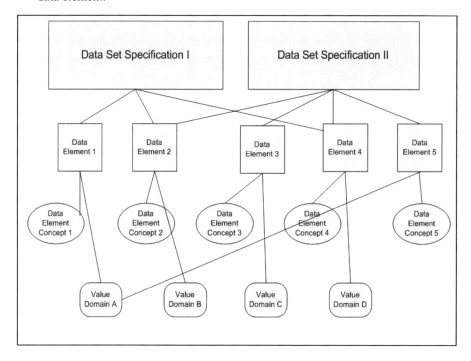

Figure 2 Metadata Structure Summary

The Australian Institute of Health and Welfare provide access to national metadata for health and welfare. The example used comes from that metadata collection.

3.2 Development of Metadata

When data was collected in manual systems information was generally very free format, codes are indicated by tick boxes and when you need to say something that the form doesn't cover, it can be written in the margin. This freedom often disappears when you move to a computerised representation of information. To ensure that information can still be represented accurately, be relevant, consistent and understood the concept of detailed descriptions of what the data actually represents and how it is recorded in the computer system have become essential. This is particularly true in rich and complex data environments such as you find in health care.

The process of deciding what data format to use and understanding the data required for collection requires an understanding both of the actual data collected and of the way the data is and could be used. Historically development of detailed data dictionaries were only undertaken by national or state health data collections, where they made clearer the data intended to be included in data for administrative, epidemiological or other data capture and comparison. Healthcare today has data collection in local systems, within hospitals. A local hospital near me did a recent study that identified that they had more than 300 individual databases collecting information for different purposes. The unfortunate thing about these collections is that they are generally not linked to and thereby optimizing the value of data already in the hospital system, and are not comparable to data collected in any other system.

The development of metadata to define and describe data collected is increasingly relevant at all levels of health care. The introduction of the concept of an electronic health record, sharable between different health care providers, and as a source for reporting of health status and activity to state, national and professional bodies requires accurate and clearly understood data specifications. This new approach to data requires that the data specifications be universal throughout healthcare.

For example: Data recorded in a person's record at the local hospital needs to be able to be extracted to:

- Inform their local General Practitioner about their medications and treatment after they leave the hospital
- Inform the district nurse about care required at a visit
- Report to the State about services provided
- Report to the public health care system about disease trends in the community.

This cannot be achieved if the data is stored / collected in different ways in every system. Standardised data components and structure are an essential to achieve this level of communication in a safe way.

3.3 Metadata Registry

Australia's approach to metadata registration has long been to standardise nationally and to make available the content of the registry. Early in the 1990's the Australian Institute of Health and Welfare developed the first national health data dictionary. In 2005 this dictionary was converted to an online Metadata Register [5]. The provision of an open to anyone, easy access mechanism to access information about health data has increased the use of metadata and given a mechanism that supports re-use and improved understanding of health data. Other countries such as Canada and the UK are following a similar trend to the development of national metadata and to ensure free and easy access to this descriptive tool.

4. Data Set Specification

Data sets are groups of individual data elements used for a specific purpose. Simple examples of data sets used in health care include the data required for reporting an episode of inpatient care to the state/national health data collection. Morbidity and mortality data have been collected for many years and have always included information about the individual (the person) the event (the inpatient stay) and the disease/s. Some of the data elements specific to this type of collection include:

Person information: age at admission

Event information: date of admission, date of discharge, length of stay

Disease: disease underlying the reason for admission to hospital.

Data Sets include specifications of data elements. The nature of health care means that data sets for different purposes will often share data elements, even if the data is collected by different organisations in different ways, the actual type of data will be consistent. This is called data element re-use.

For example: the Morbidity data set includes details on the person's sex and age. The Cancer Registry system also includes data on the person's sex and age. The availability of standardised data elements to 'pick from' reduces the effort in the development of standardised data and ensures the ability to compare data collected in one system to that in another, thereby improving the value of each individual data collection.

Examples of common data sets collected in many countries around the world include:

- Mortality – data about people who have died, including the disease or situation responsible for their death
- Morbidity – data about people and disease, usually from people treated in hospitals
- Cancer Registration – data about people diagnosed with cancer.

These data sets serve our communities through the identification of disease trends and details about where and to whom diseases occur. Public health initiatives such as anti-smoking campaigns, breast cancer screening programs are all influenced by these data. The provision of health services and the resourcing of those services are also informed by these data collections as they detect the geographic area where diseases are occurring and allow planners to develop strategies to reduce and treat diseases effectively. These data sets also support clinical research by supporting the analysis of changes in disease and treatment patterns. These data collections are made up of many data elements. During 2008 the Australian Admitted Patient Care National Minimum Data Set Specification included 36 different data elements [5].

5. Data Elements

The concepts in a manual form are generally easy for a person to understand and use, though we don't always use forms consistently. A computer is neither as flexible, nor as imaginative as a person. A is not able to identify context just by looking at the data element and the position of the data on a form. The person sees the data element as a part of a form and a record of a person, a computer cannot do that without a defined structure. In a manual system it would also be easy to indicate multiple tests in the test ordered space on the form. In a computer environment, the ability to record more than one of a data element needs to be specified and understood by the technical designers before the system is developed as they can affect the whole design of the system and the screens used to collect and present your data.

Example: A practitioner orders 3 different tests for a person in the manual record by entering short and simple instruction which, when read by the attending nurse is actioned and followed through. For a computer to action and follow through such a set of orders, there is a need to understand each individual data element component of that order. The date of the order, the provider making the order, the patient to whom it relates, the test being ordered, any additional information about the patient relevant to the test.

Data elements are the principle components of any data collection. In computer systems full dictionary like descriptions of data elements details are used to describe all of the characteristics of that data element. The descriptive information indicates an agreed meaning and the representation (e.g. codes) to be used when collecting or presenting this data. Each data element is described using attribute such as those shown in Table 1.

Table 1 Data Element Attributes

Attribute	Description of Attribute	Example [3]
Name	(the name of the data element) – this should be unique to that there can be no misunderstanding of the element to which people refer	Episode of care-behaviour-related risk factor intervention, code NN
Short Name	A name that is meaningful to purpose but short enough to be of practical use	Behaviour - related risk factor intervention
Data Dictionary / Metadata registry identifier	Unique ID used to reference this data element.	270165
Definition	A definition of the data element used to explain the concept and content of the element.	The intervention taken to modify or manage the patient's behaviour-related risk factor (s), as represented by a code
Data Element Concept	A description of the concept being described	Episode of care—behaviour-related risk factor intervention (see section 7)
Area of relevance	In a complex metadata register, data elements may originate or relate specifically to one or more domains. In the Australian example data is defined for use in health, welfare and the community.	Health
Status	The status of this definition, it could be a standard, or a proposed standard, or it could be an out of data definition that has been 'retired'.	Standard 01/03/2005
Guide for use	Information about how this item is to be collected	More than one code can be recorded
Source (submitting organisation)	The organisation responsible for developing and maintaining this specific data element	Cardiovascular Data Working Group
Related metadata references	Metadata which use or are related to this data element. This would include the relationship of length of stay to admission/discharge dates from which it is calculated	Supersedes Behaviour-related risk factor intervention, version 1, DE, NHDD, NHIMG, Superseded 01/03/2005.pdf (18.62 KB)
Implementation in Data Set Specifications	The data set/s in which this data element is used	Cardiovascular disease (clinical) DSS Health, Superseded 15/02/2006 Cardiovascular disease (clinical) DSS Health, Superseded 04/07/2007

Each data element is defined using two components, the concept itself and the code/s or format in which the content of the item is described.

6. Data Element Concept

The Data Element Concept describes the meaning of the data collected, the thing about which you intend to talk. Data element concepts are also uniquely identified, a process that supports computer reference to the specific concept. Data element concepts are also described with a status and definition. The attributes of a given concept are also defined in details. Table 2 provides an example of the data element concept attributes associated with the data elements defined in Table 1.

Table 2 Data Element Concept Attributes

Attribute	Description of Attribute	Example [3]
Name	(the name of the data element concept) – this should be unique to that there can be no misunderstanding of the element to which people refer	Episode of care—behaviour-related risk factor intervention
Data Dictionary / Metadata registry identifier	Unique ID used to reference this data element concept.	269626
Definition	A definition of the data element concept, the thing being collected in this data element.	The intervention taken to modify or manage the patient's behaviour-related risk factor(s).
Area of relevance	In a complex metadata register, data elements may originate or relate specifically to one or more domains. In the Australian example data is defined for use in health, welfare and the community.	Health
Status	The status of this definition, it could be a standard, or a proposed standard, or it could be an out of data definition that has been 'retired'.	Standard 01/03/2005
Context	The environment or discipline to which this data element is used, and rules related to tit's collection and meaning.	Public health, health care and clinical settings: To enable analysis of the interventions within an episode of care, in relation to the outcome of this care, especially when linked to information on risk factors. The recording of Clinician's management interventions is critical information for health service monitoring, planning and patient outcomes. It is a major descriptor of the care provided throughout an episode of care.

The data element concept may be divided into components as in this case where the component has a specific relationship. The data element occurs in relation to an episode of care. This is called the object of the data. This object has its own data element definition (*'a period of health care with a defined start and end'*). The data element concept also has a property of the object, something that defines an attribute of the object. In this case the episode of care object has the attribute of *'behaviour related risk factor intervention'* described as *'the action taken to address a behaviour-related risk factor'* [3].

7. Value Domain

Each data element is represented by a value domain – a set of values or rules used to record information in this data element.

Table 3 Value Domain

Attribute	Description of Attribute	Example [3]
Representation Class	Describes the way in which this concept is represented, code, text, number, date etc.	Code
Data Type	Described using traditional computer based data types. These include concepts such as String, Integer, Boolean. In healthcare data types have been re-defined to more accurately represent the wide range of concepts used in health care. These data types include concepts such as coded value (a defined set of codes), identifier (a code that uniquely identifies, a name. [6]	String
Format	The format structure of the data in the computer, it can indicate N= numbers, A= alphanumeric.	NN (two numbers)
Maximum character length	The maximum size of the data element. This definition assists in design of screens and reports, ensuring that there is sufficient space to represent the concept	2
Permissible values	The code set – the values that are permitted, and a description of each of these	01 No intervention 02 Information and education (not including written regimen) 03 Counselling 04 Pharmacotherapy 05 Referral provided to a health professional 06 Referral to a community program, support group or service 07 Written regimen provided 08 Surgery 98 Other
Supplementary values	Values that do not indicate information about the concept – they include mechanisms to indicate the unknown.	99 Not stated/inadequately defined
Guide for use	Information provided to assist accurate data collection	**CODE 01** No intervention Refers to no intervention taken with regard to the behaviour-related risk factor intervention-purpose. **CODE 02** Information and education (not including written regimen) Refers to where there is no treatment provided to the patient for a behaviour-related risk factor intervention-purpose other than information and education. **CODE 03** Counselling Refers to any method of individual or group counselling directed towards the behaviour-related risk factor intervention-purpose. This code excludes counselling activities that are part of referral options as defined in code 05 and 06.

Table 4 Value Domain (cont'd)

Attribute	Description of Attribute	Example [3]
Guide for use	Information provided to assist accurate data collection	**CODE 04** Pharmacotherapy Refers to pharmacotherapies that are prescribed or recommended for the management of the behaviour-related risk factor intervention-purpose. **CODE 05** Referral provided to a health professional Refers to a referral to a health professional who has the expertise to assist the patient manage the behaviour-related risk factor intervention-purpose. **CODE 06** Referral to a community program, support group or service Refers to a referral to community program, support group or service that has the expertise and resources to assist the patient manage the behaviour-related risk factor intervention-purpose. **CODE 07** Written regimen provided Refers to the provision of a written regimen (nutrition plan, exercise prescription, smoking contract) given to the patient to assist them with the management of the behaviour-related risk factor intervention-purpose. **CODE 08** Surgery Refers to a surgical procedure undertaken to assist the patient with the management of the behaviour-related risk factor intervention-purpose.

Just as a data set may use data elements that have been used in other data sets, data elements may be described by value domains that also describe other data elements. A simple example of this is the value domain used to describe diagnosis in healthcare, particularly for reporting, aggregation and analysis of health trends and health care, the International Classification of Diseases. Some of the value domains used to capture information in data elements using this classification, a set of codes and the descriptions and instructions on how to use those codes are:

- Activity Type – the type of activity being undertaken when injured
- Neonatal Morbidity – condition diagnosed in infancy
- External cause – external cause of injury, poisoning or other adverse effect
- Diagnosis – description of specific diseases, injuries and symptoms
- Place of occurrence – the place where the external cause of injury, poisoning or other adverse event occurred.
- Pregnancy/childbirth and puerperium – maternal diseases, conditions, illnesses, complications associated with pregnancy and childbirth events.
- Primary site of cancer – the site of origin of a tumour, as oppo9sed to the secondary or metastatic site/s.
- Vascular condition
- Non-admitted patient injury event activity
- Human intent in injury
- Non-admitted patient external cause[3]

This approach to the specifying of the way a data element is described not only makes it easier to develop the data item, as there is no need to constantly come up with new ways of describing things, but also improves the value of the data you capture. Data is more valuable as it is possible to compare data collected in one data element to that collected in another.

For example: it is possible to look in the diagnosis data element to see the number of admitted episodes of care for a specific primary site of cancer and compare the occurrence of the cancer in the community (which is measured by the Cancer Registry Data Set) with the services provided in hospitals to a given type of cancer (the admitted episode diagnosis). The same value will be used to describe the cancer in each case.

7.1 Codes

Some data elements are represented with 'free text' value domains, where you can enter anything in plain language. The difficulty with this is that though people can read and understand this information, it is difficult to find similar information and analyse what is present in a health record. Therefore the information collected, though it may meet the core purpose of supporting patient care, is of little value for other purposes, unless a person reads the information and manually codes it.   Codes are the *"controlled representation of a concept or group of concepts.   Codes may be alphabetic, numeric or combinations of these and are constrained in meaning and use. The code may be structured to indicate a hierarchy"* [1]. A code may represent something simple:

> M = male
> F = female

Or something more complex like a disease "J12 – Viral pneumonia, not elsewhere classified" [7]. A code need not have meaning but many do, such as BPH – benign prostatic hypertrophy, or are able to be broken down into parts such as a code like Viral-Lung-NEC.

It is important that codes, whatever they represent have only one meaning in the set of codes in which they are used throughout the life of that code set. For example if you use the code 123 to mean Dr Smith and Dr Smith leaves the organisation it would be confusing to allocate the code 123 to Dr Jones. If you did this it would not be possible to automatically identify whether Dr Smith or Dr Jones treated a given patient.

Some codes occur within classification systems. These systems are designed to count or group information about a given topic. The International Classification of Diseases is an example of such a system widely used in health care.

Code sets can be sub-sets of broader, more general coding systems. For example the cancer codes used to describe the primary site of a cancer are a sub-set of the total codes available in ICD-10. So a value domain may be a constrained (limited) set of codes from a broader group for a given purpose.

Code sets should be able to represent every concept in the data element. For this reason they will usually have two special values – Other, and Unspecified (or not elsewhere classified). These are important values that support the collection of quality, complete information. Other allows the user to indicate that there is not a specific code that covers the idea or situation that occurred, while unspecified indicates that the user did not have sufficient information to indicate which specific code was relevant. If you do not offer these alternatives at the point of data collection the user will be forced to guess, or select something from the codes offered, even if they know that what they are entering is inaccurate, thereby degrading the value of the whole data collection.

Code allocation is achieved in many ways. For simple code systems it can be selection from a list or tick boxes. This approach, though simple works well for very short lists of alternatives, when the list gets longer, say over 10 alternatives people are very poor at selecting the right option from the list. Alternative mechanisms to collect data should be considered in this instance. Context based natural language processing alternatives to data collection are being developed.

For some complex data collections such as hospital based treatment of diseases a process of manual data extraction and coding has occurred for many years. This information is obtained by either the doctor assigning codes to the episode of care when the patient is discharged (generally resulting in poor quality data), or by specially trained people reading the record after discharge and allocating codes to represent diseases and treatments during the patient's stay. This is a costly and highly skilled data collection process, but the value of the information obtained is considered worth the investment.

In the electronic health record environment both the value of the free text data for direct clinical care and the manual data extraction process are being challenged.

Computer systems are able to compare codes for symptoms and diseases to those conditions that may contraindicate the use of a particular medication. They are also able to look up instructions on best practice pathways for given conditions in patients and to remind professional health care staff about dangerous, or advantageous practices – and thereby improve the care provided to the individual. This process requires data to be coded. If the patient's record has coded (computer readable) information AND the best practice or drug contraindication information has also been coded, the computer can automatically compare them and provide feedback to the care provider.

The development of systems that can automatically extract data from electronic health records for reporting is also being undertaken and is likely to reduce the need for manual data extraction significantly over the next 10 years.

7.2 Terminology

Unlike codes, that group and categorise information, terminological systems in health care seek to represent precise and concise information about an element of healthcare. The most extensive terminology in healthcare is the Systematised Nomenclature of Medicine – Clinical Terms (SNOMED-CT)

e.g. 75570004 Viral Pneumonia

These systems differ from code systems to in that they do not include concepts such as other and not otherwise specified – they are always concise. They are also different, as they are not simple lists of coded values. Each concept can be defined by the attributes of the concept. In the case of viral pneumonia for example the concept is defined as:

Viral Pneumonia (disorder) is a
  Viral respiratory infection
  Infective pneumonia
  Has a causative agent of
   Virus
  Has associated morphology of
   Inflammation
   Consolidation
  Has finding site of
   Lung structure

Qualifiers can be added to the description of the concept such as severity(moderate), episodicity (first occurrence) and clinical course (gradual onset). The next chapter describes these concepts in more detail.

7.3 Governance (Agreement)

Whether defining data elements, codes or terminology to be used it is essential that the content, meaning and usage are known and agreed by all. There is little point in a government agency agreeing to collect 'size of head – if this is of no value to the clinical treatment of the patient – as the busy clinical staff in the organisation will concentrate their data collection efforts upon direct patient care rather than on collection of administrative data'. Collection of accurate information is dependent upon information being of value to those that have to collect it. Agreement and understanding of that data collection process is essential. A process for agreement on data content in systems is essential, whether in a single general practice or district nursing system, or in a more extensive state wide data collection. This agreement has become even more important in the last few years as health care organisations strive to share health data to support improved patient care and more efficient systems.

8. Information Model (Context)

Today there is recognition that to understand the meaning of the data in a field there is often a need to understand the relationship between that field and its content to other data in the system.

For example: A record indicates that a person has 'a painful hip'. This could represent many concepts, and be clinically indicative of a wide range of problems. When you also have the information that this statement was recorded in a field for adverse reactions to injection, and that the injection was received earlier that day, the issue is much clearer, and would probably require little intervention other than ongoing observation.

The relationship between the instances of the data – this particular entry for this person at this time, is dependent upon the reason for recording the information. These are relationships that are represented using information models that graphically represent the structure of information and the content that can be recorded in each of those structures. The simplest of these is a data model. Data models indicate the simple relationships between elements of data. More information on context is provided in chapter 8.

9. Other Representational Forms (Pictures and Icons)

Information is provided through headings and data elements, the content of those data elements, but also through the use of colour and pictures in computer systems. Test results that are out of the normal range are often shown in RED to highlight the need to review the results. Pictures are used to indicate actions or information, refer to Figure 3 as an example.

Figure 3 Icon for Blind

These tools are valuable to aid fast and simple communication, but they must be consistent. If the use of colour or graphic representation or icons are inconsistent, or unclear they can be of great danger in communicating health information [8].

Conclusion

It should now be evident that the use of our health language in information systems requires a thorough understanding of the complexity of representing health concepts such that the meaning of these concepts is expressed clearly and safely. Only then is it possible to make safe use of information collected, processed, stored and presented by health information systems. This chapter has provided you with an overview of the purpose and means of defining health information concepts and their relationships as well as the difference between actual patient information and information structure and metadata

References

[1] *AS5021: 2005* Standards Australia, *The Language of Health Concept Representation*. 2005, Sydney: Standards Australia IT14.
[2] *HB291-2007* Standards Australia, *Health Informatics - Guide to Health Data Development*. Vol., Sydney: Standards Global Inc.
[3] Australian institute of Health & Welfare (AIHW). *MetaData Online Registry (Meteor)*. 2004 [cited 10 November 2005]; Available from: http://meteor.aihw.gov.au/content/index.phtml/itemId/181162
[4] *ISO/IEC WD 11179-3 Information Technology - Metadata Registries (MDR) - Part 3: Registry metadata and basic attributes*. 2004, International Organisation for Standards ISO TC215.
[5] METeOR. *Admitted patient care NMDS 2008-2009*. 2008 [cited 15 May 2008]; Available from: http://meteor.aihw.gov.au/content/index.phtml/itemId/361679.
[6] ISO/DIS 21090 Health Informatics — Harmonized data types for information interchange ISO TC215, 2008, International Organisation for Standards: Genève.
[7] National Centre for Classification in Health (NCCH), *The International Statistical Classification of Diseases and Related Health Problems, Tenth Revision, Australian Modification - 4th edition (ICD-10-AM)*. 5th ed, ed. National Centre for Classification in Health. 2004, Sydney: National Centre for Classification in Health.
[8] *HB: 306-2007* Standards Australia, *User interface requirements for the presentation of health data*. 2007, Sydney: Standards Global, Australia

Review Questions

1. Give examples of a health concept and different ways in which that concept could be represented.
2. Why should data collected in systems be clearly defined, and who should be responsible for this task?
3. What is the difference between a code system and a terminology?
4. What purpose does the clear specification of a data element and value domain have to support direct patient care?

70

Health Informatics
E.J.S. Hovenga et al. (Eds.)
IOS Press, 2010
© 2010 The authors and IOS Press. All rights reserved.
doi:10.3233/978-1-60750-476-4-70

7. Clinical Terminology

Heather GRAIN[1] A.Dip MRA, RMRA, GD DP, MHI, FACHI
Academic Fellow Austin Health, Director E-Health Education and Director Pavillion Prime Care, Melbourne, Australia

Abstract. This chapter gives an educational overview of:
- What a clinical terminology is.
- How clinical terminology is constructed and used
- The concept of mapping terminologies
- Why clinical terminology is an essential component of electronic health records and clinical decision support systems
- The issues that relate to good use of terminologies and the need for governance and standardisation to support health information quality and the linkage to safe/consistent clinical decision support.

Keywords. Terminology, Information Science, Information Management, Health Information Systems, International Classification of Diseases (ICD), Health Care Systems, Logical Observation Identifiers, Names, and Codes (LOINC)

Introduction

Clinical terminologies have existed for centuries as the language of healthcare. Like any language, the language of healthcare has developed over many years from a mixture of languages. The need for detail, the complexity of health care and the rapid extension and expansion of the knowledge and processes in healthcare, as well as the different terms and ideas expressed by different professional groups means that healthcare has millions of different concepts to be described. "it has been estimated that there are between 500,000 and 45 million different concepts" to be accurately and consistently described [1].

However when we talk of clinical terminology in health systems today, the requirement is to have an approach that allows the computer to 'understand' the term being used and to be able to use that understanding to assist the processes of health care and the understanding of activities in the health care system. Discussion of this topic is often confused by the language that surrounds it. What is a vocabulary? Is it different to a terminology?

The description of computer processable terminologies and the representation of knowledge are developing and the agreed understanding of the way the components and concepts are described is still emerging. A brief description of the terminology used to describe terminology is helpful to appreciate both the complexity and the simplicity of the ideas inherent in these systems. Definitions of concepts frequently misinterpreted are provided in Box 1. This is followed by further explanations.

There is a general language of healthcare, but there are also special variations that are specific to different professional groups or clinical specialties. Terminology is the

---

[1] Corresponding author: heather+lginformatics.com

term usually used to indicate a computable terminology, one that can be referenced by computers and used to support processing and decision making. The reference terminology provides a link between the formal computable reference terminology, which is complex and not necessarily something that clinical staff would actively use in the work place. The reference terminology describes the unique concepts of health care and the preferred (canonical) term used to describe that concept, as well as all the other terms used to describe the concept, including the terms used in different languages. Local expressions can be used to describe a concept or specific definitions can be selected to be used in local or domain specific instances (the interface terminology). It is common for a terminology to include the reference elements and the interface components together in one system. It is also common that the reference terminology provide mechanisms for grouping or aggregating ideas together for reporting or decision support.

Box 1 Definitions of Common Terminology Related Concepts

Vocabulary	A set of terms belonging to one special language or culture [2]
Reference Terminology	"A reference terminology is a terminology designed to uniquely represent concepts. It does this by listing the concepts and specifying their structure, relationships and, if present, their systematic and formal definitions. It normally contains a unique identifier, a rubric and may contain reference to alternate terms to the preferred term (which may be conceptualized as an interface term (interface terminology)and it may contain maps or pointers to aggregate terminology." [2]
Interface Terminology	"A maintained set of unique identified terms designed to be compatible with the natural language of the user." [2]
Aggregate Terminology	"A grouping of similar concepts, for particular purposes, using relationships that may be hierarchical and/or uni- or multi-dimensional" [2]
Clinical terminology	'the component of health language used at the point of care for the purpose of clinical management of subject(s) of care" [2]

The interface terms relate to a given unique concept in the reference terminology and could be considered similar to a synonym used for a specific situation. For example a term used to explain a condition to a patient may be different to the term selected for presentation on a screen to a clinician. A report for the patient might describe their condition as a blockage of a blood vessel of the heart, while the clinician might see AMI on their patient problem screen. Aggregate terminologies are often classifications for statistical, epidemiological and administrative use that group together concepts according to a defined set of rules and structure for a specific purpose.

It is important to recognize that the definitions provided here represent the conceptual usage of terminologies, rather than the actual products that contain the terms and references. Products used to represent clinical concepts often have a mixture of these concepts. For example the International Statistical Classification of Diseases and Related Health Problems, Tenth Revision, Australian Modification (ICD-10-AM) has an index section which represents individual concepts (similar to a reference terminology or interface terminology), while the tabular list groups the concepts as an aggregate terminology.

1. The Relationship Between Clinical Terminology and the Deliverables of Electronic Health Record (EHR) Systems

EHR systems promise:

Clinicians
- a record where information is easier and faster to find.
- an information system with information that can provide clinical knowledge when it is needed and advice upon best practice through clinical pathways and clinical decision support systems.

Administrators and Governments
- a source of more accurate information from which service provision, epidemiological, research and administrative knowledge can be gained and decisions made.

Patients, Carers and other Consumers of Health Care
- the ability to access their health information and to understand that information so that they are able to be more pro-active in their own health care.

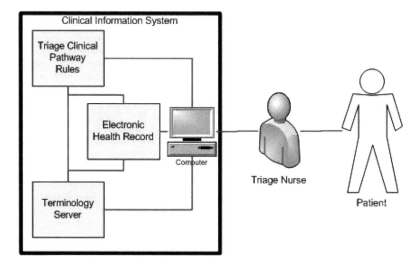

Figure 1 Where Terminology Fits in the System

Figure 1 shows an outline of the processes used in clinical information systems and the place of terminology in those systems. In this example a patient arrives at the emergency department where they are seen by the Triage nurse. The nurse enters details of the patient's condition indicating that they have a ?# tib/fib. The computer system identifies the unique concepts represented by this statement.

414293001 – fracture of tibia and fibula (disorder)
Qualified by
415684004 – suspected (Qualifier Value)

Having stored these concepts in the patient's electronic health record in the triage presenting condition field, the computer can be used to identify if there are any clinical instructions that have been established for this condition. At this hospital there is a rule that says any fractures or suspected fractures presenting to emergency are to be x-rayed, so that the results of x-ray are available to the clinician as soon as possible, thereby speeding up the process of diagnosis and reducing patient waiting times. The rules for this clinical pathway have been stored in the computer and they could look like:

If Presenting Condition is a 72704001 – Fracture order x-ray.

Then the clinical terminology system is built with relationships that can be used to group and identify clinical components. The definition of a fracture of tibia and fibula is shown in Figure 2.

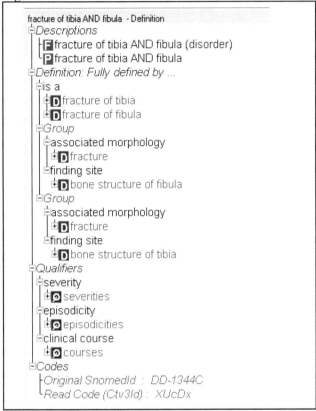

Figure 2 Definitions and Relationship Example

Figure 2 shows that there are two descriptions for the condition and that the condition is defined by being a fracture of the tibia, a fracture of the fibula, that it is a fracture and has a finding site of bone structure of tibia, and of fibula. Using this structure the computer is able to apply the rule saying that if the condition is a fracture (which this is – see associated morphology in Figure 2) an x-ray should be ordered. The order will represent the presenting condition in clear, accepted terms (the definition that has been determined as the one to be used in the organisation) so the order would be:

X-Ray of Tibia and Fibula (the body structures)
Presenting Condition: Fracture of Tibia and Fibula, Suspected

A clinical terminology therefore not only represents the concept but is able to support a computer identifying the attributes of the concept being described. This chapter explains both what a computer processable clinical terminology is and how it is used to support improved health care systems. A computable terminology uses the attributes of a disease, or procedure to uniquely define that concept and to indicate the relationships between different terms.

2. What is a Clinical Terminology?

Clinical terminologies have been developed in different areas of health care. The College of American Pathologies first published the Systematised Nomenclature of Pathology (SNOP) in 1965 [3]. This base was widely used and well accepted in the medical community and has been extended since then and has evolved into the most extensive clinical terminology with more than 300,000 concepts and 900,000 descriptions of those concepts and is now called the Systematised Nomenclature of Medicine – Clinical Terms (SNOMED-CT). This terminology is available in Spanish as well as English. Other common terminologies in use include the Logical Observation Identifiers, Names, and Codes (LOINC) developed at the Regenstrief Institute for Health Care in 1994 to represent clinical data from hospital laboratories [4].

These systems are not designed to be used by looking up codes in books, rather they are intended to be automated. To support this automation they have a structure upon which computers can react. The examples used in this chapter are from SNOMED-CT as this is now an international standard for clinical concept representation. The principles discussed here are true of any quality terminologies, though the specific structure and content vary.

2.1 Concepts

Clinical terminology provides a system that uniquely identifies each concept in health care. A concept is not the name we know the thing by, but the thing itself.

Using an example from the Systematized Nomenclature of Medicine – Clinical Terminology (SNOMED-CT) the idea of a headache is uniquely identified using a unique code (25064002). There are 8 different English words or descriptions used to describe the idea of a headache, each of which can be uniquely identified too as shown in Box 2.

Box 2 The Concept and Description for Headache

Concept ID	Descriptions – Description Identifier
25064002	F Headache (Finding) - 755191011
	P Headache – 41990019
	S Cephalalgia – 41993017
	S Cephalgia – 41994011
	S Cephalodynia – 41995012
	S HA – Headache - 1224414017
	S Head pain – 41992010
	S Pain in head – 1224415016

The concept identifier is unique. The concept of headache can be divided into other forms of headache, and more extensive versions of the concept may arise over time. Any variation in the thing being described results in a new concept being defined. A concept is NEVER changed. It can be 'marked' as out of date and no longer used, but it is never removed from the terminology. This means that health information stored in a patient's medical record 5 years ago would have concept identifiers that can be described accurately as they were at the time, even if the concept is now understood to be a different type of thing. This makes the terminology 'history proof' and able to represent health information in a legally and historically accurate way even though clinical knowledge may change over time. Each concept may have many terms used to describe it. Each term has one description however that describes not only the concept, but the context in which it is intended to be unambiguous. This is called the Fully Specified Name and is sometimes displayed with an F in front of it. In Box 2 the *Fully Specified Name* is Headache (Finding). While the *Preferred term* – the term used in a clinical record is Headache. Other names used to describe the concept are also included. These other descriptions may be used when searching for a concept, or may be used when displaying or collecting information in a given context (when presenting information to patients the term cephalgia would not be used, while in an emergency department or where limited space is available HA might be displayed as sufficient to represent the idea concerned. Irrespective of the description used, the concept is always the same and always stored as the unique identifier for the concept in this case: 25064002.

2.2 Concept Hierarchy and Relationships

Clinical terminology has multiple axes by which a concept can be identified and retrieved. These axes assist in defining a specific concept and also assist in finding like concepts. For example if you were to search for all the conditions that include a finding of pain, headache would be included. The computer is able to find all the cases that include pain because of the multiple axes and relationships inherent in the system.

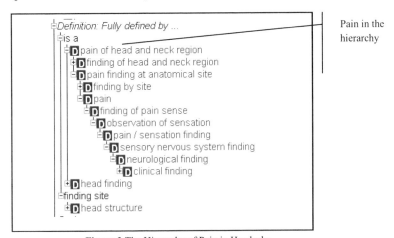

Figure 3 The Hierarchy of Pain in Headache

Figure 3 shows how the terminology links headache to pain through the hierarchies of the system. The system defines a headache as being pain of the head and neck region and a finding of the head. If you follow the hierarchy of the pain component of headache, 3 levels up from headache is the concept of pain. This represents that a headache, is a pain of the head and neck region, which is a pain finding at an anatomical site (and a finding of the head and neck region), which is a pain (and a finding by site). Each indentation along the display represents a less specific concept of which this concept is an example (into which group this concept falls). Each concept may, and usually will fall into more than one 'group'. All conditions that are expressed as a pain finding could be found through this hierarchy, just as all the fractures can be found.

These relationships are held in the computer in tables of relationships showing the parents of a concept. The example in Figure 4 uses terms rather than the unique identifiers to explain the idea of relationships. Relationships of different types occur and it is these relationships that can uniquely identify a concept. In the case of headache, there is no other condition that is a finding of head, and pain of head and neck region, with a finding site of head structure it is for this reason that this condition is considered a Fully Defined Concept.

Figure 4 shows the relationships between headache and its parents (the concepts of which headache is a member). By following this string of relationships it is possible to navigate up and down. If you were looking for a neurological finding – the answers you receive from the computer system would include headache, if you searched for conditions with a finding site of head, it would also include headache. It is this flexibility which provides the power of clinical terminologies. It should be noted that two of the hierarchies of headache lead to the parent of clinical finding. The entire system of SNOMED-CT uses a hierarchical system in which a concept may be linked to multiple hierarchies and thereby indicate the relationships between one concept and another.

SNOMED-CT not only uniquely identifies, concepts but also the relationships between them. A patient situation may take many different elements to describe it effectively. For example: Gradual onset of (61751001) Cellulitis of Leg (238402004) due to (42752001) Staphylococcus Aureus (3092008). Each of these concepts fit into different places in the hierarchy.

> Gradual onset of (qualifier)
> Cellulitis of Leg (disorder)
> Due to (attribute – Linkage concept)
> Staphylococcus Aureas (organism)

There are 15 top level concept hierarchies in SNOMED-CT under which all concepts reside and which are used to assist in retaining and representing meaning. These are described briefly in Table 1 [5].

The hierarchy within which a term occurs changes the meaning intended. For example the term liquid can be used as a finding to indicate that something is found to be liquid, or as a substance, or as a qualifier on a dosage of a drug, where the form of delivery is liquid. It is for this reason that simply finding the right word in a terminology is not sufficient; it has to be the right concept as represented by the word in a given situation (which requires the hierarchy to ensure clarity and accuracy of meaning).

2.3 Representing Concepts

Concept Identifiers can be stored in clinical systems, or sent in messages to represent ideas in a way that a computer can process. However no terminological system will ever represent every single idea in a domain. For this reason concepts are built so that ideas can be joined together to represent more specific or new concepts.

2.3.1 Pre-coordination

Many of the terms in SNOMED CT represent 'joined ideas'. For example the concept of Cellulitis of Leg (238402004) is a single concept with a unique identifier. This is called pre-coordination where the concepts, in this case of cellulitis and of leg (as the finding site) have been gathered and are represented as a single entity. Think of it as pre-packaged ideas. These ideas are those that occur commonly and have been joined together to make access and management simpler, it is easier to use one identifier than it is to use two. It is important to recognise, however that terms can be 'built to order'.

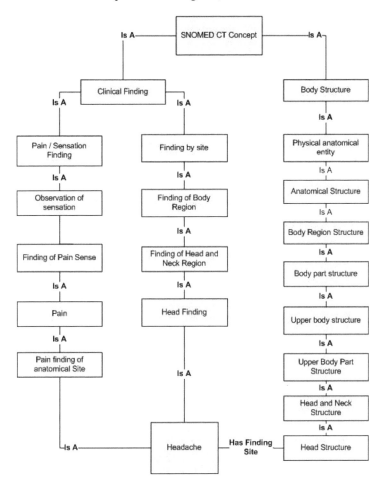

Figure 4 SNOMED CT Relationships Between the Concept 'Headache' and its Parents

Table 1 SNOMED-CT concepts

Hierarchy Name	Description	Examples
Body Structure	Normal and abnormal anatomical structures. Abnormal structures include morphological abnormalities.	Normal: Head, Femur, Entire Skin of Hand, Erythrocyte Abnormal: Intraductal carcinoma, non-infiltrating, cutaneous plaque, fracture
Clinical Finding	Includes concepts that result from an assessment or judgement. This group includes disorders which are concepts where there is an underlying pathology. Findings are often called observations.	Generalised oedema, fever, nausea. Disorders: Subdural Haematoma, Migraine, gastroenteritis
Environment or Geographical location	Types of locations and actual named locations.	Home, school, staircase, football field, Australia

Table 1 SNOMED-CT Concepts (cont'd)

Hierarchy Name	Description	Examples
Event	Occurrences that impact upon health status, result in injury. It does not include procedures or intervention which is intended events undertaken in healthcare.	Fall, motor car accident, death, birth, legal intervention
Observable Entity	Processes or things that can be observed or measured.	Range of Movement, acoustic feature of mass, body temperature
Organism	All organisms including micro-organisms and infectious agents, fungi, plants and animals.	Staphylococcus Aureus, Shellfish, Dog, HIV
Pharmaceutical / Biologic Product	Products used in healthcare including herbal medicines.	Penicillin (a class of antibiotic), Beta-Blocking Agent,
Physical Force	The forces of nature and mechanisms of injury.	Motion, friction, gravity, electricity, magnetism, sound, radiation, heat, cold, humidity, air pressure.
Physical Object	Natural and man-made objects, including devices and materials	Tennis Ball, Boat, Wheel Chair, Prosthesis, furniture, Dagger.
Procedure	Includes all operations and interventions in healthcare. All intended activities performed in provision of healthcare	Appendicectomy, Arm Injection, Catheterisation, Physical Therapy, peer review
Qualifier	Represents concepts used to make more specific any of the other categories included here. These are considered to be attributes describing the concept defined.	Suspected, Episode (1st, 2nd), Severity
Situation with explicit context	Context dependent situations. Where the situation changes the meaning of the concept being described	If the concept of colon cancer is recorded in a patient record, the meaning seems clear, however if it is recorded in the situation of family history, the meaning is very different. Family history is an example of a situation. Other examples of situations include outbreaks, risk factors and partner dying.
Social Context	Indicates social information relevant to a situation, explaining something about who is the subject of the information.	Community, Group, Family, Occupation.
Specimen	Indicates a concept that has been obtained for examination or analysis	Biopsy sample, Cytological material, scrapings, microbial isolate specimen
Staging and Scales	Represent measures of disease stage or process progression	Gleeson Grading System for prostate cancer. The concept can be associated with an actual value (a measure). The combination explains the quantity (the measure) and what has been measured (the staging/scale).
Substance	Includes chemicals, drugs, proteins as well as functional or state of substances.	Water (an example of a liquid substance) Acid,
Miscellaneous items, used to maintain and manage the concepts and their relationships		
Record Artifacts	Indicates whether this is the current version of the concept, or where a concept has been replaced by more recent knowledge the new structures used.	

Table 1 SNOMED-CT Concepts (cont'd)

Hierarchy Name	Description	Examples
Special concept	Indicates how a concept is used or accessed.	Inactive Navigational – provide pathways for access to specific concepts. These pathways can be specific to a given purpose or group of concepts (SubSet).
Linkage Concepts	The representation of a link between one concept and another. There are links that can define a concept. These linkages represent attributes of a higher level concept.	Defining Linkages The concept of a fracture of the humerus is fully defined by linkages to: Is A – injury of upper arm Is A – fracture Associated Morphology – Fracture Finding Site – Bone structure of humerus

2.3.2 Post-coordination

Where a term doesn't exist in the terminology it can be created by joining concepts together to represent the idea. For example:

128045008 = Cellulitis (disorder)

61685007 = Lower extremity = lower limb structure (body structure)

Therefore cellulitis of leg could be represented as

128045008+61685007

This is called Post-Coordination. The capacity to build concepts in this way is one of the strengths of a terminological system such as SNOMED-CT. However when representing clinical information it is important that the information be represented consistently and that consistency is highly supported by pre-coordination of the terms.

3.   Providing Access to Information

Clinical terminologies are extremely complex and often very large. It is not practical to expect clinical staff to search the entire terminological system to obtain the specific concepts required to represent patient information and care. A range of approaches are used to assist implementation and the use of clinical terminologies.

There are clinical terminology browsers that assist those who develop clinical terminologies to find the required concept and the ID and Descriptions relative to that concept. Those who govern terminologies provide tables of data that contain the concept ID's, Descriptions, Relationships used by local computer systems to display descriptions and to query to find concepts by their characteristics or attributes. The most common approach to simplifying selection of terminological concepts for recording health information is the use of Sub-Sets.

Once a concept ID has been stored in the computer system to represent a concept or group of concepts, the benefits of a terminology are obtained through the ability to query the information held. For example: to query what type of disorder is being recorded or the organism causing a condition and to use that information to provide best practice information to clinicians, or to further analyse the information for public health, administration or other related purposes. These processes require the use of a terminology server which can process and analyse the 'meaning' or definitional elements of a concept and the relationships between those concepts. Terminology servers also provide facilities to indicate greater specificity through access into the hierarchy of the terminology by providing a 'starting point' for lookup. For example the user might enter or select Asthma and be given a list of sub-types or more specific concepts that all fall within the disorder of Asthma.

3.1 Reference Sets

It is neither feasible nor desirable to expect clinical staff to search a clinical terminology and to select the right concept for the right situation. To make implementation simpler and data capture more accurate, sections of a terminology can be selected and presented as a purpose specific term set. This hides some of the complexity of the terminology from the user, while supporting full functionality for analysis and querying information stored in a clinical record. In the past these were called sub-sets of the terminology, but today they are called reference sets.

Reference sets are developed by people skilled both in the clinical domain concerned and in the terminology. The sets include terms that represent the concept accurately (concepts from the right section of the hierarchy) relevant to a specific context and purpose. They reduce the number of potential terms from which clinicians choose.

4. Mapping

As data representations, codes, unique identifiers of concepts in terminologies and the way we use information change, the way we group and classify information also changes. The ability to convert information collected in one form to an alternative representation or classification system is needed if data aggregation and reporting, and comparison of data over time are to be achievable.

Mapping is the mathematical process that provides a mechanism of going from one way of representing a concept to another

4.1 What is in a Map

A map provides a computer with a means of taking data represented in one system and converting it to be expressed in another. For example you might want to describe a concept in SNOMED-CT and to be able to convert that SNOMED-CT concept to a concept in the International Statistical Classification of Diseases (ICD). In the simplest case a map is a table that identifies the value in one system and the corresponding value in the alternative representational system.

Table 2 gives an example of simple mapping for SNOMED to ICD concepts. This is an example where you are linking from a detailed concept representation to a less detailed (aggregate) representation.

Table 2 Mapping of Simple Concepts SNOMED to ICD

Term	Snomed-CT concept ID	ICD-10 Code
Vomiting	422400008 – Vomiting (disorder)	R11 Nausea and vomiting
Nausea	42222587007 - Nausea (finding)	
Vomiting and Nausea	16932000 – Nausea and Vomiting (disorder)	

In this instance the mapping or relationship is straight forward there are many Concept ID's to one concept ID (Figure 5)

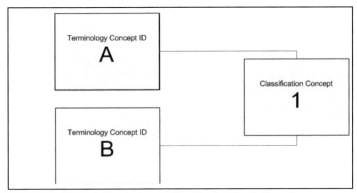

Figure 5 Terminology to Classification Simple Example

However the concept of mapping from one representational form in clinical terminologies and classification is not usually as straight forward as it may seem. There are many cases where the concepts are not as simply or cleanly converted from one concept representation to another. In the cases above there are no 'rules' these conversions or mappings are true in all cases.

In the case of gastroenteritis the situation is not as clear. Table 3 shows examples of this problem.

Table 3 Mapping - More Complex Example

Term	SNOMED-CT	ICD-10-AM*	Problem
Urinary Tract Infection	25374005 – Gastroenteritis (disorder)	O03.3 with obstetric spontaneous abortion O86.2 Urinary tract infection following delivery N39.0 – Urinary Tract Infection, site not specified	Additional logic is required to determine which code is appropriate. There are also rules in the coding standards that indicate: "do not code the following: N39.0 Urinary tract infection, site not specified, when only microbiology results show organism(s) have been cultured" [6].
Patient had heart attack during laparoscopic appendicectomy, surgery not completed.	51316009-Laparoscopic appendectomy 385660001 - Not done 57054005 - AMI 74477009 – exploratory laparotomy	30373-00 – Exploratory Laparotomy	While SNOMED-CT can represent the story of what occurred, a single simple map is not able to represent the complexity of decisions that indicate the morbidity reporting requires only the procedure (as far as it progressed).

ICD-10 AM = International Classification of Diseases, tenth revision, Australian Modification

Though it is possible to develop computer based programs that can query other fields of data in the record and determine which of the codes applies in a fully automated way this is not normally what is included, particularly in the traditional mappings used by government agencies to support reporting processes and practices.

4.2 Limitations of Mapping

Maps are useful tools, however it is important to understand their limitations. Maps are built for a specific purpose and often assume a specific context. For example maps from SNOMED-CT to ICD have been developed and are being extended to include

ICD-10-AM. These are simple maps to provide a 'best' solution. These maps generally support reporting of morbidity data to government agencies.

Though such reporting is seen to support public health as well as service planning their utility is constrained by the fact that these reporting systems also generate data used for fiscal reporting and because of that have restrictions placed upon them as to what may be included in the collection. These exclusions may impact utility of the data for other purposes. For example: The Australian Coding Standards [7] indicate that :

"postoperative atelectasis documented in clinical record and noted on chest x-ray results, two days following abdominal surgery which resolved spontaneously without treatment" The instruction is not to include this in the data collection as it doesn't meet the definition of data to be included.

Though this data may be highly relevant to a specific study, or to the nursing workload requirements at an individual site, the information may adversely impact upon the fiscal re-imbursement of more complex cases (as it may seem to be more complex than it is), or if coded may indicate an ongoing clinical problem which does not exist. All classification and data collection systems make choices like this one to support the quality and usability of the data they collect. More details regarding the link between ICD-10-AM and fiscal re-imbursement (based on casemix) is presented in chapter 25 on resource, quality and safety management.

5.   Relationship to Context

The meaning of a term is often dependant upon the context in which the term is used. Some terminologies attempt to describe context (the field or situation to which the content relates) as well as content (the term). The complexity of clinical terminology required to represent the concepts of medicine are significant. If the terminology also attempts to represent all of the contexts of medicine as well the size and scope of the system, particularly if the policy is to create pre-coordinated concepts to support consistency, the system will grow exponentially. This is of concern to those attempting to develop and manage electronic health records in a standardised way.

Historically there has been no option but to use the terminology to represent context as there has not been a standardised approach to context. However this is no longer the case as both the work of the OpenEHR Foundation and of HL7 are moving towards standardised representations and reference-able representations of context. The question can be asked, whether the terminology should attempt to manage content as well as context? This is a difficult area, largely contributed to by the lack of cross over between the skills and interests of the terminologists and the modellers, but it is a problem being considered internationally.

6.   Governance

If the health care system requires the ability to share and compare health information electronically, and if there is a need to build consistent, re-usable, safe clinical knowledge and decision support systems, terminology, and more importantly its use, must be managed and standardised.

The International Health Terminology Standards Development Organisation was established in 2007 to support the international standardisation and development of SNOMED-CT [7]. These members of this organisation are countries and include the Charter Members (original founders) Australia, Canada, Denmark, Lithuania, Sweden, The Netherlands, New Zealand, the United Kingdom and United States of America. The governance structure of the organisation includes a General Assembly and committees on Content, Quality, Technical and Research and Innovation activities. This organisation is responsible for updates to and release of SNOMED-CT and is working on the development of purposes specific reference sets and mappings.

SNOMED-CT is updated to meet the needs of users around the world and revisions are released twice a year [5]. Prior to release, the content undergoes a quality assurance process and then pre-release to members for broader review before the final files are generated and distributed for use in computer systems around the world.

References

[1] ISO *17115:2007 Health Informatics: Vocabulary of Terminological Systems*. ISO TC215: Geneve
[2] *AS5021-2005 The Language of Health Concept Representation*. Standards Australia IT-14, Sydney. Available from http://www.e-health.standards.org.au/
[3] Stanfill, M., *Systematized Nomenclature of Medicine Clinical Terms (SNOMED-CT)*, in *Healthcare Code Sets, Clinical Terminologies, and Classification Systems*, K. Giannengelo, Editor. 2006, American Health Information Management Association: Chicago, Ill. p. 101-123
[4] Scichilone, R., *Logical Observation Identifiers, Names, and Codes (LOINC)*, in *Healthcare Code Sets, Clinical Terminologies, and Classification Systems*, K. Giannengelo, Editor. 2006, American Health Information Management Association: Chicago, Ill. p. 149-156.
[5] IHTSDO, *SNOMED-Clinical Terms User Guide*. 2007, Copenhagen: IHTSDO. Refer also http://www.ihtsdo.org/
[6] National Classification Centre for Health (NCCH) International Classification of Diseases (ICD)-10-AM v6 2008 http://nis-web.fhs.usyd.edu.au/ncch_new/2.12.aspx viewed November 2009
[7] National Classification Centre for Health (NCCH) International Classification of Diseases (ICD)-10-AM v6 2008 Australian Coding Standards http://nis-web.fhs.usyd.edu.au/ncch_new/2.8.aspx viewed November 2009

Review Questions

1. Give examples of a health concept and different ways in which that concept could be represented.
2. Why should data collected in systems be clearly defined, and who should be responsible for this task?
3. What is the difference between a code system and a terminology?
4. What purpose does the clear specification of a data element and value domain have to support direct patient care?

Health Informatics
E.J.S. Hovenga et al. (Eds.)
IOS Press, 2010
© *2010 The authors and IOS Press. All rights reserved.*
doi:10.3233/978-1-60750-476-4-84

8. Knowledge and Information Modeling

Maria MADSEN[1] BS, BSc(Hons), GDAC, MB(IS), MACS PhD Candidate
*Lecturer, School of Management and Information Systems, Central Queensland
University, Rockhampton Qld and Director of eHealth Education Pty Ltd*

Abstract. This chapter gives an educational overview of:
- commonly used modelling methods what they represent
- the importance of selecting the tools and methods suited to the health information system being designed
- how the quality of the information or knowledge model is determined by the quality of the system requirements specification.
- differentiating between the purpose of information models and knowledge models.
- the benefits of the openEHR approach for health care data modeling.

Keywords. Model, Knowledge, Software Design, Health Care Systems, Systems Analysis

Introduction

In this chapter we discuss knowledge and information from a logical design point of view. That means that this chapter does not say anything about how to build either a knowledge base or a database. Rather the discussion focuses on the analysis and design of information from data models to knowledge models.

1.   Knowledge and Information

It is common to find authors describing the data, information, knowledge, wisdom (DIKW) continuum, or hierarchy, as a progressively more complex and more meaningful understanding of things that interest us in a given context. Sharma [1] has traced the origin of this hierarchy to T.S. Elliot who wrote the following words in *Chorus From The Rock* in 1934,

> *Where is the Life we have lost in living?*
> *Where is the wisdom we have lost in knowledge?*
> *Where is the knowledge we have lost in information?*

It is not absolutely clear if Elliot's poem was indeed the source of the hierarchy as it is used today, but these lines from the poem do eloquently describe both the hierarchy and a modern problem commonly known as 'information overload'. The availability of more and more information does not necessarily translate into more effective work practices or better decision making. As humans we are limited in our own ability to process large amounts of information and can become anxious,

---

[1] Corresponding author: m.madsen@ehealtheducation.net

frustrated, and confused if we find ourselves unable to process all of the information that we think we should [2]. Himma suggests that technologically we will find ways of processing larger and larger amounts of information, but that psychologically people need time away from information content. Himma quotes Levy (2005) saying that people need time, "to think, to reflect, to absorb, to muse." This chapter is of course concerned with some of the technological solutions to information management rather than the modern human condition per se. Even so, it is always important to remember that information systems are designed for humans to use and that the psychological state of the users is affected by the system they are using.

2. Defining Data, Information, Knowledge, and Wisdom (DIKW)

Returning now to the DIKW hierarchy, commonly data are described as 'raw' facts that are collected by an organization during its normal course of business. Information is described as data that has been processed to provide meaning. Knowledge and wisdom are not yet well defined with many competing definitions still in existence. Thus we will define these terms from an information systems perspective. Knowledge, as it is used here, can be defined as data and information used with understanding (gained through experience or from context) to make a decision under a particular set of circumstances. And finally wisdom, as used here, is defined as the use of data, information, and knowledge with understanding and intuition (gained through experience). Some examples follow, that should help to explain these definitions.

Health care data are comprised of facts such as demographic details (name, address, age, and sex for example), admission details (hospital name, date of admission, admitting physician, and insurance), and clinical details (weight, temperature, allergies, blood pressure, etc.). Taking temperature as an example, we can see that a single temperature reading taken on admission and recorded in a patient record doesn't tell the clinician much about the patient's progress. But a series of temperatures taken every half an hour and displayed graphically tells the clinician how the patient has progressed over several hours and can be used to determine the effectiveness of medication given or treatments performed to bring the temperature back into a normal range. Thus temperature data has been transformed into clinical information by plotting temperature against time. Data and information are closely related and information modelling is, for all intents and purposes, data modelling. Both data and information are facts about things that are in the past.

Now consider a collection of such temperature/time data alongside other clinical data and information about the effectiveness of temperature lowering medications and treatments and we now have a foundation for decision making about how to manage elevated temperatures in a variety of contexts. The task of retrieving, collating, and making this type of data and information available to clinicians when they need it, is the basic task of knowledge management. This is not to say that simply making these things available is in itself creating knowledge. There is no 'knowing' if the person viewing the information has no understanding of what it means or how it can be used to make decisions. Knowledge is information which, when understood through experience in the context of prior knowledge, can be used to make decisions about a current situation. Knowledge therefore is about the present.

Only in the area of intelligent decision systems is there an attempt to emulate the decision making ability of a human expert thereby automating knowing and decision making. Decision support systems are covered in greater detail later in Chapters 22 and 23.

Much has been learned about data, information, and knowledge management over the past three decades. Data and information management are now commonly used and understood. Knowledge management has also become quite common as organizations realised that they could gain competitive advantage by further exploiting the data that had already been collected. Far less research work has been done on the topic of wisdom, but there are some authors who are investigating and thinking about the transition from knowledge to wisdom and what this means for the practice of knowledge management [3].

Wisdom is about using knowledge to make strategic decisions for the future. Wisdom encompasses a decision maker's ability to make intuitive judgements to particular situations and to conceptualize future contexts and consequences. For example, clinical knowledge (evidence) may advise a standard treatment, such as antidepressants, to treat depression in most patients. But an experienced and wise clinician may decide not to follow that advice given his/her understanding of the circumstances of a particular patient's case because he/she intuitively believes that the recommended treatment will not work for this patient in these circumstances. If asked to explain the reasoning for such a decision it may be impossible for the clinician to explain other than to say it was an instinctive decision or that it was based on experience.

Another controversial but useful example is euthanasia. A wise clinician is able to decide when further intervention to keep a patient alive is no longer the correct or appropriate course of action. Such decisions are made every minute of every day in hospitals around the world. In the case of euthanasia however, there remains much debate and controversy over whether or not the patient can be allowed to decide for themselves when it is time to die. Some people, clinicians included, have a moral belief that it is correct and appropriate to assist patients to end their own lives in order to prevent them experiencing further pain and suffering. Other people hold just as strongly to the opposite belief in exactly the same context. In order to make such a decision requires wisdom, by our definition, irrespective of which decision is made. Thus to be wise, from an information systems perspective, is not necessarily to be correct. There are no absolute truths in decision making. Decisions can only be judged as 'good' or 'bad', successful or unsuccessful, after the outcomes are known. When the decision has moral and ethical dimensions as substantive and deep seated as those surrounding euthanasia, there is unlikely to be general agreement about what is the right and proper course of action. It is precisely for this reason that most societies have laws that take the power to make such decisions out of the hands of the individual. Since wisdom is not yet well understood it will not be discussed any further in this chapter.

Finally it should be said that the divisions between data, information, knowledge, and wisdom in the hierarchy are not discreet. The transitions between one conceptual level and the next are largely defined by the needs and experience of the decision maker. What is widely agreed is that the quality of decisions is dependent on the quality of the knowledge available to the decision maker at the time the decision is made, which in turn is dependant on the quality of the data that has been collected and stored in the first place.

Data, information and knowledge quality is based on the quality of the design of the technologies from data retrieval and storage at the back end to collection and presentation at the human-machine interface.

2.1 Why Model?

To design is to model. McNeill [4] defined a model as an abstraction of reality, representing those features that we consider important for the purposes of the model, and ignoring those that we consider unimportant. But what is the purpose of a model? By focussing on the important features, the model helps us to gain a better understanding of the underlying reality. We can use the model to make generalisations, to categorise and classify, to simplify, to organise, and to predict. Models help us to clarify our grasp of the subject modelled, and help us communicate our ideas to other people. Models can take many forms but in this chapter we will focus only on modelling techniques used to model information and knowledge. Models can be static, used once for their purpose, or they may be reused time and time again. Models may be permanent, reflecting they are of reality well enough for continued use, or they may change and evolve as the understanding of the underlying reality changes and evolves. Models are often composite or layered. A composite model may consist of a number of interrelated sub-models, each of which highlights a different aspect of the reality being modelled. A layered model has a sequence of similar models, with the top level showing only the most significant features and generalities, and the subsequent levels, each introducing features and details less important than shown on higher levels.

The modeling process begins when somebody realises there is some facet of reality that they need to understand better or to communicate to others. An initial model is constructed showing a few of the more important features that we are interested in. The model is checked against our understanding of the situation being modelled, and additional features are slowly added to make the model more complete. Modelling is typically an iterative and evolving process, starting with very simply, basic models that are well understood but tell us little, and gradually changing through progressive refinement into more complex models that are somewhat harder to understand but tell us much more. Details and features needed for better understanding are gradually added, and errors and unnecessary complexities are removed when discovered. Each stage of the model is tested against what is already known, and sometimes experimentation is used to verify implications of the model. Although models can be developed by individuals, their strength, robustness and applicability are improved if tested, verified, and validated by groups.

Information and knowledge modelling are the means by which information and knowledge resources and requirements are analysed during the development of a health information system or the upgrade of an existing health information system. The models produced are representations of how the information and knowledge will be stored electronically. Just as paper-based files are easier to find and use if they are stored under a recognised and clearly specified filing system, a systematic specification for the structure and storage of electronic files and their contents improves the performance of the information system. Moreover, the way in which the files and filing system are structured determines the logic required to access and use their contents and this is discussed later in the chapter. If in a paper-based system, X-Rays for patients whose surname starts with the letters 'A' through 'C' are stored in the X-Ray department, but those for surnames from 'D' through 'E' are stored in the

Emergency department and the rest are stored in a disused room on the Maternity ward, it would be very difficult and time consuming to find a file when it was needed. This is an example of a very poorly structured and implemented manual health information system. The efficiency and effectiveness of a health information system, whether manual or electronic or hybrid of these, is dependent on the structural design of the system.

An electronic filing system, or database, is more complex to design than a manual system because all aspects of the system must be specified within the system. For example, if a clinician picks up a patient file and wants to write orders for a particular medication, the file doesn't need to have been specially designed to be able to store the order. The clinician simply picks up the folder, finds the correct page and writes the order. But if a clinician accesses an electronic patient record via a computerised physician order entry device, the computer system must have been programmed to store the data, access certain files, retrieve the data, display the data, accept the new input data in a pre-determined format, update the stored file with the new data including the clinician's details (ID at the very least), the date must be captured or entered and stored, and to handle all other data and functions that are relevant to this one action.

Because of the complexity of these tasks, information systems development requires attention to detail. It often takes a team of people who are each expert in a particular area of the development process to complete a full information project. It is for these reasons that modelling is an essential task in information systems analysis, design and development a process described from a requirements perspective in chapter 12.

2.2 Information Modeling

There are different types of models for each part of a computerised system just as there are different types of models for each part of any other complex artefact. In the design of a large cruise ship for example, different designs are created for the ship's structure, its electrical system, its navigation system, its communications system, and for the human spaces, such as dining rooms and sleeping quarters. We accept, in the case of a large ship, that it is unlikely that the same design technique could be used for each of these different parts of the ship. Likewise it is not possible to use one design technique for all of the parts of an information systems infrastructure. There are modelling techniques for every part of an information system. Since computing is a relatively new field of engineering and because computing technologies change so rapidly, it is not possible to say that one modelling technique is definitively better than any other. The selection of a modelling technique is based on a number of factors including, the analysts' preferences, the type of system or application being designed, and the existing system design, if any. Each modelling technique is based on a set of principles and rules (logic) that dictate what the model represents. The rules of each technique must be followed if the model created is to be an accurate and meaningful representation that can be translated into a functional and functioning electronic artefact such as a health information system. Before one can follow the rules, one must know what those rules are and how they are to be applied.

3. A Brief History of Information Modeling

Early computers were programmed to perform calculation tasks with code that consisted of binary instructions that were not human readable. Eventually, as computers became more sophisticated, more powerful, and more widely used, the binary instructions gave way to word like instructions that the computer could convert back into binary for its own use. The instructions were written by the programmer and executed by the computer in a sequential pattern from beginning to end, *sequence*. As the ability of the computer systems improved and larger instruction sets could be executed it sometimes became necessary to find a way to make the computer execute one instruction instead of another, *selection*, and to repeat one or more instructions, *iteration*. Since at the time each line of code was numbered, it was easy to tell the computer to "go to" a particular line of code and start from there. If the GOTO instruction was used frequently the trace of the program execution looked like spaghetti. Complex code with lots of goto statements came to be known as 'spaghetti code' and could be a programmer's worst nightmare especially when code needed to be modified or corrected. It could be virtually impossible to trace through code that used GOTOs to find calculation or instruction errors. Flowcharts were commonly used at this time to model the logic of the program including the backwards jumps often associated with the GOTO statement.

During the 1960s, various people and groups of people were working on ways to improve program code by using structured programs. Two competing paradigms emerged. These were procedural programming and object oriented programming. In the short term, procedural programming won the day and became the most commonly used programming paradigm for many years. It was so common, that procedural programming came to be synonymous with structured programming. It would be several decades before object oriented programming would come to the forefront of computer programming and systems design. Table 1 summarises these modeling techniques and their purpose.

The following sections provide brief descriptions and examples for several of the most common modeling techniques used in the design of information systems. In each section there is a simple example of the diagramming tool associated with that method. These diagrams have been kept deliberately simple and generic in order to highlight the similarities and differences between them.

4. Programming Logic Modeling

There are two primary programming logic paradigms, structured (procedural) programming and object oriented programming.

4.1 Structured Programming

The theory of **structured programming** by and large did away with the GOTO statement in favour of program logic that could be easily traced and proven. Mainstream structured programs were written in simple procedural programming languages such as BASIC, PASCAL, and COBOL. Ungainly jumps from one line of code to another, using GOTO statements, were banished from the good programmer's repertoire of coding instructions. Instead, orderly sets of instructions packaged into functions and procedures that could be called into execution were introduced. Many procedural programming logic modelling methods have been developed and used over time. The Nassi-Schneiderman Chart and the Structure Chart were two of the most frequently used. Flowcharts were strongly discouraged because they allowed the GOTO statement to be modelled. That is, the GOTO statement allows backward loops and ad hoc statement execution. In flow charts you can model the back ward loop and the ad hoc jumps around the code. Programmers were discouraged from using flowcharts for this reason. The diagrams used to model the program logic had to be able to represent the three key procedural instruction execution methods: sequence, selection, and iteration. One of the key aspects of procedural programming is that considerations of data design were separated from the program. At run time, the program only needed to 'know' which data files to access and how to locate the data needed. Figure 1 illustrates a simple generic structure chart.

Table 1 Summary of Information Modeling Techniques

Paradigm	System Component	Model/s	Purpose
Procedural/ Structured	Program Logic	Nassi-Schneiderman Chart Structured Program Chart	To represent the processing of data at the primitive level and the flow of data through the program
Object Oriented[2] (Object methods use procedural logic)	Objects and Object Interactions	Object Oriented Model Unified Modelling Language	To represent the collection of objects in a system along with the interactions between them
Relational	Data store (database)	Entity Relationship Diagram Conceptual Schema Diagram	To represent data at rest, i.e. as it is stored (filed) in the data store and the relationships between data tables.
Traditional	Business Processes	Data Flow Diagrams	To represent the business processes and the flow of data through the system via processes, data stores, and entities external to the system.
Ontological	Knowledge Base	Ontology	To represent knowledge using formal logic to enable reasoning for decision support.
Ontological	Shared Electronic Health Record	openEHR Archetypes	To represent clinical data to enable reuse and interoperability

If one knows the rules for drawing a structure chart, then one knows by looking at Figure 1 that: the Main Function is the first function that is executed; Procedure A executes next; Procedure A calls Procedure B next and then calls Function A into execution; control is then returned to the Main Function which then calls Function B; once Function B is finished, Function C is called; Function C calls Procedure A; then Function C calls Function A; control then returns to Main which contains the code that ends the program. Data in a procedural program is *passed* from one procedure to another as it is needed. There are different ways to pass data through the program, but the detail of *parameter passing* is outside the scope of our discussion. Data is also passed to and from the user via some peripheral device such as a monitor or printer.

---

[2] The methods encapsulated in an object are written using procedural logic. The object oriented paradigm changes the way in which the methods (or functions) are called. Methods and data belong to objects and can only be used by instantiating that object.

Data is also passed to and from data files. Today these data files are most likely to be stored in a relational database.

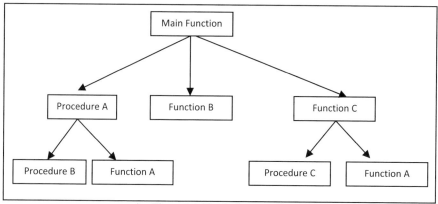

Figure 1 A Simple Structure Chart

If you do not understand the diagramming rules, i.e. the **syntax and semantics** of structure charts and you do not understand the theory of structured programming then Figure 1 could just as easily be interpreted as a class hierarchy which would be completely incorrect in this case. Without knowing the syntax and semantics of this diagram, or any diagram, the diagram has no meaning.

4.2 Object Oriented Programming

The object-oriented paradigm hinged on the notion of *encapsulation* which is the packaging of the data and process. Unlike functions in procedural programs which are processes for which data elements are defined, the classes in object oriented programs are data structures for which functions (methods) are defined. The conceptualization of data structures for which certain functions could be performed became popular. It seems that it is cognitively easier, especially for non-technical people, to visualize program functionality as data objects with functions rather than as a series of functions that work on data. Figure 2 illustrates a simple object oriented diagram.

Again, a person who understands the object oriented syntax and semantics will understand that Class A is the base, or parent, class and that all classes beneath it are types of Class A. The arrows are understood and read as *is-a* (subsumption) relationships. It is also understood that each of the sub-classes beneath Class A *inherit* both the data and methods of Class A. That means that each of the sub-classes contains datum1 and datum 2 and can use methodA1, methodA2, and methodA3. In addition, some of the sub-classes have their own specific data and methods that do not appear and cannot be accessed by any other class. Likewise, classes E and F inherit data and methods from Class B in addition to those inherited from Class A. Finally in this example, Class E does not have any of its own specialized methods and Class F does not have any of its own specialized data.

The object oriented paradigm changes the way that the functions (methods) of the program are activated to do the work required. In procedural program, discussed above, functions are called when they are needed from the main body of the program. In an object oriented program, functions can only be called after an object has been instantiated (an instance has been created). One may have a Patient object defined in an OO program, but this is just the template for a patient object. There can be no patient data, nor anything done about a patient until an instance of a patient has been created within the program. Let's say that we have a patient called Mr. Smith, we have instantiated the patient object with an instance called Mr. Smith. When we need to admit Mr. Smith we would call the Admit method for the Mr. Smith instance of the patient object. We can never call the Admit method directly for the general patient object.

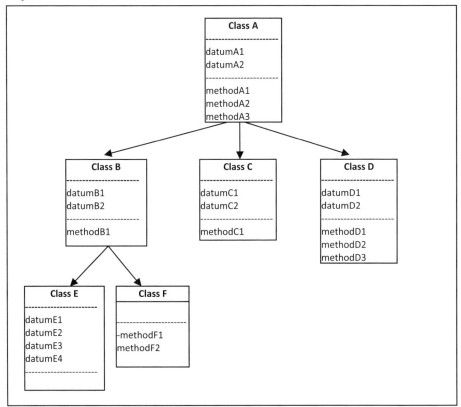

Figure 2 A Simple Object Oriented Diagram

Another point of difference is the way that the two paradigms treat data. Data in an object oriented program, like the methods, are encapsulated within the object and once again can only be accessed if that object has been instantiated. Data about Mr. Smith can only be accessed by specifying Mr. Smith's name, or Mr. Smith's age.

I suspect that as you are reading this, even if you don't already know anything about programming, you will be thinking that it makes sense that a Mr. Smith patient must exist before anything can be done in the system about Mr. Smith. It is this intuitive nature of the object oriented paradigm that has made it a popular design and programming method. Unfortunately the OO paradigm is not as successful when it is applied to database management and although some OO databases do exist, the trend appears to be to use a hybrid of object oriented programming and modelling with relational database management. Such systems are referred to as hybrid systems. The evolution of hybrid systems was inevitable since most existing legacy databases are relational in design and would have had to be replaced if an organization was to choose to implement a completely object oriented approach.

Thus in most cases, an object oriented model of an information system does not model the relational nature of the underlying database. Relational data modelling therefore remains a powerful and popular database design method.

5. Data Modeling

While programming methods were evolving so too was the need to store and use data. Early in the piece data were stored in simple sequential files. In order to access a data item in the middle of the sequence the entire file had to be read from beginning to end. This was time consuming and inflexible. Just as sequential programs gave way to structured programs, sequential data files gave way to data structures. As the need to handle larger quantities of data more efficiently increased data were organized into records, records were organized into tables, the tables were organized into databases, databases were organized into data warehouses, and eventually data warehouses were combined with other systems functions into enterprise wide systems. As with programming itself, database structures were logically conceptualized in many different ways by mathematicians and computer scientists who put their minds to these problems. There were hierarchical database structures, network database structures, relational database structures, and object oriented database structures, to name a few. By far the most widely used database structure over the past two decades has been the relational database. Relational databases are essential components in an information system and will be discussed in greater detail in Chapter 12.

Each of these database structures can be represented mathematically and/or diagrammatically. Information modelling is the representation of structured data. Diagramming is much easier than developing and reading a series of mathematical equations. It is also much easier to use a diagram to explain a database to non-technical people such as managers. Diagramming has therefore become an important tool in information systems analysis and design. Each diagramming method uses specific and carefully chosen symbols. These symbols may only be combined in ways that do not violate the rules of the underlying modelling theory.

5.1 Traditional Information Design Methods

Traditional system design refers to a combination of techniques and methods that became popular during the latter part of the twentieth century. The overall design process is known as the Systems Development Life Cycle (SDLC) and specified a series of steps to be followed and techniques to be used to build and implement an information system. Traditional information design includes methods for both data and process modelling in order to capture the requirements of data at rest (in a database) and at work (flowing through the organization).

5.2 Modeling Data at Rest

The primary diagramming tool used to represent relational databases was the Entity Relationship Diagram (ERD), although there were others available. The ERD in conjunction with normalization theory provided a very stable and manageable data storage solution for large data sets. Moreover the relational database model also provided proven mathematical methods for searching, combining, and extracting data from the database as required. The ERD required only a small set of symbols to represent complex databases.

The syntax of an ERD as with the previous diagram types is in the use of specific symbols to represent the logic of the model conceptually. The semantics of the ERD are found in the definition of the meaning of each symbol and in the overall meaning of the diagram which represents and reflects that theory of the model. Figure 3 illustrates a simple ERD. It defines three data entities, which will be implemented as 'tables' in a relational database. The attributes of each entity are the data fields, the columns in the tables. Attributes that are underlined with a solid line indicate the primary key of each table. If the underline is dashed, the attribute is immediately identified as a secondary key. When there is more than one attribute underlined for an entity, it is understood that the attributes are combined to form a 'concatenated' key. Each table is in fact a single data file containing a set of data records.

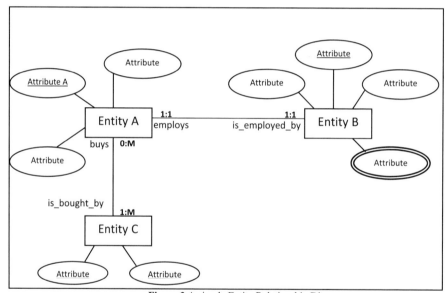

Figure 3 A simple Entity Relationship Diagram

The verbs and verb phrases alongside the relationship lines connecting entities to each other are the names of the relationships. It is clear that each relationship is bi-directional. The 0:M symbols represent the ordinality and cardinality of each relationship. For each Entity A there are many Entity C's and vice versa. We know this from the M (for Many) in the symbols. We also know that there does not have to be an instance of Entity A in the database at the time that the database is created, ordinality is 0. But we also know that there does need to be an instance of Entity C at the time that the database is created, ordinality 1. We also know that the relationship between Entity A and Entity B is 1 to 1. For each Entity A there can only be one Entity B. The double line around an attribute, as in Entity B, represents a set of this attribute.

Finally, those knowledgeable of relational database design know that there are two major violations of the rules of relationship database design in this model. First, the many to many relationship between A and C cannot be allowed to exist. Second, the set valued attribute in Entity B is also disallowed. The process by which these two violations are handled is the normalization process. The set valued attribute will be changed to a single valued attribute by creating another entity, table, that stores the multiple values. The many to many relationship will also be handled by the creation of a new entity, table, that stores the multiple instances of the relationship. It is not necessary for us to go into the details of this process here.

It should be clear at this point that even a very simple diagram encompasses a large volume of knowledge. Furthermore it should also be obvious by now that the syntax and semantics of each type of modelling is critical in representing the logic of the model correctly, accurately, and usefully.

5.3 Modeling Data at Work

As well as the model of the data required in an information system, the analyst must model the processes of the organization. Process modelling proved to be an extremely useful tool allowing organizations to re-engineer their processes to rationalize the use of data, personnel, equipment and all other resources. Unfortunately, for many workers rationalization often came to be associated with downsizing and job losses.

The primary tool used to model processes is the Data Flow Diagram. Unlike entity relationship diagrams which model data at rest, data flow diagrams (DFD) model data at work, i.e. data flowing around the various tasks and activities that must be performed by an organization to achieve its goals as shown in figures 4 & 5. Data flows include inputs to and outputs from the system to external entities such as suppliers and customers.

DFDs are drawn as a series of more and more detailed diagrams that end at the *primitive level* which is the level at which a process represents a single computer program. All DFDs begin with a *context diagram* (level 0) that represents the inputs to and outputs from the system to the external environment. The next level down (level 1) represents the main processes in the system. There should only ever be a few processes represented in each diagram. So for the diagram from Figure 5, above, there will be three DFDs drawn for the next level of detail in the system, one for each of the main processes represented at level 1. The process of *exploding* each diagram to its next level of detail continues until the primitive level is reached. A full process analysis of a system using this method could result in hundreds of separate DFDs.

In using these two methods of data design a good deal of additional information about the data needs to be recorded such as what type of data it is, where it is used in the system, and who has access to it. This type of information is really data about the data in the system. This is known as meta-data. You will not see the term 'meta-information' since information about the information in the system is more likely to be called *knowledge*[3]. Managing the meta-data was an enormous task which led to the development and use of computer aided software engineering (CASE) tools.

---

[3] When reading information systems books or journal articles it is prudent to make sure that you understand how a particular author is using a term before assuming that you know what is meant. It is unlikely that terminology in information systems is going to reach a point of stasis any time soon. Technology and information systems theories are too diverse and simply change too rapidly for the terminology to settle into some consistent lexical usage.

Figure 4 Simple Context Level Data Flow Diagram

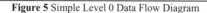

Figure 5 Simple Level 0 Data Flow Diagram

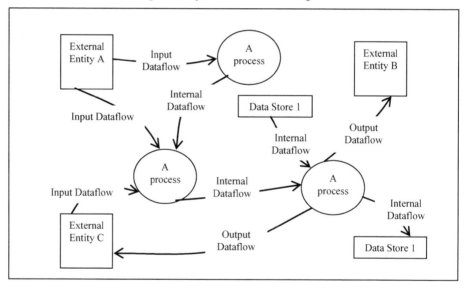

5.4 Computer Aided Software Engineering Tools

A CASE tool, or workbench[4], provides the analyst with diagramming tools, a data repository in which to store the meta-data, and usually includes programming code that checks the consistency and integrity of the design against the rules of the design method. For instance, a CASE tool will not allow you to give the same name to two

---

[4] The difference between a CASE tool and a CASE workbench is in the sophistication of the integrated development environment provided to the user. With its ability to automatically generate code in several different computer languages and many other capabilities, Enterprise Architect would be considered a workbench.

different data entities in an ERD nor will it let you 'lose' or change the dataflows from one level of DFD to the next. Many CASE tools today also include applications to generate computer program code from the models created. This is a powerful tool that enables end users to design and build their own systems. As with all end user computing however, as good as these CASE tools have become good designs are more likely to be generated through the collaborative efforts of end users and skilled information analysts.

Unfortunately, the proliferation of CASE tools further complicated the problems for end users wanting to model. Tools such as Enterprise architect include so many different diagramming tools that it can be difficult to know which is the best choice for your purposes. In addition to this the symbol sets used in a particular CASE tool for ERD, for example, may differ to the symbols used in another CASE tool. An example of this, is the representation of an ERD in MS Access. An MS Access ERD does not look like the ERD in Figure 3 above. Differences such as these are more often than not due to the programming decisions rather than modelling decisions. The attribute symbols, ovals in Figure 3, have been done away with completely. They would simply take up too much space on the screen. As it is, even a small ERD is difficult to read in MS Access. In spite of the differences the modelling theory behind the MS Access ERD is entity relationship modelling and all of the relational database design rules apply.

5.5 Unified Modeling Language (UML)

The Unified Modeling Language was developed by a group of information modelers, Grady Booch, Ivar Jacobson, and James Rumbaugh in the 1980's to fill the systems modelling gaps that could not be addressed by an object model alone and to provide modelers with a suite of the most useful modelling methods and tools selected from amongst the plethora of methods around at the time [5].

Use cases for example, allow the modeller to consider the interface, the workflow, and the data inputs and outputs required in particular tasks. An OO diagram alone does not provide this ability. A systems analyst would use all of the UML components to derive a full system requirements specification. The object model on its own simply does not provide the information that one requires to build a complete system.

6. Knowledge Modeling

Knowledge is information used in context with understanding. To computerise knowledge the understanding of the human information user has to be coded into the computer. This understanding is transformed into a set of rules that apply to the data and information. For example, the statement, 'The patient has an elevated temperature.' is a piece of information while the statement, 'If the patient has an elevated temperature then administer Panadol', is information with a rule applied. The latter statement advises a decision maker on what action to take and under what conditions to take that action. The advice is derived from the knowledge. Knowing what the data means, knowing what to do about it and knowing when to do it are cognitive processes associated with human decision making. The purpose of knowledge modelling is to provide the information and the rules necessary to emulate these processes with a computer. There are several different types of knowledge models. Some, such as those found in expert systems, are built by knowledge engineers and some are derived by computer programs, such as case based reasoners and neural networks, from existing evidence.

In recent years, formal knowledge models have come to predominate the knowledge management field. This trend is possibly due to the fact that models based on formal logic are thought to be more robust and more easily explained, maintained, and re-used than models produced following some ad hoc process. Knowledge models based on formal logic are known as ontologies.

7.   Ontology

Ontological modelling is based primarily on the representation of knowledge as a class hierarchy. This class hierarchy, without question, is similar to the class hierarchy in an object oriented diagram. Both model classes, both are fundamentally structured around the *is-a*, or subsumption, relationship, both embrace the notion of inheritance, and both use conceptual abstraction to define upper-level or base-level classes, and both use the terminology of parent and child classes.

Beyond these syntactic similarities though, the two forms of modelling are in fact significantly different. Ontological models do not represent encapsulated objects. Object oriented models do not support logical reasoning. Ontological models do not represent database designs. Object oriented models do not represent knowledge. Ontological models are based on various formal logical theories such as frames, description logics, and formal logic. Object oriented models are based on the logic of object oriented programming. The data modelled in an object are data as these need to be used in a program. It is not a representation of the best, most efficient, way to store that data, nor does it provide any rules about the meaning of these data. This topic is discussed in greater detail in the next chapter.

8.   *open*EHR Archetypes: an ontological approach to record sharing

The *open*EHR (*pr. open air*) approach to information modelling is an ontological one[6]. It is strongly based on the belief that the best way to achieve health information system interoperability that will enable the shared electronic health record is to develop information models that are independent of the information systems that will use the models.

Platform independence is not a new idea, software developers have striven to develop applications that could be used on a variety of computer equipment and operating systems without having to modify the code in any way for many, many years. Platform independence has been more or less successfully achieved by some software developers. Java is perhaps the best known example of a programming language that achieves platform independence. Platform independence means that the applications are not limited by the capacity or idiosyncrasies of the computer systems on which they are used. Eliminating specific system constraints results in the freedom to focus on the design.

*open*EHR recognized that there was a greater likelihood that a Shared Electronic Health Record (SHER) would be possible if the data and information models were platform[5], terminology, language, and location independent. That means abstracting the data concepts from common usage to higher level data concepts that are applicable across all health care systems irrespective of technology and terminology.

To achieve this level of abstraction and independence, a high level modelling language was required. *open*EHR developed the Archetype Definition Language (ADL) to address this issue. One of the desired outcomes for the *open*EHR project was that clinicians should be encouraged to design their own archetypes (clinical knowledge (constraint) models) based on their needs and their view of the world. The archetype specification guides the developer to produce an archetype that fits the *open*EHR model and therefore is, by design, shareable and reusable. Once designed the archetype is available to anyone else who had a similar need. The *open*EHR approach is to allow as many similar archetypes as people want to create to be created. All are stored in an archetype repository known as a clinical knowledge manager, a global, open source repository maintained by the *open*EHR foundation.

The theory behind the ADL is based on a formal, logical abstraction of data to higher level concepts which is consistent with ontological modelling as explained in more detail I chapter 10.[6] *open*EHR is not an isolated effort. The *open*EHR foundation works with standards organizations such as CEN TC251, ISO TC215, and HL7. But in itself *open*EHR does not adopt a standards based approach to development believing that such an approach hampers the speed and flexibility of development efforts. Furthermore, the foundation is committed to providing open source solutions to the health care community and encourages anyone who is interested to join. In its Archetype Object Model document [7[p.9]] the *open*EHR Foundation states that,

- An underpinning principle of openEHR is the use of archetypes and templates, which are formal models of domain concepts controlling data structure and content of data. The elements of this architecture are twofold.
- The openEHR Reference Model (RM), defining the structure and semantics of information, and the service models (SMs), describing service interfaces. These models correspond respectively to the ISP[7] RM/ODP[8] information and computational viewpoints. The information models define the data of openEHR EHR systems; meaning that every data instance in a system is an instance of a type defined in the Information Model. The information model is designed to be invariant in the long term, to minimise the need for software and schema updates.
- The openEHR Archetype Model (AM), defining the structure and semantics of archetypes and templates. The AM consists of the archetype language definition language (ADL), the Archetype Object Model (AOM), the openEHR Archetype profile (OAP) and the Template Object Model (TOM).

Box 1 contains Leslie's [8] list of points as the points of difference between *open*EHR and other approaches to health information semantic interoperability.

Thus the *open*EHR approach has been purposefully developed to enable EHR end users, the clinicians, to have direct input into the design of the EHR. This was achieved

---

[5]   In computer programming, platform independence was also known as **portability**, meaning that the program was portable to any computer and it would run as expected and without fault or failure.

[6]   Visit the openEHR web site at: http://www.openehr.org/home.html

[7]   Internet Service Provider

[8]   Reference Model of Open Distributed Processing

by exploiting the most appropriate information and knowledge modeling theories and practice. In this way alone the *open*EHR approach is a unique example of how a commitment to meet the needs of the user can produce an information model that is flexible, useful, and, in the words of the *open*EHR Foundation, 'future proof'. Ontological and archetype modeling is discussed further in the chapters 9 and 10.

Box 1 Points of difference between *open*EHR and other approaches to health information semantic interoperability.

1.	Open Source Initiative - … specifications are freely available under an open licence.
2.	Separation Of The Technical And Clinical Domains - The openEHR design is … is a 2 level information model. These 2 levels allow a clear separation of the technical reference (i.e. data) model on which software is based from the clinical knowledge itself. …
3.	Purpose-Built EHR - The design of the reference and archetype models support many unique openEHR features required for robust clinical record keeping, clinical business process and medico-legal compliance …
4.	Knowledge-Enabled - Clinicians are able to contribute actively and directly to the development of the clinical knowledge models that underpin their EHRs. Archetypes can be revised and versioned to reflect the rapid and varied changes in health domain knowledge.
5.	Terminology Agnostic - …connects flexibly to any or all terminologies through either archetypes or templates. … Archetypes and terminologies are not competitive, but rather complement each other.
6.	Semantic Querying - Archetypes, in combination with terminologies enable powerful possibilities for semantic querying of repository data …
7.	Language Independent - There is no language primacy in archetypes; they can begin in any language and be translated to multiple other languages. … Archetypes are currently available in English, German, Turkish, Dutch, Swedish, Farsi, Spanish and Portuguese.
8.	Sustainable Reference Model - … consists only of generic data types, structures and a small number of generic patterns, resulting in a small, stable and sustainable information model for IT people to maintain. This approach allows a clinical data repository to act as a future-proof data store, totally independent of software applications and technology change. …
9.	Ease Of Implementation - … there is little infrastructure required; the software required is small, due to being based on a compact and stable, object-oriented reference model; and the clinical models (archetypes) can be developed separately from the software application.
10.	Ongoing Development And Enhancement - Based on feedback from its international collaborators, openEHR is undergoing continuing development, with ongoing maintenance and releases of specifications and software.
11.	Governance Of Shared Content - Archetypes are created once, and if broadly agreed upon, they can become the basis of consistent sharing of data content between systems, providers and even other countries. … All systems that use the same archetypes – even across country borders and terminologies – will be able to interoperate. …
12.	Collaborative Development - … development to date has been the result of interested and motivated volunteers from a broad international community of clinicians and software engineers. … Clinical Review Boards, comprising world experts in their fields, have had oversight of the overarching strategy, process and governance. …

9. Model Quality and Requirements Specification

What does all of this mean to the clinician or the health informatician? It means that it is the responsibility of the model user, who is generally part of a design team, to make sure that they understand the modelling methods, that the models are appropriate to use for their purposes and that they clarify for themselves any minor syntactic differences (use of square boxes instead of rounded boxes for external entities in a DFD for example) between available modelling tools .

It also means that whatever modelling methods are chosen, the design of the system components and the overall system must be based on the user requirements that have been determined before the design process begins. This chapter has focussed on various diagrammatic models that are commonly used. Visual models such as these diagrams, are one way to communicate a design to others. Visualizing a design enables its evaluation against the requirements specification and with stakeholders before implementation is attempted. It is much easier to change a diagram than it is to change parts of an information system.

In an information system, all aspects of the system must be designed. Data are the fundamental building blocks of all electronic systems. The formats in which data are collected, stored, used, and displayed are fundamental to the efficient and effective functioning of an information system. Most people have heard of the *garbage in garbage out* principle. Well this still holds true for all computerised systems even the pseudo-intelligent ones. If a CPOE application, for example, has been programmed to accept dosage amounts with up to three decimal places in an input field (eg. 0.025mg) and the clinician enters 0.05mg, but all values entered into this field are sent to a field in a database table that can only store one decimal place, then the clinician will think that the correct amount was entered but a completely incorrect value (0.0mg) will have been stored. Clearly a trivial problem for the database administrator, but a potentially fatal error for the patient. The next person to access the record for that patient will not see the order correctly. In order to meet both the clinician's and the patient's needs the solution to this problem is not to restrict the input field at the user interface to one decimal place so that it matches the database, but rather to extend the corresponding field in the underlying database table to three decimal places.

An information model is not a fictional creation of a systems analyst. It is the result of a thorough systems analysis of user and organizational needs that leads to a completed requirements specification. There are many different ways to conduct a systems analysis including the traditional systems development lifecycle, rapid application and design, prototyping, and joint application design. The decision about which method to use is up to the analyst and should be made with consideration to the project scope, time constraints, and resource availability. It may be that a combination of methods are used for different parts of the analysis. Prototyping might be beneficial when designing the user interfaces because user's are able to try the forms and applications and give specific feedback. A traditional SDLC approach might be used to do a thorough analysis of the data and process requirements. Chapter 12 provides a more detailed discussion of health information systems and requirements specifications.

10. Conclusion

At the heart of all information systems is the data that is input and output at the user interfaces. Data at rest in an information system is of little value. It may even become a liability if it is not used. Data are put to work when they are transformed into the information required by the users, clinicians, managers, and patients. Information is a valuable asset to an organization. Even more valuable to an organization is knowledge which is information combined with the understanding of experienced decision makers that is made available to others. Access to knowledge can enable a less experienced decision maker to make more effective and timely decisions. Critically neither information nor knowledge has any value if it does not provide the users with what they need to do their jobs.

It is therefore important that an information model is based on the needs of the users and the organization. These needs are identified in the requirements specification which is an outcome of the systems analysis process. It is also important that a modelling method is used that is suitable for the system being designed. For example, if there is a decision support system to design, then an ontology would be a good modelling choice. If there is a relational database to design then an entity relationship diagram would be the model of choice. Selecting an Object model to design a relational database is not a particularly good idea because the translation of the object model into a relational database implementation is not straightforward and may lead to confusion and a poor outcome.

If user requirements are not addressed in the design and the design is not communicated back to the users for evaluation prior to implementation, the successful function and adoption of the information system is at risk.

The *open*EHR approach to clinical data modelling for the purposes of enabling the SEHR is to put the design activity into the hands of the clinician. They have accomplished this by providing a data structure, the archetype, that is both stable in its overall design and flexible having only a few basic, mandatory fields. The designer of a new archetype thus has the freedom to design it to suit their needs while being confident that the overall structure of the archetype will always be compatible and semantically interoperable with all other archetypes.

References

[1]   Sharma, Nikhil. 2008. The origin of DIKW Hierarchy. *The Origin of the "Data Information Knowledge Wisdom" Hierarchy.* http://www-personal.si.umich.edu/~nsharma/dikw_origin.htm cited May 9, 2008).
[2]   Himma, Kenneth. 2007. The concept of information overload: A preliminary step in understanding the nature of a harmful information-related condition. *Ethics and Information Technology* 9, no. 4:259-272. http://dx.doi.org.ezproxy.cqu.edu.au/10.1007/s10676-007-9140-8 cited May 9, 2008).
[3]   Zeleny, Milan. 2006. Knowledge-information autopoietic cycle: towards the wisdom systems. *International Journal of Management and Decision Making* 7, no. 1:3-18. http://inderscience.metapress.com/app/home/contribution.asp?referrer=parent&backto=issue,1,8;journal ,11,25;linkingpublicationresults,1:110876,1 cited May 16, 2008.
[4]   McNeill R R Database in Hovenga, Kidd, Cesnik (Eds) Health Informatics: an overview. Churchill Livingstone, Melbourne 1996
[5]   Roff J.T *UML A Beginner's Guide* McGraw-Hill/Osborne 2003
[6]   *open*EHR Foundation : http://www.openehr.org/home.html
[7]   Beale, Thomas, ed. 2007. *The Archetype Object Model.* 1st ed. The openEHR Foundation http://www.openehr.org/releases/1.0.1/architecture/am/aom.pdf cited February 17, 2007.
[8]   Leslie, Dr Heather. 2008. OpenEHR: The World's Record. *Pulse+IT Magazine* http://www.pulsemagazine.com.au/index.php?option=com_content&task=view&id=239&Itemid=1 cited May 16, 2008.

Review Questions

1.   What is the purpose of information modelling?
2.   How does the *open*EHR approach to clinical data differ from previous modelling and design approaches?
3.   How would you select the appropriate modelling tool to use if you were asked to participate in the development of a new CPOE application?

4. Why is it important to base an information model on the requirements of the people who will be using the information?
5. Are the classes in an object oriented model different to those in an ontology? If so, how and why are they different?

Health Informatics
E.J.S. Hovenga et al. (Eds.)
IOS Press, 2010
© *2010 The authors and IOS Press. All rights reserved.*
doi:10.3233/978-1-60750-476-4-104

9.   Health Care Ontologies: Knowledge Models for Record Sharing and Decision Support

Maria MADSEN[1] BS, BSc(Hons), GDAC, MB(IS), MACS PhD Candidate
Lecturer, School of Management and Information Systems, Central Queensland University, Rockhampton Qld and Director of eHealth Education Pty Ltd

Abstract. This chapter gives an educational overview of:
- The difference between informal and formal ontologies
- The primary objectives of ontology design, re-use, extensibility, and interoperability.
- How formal ontologies can be used to map terminologies and classification systems.
- How formal ontologies improve semantic interoperability.
- The relationship between a well-formed ontology and the development of intelligent decision support.

Keywords. Terminology, Classification, Ontology, Decision Support Systems-Clinical, Knowledge, Semantic Interoperability

Introduction

The topics of knowledge modeling and ontology were introduced in Chapter 8. You learned that an ontology is one type of knowledge model. In this chapter we explore knowledge modeling in greater detail. Knowledge modeling is part of the knowledge representation stage of the complete knowledge engineering process. An ontology is a particular type of knowledge representation. It is not our purpose here to explain knowledge engineering in full. This chapter is concerned with ontologies as knowledge representations that improve semantic interoperability and enable the sharing of electronic health records.

We begin with a little background information about communication and knowledge. Then we will revisit ontology engineering in some detail with a focus on semantic interoperability. Finally we look at how formal ontologies are used in health care.

1.   Background

Knowledge representation theories can be daunting with many unfamiliar words, such as ontology, subsumption, mereology, and others. The ideas can seem somehow

---

[1] Corresponding author: m.madsen@ehealtheducation.net

divorced from our everyday lives and work. But the reality is that we are what we are because knowing is a uniquely human capacity. In the 16th century the French philosopher, scientist, and mathematician Renee Descartes famously stated, "Dubito ergo cogito; cogito ergo sum." Translated from the Latin this statement reads, "I doubt therefore I think; I think therefore I am." Humans create knowledge.

Computers do not do anything unless they are programmed to do so and up until now there are no computers that are programmed to think for themselves[2]. Computers therefore do not *know* anything. Knowledge representation is the process of finding a way to create computer programs that can at least help us to manage knowledge so that it is accessible and preserved.

2. General Communications

As human beings we communicate ideas, feelings, and facts by using concepts. If, while we are eating a meal, I say to you, "Please pass the salt.," you will know immediately what I mean and you will respond in some way to my request. In that sentence I have used concepts that we both understand to express my needs. I have, therefore, communicated my needs to you.

Each of the words (terms) in the sentence is a concept. Only one of these words, however, is absolutely essential and that is the word "salt" because it identifies what I want. The meaning, or **semantics**, of my sentence is conveyed by the words. The accepted structure, or **syntax**, of my sentence is constructed by using all of the words in the sentence in a very specific order according to the rules, or **logic**, of the English language.

Computers are still as yet incapable of making good sense out of natural language. If we want our computerized information systems to be able to handle clinical knowledge, which is far more complex than the sample sentence above, then it is necessary to structure this knowledge into a form that can be used by a computer program, i.e. to create a logic other than natural language construction. While doing so it will be necessary to choose only essential concepts. If we were coding the sample sentence, for example, we would not bother with the word 'the' as this term is not essential to the meaning we wish to convey.

3. Health Data Communications

If patient records are exchanged between two organizations that have health information systems (HIS) using exactly the same terminologies, classifications and database structures then the information in the records would be able to be exchanged in a meaningful way and the two systems would be interoperable. For example, a hospital has to send discharge summaries to an aged care facility for Mr. Smith. If the two HIS are interoperable then the hospital will be able to extract and send Mr. Smith's details electronically to the aged care facility without having to do anything to it and the aged care facility will be able to simply update their database with Mr. Smith's details as they were received. Wonderful!

---

[2] There are some computerised artefacts that emulate human interaction (mostly toys) but this level of function is still a long way from being true independent thinking.

Unfortunately, there are very few health care systems that enjoy this level of interoperability even different systems within one health organization are unlikely to be interoperable. This is not a problem that is unique to health care organizations. It was the lack of internal interoperability of information systems that led to the development of what are known as Enterprise Wide Systems. The premise for having an enterprise wide system was to connect all of the information systems within one organization so that the best use could be made of the data, information, and knowledge that already existed but was previously inaccessible due to poor or non-existent connectivity.

If, as is normally the case, the two facilities, or two departments, use different terminologies and different database structures then much work will need to be done before Mr. Smith's details can be exchanged successfully. To solve the terminology differences a reference terminology may be required to aide in the translation of terms from the sender to their analogs in the receiver's terminology, just as Descartes' quote was translated from Latin to English earlier. This goes some way to solving the interoperability problem but there is still the matter of the database structures. The data, now containing terms that can be understood by the receiving system, will be in a structure that does not match the structure of the receiver's database. This means that the data cannot simply be added to the database but rather will have to be restructured first. Each time the data are manipulated there is a chance that errors will be made. The translation and restructuring also takes valuable computer processing time and resources. Such exchanges are neither effective nor efficient but will remain necessary until interoperability is achieved.

4.   Preserving Specialized Knowledge for Reuse

As well as using concepts to communicate with each other, humans are also very good at organizing concepts so that they can be learned and used by others. An unabridged dictionary, for example, provides us with an exhaustive list of words for a particular language along with the various meanings that these words are used to convey. Such a list is useful for general purposes of communication but not very useful if we want to communicate about more highly specialized knowledge domains such as medicine. In specialized domains in addition to the words that exist in the general language there are also specialized terms that are only used within those domains. Terminologies are collections of these specialized terms. When the terms are highly related to each other a terminology can be further refined by classifying terms into a hierarchy of related terms. There are many ways in which a classification can be made and most classification systems have evolved out of the needs of those who use the terms.

In health care the ad hoc evolution of classifications has resulted in a plethora of classification systems and terminologies that are related but not entirely similar. Terms may have several different meanings across classifications, there may be multiple terms with the same meaning within a classification, and some terms may have no meaning outside of the local domain in which the classification was developed. In other words, the semantics of one classification is often incompatible with the semantics of others.

If, as in health care, a need arises to share information between the domains, it may be difficult or impossible to do so without first mapping the terms in one classification with the terms in the other. The mapping of one to the other is often carried out manually because humans are much better than computers at filling in gaps, solving problems, and making sense out of incomplete information. In fact, most computer programs cannot make sense out of incomplete information. There are many different methods that can be used to map one ontology to another. Noy [1] describes some of these methods and the interested reader is advised to view her presentation as an introduction to the topic of mapping and alignment. The methods discussed by Noy are also applicable to terminology mapping in health care.

5.   Formal Ontology

To build a computer system that can make some sense out of a classification system, the domain knowledge has to be structured in a very precise, computer useable syntax. At the same time the meaning, i.e. the semantics, of the concepts as they relate to the particular domain must be retained. A precise syntax that represents the semantics of a knowledge domain is a **formal logic.** The logic is the set of rules that constrains the classification of concepts and the assertion of relationships between them. The logic is formal because it is based on a precise, mathematical, syntax. A knowledge representation (model) designed using a formal logic can be coded into and worked on by a computer. Fig. 1 depicts a continuum of ontology types from least to most formal.

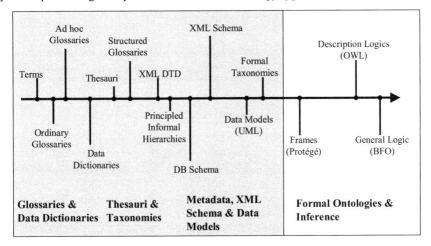

Figure 1 Ontology Types and Languages (adapted from [2])

Health care is replete with clinical terminologies and classification systems that fall outside of the Formal range, white area of Fig. 1. Such informal ontologies[3] do not enable decision support and are not inherently interoperable. This does not mean that they are not useful for the purposes for which they were designed, clearly they are.

In this chapter, we are interested in formal ontologies as knowledge models that do enable decision support and do provide semantic interoperability. Table 1 synthesizes and summarizes the formal ontological modeling concepts discussed in this chapter. Box 1, below, lists five key criteria that distinguish well-formed, formal ontologies.

---

[3]   **NB:** Bittner states that 'informal ontologies' are not true ontologies.

Granularity	Knowledge Type	Number of Concepts	Level of Abstraction	Scope of Problem Domain	Changeability	Comments
Coarsest	Intentional	Few	0	Universal	Unchanging	Timeless
Coarse	↑	↑	1	Discipline Specific	Unlikely to change	Longitudinal stability
Medium			2	Specialization Specific	May change with new knowledge	Medium to long term stability
Fine	↓	↓	3	Problem Context Specific	May change with change in context	Short to medium term stability
Finest	Extensional	Many	4	Location & Implementation Specific	Fluid, likely to change with needs & practices	May describe this as "agile" High flexibility can be changed as needed.

Table 1 Characteristics of ontologies at varying levels of granularity

Box 1 Objective Design Criteria for Formal Ontologies.

Gruber [8] suggests five objective design criteria based on the purpose of the ontology:
- **Clarity** – all terms should be objectively, fully and carefully defined,
- **Coherence** – the structure of the ontology should not give rise to inferences that are inconsistent with the already stated definitions,
- **Extendibility** – the structure should be able to accommodate additions that support sharing and re-use.
- **Minimal encoding bias** – the design should not be determined by the coding used, for example a Protégé ontology should be equally as valid when used in XML format as when it is used within Protégé, and
- **Minimal ontological commitment** – the ontology should not try to define everything in the domain. It should cover only concepts essential to enable knowledge sharing in that domain.

Although Gruber's design criteria seem sensible and reasonably straight forward, they are not always easily achieved. Formal ontology design requires creative insight that is more akin to the arts than to computer science. There is as yet no single widely accepted methodology for engineering an ontology. Noy [1 p.9] states that, "Ontology is not a reality it is a subjective representation of it (Different designers have different views); Different tasks and requirements for applications; Different conventions ..." Thus even formal ontologies may fail to be truly interoperable with each other. Until such time as the wider ontology engineering community agrees on some basic modeling conventions, i.e. a methodology, the situation is unlikely to improve as ontologies are relatively easy to develop.

6.   Knowledge Acquisition

Before knowledge can be represented in any useful way, essential domain concepts and knowledge sources must be identified. The process of discovering those concepts that are essential in a clinical context, the relationships between them, and the rules associated with their meaning is known as knowledge acquisition.

Knowledge exists in two basic forms, tacit and explicit. Explicit knowledge is knowledge that can be easily communicated. It is, hopefully, the type of knowledge that the authors are imparting to you in this book. It can be captured, codified, and communicated. Tacit knowledge, on the other hand, is the knowledge that humans acquire over a lifetime of experience. It is a deep understanding of the complexities of a given problem that comes from experience. This type of knowledge is very difficult to communicate and that makes it difficult to elicit from those who have it, the domain experts. Tacit knowledge is not only a problem for knowledge engineers, but can also be a problem for systems engineers when they try to elicit user requirements during a systems analysis. Many people simply are not able to articulate what they do when they do their work, much less why they do it.

There are methods that can assist the elicitation process. One of these is *protocol analysis* which requires a person to talk through the steps in their work while they are carrying out the various tasks. The person is asked to describe and explain what they are doing while they are doing it. The analyst may provide the person with a voice recorder and may also observe the person at their work. Observation can be useful, but having an observer present can also change the way that a person actually performs the tasks. As you can see this is an area fraught with difficulties and is one of the impediments to the development of knowledge based systems. The difficulty of knowledge acquisition can be the source of design flaws in the development of any information system. Appropriate methods of knowledge acquisition and elicitation should be selected during the project planning phases of systems development as illustrated in Fig. 2.

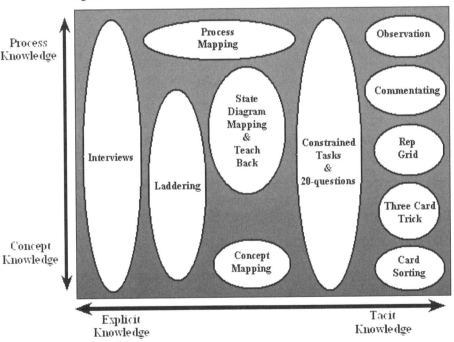

Figure 2 Knowledge Acquisition Techniques for Specific Types of Knowledge [3]

7.   Granularity

Knowledge can be conceptualized as either intentional[4] and extensional. For our purposes, the "***extension*** of an idea is 'the collection of all the objects falling under it' Bolzano as explained by Sebestik [4[p.46]]. It is this process of identifying the aggregation of concepts under a common parent class, that is more commonly referred to as *concept abstraction*. As the opposite of extension, intentional knowledge is specific instances of things that exist. These definitions are consistent with our view of ontological engineering which is dependent upon the use of high level concepts (classes) under which more specific things can be aggregated according to the formal logic being used. This process of concept aggregation results in a hierarchy of domain concepts from most general to most specific.   The levels of abstraction are the *granularity* of the ontology, Fig. 3.

Although Fig. 3 makes the levels appear to be quite separate and discrete they are not in any way discrete. For example, if the knowledge domain, or universe of discourse, was in fact universal reality, then the BFO would be a domain ontology. This is a trivial observation with respect to our current discussion, but highlights the subjectivity and sensitivity of assigning levels in context of the knowledge domain of interest. The levels in Fig. 3 are also indicative of the intended purpose of the ontology described. It follows that, conceptually, formal ontologies can be themselves classified as belonging to different levels of abstraction.   Such a classification of ontologies would itself be an ontology, a **meta-ontology**.

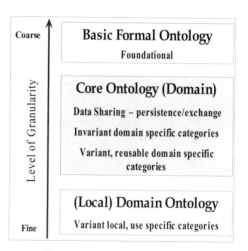

Figure 3 Ontological Levels: [5]

8.   The subsumption hierarchy

Concepts may belong more or less to any level depending on how the concepts are defined. The level at which concepts are defined within an ontology is entirely

---

[4] Note: The use of the term 'intention' here is not the same as the common English usage of the term.

dependent on the knowledge domain being modeled and the decisions made by the ontology engineer.

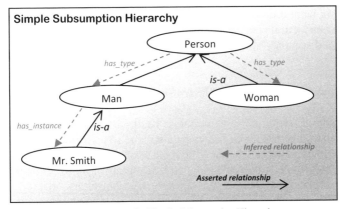

Figure 4 Example of a Simple Subsumption Hierarchy

9. From Ontology to Intelligent Decision Support

Decision support is based on the timely access to data, information, and knowledge in order to make a well informed decision. The trend in decision support continues to be toward developing ever more highly automated software that takes the decision making activity away from the human user altogether. So at one end of the spectrum we have decision support with human decision making and the other end of the spectrum we have decision support with machine decision making. The decision support systems in the mid-range of this spectrum are the systems that are of particular interest with respect to ontological engineering. These systems are known as knowledge based systems, or expert systems, or intelligent decision systems. Decision support systems are covered in more detail in Chapters 22 and 23.

Decision support is enabled by formal ontologies because a well-formed knowledge model can be reasoned over by an inference engine (or reasoner[5]) which means that the knowledge can be used by a computer to arrive at a decision. The hierarchical model produced through the concept abstraction process, discussed above, is the *asserted* knowledge model. But new facts can also be *inferred* from those that are asserted. Box 2 illustrates assertion and inference in a simple knowledge model.

The concept 'Man' is an extension while the concept 'Mr. Smith' (if he really exists) is an intention. In our knowledge model we assert that **Mr. Smith** *is-a* **Man**. And we assert that **Man** *has-sex* **Male**. Then we can infer that **Mr. Smith** *has-sex* **Male**. This is the basis for deductive reasoning over a knowledge base. If we have also coded into our knowledge base that the class **Man** is exclusive of all members of the class **Woman**, then we can also deduce from our model that to state that **Mr. Smith** *is-a* **Woman** is false. This logic is *inferred* by the computer from our model.

Box 2 Example of Assertion, Reasoning, and Inference in a Formal Ontology

---

[5] A computer application designed to "read" through a knowledge base and arrive at a decision by applying a set of decision rules that are stored in a rule base. An intelligent decision system consists of a database, knowledge base, rule base, inference engine, and a human interface.

The quality of an ontology, is manifest in its use as part of a knowledge based system, i.e. a reasoning system. The subsumption hierarchy is traversed by the inference engine, one node at a time, from root to leaves, as it tests the relationships against the domain rules that have been coded. An ontology that is concise, consistent, and which can be traversed both down and back up[6] the hierarchy will improve the efficiency and accuracy of the reasoner results.

10. Ontology and the Shared Electronic Health Record

The exchange of health information across health information systems using disparate computer platforms, terminologies, and data models is a major impediment to both the efficient delivery of health care and the realization of the lifelong health record. HL7[7] messaging as a means of packaging and delivering health data from one place to another has been very successful for those organizations that have managed to implement the messaging system. HL7 however has some problems including a large number of different versions which should be backwards compatible but are not necessarily so dependent on how well the implementers have followed the HL7 recommendations. HL7 messaging thus enables sharing of certain types of health information but is not a Shared Electronic Health Record (SEHR). On the other hand the *open*EHR Foundation has set out to develop an infrastructure that will enable a true SEHR that is platform independent as explained previously in chapter 8. The *open*EHR archetypes are information "containers" that have a standard, well defined, unchangeable structure within which a clinician can create their own version of a record or data item that will meet their particular need. The governance of the repositories has itself been tackled as an ontological problem space [6]. Garde et al.[6 p.7]) state that, "A formal OWL Archetype Ontology can provide the necessary meta-information on archetypes for Domain Knowledge Governance and also support reasoning to automatically find similar archetypes."

For the shared electronic health record, *open*EHR provides a foundational ontology, a development methodology with an integrated development environment, and a knowledge governance model. The *open*EHR approach is discussed further in the next chapter.

11. Uses and Limitations of Ontologies

Ontologies can not only be designed in a variety of ways, but they can also be used in a variety of ways. Ontologies can be created specifically for human use (eg. decision support) or for computer use (eg. intelligent agents/bots). Ontologies can be high level models of reality[8] or low level models of some specific clinical context[9] or at various levels of abstraction in between these bounds. Ontologies can be used as reference

---

[6] Bidirectional traversal of the subsumption hierarchy is achieved by asserting relationships and their inverses where possible.

[7] HL7 (Health Level 7) is an international standards development organization specializing in health care messaging standards, http://www.hl7.org

[8] Foundational ontologies such as the Basic Formal Ontology from IFOMIS, http://www.ifomis.org/bfo

[9] Domain ontologies such as the Gene Ontology (GO), http://www.geneontology.org/

models that aid in the mapping of one ontology to another when the semantics are not naturally interoperable, for example the Unified Medical Language System (UMLS).

Ontologies can be very useful but ontologies will not be the magic bullet that solves the interoperability issue until there is some common consensus on how to build them consistently. This does not necessarily mean that there needs to be an international standard developed to control how all ontologies are built, but rather a hope similar to that expressed by Uschold [7 p.3],

> A long range goal is to ... [have] a coherent framework which might be in the form of a handbook. Such a handbook should clearly characterise the dimensions of variation for ontologies and give guidelines for how to build any given ontology, matching the particular circumstances with appropriate methods. The main barrier to the production of such a coherent unified framework embracing all of these techniques and methods for building ontologies is that *there is no clear indication of how general the individual techniques and methods reported to date are.* Consequently, in a given set of circumstances, there are no guidelines for deciding what techniques and methods are likely to apply.

This statement by Uschold is perhaps even more relevant today than it was in 1996 given the explosion of ontology development and ontology engineering tools in recent years.

In the area of medical ontologies, the Institute for Formal Ontology and Medical Information Science (IFOMIS) researches and develops formal ontologies based on their own foundational, universal, Basic Formal Ontology (BFO). While the IFOMIS group has not yet published a universal ontology engineering methodology, their activities provide valuable and practical insights into good, if not best, ontology engineering practice.

With respect to health care records, a true shared electronic health record will remain little more than an idea unless a formal methodology, such as openEHR, is accepted and adopted globally by clinicians, vendors, and regulatory authorities.

12. Future directions

If health care is to be sustainable in an environment of rising costs and consumer demand, health care systems are going to have to become more efficient. One way of achieving efficiency is to make better use of the data, information, and knowledge that already exists within the system. Enabling the shared electronic health record is essential to promote sustainability in the sector and it is more likely to become a reality if there is a consistent approach to the modeling of clinical information. A formal ontological approach to clinical information and terminology modeling promises to provide the mechanism by which truly interoperable EHR can be built. The benefits of ontology based SEHR is that they will naturally enable decision support including intelligent decision support, information exchange, the provision of web services and improved knowledge governance. The ontological approach should also save time and money, as evidenced by the experience to date of *open*EHR archetypes, because formal, well-defined ontologies are extensible and reusable.

References

[1]   Noy   N,   Stanford   University   -   *Ontology   Mapping   and   Alignment   2005.*
        http://dit.unitn.it/~accord/RelatedWork/Matching/Noy-MappingAlignment-SSSW-05.pdf (cited May
        19, 2008).
[2]   Bittner, Thomas. 2005. Some comments on Granularity Scale & Collectivity by Rector & Rogers.
        Workshop presented at the *Workshop on Ontology and Biomedical Informatics,* Rome.
[3]   Milton, Nick. 2003. Knowledge Acquisition. *Epistemics.* http://www.epistemics.co.uk/Notes/63-0-
        0.htm cited 2 October 2008
[4]   Sebestik, Jan. 2007. *Bolzano's Logic.* Ed. Edward N. Zalta. 2007th ed. The Stanford Encyclopedia of
        Philosophy.
[5]   Madsen, Maria. 2006. A health information privacy ontology: toward decision support for compliance
        assessment, In Johanna Westbrook, Joanne Callen, George Margelis, James Warren (Eds) *HIC 2006
        Proceedings.*   Health   Informatics   Society   Australian   (HISA),   Melbourne.
        http://search.informit.com.au/documentSummary;dn=951939275357684;res=IELHSS
[6]   Garde, S, EJS Hovenga, J Gränz, S Foozonkhah, and S Heard. 2007. Managing archetypes for
        sustainable and semantically interoperable electronic health records. *electronic Journal of Health
        Informatics* 2, no. 2. www.ejhi.net
[7]   Uschold, M. 1996. *Building Ontologies: Towards a Unified Methodology.* Technical. Artificial
        Intelligence Applications Institute, University of Edinburgh, Scotland.
[8]   Gruber, T.R., 1995. Toward principles for the design of ontologies used for knowledge sharing.
        International Journal of Human-Computer Studies, 43(5/6), 907-928.

Review Questions

1. Is SNOMED CT a formal or informal ontology? Explain your answer.
2. What is semantic interoperability and how do formal ontologies improve it?
3. How does openEHR use ontological modeling to both design and manage archetypes?
4. Ontologies can be designed at various levels of granularity. What does this mean and how does it apply to the shared electronic health record?
5. Explain what is meant by terminology mapping and explain why this is sometimes necessary?

Health Informatics
E.J.S. Hovenga et al. (Eds.)
IOS Press, 2010
115
doi:10.3233/978-1-60750-476-4-115

10. Sustainable Clinical Knowledge Management: An Archetype Development Life Cycle

Maria MADSEN[1] BS, BSc(Hons), GDAC, MB(IS), MACS PhD[ab] Candidate, Heather
LESLIE MBBS, FRACGP, FACHI[c], Evelyn J S HOVENGA RN, PhD (UNSW),
FACHI, FACS[b], Sam HEARD , MBBS, FACHI[c]

[a] *School of Management and Information Systems, Central Queensland University,*
Rockhampton Qld, Australia
[b] *eHealth Education Pty Ltd, Melbourne, Australia*
[c] *Ocean Informatics Pty Ltd, Melbourne Australia*

Abstract. This chapter gives an educational overview of:
1. The significance of having a formal ontology of health care data.
2. How *open*EHR has used an ontological approach to designing an electronic health record.
3. The phases of archetype development and key steps in the process.
4. The openEHR architecture and integrated development environment.

Keywords. Medical Record Systems-Computerised, Systems Analysis, Systems Integration, Model, Software Design, Knowledge, Information Science, Terminology, Documentation, Archetypes, Clinical Domain Models, Ontology

Introduction

We have seen from the previous chapter, that the adoption of formal ontology engineering principles improves the consistency, extensibility, and interoperability of the knowledge models produced. A primary concern for the future of health care management and delivery is the mobilization and efficient utilization of health care data. Effective and efficient use of health care data depends on the development and adoption of a shared (or shareable) electronic health record (SEHR). From its inception, the *open*EHR Foundation approached the problem of health care data sharing and reuse as a logical information modeling problem. In the *Origins of openEHR,* Ingram [1] states that,

> So many systems describe themselves as electronic healthcare records and yet share little common concept of what such an entity is and what it is for. ... Confused and confusing arguments have persisted about esoteric models of ill-defined clinical terminology, processes and communications. Continuing reinvention of wheels at these levels of abstraction has inhibited progress.

---

[1] Corresponding author: m.madsen@ehealtheducation.net

The *open*EHR archetypes were the outcome of a long term systems development project. It was recognized that health records had a hierarchical structure with a record for each patient that would hold information in a series of compositions or documents generated from each health care event. In turn, entries for tests, treatments, and notes comprise the compositions – the unit of contributing clinical documentation to the record. This hierarchical structure is reflected in the design and implementation of the *open*EHR archetypes. But the archetypes are only part of the solution in as much as they provide a standard clinical content specification that can be used in any health care environment and context. A second part of the design problem was how to represent all of the different types of health care and personal data that make up the record. The ontological engineering approach taken by the *open*EHR foundation was to design a logical record architecture for a **universal, shareable electronic health record**, not a database.

A universal, shareable data model for the health care record is precisely the type of problem space with which applied ontology is concerned. We have seen already in the previous chapter that the key elements of a useful ontological design are semantic interoperability, extensibility, and re-usability. Furthermore we have learned that these characteristics are achieved by the process of concept abstraction according to formal ontology principles. Formal ontology is about modeling some section of reality, i.e. the universe of discourse or domain, using first order logic[2]. We have also seen that ontologies can be categorized according to their granularity and that the level of granularity is related to the distance the concepts are away from a particular reality.

There are at least three identifiable levels of ontology [2]. At the topmost level there are foundational ontologies that are universal and contain a few, highly abstract concepts that are applicable across *all* domains. The IFOMIS Base Formal Ontology is a foundational ontology [3]. In the middle there are core ontologies which are more granular than foundational ontologies, i.e. contain more concepts, and these concepts are applicable across a fairly broad domain, such as health care. At the bottom most level lie the domain specific ontologies which contain the most concepts and these concepts are highly localized and subject to change. One might create an ontology that has within it all three of these levels of granularity. Exactly what type of ontology is required is dependent upon the scope of the domain that is to be modeled.

In this chapter we explore in greater detail the way in which the *open*EHR Foundation adopted, and applied formal ontology engineering principles to the problem of the universal electronic health record. We begin with an overview of the knowledge domain and the *open*EHR approach. Next we consider a formal ontology engineering framework as it relates to the development approach used by *open*EHR. We then discuss the *open*EHR archetype development process, which evolved from the experiences of archetype developers, in the context of the traditional software development lifecycle. Finally, we see how *open*EHR proposes to manage and maintain the archetype repository.

---

[2] First order logic is a method of deductive reasoning using propositions and quantification that results in unambiguous statements about the universe of discourse.

1.   The knowledge domain and the knowledge of interest

There are many health related knowledge domains; many of these consist of various aspects from multiple knowledge domains. Each knowledge domain has a theoretical or philosophical foundation from which the relationships between the major concepts may be determined. This also guides the level of data granularity required to truly represent all concepts within the knowledge domain thus determining which terminologies or data sets or classifications are best suited for data communication purposes in whatever form. This concept is shown graphically in Figure 1.

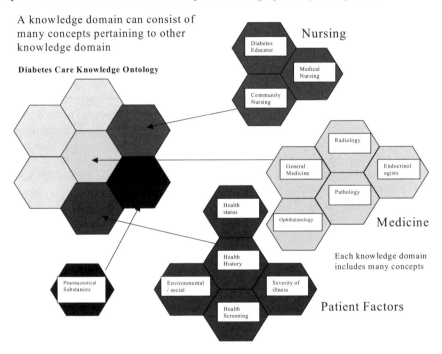

Figure 1 A Diagrammatic Representation of Relationships Between Various Medical Domains.

Kent [4] notes that 'ontology sharing facilitates interoperability between online knowledge organisations' and that 'ontology supplies the content, consisting of the entities, relations and constraints in the application domain'. He then goes on to demonstrate how ontology sharing is able to be formalised within the conceptual knowledge model of Information Flow, the logical design of distributed systems, as originally described by Barwise and Seligman in 1997 [5].

2.   The *open*EHR: Ontologically Engineered to be Flexible and Future Proof

It has been established that for e-health records to be an effective contributor to a sustainable health system and quality care we need to adopt a standard structure for such records. The Australian Good Electronic Health Record (GEHR) project first introduced the idea of the two-level model architecture. This work has been updated, further developed and brought under the auspice of the *open*EHR Foundation – a non-profit organization that holds the copyright and issues the 'open source' license for the *open*EHR specifications. The first level of the model consists of an invariant reference model and schema, and the second a variant model, consisting of clinical content models known as archetypes.

The separation of these two levels enables sustainable software and self adapting systems to be constructed. The adoption of ontological 'layering' progressively separates more specific and changeable concepts into modular layers allowing a division of what is hard wired into software and what is knowledge only available at runtime. Standards need to reflect these separations.

Archetypes need to be ontologically and semantically sound to enable their content to be reliably computer processed and thus enable semantic interoperability between systems to be realized. The archetype methodology has been incorporated as part of the basis of the European standard for EHR extracts [6]. As a result, archetypes, providing a relatively simple means to specifying clinical content, are increasing in popularity and uptake globally as a form of electronic clinical knowledge management; thus it is important to understand the archetype development life cycle.

In addition to archetypes structuring clinical content, every term in an archetype can be 'bound' to one or many terminologies, where appropriate, to facilitate accurate exchange of clinical data.   Archetype data elements can also be bound to terminology subsets of potential meaningful values.

The terminology of choice for many nations is SNOMED CT; issues arise in that not all clinical concepts can be represented in this terminology and this terminology has only been translated into a few languages. Hence there is a need to adopt terms from other terminologies where appropriate. There is a strong interdependency between vocabulary used in messages and the information model as expressed by the message structure used. For example the most commonly used vocabulary within HL7 messages are the LOINC codes. The LOINC[3] database is a no-cost database of over 35,000 names and codes that identify laboratory, clinical, and HIPAA attachment variables, maintained by the Regenstrief Institute.

Clinical content models require structured terminology to enhance interoperability – structured content alone is powerful but not enough to represent clinical information. Likewise, terminology alone cannot represent clinical content and shared EHRs. Beale & Heard [7] note that:

> "Archetypes and templates also act as a well-defined semantic gateway to terminologies, classifications and computerised clinical guidelines. The alternative in the past has been to try to make systems function solely with a combination of hard-wired software and terminology. This approach is flawed, since terminologies don't contain definitions of domain content (e.g. "microbiology result"), but rather facts about the real world (e.g. kinds of microbes and the effects of infection in humans)".

Many experts in the field believe that archetypes make comprehensive clinical terminologies workable as they are the missing link between the terminology and the application system that requires the definition of structured data. Terminology structure determines the ease with which practical and useful interfaces, for term navigation, entry, or retrieval can be supported [8]. Cimino [9] indicated that existing controlled medical terminologies are evolving from simple code-name-hierarchy arrangements

---

[3] For details refer http://loinc.org/

into rich knowledge based ontologies of medical concepts. Elkin, Brown and Chute [10] have provided a guideline with the principles needed to construct useful, maintainable controlled health vocabularies. More detail about health information concepts was covered in chapter 6.

2.1 The openEHR Archetype Ontology

As we stated above, the problem space for *open*EHR was to model health care data in such a way that it would be useful for the purposes of implementing a shared electronic health record. The domain for *open*EHR to consider was the shared electronic health record (SEHR). Since the SEHR domain is not universally applicable to *all* other domains it is not a foundational ontology. Neither is it a localized, domain-specific ontology because, for example, it was not to be a model of the SEHR for the Royal Brisbane Hospital. Thus, the *open*EHR ontology fits our definition, as presented in the previous chapter, of a **core ontology** of health care data. The *open*EHR ontological levels and the corresponding models are presented in Table 1.

Table 1 openEHRs' Ontological Levels in Health and Corresponding Models

*open*EHR Architecture Level	Ontological Level	Definition	*open*EHR Corresponding Model
Not within scope of *open*EHR core ontology	Level 4 – variant Local & use-specific	Use context-specific concepts eg. asthma note or ante-natal exam	Locally defined semantic templates where archetypes act as re-usable components and form a basis for defining re-usable screen elements.
Level Two Variant	Level 3 – variant Re-usable domain concepts	Atomic domain concepts eg lab result, patient, apgar score or BP measurement using data types that are subtypes of data_value to satisfy clinical needs. Eg coded text, quantity, ratio, multimedia	Archetypes bound to terminology/ontology defined in terms of domain base concept model concepts able to form the basis for querying and other semantically meaningful data processing.
Level One Invariant	Level 2 – invariant Domain concepts	Base ontological commitments of domain eg observation, subject of care, protocol	Domain Base Concept Model – the base ontology for archetypes (eg *open*EHR reference model and schema).
	Level 1 – data-sharing Persistence/ex change	Minimal ontological commitments – sufficient for recording and sharing eg composition, committer, attestation	Persistence information model that enables 100% bidirectional mapping to the domain base concept model and exchange information model.
	Level 0 – foundational	Object meta-model (objects, attributes etc) with built-in data types.	Object, attribute, string, Boolean, character, date, time

Source: Based on [11] Ontological Principles of Information Modeling for Future-Proof Systems v.12

There are two issues that need clarification with respect to Table 1 above. First, it should be noted that in Table 1, the foundational level is stated to be the *object meta-model*. In this case the objects[4] referred to are high-level categories of data, i.e. classes of data relevant to health care. The foundational level in the *open*EHR model is not

---

[4] These are not analogous to objects as found in object-oriented modeling.

foundational for a universal ontology. Rather, the *open*EHR designers viewed the foundation of the shared electronic health record problem as the universe of computer programming. Thus the foundational ontology is comprised of basic, universally accepted computer and mathematical concepts, such as *object* and *integer* respectively. Theoretically, one could merge this *open*EHR ontology with a truly foundational ontology such as the IFOMIS BFO without too many problems[5]. Secondly, it should be noted that Level 4concepts as they appear in Table 1 are expressed in the *open*EHR development environment as templates. While templates are indeed part of the development and implementation environment of *open*EHR, the detail captured in a template is localized and highly specific for local concepts. From an ontological perspective this level of detail is not within the scope of the *open*EHR core ontology. The concept of the *open*EHR 'template' is part of the *open*EHR ontology, but the detail captured by a particular instance of a template is not. Thus anyone contemplating developing archetypes or templates must be aware that the *open*EHR ontology and tools provide a consistent, interoperable platform but it does not ensure that you will include the correct detail in your template. It is up to the developer to make sure that they have analysed their needs fully before embarking on the development process. The following section provides a stepwise explanation of the development methodology recommended by *open*EHR..

3. An Ontology Development Methodology and the *open*EHR Approach

It is unlikely that the contributors to the *open*EHR project intentionally followed any particular ontology engineering methodology since none exists. Rather they have followed a well planned and careful information modeling process using ontological modeling as the most appropriate method for their task. None-the-less we can see that the process that was followed and the methods that were used resulted in outputs that are remarkably consistent with the outputs one might expect from a systematic and iterative ontology engineering process such as that proposed by Little [12]. Table 2 is based on Little's six step process [12 [p.4]] that form a basic methodology framework albeit devoid of method.

The success of *open*EHR thus far demonstrates the usefulness of formal ontological principles when applied to the shared electronic health record. The developers of the *open*EHR specifications have applied formal ontology principles throughout the project. This has resulted in a modularized and integrated architecture comprised of a set of well defined, integrated, artefacts that contribute to the overall robustness and flexibility of the *open*EHR approach.

3.1 openEHR Ontological Structure

The highest level information model includes a class identified as 'versioned_composition' where compositions are defined as "the containers of all

---

[5] IFOMIS has tested the HL7 RIM against the BFO (Vizenor, Smith , and Ceusters 2004). The HL7 RIM was shown to suffer from a number of internal inconsistencies. To be fair, however, the HL7 RIM is an object model not an ontological model and one could not sensibly expect it to merge neatly with a formal foundational ontology such as the BFO.

clinical and administrative content of the record". This is where the main EHR data are located [13]. Each Composition consists of Entries organised by Sections within the Composition. Each Entry consists of its own ontology of clinical information as described by Beale and Heard [14 p.762]. This formed the basis for their Clinical Investigator Record ontology (Figure 2) that provides the basis for the Entry classes in the *open*EHR reference model. This model has proven to be semantically robust and a successful basis for defining clinical content models (archetypes).

Table 2 Little's Ontology Engineering Process (LOEP) Showing Respective openEHR Components.

LOEP steps	LOEP outputs	*open*EHR component
1. Develop a sufficiently large and representative lexicon of terms [for the knowledge domain]	1) a shared lexicon of terms which both denote and connote the wide range of items (physical and non-physical) within a given domain	GEHR project Analysis of existing terminologies, standards, and health care databases
2. Develop a set of metaphysically-grounded upper-level (abstract) categories.	2) A formal structure capable of capturing the relations between those lexical items;	Archetype definition language Reference model terminology Archetype internal terminology
3. Develop a sufficiently large set of region-specific (lower-level) categories.	3) a methodology for checking the consistency and comprehensiveness of those lexical/categorical items;	Binding to external terminologies as needed
4. Diagram formal relations between terms/categories.	4) a sufficiently complex artificial system capable of querying information within a given domain and inferring new (and possibly more complex) relations within that domain.	Archetype Object Model Template Object Model
5.Develop/find a computational framework capable of capturing all items in 4.	Not specified by Little	*open*EHR Architecture Service Model (SM)
6. Develop methodologies for evaluating the ontology.	Not specified by Little	Open source – feedback from users Ongoing collaboration with recognized standards organizations Governance policies, procedures, and mechanisms

The CIR ontology then becomes the basis for any clinical domain ontology focusing on those aspects that significantly vary from these generic ontological attributes. For example a history consisting of observations and actions is a necessary part of any EHR. As a consequence a standard set of archetypes are needed to enable such data to be collected, computer processed and retrieved. Generic archetypes can be developed to capture common clinical concepts such as diagnosis or symptom. However each clinical specialty is expected to have its own additional set of data requirements pertaining to that specific ontological domain. In order to extend the generic CIR ontology to any specialist domain, either standard archetypes need to be modified or new archetypes need to be developed to reflect the specific data needs of the new domain, as described in the following sections of the Archetype Development Process.

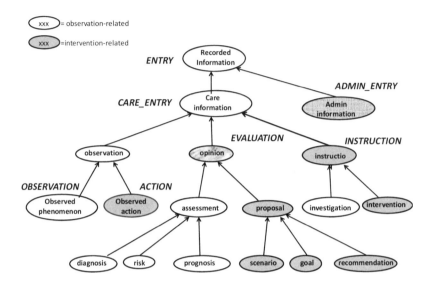

Figure 2 The Clinical Investigator Record (CIR) Ontology

Archetypes are ideally designed as maximal datasets for a universal use case, when interoperability is the goal. Good design will ensure that each archetype can capture all of the data for a given clinical concept no matter what the use-case, specialist domain or health professional's role – even including consumer self-recording. The *open*EHR Clinical Knowledge Manager is an international repository of archetypes, which supports the authoring, review and publishing process of archetypes. It has designed according to the ontology structure as presented in Fig 2 as well as enabling ontology-based searching via clinical specialties, clinical purpose, health professional roles and available language translations.[6]

4.   *open*EHR Archetype Development Life Cycle

The *open*EHR methodology has specifically been designed for clinicians to create the archetypes that capture their clinical recording requirements and workflow – effectively shaping their own EHR systems. It is also true that these clinical models need to capture the relevant elements of the softer side of medicine, sometimes known as 'the art of clinical practice', that is directly relevant to patient care. Medicine is not an exact science that can be distilled into a spreadsheet or managed purely by a terminology, but archetypes can provide context for data that support the clinical decision making process. The models need to be designed with a balance between formally structured clinical content that will be computable and critical for inferencing, with an allowance for an amount of free text to enable clinicians to capture the nuances and subtleties of their interaction with a patient that cannot be structured. In truth, modeling to maximise re-use and interoperability probably requires some expert informatics background knowledge, but should not deter interested clinicians from

---

[6] *open*EHR Clinical Knowledge Manager available at http://www.openehr.org/knowledge

participating; if not involved in design, certainly they are absolutely critical to the review and publication of agreed and approved sets of archetypes. Rigorous design and governance of archetypes are required to support and facilitate sharing of archetypes and semantic interoperability.

Archetypes as representations of clinical data require Clinicians as the knowledge experts to be at the core of design and publication. However other expert input is essential for appropriate and useful archetype development and may include any or all input from terminology, technical modeling, messaging and/or user interface expertise. The primary aim of an EHR is to support the provision of quality patient care, and so archetypes need to:

- Accurately reflect the needs and requirements of high quality, hands-on, clinical care delivery;
- Leverage existing best-practice guidelines and work processes;
- Complement and leverage the value provided by terminology and data models in use;
- Are modeled in a strategic, measured and consistent manner;
- Provide context for data that support the clinical decision making process
- Maximise the potential re-use of the model output; and
- Maximise potential for interoperability.

Complex clinical content such as an antenatal visit can be broken up into smaller chunks where each component clinical concept is modeled separately, for example, measuring fetal heart rate, blood pressure and an order for an ultrasound. The whole concept then needs to be represented by the drawing together each of these component archetypes into a single template that represents the antenatal visit as a whole. It is not uncommon for a clinical encounter to be composed of 50-100 separate archetypes.

Creation of templates does not require the same rigorous design that is needed for the archetype. Templates are aggregations of archetypes that are for a specific use-case, domain, location or specialty. As stated previously, each archetype should comprise a maximal data set. This will assist in minimising the overlap between archetypes and simplify archetype governance. In an ideal world, all archetypes are governed globally via an international repository of authorised and standardised archetypes. In reality, there will be many options, but the initial instance of the *open*EHR Clinical Knowledge Manager will be a keystone in supporting additional levels of governance to occur in repositories at the national- or enterprise- levels. These repositories can draw archetypes from the international sets, create their own to meet local data needs and potentially contribute these back to the international repository. It is common sense that the greater the number of archetypes that can be shared ubiquitously, then the greater the potential for health information system interoperability. A template library is also planned as a feature of the international *open*EHR Clinical Knowledge Manager. Templates do not require the same design or governance rigour as archetypes and can be modified to suit specific purposes without compromising system interoperability.

Prior to commencing the actual archetype development process it is necessary to:

- undertake an initial data analysis,
- develop a modeling process plan,
- engage with end-user clinicians to ensure a sound understanding of their information requirements and also to

- consider potential screen layout, workflow, terminology use, clinical decision support querying requirements, GUI design, software application design, terminology and technical standards implications.

Model development needs to be co-ordinated with clinical end-users, technical and terminology experts as well as with vendors and a governing authority.

4.1 Proposed Archetype Development Process

Through the ongoing work of *open*EHR contributors and pioneering clinicians from around the world many archetypes have already been developed. This experience has enabled the *open*EHR group to begin to define a working methodology for the archetype development process as shown in Figure 3.

We have fitted the *open*EHR development process to the stages of the traditional software development life cycle (SDLC). This results in the following iterative process which might be described as the 'ideal' archetype development life cycle (ADLC).

4.1.1 Planning Phase

Content gathering
- ° Initial gathering of paper-based forms used in clinical practice can be performed by any clinician or administrative support personnel working within the clinical domain being modeled.
- ° Content should come from as many sources as possible to support the premise of 'a maximal data set for a universal use-case'. Rather than starting from scratch, content should be sourced from relevant existing content in all formats and styles, clinical practice guidelines and recommendations from authoritative bodies and national programs, current EHR applications and clinical tools, national/international bodies of excellence, data dictionaries, journals/text books, and the internet.
- ° Content format will vary and should – include existing paper content and electronic representations of paper forms, electronic spreadsheets and databases,
- ° Direct content gathering engagement with clinicians is ideally facilitated by a Health Informatician, bridging the gap between grassroots clinicians and the technicians. Content gathering in isolation from the archetype development requirements process will not result in archetypes that are fit for purpose. Content should be gathered in the context of how that content will be applied in a clinical application, how terminology might be leveraged, understanding clinical workflow, how decision support might be utilised and how the models might interact with the graphical user interface design.
- ° External parties who are engaged in gathering and distilling content from end-users should have basic training in *open*EHR methodology, including archetypes and templates, to optimise the content gathering process.

Clinician engagement
- ° At least one of the modelers, preferably a health informatician, should lead and coordinate direct liaison with the clinicians/experts to ensure that the archetype and template models under development are in alignment with the clinical user requirements.

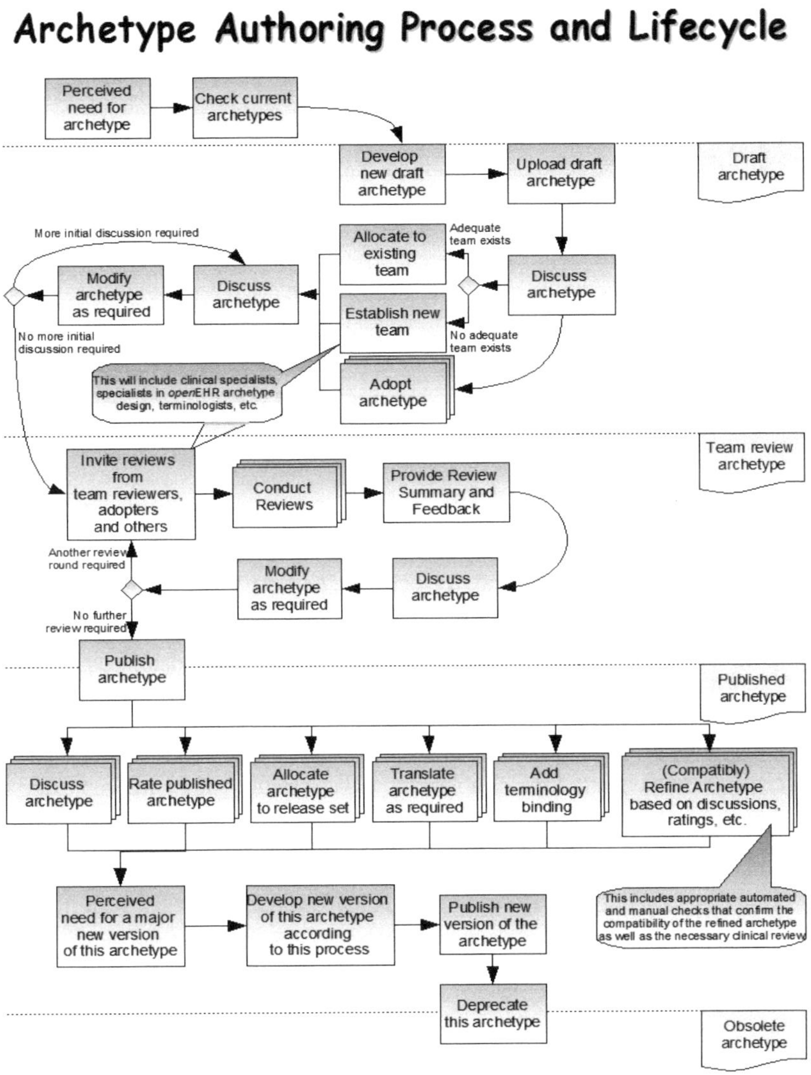

Archetype Authoring Process and Lifecycle

Figure 3 Archetype Authoring Process and Life Cycle [15]

4.1.2 Analysis Phase

Data analysis and consolidation

  ○   Content analysis should ideally be led by a health informatician, identifying
       potential gaps and directly engaging with the clinician/experts to ensure that the
       material provided to the clinical modelers for archetype authoring is accurate,
       correct and appropriate for modeling.

○   Ideally, analysis is also needed to review current workflow processes, for example, identifying that a current paper-based or manual process may need to be reviewed or enhanced as part of the transformation to a computer-based activity within an EHR.

○   The domain knowledge and skills of the archetype modelers should influence the ideal format and method of final content delivery to modelers. There is some danger of content loss or creation of potential misunderstandings when the clinical information is 'distilled' or transformed eg from a variety of sources into a single spreadsheet – in many ways analogous to the gradual loss of information integrity exchanged in the childhood game, 'Chinese Whispers'.

•   Clinician modelers can be more adaptive to a variety of formats and also be able to identify potential content gaps and fill them as required.

•   If the modeler has little or no clinical knowledge, the analysis must present the content in such a way that requires no interpretation.

Draft modeling estimate

○   In an ideal modeling scenario, once the scope of a project has been suggested, there is a need for experienced clinical modelers to conduct a review of existing archetypes in order to:

  •   determine where content is already developed,
  •   define where modifications to archetypes need to be made, and
  •   decide where new archetypes need to be created.

Knowledge of the current available archetypes or access to an index of archetypes and their attributes will assist with possible existing archetype identification.

○   Identification of the number, type and complexity of the archetypes that need to be modified and created must be estimated, plus identify any gaps in knowledge or other problems that need to be referred back to the client or to content domain experts. The Clinical Knowledge Manager repository will perform a key function here.

○   Modifications to good quality and thoughtfully designed archetypes can be relatively simple and straightforward (thereby creating a new revision which is backwardly compatible), although if archetypes have not been well designed in the initial development or content requirements are radically different, modifications may require major changes require a new version of the archetype (which is not backwardly compatible). Revisions have a significantly smaller flow-on effect to models that have been implemented in systems, in comparison to the creation of new versions of archetypes, and so creating a model such that it is relatively easy to update an archetype by revising should be encouraged for efficiency and maximising Return On Investment (ROI).

4.1.3 Requirements Specification Phase

Collaborative requirements meetings – these can be electronic or face-to-face and should ideally include health informaticians, clinical modelers, technical modelers, user interface experts, vendors and terminologists – to determine issues around content related to each expert area.

○   Quality clinical models require input from a number of domain experts – the common four will consist of health informaticians, terminologists, vendors and technical modelers. User interface input could also be considered as a participant at this point in archetype development. The end model will benefit from collaborative input through the development process. This input should start early, and include specifying the information that is required from end-users that is necessary for each domain.

° Terminology plays a key role within archetypes and templates, and the availability of suitable codes within a terminology can have significant impact on the archetype development. Content that requires structured values will utilise terminology subsets where available or may have to be modeled explicitly within the archetype as an internal code set. Ongoing discussion and research continues around the optimal approach to modeling the 'grey zone' - the name given to that area of overlap between structured content that should clearly be archetyped and the other end of the spectrum in which the content should unambiguously be bound to terminology.

° Early discussion with vendors to determine application requirements should be a strategic part of model planning - this usually impacts at a template design level rather than impact directly on archetype design.

° Further collaborative meetings should occur progressively through model development, in proportion to the complexity of the clinical concept being modeled.

Clarify content questions and other issues with end-users

° At least one of the modelers should have direct and consistent engagement/liaison with the clinicians/experts so as to ensure models under development are in alignment with the clinical user requirements.

° Modelers and the clinical users should have direct interactions during both the data analysis phase and iteratively during the modeling process.

Create a modeling plan

° An estimate of the potential modeling workload largely needs to be based on an analysis of the numbers of archetypes that can be re-used, those requiring modification and new archetype creation in order to create the final templates to encompass the agreed project scope.

4.1.4   Design Phase (Archetype Design)

Create clinical models

° Creation of the clinical models should be driven primarily by the clinicians. The structure and language of the models should reflect the primary purpose of the clinical content i.e. capture, display and querying of clinical information in delivering clinical care to a patient.

° Terminology, user interface requirements and technical modeling expertise should be closely aligned and support and shape the way that the clinical content is modeled.

Add Terminology

° Terminology subsets can largely be determined in parallel with model development.

- ° Single codes from one or many terminologies can be bound to any data node, internal code or event in an archetype where these can be universally agreed.
- ° Terminology subsets will usually be bound in templates on a use-case basis. They should only be bound to archetypes where they will be universally applicable, and to date there are few examples of this.
- ° Multiple subsets for multiple terminologies can be bound to any single node in a template.

4.1.5 Testing, Evaluation, Review Phase

Content and terminology review iterations
- ° Clinician end-users and archetype reviewers should receive introductory training on *open*EHR modeling. A sufficient overview of *open*EHR and archetypes and templates can be delivered in a one hour session, and will equip the reviewers to give informed and meaningful feedback at content review.
- ° Review of the terminology subset should be included in the context of the complete clinical model review. It is only when the subsets can be viewed that a clinician user or reviewer can see if all content is captured adequately and correctly.
- ° Iterative content reviews should continue until the users and reviewers can approve that the content has been captured comprehensively and in correct context.

Modeling Review
- ° Despite modeling guidelines, best practice advice and examples, it is inevitable that there will still be potential variation in the style and structure of the models created by different modelers. It is worth taking time for the team to review the models that have been created to ensure that they have a consistent approach – this includes structure; phrases; consistent descriptions, use and misuse; use of keywords; linking between archetypes; and binding to terminology – all of which will improve the potential for the models to have a cohesive and consistent style, and maximal usability. Submission of the archetype to the Clinical Knowledge Manager will ensure that the model undergoes a review ensures alignment with consistent archetype modeling methodology.
- ° There may also a need to make sure that the models are aligned with other modeling work. Once the clinical information is captured, refined and modeled, the technical modelers can provide feedback regarding alignment with parallel work that is progressing in other modeling work, for example HL7.

4.1.6 Delivery Phase

Model signoff - As soon as there is approval from each of :
- ° Users and reviewers regarding the clinical content, including terminology binding, and
- ° Technical model alignment
- ° then the draft models can be signed off and formally 'published' for public availability.

Handover to vendor

○   Vendors will be able to directly access clinical models from a central repository of published and approved archetypes and templates.

○   Health informatician involvement may facilitate handover to the technicians implementing the models in the vendor application.

4.1.7 Maintenance Phase

Governance of archetypes used in a given project needs to be established to ensure the management of authoring and versioning processes. These archetypes can be kept at a local level, or can be promoted for use on a wider level but pushing to a national or international repository.

Governance through the ontology-based openEHR Clinical Knowledge Manager repository has commenced in Q3 of 2008.

5.   The *open*EHR Integrated Development Environment (IDE)

In order to support the vision of "flexible and future proof electronic health records", *open*EHR has also developed and made available the tools required for archetype development. The toolset as listed at the *open*EHR web site[7] at the time of writing includes:

- **Archetype Editor**: a tool to author archetypes
  - ○ The Ocean Archetype Editor (Ocean Informatics - open source, .Net platform)
  - ○ The Linkoping Archetype Editor (Linkoping University - open source, Java)
- **Template Designer**: a tool to create templates based on archetypes
- **The Ocean Template Designer** (Ocean Informatics - .Net platform)
- **openEHR Clinical Knowledge Manager:** a web-based shared knowledge management environment for archetypes and templates based on an OWL[8] ontology (Ocean Informatics – licensed to the openEHR Foundation for public use)
- **Archetype Workbench:** a tool to test and maintain the correctness of a set of archetypes and their relationships (Ocean Informatics – open source).

In addition to this toolset the *open*EHR Foundation provides interested users with all of the specifications and relevant supporting material required under an open source licensing agreement.

The most recent tool included in the *open*EHR IDE is the Clinical Knowledge Manager (CKM)[9]. The CKM enables:

- Searching for existing archetypes for re-use or modification.
- New archetypes to be submitted for *open*EHR community review

---

[7] www.openEHR.org

[8] OWL – Web Ontology Language (see http://www.w3c.org)

[9] http://openehr.org/knowledge/

- Archetypes in draft and published states to be downloaded and used by any registered users.
- Volunteer teams of editors and reviewers to participate in the revision and publication phases
- Administrators to form release sets of archetypes comprising known versions and revisions.

The Archetype Editorial Group has oversight to the team reviews within CKM. Ultimate governance of *open*EHR archetypes within CKM are under the jurisdiction of the *open*EHR Clinical Review Board.

Fig. 4 shows the Search screen of the CKM for the example of searching for existing blood_pressure archetypes. Fig. 5 shows a Mind Map view of the blood pressure archetype.

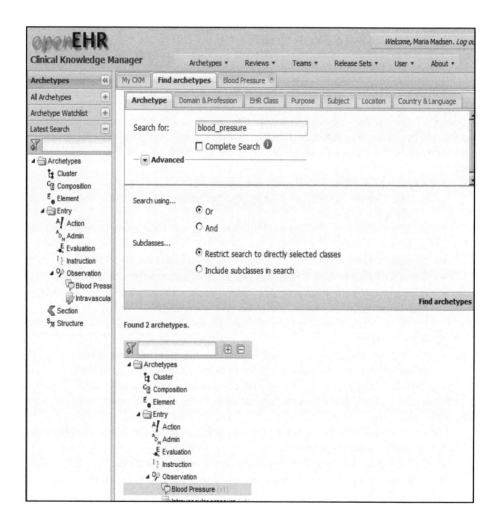

Figure 4 openEHR CKM Search Interface (Source: openEHR 2008)

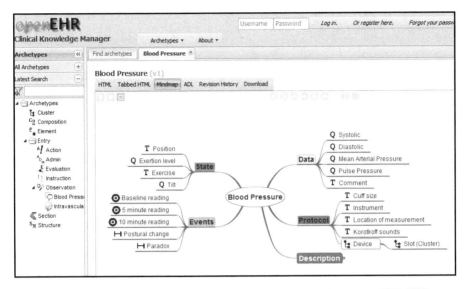

Figure 5 openEHR CKM Mind Map of Blood Pressure Archetype (Source: openEHR 2008)

6. Conclusion

This chapter has argued that having a formal ontology of health care data is a significant contribution to the ability to have information systems that have the potential to be fully semantically interoperable so that the full benefits of available technologies may be realized via the adoption of the *open*EHR architecture and an integrated development environment. The *open*EHR foundation has used an ontological approach to designing an electronic health record, this was explained in some detail. However the use of ontology represents only part of the solution, there is also a need for systems to be compliant with the right set of technical standards. That is the topic of the next chapter. Adoption of the many steps detailed as being part of the archetype development life cycle enables clinicians and others to become involved in archetype development.

References

[1]   Ingram, David. 2002. *The Origins of openEHR* - openEHR :: future proof and flexible EHR specifications. *openEHR*. http://www.openehr.org/about/origins.html#dsy20-OE_openehr .
[2]   Gangemi, A, F Fisseha, J Keizer, I Pettman, and M Taconet. 2004. A Core Ontology of Fishery and its use in the Fishery Ontology Service Project. *First International workshop on core ontologies. EKAW Conference CEUR-WS* 118.
[3]   IFOMIS. 2008. Institute for Formal Ontology and Medical Information Science (IFOMIS). *Institute for Formal Ontology and Medical Information Science*. http://www.ifomis.uni-saarland.de/ .
[4]   Kent, RE 2000, The information flow foundation for conceptual knowledge organisation, in *Proceedings of the 6th International Conference of the International Society for Knowledge Organisation (ISKO)*, Toronto, Canada.
[5]   Barwise, K, J. & Seligman, J. (1997) *Information Flow: the Logic of Distributed Systems* Cambridge, University Press

[6]   ISO/FDIS 13606-2: 2008 *Health Informatics: Electronic Health Record Communication* - Part 2 Archetype interchange specification.
[7]   Beale T, Heard S. *open*EHR Release 1.0: *Archetype Definitions and Principles.* 2006. Available from:
      http://svn.openehr.org/specification/TRUNK/publishing/architecture/am/archetype_principles.pdf
[8]   Elkin PL, Tuttle MS, Keck K, Campbell K, Atkin G, Chute CG. The role of compositionality in standardized problem list generation. In: Cesnik B et al., editors. *Proceedings of MEDINFO 98, 1998.* p. 660-664.
[9]   Cimino JJ. Terminology tools: state of the art and practical lessons. *Methods Inf Med 2001; 40 (4):* 298-306.
[10] Elkin, Brown and Chute, Guideline for Health Informatics: Controlled Health Vocabularies - Vocabulary Structure and High-level Indicators In: Vimla L. Patel, Ray Rogers and Reinhold Haux (Eds) *MEDINFO 2001 Proceedings of the 10th World Congress on Medical Informatics*, IOS Press, Amsterdam
[11] Beale T (with contributions from Lloyd D, Heard S, Kalra D), Ontological Principles of Information Modeling for Future Proof Systems v.12. *Presentation at the CEN TC251 meeting May 2005*, Berlin.
12]   Little, E. 2003. A proposed methodology for the development of application-based formal ontologies. In , 94: *Deutsche Bibliothek.* http://ftp.informatik.rwth-aachen.de/Publications/CEUR-WS/Vol-94/ki03rao_little.pdf.
[13] Beale T, Heard S, Kalra D, Lloyd D (Eds) *open*EHR *Reference Model Release 1.01 EHR Information Model* 2007 p.22 http://www.openehr.org/releases/1.0.1/architecture/rm/ehr_im.pdf
[14] Beale T, Heard S, An ontology-based Model of Clinical Information In: Kuhn K, Warren J.R, Leong TY (Eds) *Medinfo 2007 Proceedings of the 12th World Congress on Health (Medical) Informatics.* IOS Press, Amsterdam.
[15] *open*EHR. 2008. openEHR Clinical Knowledge Manager viewed November 2009. http://okm.oceaninformatics.com:8080/okm/ .

Review Questions

1. What factors differentiate the *open*EHR approach to problem of the shared electronic health record from previous approaches?
2. What is meant by the two-level model architecture in relation to the *open*EHR?
3. Explain how data concepts can belong to more than one knowledge domain?
4. Explain how the *open*EHR archetype ontology fits the definition of a core domain ontology.
5. Describe the Clinical Knowledge Manager in terms of its function in the governance of the archetype repository and as an OWL-based ontology.
6. Ideally archetypes are designed and used by whom?

Health Informatics
E.J.S. Hovenga et al. (Eds.)
IOS Press, 2010
doi:10.3233/978-1-60750-476-4-133

11. National Standards in Health Informatics

Evelyn J S HOVENGA, RN, PhD (UNSW), FACHI, FACS

Director, eHealth Education, Consultant, openEHR Foundation, and Honorary Senior Research Associate, Centre for Health Informatics & Multiprofessional Education, University College London, Honorary Academic Fellow, Austin Health, Melbourne, Adjunct Professor, Central Queensland University Rockhampton, Queensland, and Victoria University, Melbourne, Australia

Abstract. This chapter gives an educational overview of:
- The relationship between standards and a national e-health strategy
- National and international standards development processes
- The Development of a national HI standards roadmap
- The benefits of standards adoption

Keywords. Health Care Systems, Standards, Medical Informatics, Health, Medical Record Systems-Computerised, Software Design, Computer Communication Networks, Systems Integration, Information Systems, Interoperability

Introduction

Chapters 3 and 4 have essentially provided an overview of national health care business drivers shaping any national e-health strategy and associated implementation priorities. One common driver is the desire to implement personal or patient centred e-health records and systems. There is a general acceptance that the development and adoption of suitable technical standards is key to realising this objective. For example national standards development organisations work closely with their Governments who have adopted an e-health implementation strategy, to develop standards based on Government priorities enabling them to meet their strategic needs. The European Union's e-health action plan [1] identifies practical steps to achieve their vision to address common challenges via a common approach including legislation and standards to achieve interoperability enabling e-health to improve health and healthcare through the use of information and communications technologies (ICT) by 2010.

1. Why Are Standards Important?

Meeting system connectivity and interoperability requirements to enable systems to communicate effectively and efficiently with each other requires the adoption of technical standards. In particular standards are needed to facilitate interoperability between clinical information systems within and between healthcare organisations. This enables the exchange and aggregation of clinical (point of care) information documented by several health care providers' within any number of clinical information systems for each patient treated. Most if not all national e-health strategies aim to support the widespread adoption of electronic health records (EHRs) requiring data input from any number of different providers each using their own systems, so system connectivity and interoperability is a key requirement. Electronic patient records pertaining to each episode of health care may also be used to ultimately produce an electronic health record containing all health related information from birth to death for all individuals. Such records are particularly valuable for patients with chronic health related conditions. By now you should have a fairly good picture of what EHRs are likely to look like and the functions they are expected to provide to benefit the many potential users.

Another fundamental purpose of standards is to facilitate the aggregation of clinical information by patient type for secondary purposes such as practice evaluation, outcome, information and decision support systems, evaluation, quality and safety, benchmarking, monitoring, health policy development, resource management and more. The standard data elements available to be extracted from EHRs, as well as system architectures and database design adopted determine how well these systems can be used for the purpose of knowledge discovery.

The health industry is still dealing with a situation where information systems only partially serve user needs and where the needs of collaborating populations of users are not served well at all. Achieving national health system interoperability requires the adoption of a number of health informatics standards. Such standards need to be governed and managed by a national entity to ensure national consistency and in many instances international consistency is highly desirable. A national standards framework needs to be tailored to meet transitional requirements based on current systems and technology infrastructure to maximise existing system functionality as well as prepare for a future vision.

First we'll define system interoperability, as this is the concept that the adoption of standards needs to achieve. This will be followed by a description of standards development entities and processes. Finally an analysis of the types of standards within a national health informatics infrastructure required to enable the realisation of the national health business needs and a national e-health vision is presented. Many standards have already been developed, many are currently under review and being updated, others are to be developed. It isn't possible to even mention all of these here so the focus throughout is on standards that relate directly or indirectly to electronic health records as these are viewed as being fundamental to our ability to optimally realize the benefits that may be gained from the use of the best available information and communication technologies.

2.   What is System Interoperability?

Interoperability from a software engineering perspective was presented in Chapter 5. It was noted that the IEEE interoperability definition only mentioned data and information transfer and that knowledge transfer was outside the scope of mainstream interoperability solutions but that this is an area of active research. A lot of progress has been made in this regard as detailed in the previous chapters. Here we focus on interoperability relative to meeting health business needs and build on previous chapters regarding reliable semantic knowledge exchange to achieve semantic interoperability using the *open*EHR two level software engineering approach.

The Australian Government Interoperability Framework has three parts, the Information Interoperability Framework, the Technical Interoperability Framework; and the Business Process Interoperability Framework as represented in the Figure 1. This fits with the IEEE definition.

Interoperability Definition
The ability to transfer and use information in a uniform and efficient manner across multiple organizations and information technology systems.

Interoperability Focus Area		
Business Process Interoperability Framework Supporting the path from process awareness to standardised processes to interoperable processes to enhanced networked capability, depending on agencies' need.	**Information Interoperability Framework** Plan to share information principles for the management of government information Authoritative data sources, Protocols for shared/re-use of information across public and private sector. Legal policy and administrative requirements. Information lifecycle management	**Technical Interoperability Framework** Harmonisation of standards for transport, messaging, description, discovery and security.

Figure 1 - The Australian Government Information Interoperability Framework [2]

The complexity of system interoperability becomes evident when we examine the literature to identify a clear meaning. There is no consensus about defining interoperability. That is probably a direct result of an overall poor understanding of this concept. There are also a variety of views about the degree of interoperability required. For example HL7 have developed an Interoperability Model that establishes an industry consensus view of "What is EHR Interoperability?" based on extensive research about this concept definition and usage. It provides a reference list of characteristics of (and requirements for) interoperable EHRs. The EHR Interoperability Model (EHR/IM) conformance criteria permit EHR records to be validated (vis-à-vis the interoperability characteristics) at points of EHR record origination, transmission and receipt. This EHR/IM forms the basis for the US EHR certification as discussed in chapter 4. According to the HL7 website the EHR/IM is a draft standard for trial usage and may be profiled to meet the specific needs of care settings, regions, implementations and uses. Many argue that the use of messages alone cannot create records. Compliance with this draft standard only enables technical system communication using syntactical messages in accordance with the IEEE definition.

Walker et al [3] and Elkin et al [4] have described interoperability for the health industry in a manner that assists the reader in understanding this concept more comprehensively. One used a taxonomy as the basis for assessing the value of interoperability, the other developed an ontology to describe this domain. Both demonstrate agreement that there are different levels or degrees of interoperability determining functionality. Walker et al [3] described a four level functional taxonomy of interoperability reflecting the amount of human involvement required, the sophistication of IT, and the level of required standardization to form the basis, to assess the value of electronic health care information exchange and interoperability, as shown in Table 1

Table 1: Four Level Functional Taxonomy of Interoperability [3]

Level 1	Non electronic data – no use of IT to share information (examples: mail, telephone)
Level 2	Machine-transportable data – transmission of non-standardized information via basic IT; information within the document cannot be electronically manipulated. Examples: fax or Personal Computer (PC), based exchange of scanned documents, pictures, or Portable Document Format (PDF) files
Level 3	Machine-organisable data – transmission of structured messages containing non-standardized data; requires interfaces that can translate incoming data from the sending organization's vocabulary to the receiving organization's vocabulary; usually results in imperfect translations because of vocabularies' incompatible levels of detail. Examples: e-mail of free text, or PC-based exchange of files in incompatible/proprietary file formats, HL7 messages
Level 4	Machine-interpretable data – transmission of structured messages containing standardized and coded data; idealized state in which all systems exchange information using the same formats and vocabularies. Examples: automated exchange of coded results from an external lab into a provider's Electronic Medical Record (EMR), automated exchange of a patient's "problem list".

There is another way to differentiate between levels and degrees of interoperability. Elkin and his colleagues explain three levels, syntactic, semantic and pragmatic. These three levels of interoperability were described as follows:

"Syntactic Interoperability deals with interoperable structures. Semantic Interoperability deals with the interoperability of a common shared meaning. Pragmatic Interoperability deals with the external constraints on the system. This last category takes into account the level of granularity needed for common understanding and the complexity or difficulty required to achieve a certain level of interoperability" [4 p.725].

These three levels formed the foundation of the development of an ontology of interoperability. Each level was assessed as supporting specific application needs and is described in terms of functionality resulting in various degrees of interoperability within each of these levels. Each of the three levels was analysed into a series of system application requirements that may be met thus further scaling the degrees of interoperability. Syntactic interoperability suits those software applications dependent only on interoperable structure, whereas semantic interoperability is essential for those applications that are dependent upon the ability to process "common shared meanings" via the adoption of data standards or a standard health language. This ontology was then used as evaluation criteria for any existing HL7 compliant system to assess compliance. None of the systems evaluated were able to meet the highest semantic interoperability level.

This difference between the syntactic and semantic levels may be described in terms of the connectivity provided by the Internet versus that provided by the World Wide Web. The Internet transfers packets of information from one computer to another anywhere in the world (structure) but the world wide web is about identifying content, documents, sounds, videos etc. via programs that communicate between computers connected via the Internet using Hypertext Markup Language (HTML) (common shared meanings) mostly accessible to anyone including search engines such as Google [5 p.60] although this is not true semantic interoperability; it is getting closer through the use of synonyms, homonyms etc. but remains incomplete and insufficient in semantic terms.

Within the health industry we find that many existing clinical applications are able to send or receive messages from another using a standard format (structure) as defined by standard HL7 messages. They may also incorporate a standard terminology to define common clinical concepts that are incorporated within those messages but this still best equates to syntactic interoperability. Six degrees of interoperability were identified within the syntactic interoperability level and described ranging from "simple headings" to "fixed and formatted hierarchically organized fields with possible structural links" indicating non-hierarchical relationships between concepts [4 p.728].

Semantic interoperability is required for the reliable transfer of clinical data as this is where the meaning of the data must be retained to validly enable the transferred data to be processed by the computer and used for decision support systems as explained in previous chapters. Eleven degrees of interoperability were identified and described for this level ranging from "free text transfer" to the ability to transfer a formal representation of knowledge using higher order logics which can fully support context described as a "model based knowledge representation coordinated semantically nationally standard detailed coding system allowing post-coordination with support for context" [4]. Chapter 7 described these concepts in some detail. Walker's interoperability level 4 does not meet the most optimum degree of semantic interoperability as described by Elkin et al [4] whose ontology is more comprehensive but both agreed that semantic interoperability must be achieved to realise the greatest benefits from an e-health strategy implementation.

Irrespective of whether Walker's taxonomy or Elkin et al's ontology for interoperability is adopted, all healthcare applications need to establish the functions they need to be able to perform so that the required degree and level of interoperability can be established enabling the identification of which standard they need to be compliant with. Each nation needs to first of all establish its unique health business requirements followed by the establishment of a national health informatics standards framework as well as a national health language framework. Both frameworks need to be supported by a national governance process to ensure that all health systems are compliant with the required technical and health language standards. Software applications within individual organisations need to be able to meet national business requirements as well as their own specific business needs.

In 2003 HL7 developed the HL7 EHR System Functional Model that provides a reference list of over 160 functions that may be present in an Electronic Health Record System (EHR-S) [6]. The function list is described from a user perspective with the intent to enable users to apply a consistent expression of system functionality. This functional model is now being considered for adoption as an ISO standard.

Today's most significant cost drivers are the number of technical interfaces that need to be developed and maintained. As Walker et al [3] demonstrated, this cost is significantly higher to achieve his defined level 3 interoperability than for systems designed to achieve level 4 semantic interoperability. This suggests that a suitable business case to support standards development activities as a component of the national e-health strategy implementation fully justifies such an investment.

Standards enabling semantic interoperability so that all functional needs can be met need to be applied to support a genuine need and to realise a projected net gain. In September 2008 the European Union published the final draft of the eHealth-INTEROP Report in response to EU Mandate/403-2007.

3.   Standards Development Organisations (SDOs) – Structure and Activities

The key health informatics standards development organisations (SDOs) are Health Level Seven (HL7) ,whose standards need to be approved by the American National Standards Institute (ANSI), the International Organisation for Standards (ISO) Technical Committee (TC215) and the European Committee for Standardisation of Health Informatics (Comité Europanéen de Normalisation - CEN/TC251). There are many others of significance such as the Clinical Data Interchange Standards Consortium (CDISC), the International Health Terminology Standards Development Organisation (IHTSDO), the Object Management Group (OMG) and more. The *open*EHR foundation is not a SDO but has developed specifications based on extensive research. These are made available freely together with their open source software and tools. These specifications and implementation experiences have influenced standards developments.

The work in progress by all of these committees is frequently at the cutting edge of development requiring contributions from many international experts. It is only by means of this collegial teamwork that a suite of suitable standards can be developed and maintained. All Standards Australia projects and publications are listed at their eHealth website[1]. Each ISO TC215 member country needs to have a good overview of its health informatics directions and need for standards as this influences these international developments. Indeed those countries that are well advanced provide considerable international leadership. Furthermore standards developers need to be aware of the "big picture" requirements to ensure that all standards are compatible and in harmony with each other. This is not an easy task as the amount of work being undertaken by the many groups identified is extensive. For example in early 2008 the standards and technical reports under review or development by the three primary international standards organisation that need to be harmonised numbered over 200. This harmonisation work is critical as the adoption and compliance with sets of incompatible standards are of little value as it compromises our potential to realize true interoperability needed to support EHRs.

There is also a realisation that there is an increasing need for several different groups to work closer together on specific projects. There is much to be gained from adopting a multi-expert team approach to standards development. The total number of health informatics standards required is extensive. In addition to the need to achieve semantic interoperability other standards needed for EHRs to be effective are to do with security and authentication, back-up and archiving, messaging and communication. It isn't possible to cover all standards published and under development here so coverage in this chapter is selective with a focus on the most crucial and also the most controversial standards development work.

3.1 Health Level Seven (HL7)

Health Level Seven (HL7)[2] is a very large and active not-for-profit volunteer organisation and is one of several American National Standards Institute (ANSI)-accredited Standards Developing Organisations (SDOs) operating in the healthcare arena. It began in the USA in 1987 and was accredited by ANSI in 1994.

---

[1] http://www.e-health.standards.org.au

[2] http://www.hl7.org

This organisation now has many international affiliate members. Widespread adoption of HL7 messaging standards version 2.x has proven to be very cost effective for the health industry. HL7 messaging standards are essentially instructions for software engineers. This version represents standards enabling syntactical interoperability, that is each field is identified in a standard sequence separated by a vertical bar | . Such messages look like the one presented in Figure 2 [8]:

The V2.4 representation of the use-case is a ORU^R01 message. The syntax encoding is based on the *classic* HL7 v2 syntax, commonly referred to as the vertical-bar syntax.

MSH|^~\&|GHH LAB|ELAB-3|GHH OE|BLDG4|200202150930||ORU^R01|CNTRL-3456|P|2.4<cr>
PID|||555-44-4444||EVERYWOMAN^EVE^E^^^^L|JONES|19620320|F|||153 FERNWOOD DR.^
^STATESVILLE^OH^35292||(206)3345232|(206)752-121||||AC555444444||67-A4335^OH^20030520<cr>
OBR|1|845439^GHH OE|1045813^GHH LAB|15545^GLUCOSE|||200202150730|||||||||
555-55-5555^PRIMARY^PATRICIA P^^^^MD^^||||||||F|||||444-44-4444^HIPPOCRATES^HOWARD
H^^^^MD<cr>
OBX|1|SN|1554-5^GLUCOSE^POST 12H CFST:MCNC:PT:SER/PLAS:QN||^182|mg/dl|70_105|H|||F<cr>

Figure 2. HL7 Message Structure Example

Note the standard sequence of the various segments and in particular note the last couple of OBX segments in the message. These segments reflect the results of the liver function test and represent a form of clinical data (content). Limitations of HL7 v2.x, are identified as:

- too much optionality
- no explicit information model
- events and profiles not unambiguous
- terminology/vocabularies/code sets not tightly defined
- not object-oriented.

This means that even systems that are compliant with these HL7 standards are likely to have various difficulties in communicating with each other.

HL7 has a number of technical committees, and special interest groups that collectively manage a vast number of projects. They meet several times each year. As from March 2005 HL7 is working collaboratively with the OMG to build a set of healthcare domain software components and services interface standards to promote interoperability across health care provider organisations and health related software products. You need to visit their website[3] frequently to get the latest news and to become familiar with the many committees, their projects and progress.

3.2 International Organisation for Standardisation (ISO TC215)

ISO TC215[4] was established in 1998 to achieve compatibility and interoperability between independent systems to ensure compatibility of data for comparative statistical purposes, reduce duplication of effort and redundancies. The ISO TC 215 has several working groups. Each of these has a convener and each is administered by a member Standards Organisation.

ISO TC215 provides opportunities for cooperation with similar committees in 22 countries who are also ISO members and 16 countries who have observer status. There is an agreement (known as the 'Vienna Agreement') between the ISO and CEN TC251

---

[3] http://www.hl7.org
[4] http://www.iso.org/iso/iso_technical_committee?commid=54960

for technical cooperation, when it suits both, to maximise the efficiency of standardisation. ISO's national members participate in standards development work undertaken internationally. ISO's work results in international agreements that are published as International Standards or Technical Reports. It begins with an approved work item (AWI), this becomes a working draft (WD), then a committee draft (CD) followed by a draft International Standard (DIS) and a final draft International Standard (FDIS) up to the point of publication. The reference number associated with each project indicates its status by the prefix that indicates the international standardising organisation with project responsibility, an indication of the current stage of the document and a reference number for the project itself followed by an indication of the version of a document and the date it was published. ISO TC 215 now has a sub-committee with representation from the three primary standards development organisations responsible for the harmonisation of standards between CEN TC251, HL7 and ISO TC215. ISO also works closely with the International Electrotechnical Commission (IEC); they produce joint ISO/IEC standards. You can view the list of ISO TC215 publications and work in progress at its website[5].

3.3 European Committee for Standardisation of Health Informatics (CEN/TC251)

In Europe, regional standardisation takes place within a legal framework [9]. This governs the behaviour of those making technical regulations and those making standards. This Directive also formally sets out the relationship between those who will initiate legislation represented by the ministries of the member states and the standardisation bodies. Areas of European standardisation to support its policies and propose mandates to CEN and its partners may be identified by a Standing Committee established by the Directive. More than two thirds of CEN's work is not based on mandates from the Commission. All work items are published twice per annum in CEN's work program. European standards and Technical Specifications are drafted following the same rules as ISO/IEC. The CEN/ISSS—Information Society Standardisation System provides a comprehensive and integrated range of standardisation oriented services and products.

3.4 Other relevant standards organisations

Clinical Data Interchange Standards Consortium (CDISC)
CDISC is a global, open, multidisciplinary, non-profit organization with a mission to develop and support global, platform-independent data standards that enable information system interoperability to improve medical research and related areas of healthcare. Their standards are freely available via their website[6].

International Health Terminology Standards Development Organisation (IHTSDO)
IHTSDO[7] is a relatively new international not-for-profit organization standards development organisation based in Denmark. Established in 2007, it has acquired the intellectual property rights of one of the most important clinical terminologies, the SNOMED Clinical Terms (SNOMED CT®) terminology and its antecedents, from the

---

[5] http://www.iso.org/iso/iso_catalogue/catalogue_tc/catalogue_tc_browse.htm?commid=54960

[6] http://cdisc.org/

[7] http://www.ihtsdo.org

College of American Pathologists (CAP). The IHTSDO seeks to improve the health of humankind by fostering the development and use of suitable standardized clinical terminologies, notably SNOMED CT, in order to support safe, accurate, and effective exchange of clinical and related health information. The focus is on enabling the implementation of semantically accurate health records that are interoperable.

Object-Management Group (OMG)

The Object-Management Group (OMG)[8] is a computer industry consortium that develops enterprise integration standards for a wide range of technologies. Its middleware standards and profiles are based on the Common Object Request Broker Architecture (CORBA/CORBAmed) that defines standardised interfaces to many health-care "Object-Oriented Services," across most usual platforms, and is available in the public domain.

American National Standards Institute (ANSI)

ANSI[9] a not for profit organisation facilitates the development of American National Standards (ANS) by accrediting the procedures of many US based standards developing organizations (SDOs) including HL7. ANSI is the US member body to the ISO TC215. ANSI has a Healthcare Informatics Standards Board (ANSI HISB) that provides an open, public forum for the voluntary coordination of healthcare informatics standards among all United States' standard developing organisations. ANSI accredits US Technical Advisory Groups (TAGs) to represent ANSI at specific ISO Technical Committees. Each US TAG has the responsibility to develop consensus relative to the position of the US in connection with ISO standards. In 2005 the Healthcare Information Technology Standards Panel (HITSP) was founded to serve as a cooperative partnership between sectors. Panel members work together to define the necessary functional components and standards – as well as gaps in standards specifically to enable and support widespread interoperability among healthcare software applications for the United States. This panel does not develop standards, its priorities are established by the American Health Information Community. ANSI sponsors HITSP.

ASTM International

ASTM[10] International, formerly known as the American Society for Testing and Materials, is a not-for-profit organisation that provides a global forum for the development and publication of voluntary consensus standards for materials, products, systems, and services. ASTM Committee E31 on Healthcare Informatics develops standards related to the architecture, content, storage, security, confidentiality, functionality, and communication of information used within health care and healthcare decision making, including patient-specific information and knowledge.

A unique volume from ASTM E31 includes eight standards on Standards for Security and Electronic Signatures in Healthcare and complies with the security requirements identified in the United States of America *Health Insurance Portability and Accountability Act (HIPAA)* of 1996 (pp. 104–191). It offers protection of an individual's health information when the information is electronically housed or transmitted over telecommunications systems. The digital signature component is

---

[8] http://www.omg.org/

[9] http://www.hitsp.org

[10] http://www.astm.org/COMMIT/COMMITTEE/E31.htm

multi-faceted and addresses message integrity, user authentication, and non-repudiation. It covers:
- authentication and authorization of health care information
- confidentiality, privacy, access and data security principles
- digital signatures
- internet and intranet security
- access privileges
- individual rights.

DICOM Digital Imaging and Communications in Medicine
The DICOM[11] standards committee originated as a joint committee between the American College of Radiology (ACR) and the National Electrical Manufacturers Association (NEMA) in 1983. DICOM is now a standards development organisation administered by the NEMA Diagnostic Imaging and Therapy Systems Division. It exists to create and maintain international standards for communication of biomedical diagnostic and therapeutic information in disciplines that use digital images and associated data. DICOM is a cooperative standard. Its goals are to achieve compatibility and to improve workflow efficiency between imaging systems and other information systems in healthcare environments worldwide. There are 21 working groups where each has taken on the responsibility for a specific aspect of the DICOM standard.

HIBCC—Health Industry Business Communications Commission
The Health Industry Business Communications Commission[12] is an ANSI accredited organisation that develops appropriate standards for information exchange among all health care trading partners to facilitate electronic communications by providing leading bar-coding and e-commerce standards.

IEEE—Standards Association
The IEEE standards association[13] is another accredited organisation under the ANSI procedures. Its standards are developed through worldwide participation and may be submitted to any national standards body for recognition as its national standard. It is represented on some, and has assumed administrative responsibility for, a number of US based technical advisory groups (TAGs) facilitating participation in ISO and the International Electrotechnical Commission (IEC). The IEEE SA directs its registration authority which is recognised by ISO/IEC as the authorised registration authority to provide a world-wide service.

IEC—International Electrotechnical Commission
The IEC[14] prepares and publishes international standards for all electrical, electronic and related technologies including electronics, magnetics and electromagnetics, electroacoustics, multimedia, telecommunication, and energy production and distribution, as well as associated general disciplines such as terminology and symbols, electromagnetic compatibility, measurement and performance, dependability, design and development, safety and the environment. One of its objectives specifically relevant to EHR systems is to establish the conditions for the interoperability of

[11] http://dicom.nema.org/
[12] http://www.hibcc.org/
[13] http://standards.ieee.org/
[14] http://www.iec.ch/

complex systems. It promotes international cooperation through its members and manages a number of conformity assessment and product certification schemes. The Joint ISO/IEC technical committee one (JTC 1) is responsible for general IT standards and has produced a number of standards relevant to health care.

EDIFACT—Electronic Data Interchange for Administration, Commerce and Transport
The UN/EDIFACT Committee[15] is managed by the United Nations/Economic Commission for Europe who appoint rapporteurs for each global region. Its objective is to maintain a previously developed single international EDI standard flexible enough to meet the needs of government and private industry. It has its own rules for electronic data interchange for administration, commerce and transport.

4. What Standards are Required to Achieve Semantic Interoperability?

Achieving semantic interoperability between all health systems is a major challenge but essential to enable EHRs to be realised. The key standards that nations need to agree to adopt to enable them to meet this vision were identified in table 1, chapter 4 as the e-health record structure/architecture/information model, set of clinical content models and terminology, unique patient, individual and organisational provider identifiers.

To date there is no international consensus about which standards are most appropriate. Many standards are incompatible with each other. This makes it difficult for any nation to develop their national standards framework. Late 2007 three key SDO's, HL7, CEN TC251 and ISO 215 agreed to work together via a joint committee within ISO to overcome this problem. However there is a view that we'll never reach consensus about a standard e-health record architecture or data model despite agreement that is the ideal to enable semantic interoperability at the highest level to be realised. Another view is that once clinical expert movers and shakers realise the significance they can insist that the architecture they view as being best able to meet their clinical needs is adopted by simply placing such a requirement in the tender documents. The software vendors would need to follow in such circumstances or lose market share.

Similarly a number of experts have spent many years exploring how best to harmonise data types. This has almost been achieved, it is an active work item for the Joint Committee. These key standards are the most complex and difficult to develop in a manner that suits all stakeholders. Consequently it has taken a lot of effort and time to gain international consensus. There are a number of possible technical solutions a nation can adopt as a component of its e-health implementation strategy. Only the more common and perhaps controversial options for standards compliance selection as these relate to EHRs are presented here.

4.1 e-Health Record Architecture (Information Model)

Prior to developing a suitable e-health record architecture, there needs to be a consensus about an EHR definition and its architectural and functional requirements.

---

[15] http://www.unece.org/trade/untdid/welcome.htm

4.1.1 EHR Definition

A recent literature review undertaken by Hayrinen et al [10] revealed that most failed to separate EHRs (the records) from EHR systems. These authors concluded that "studies focusing on the content of EHRs are needed, especially studies of nursing documentation or patient self-documentation" and noted that there is a need to "take into account all the different types of EHRs and the needs and requirements of different health care professionals and consumers in the development of EHRs" [10 p.292]. Lobach and Detmer [11] identified two research challenges, 1) rigorous evaluations of EHR systems and 2) a need to determine how to take full advantage of the potential to create and disseminate new knowledge that is possible as a result of data captured by EHRs. These need impact on national health policy and suggest actions needed for "those who are interested in changing the landscape of EHR development, research and implementation" [11 p.S104].

Some of these challenges had already been identified by members of various standards development teams and resulted in ISO-TR20514:2005, a technical report that defines a basic generic EHR as well as describing sharable, non-sharable and integrated EHRs and EHR systems.

4.1.2 EHR Architecture (Information Model) Requirements

For an EHR to meet the functional requirements associated with each EHR definition it is essential that a detailed set of user and technical requirements be agreed upon. The ISO/TS18308:2004 technical specification details these. The Standards Australia Health Informatics Committee IT-14 has overseen the conversion of this standard into an Australian Standards AS ISO/TS 18308-2005: Health informatics—Requirements for an electronic health record architecture. You can download this in a pdf format[16]. The openEHR foundation has published a review of their specifications relative to this standard that shows their degree of conformance. This document is available from their website[17].

The principal definition of an electronic health record architecture (EHRA) as used in the Australian standard AS ISO 18308—2005 Health Informatics—Requirements for an electronic health record architecture is: "the generic structural components from which all EHRs are built, defined in terms of an information model". This standard also includes the following description of the EHR architecture stating that: .....it:

> "should be broadly applicable to all healthcare sectors, professional healthcare disciplines, and methods of healthcare delivery. A "consumer" or "personal" EHR should be able to conform to the same EHR architecture as a more traditional EHR used by providers such as medical specialists, nurses, general practitioners and providers of allied health services. The same EHR architecture should be applicable to all variants of the EHR, regardless of whether these are called an EMR, EHCR, EPR, CPR, PHR or whatever. An open standardised EHR architecture is the key to interoperability at the information level".

Other relevant standards to consider are 1) the ISO/IEC 10746-1:1998 standard reference model—open distributed processing (RM–ODP), the openEHR specifications are compliant with this general ICT standard, and 2) the ISO/TR 17119: 2005 technical

---

[16] http://www.saiglobal.com/shop/script/Details.asp?docn=AS0733764436AT.
[17] http://www.openehr.org/svn/specification/TRUNK/publishing/requirements/iso18308_conformance.pdf

report titled Health Informatics Profiling Framework. The latter provides a standard method for defining and classifying artifacts such as models, standards and documentation within the domain of health informatics to facilitate highly complex systems to become conceptually manageable. This report has adopted a strong systems approach as the basis for classification of health informatics artifacts. The who, what, how, why, where and when perspective adopted by this framework is potentially useful for system developers. One needs to recognise that each standard includes comprehensive references to many other relevant standards.

4.2 EHRs Linking with Clinical Systems

The process of the development of standards for the EHR architectures made it apparent that there was a need for standards defining EHRs and its architectural requirements. This explains the order within which all of these activities have taken place over time. Indeed standards development work is a journey of discovery. There is also a need to consider the hardware used to establish interoperability among multi-vendor equipment which is available from many different sources. Just like the banking industry with its ATM cards, the health care industry needs to be able to perform transactions with its own EHR. For example, there are many different type of storage devices (smart cards, USB memory cards/tokens, PC memory cards, magnetic strip cards, zip disks, floppy disks, CDs, DVDs) which all can realistically be used to carry and store an individual's EHR. These devices need to be compatible with the GP's, the hospital's, the specialists and perhaps even the patient's own computer system (for Read and/or Write functions). This was not the case with the Australian Public Key Infrastructure, recently implemented within the GP sector, where USB tokens were used (USB were only standardised on computers purchased since 2002). Such limitations may hinder the progress of EHRs, as it can be perceived to cost more to purchase one hardware device for only a single purpose. In addition, the growth in this area is fast; therefore it is also not realistic to be locked into a hardware which can be superseded by another in less than six months.

4.3 CEN/TC215 and openEHR Activities via EHRcom

The European Committee for Standardisation of Health Informatics (CEN/TC251)[18] has been working with the *open*EHR foundation via a taskforce (EHRcom) since late 2001 to jointly work on the updating of the CEN 13606 EHR standard from a 4 part to a 5 part standard by adopting the *open*EHR two level modeling approach requiring the incorporation and use of archetypes drawing on the parallel implementation and live use within EU Projects (Synapses and SynEx) and through the Australian Good Electronic Health Record project. This work has progressed to an ISO standard. However the information model (IM) of this standard is not as comprehensive as the IM developed by the *open*EHR foundation so has limited functionality. The EHR communications standard proposed by the CEN/*open*EHR Task Force is to produce a rigorous and durable information architecture for representing the EHR in order to support the interoperability of systems and components that need to interact with EHR services. That is this five part standard is about:
  1.   discrete systems or as middleware components;

---

[18] http://www.europacs.org/cen.htm

2.   access, transfer, add or modify health record entries;
3.   use of electronic messages or distributed objects;
4.   preserving the original clinical meaning intended by the author;
5.   reflecting the confidentiality of that data as intended by the author and patient.

This is arguably the single most important standard requiring international consensus as it defines a consensus for the exchanges of EHR extracts between different systems [12]. You can read more about this ISO 13606 standard at the *open*EHR website[19].

4.4 *open*EHR's Key Features

A major strength of the *open*EHR approach is that its information model is ontologically sound as described by Beale and Heard [13 [p.760]] unlike for example the HL7 v.3 RIM [14]. The *open*EHR structure is based on a separation of domain knowledge and technical development as shown in Figure 3 whereas other approaches often mix up domain content development/maintenance and technical development.

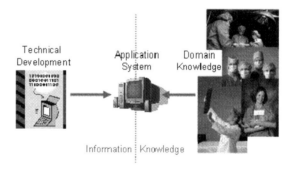

Figure 3: The Separation of Domain Knowledge and Technical Development Using the openEHR Approach.

This separation is achieved by introducing a two-level-modelling approach. The first level of the *open*EHR approach is the reference information model, which is pared down to the minimum to support the medico-legal requirements and record management functions. This ensures that clinicians can always send information to another provider and receive information, which they can read – thus ensuring data interoperability. The second level is constituted of formal definitions of clinical content in the form of *open*EHR archetypes. These archetypes can be shared between systems and clinical content of archetype instances can then be processed by the receiving provider – thus enabling semantic interoperability as described in previous chapters. One archetype models or represents one clinical or other domain specific concept by constraining instances of the *open*EHR information models to express a valid structure, valid data types, and values. *open*EHR uses archetypes to model the clinical content of EHRs completely separate from any technical design issues for an EHR system. Consequently, only the first level needs to be implemented in software, thus significantly reducing the dependency of deployed systems and data on variable content definitions. By clearly separating the three categories - information models, domain content models, and terminologies - the *open*EHR architecture enables each to

---

[19] http://www.openehr.org/standards/cen.html

have a well-defined, limited scope and clear interfaces. This limits the dependence of each on the other, leading to more maintainable and adaptable systems.

The more comprehensive IM developed by the *open*EHR foundation has adopted four levels of information organisation:

1. The cognitive **user interface** – a flexible approach to data capture and viewing
2. **Templates** - the data capture sets for each step – process-oriented, may be *ad hoc*
3. **Archetypes** - standardised semantics of the data points in data capture sets
4. The **reference model** - standardised data representation, enabling interoperability

This IM enables a standardised **querying** capability and the adoption of standardised interfaces to **terminology** for inferencing. They have also developed a specifications roadmap which is available at their website[20]. A variety of vendors use the *open*EHR approach for various products, for example the Australian company Ocean Informatics Pty Ltd. is using the *open*EHR work to produce a variety of middleware products as detailed at their website[21].

4.5 HL7 v3 Reference Information Model (RIM)

HL7 has developed another Reference Information Model (RIM) known as the HL7 v3 Meta-model that is described at the HL7 website[22] as an object model created as part of the Version 3 methodology. The RIM is a large pictorial representation of the clinical data (domains) and identifies the life cycle of events that a message or groups of related messages will carry. It is a shared model between all the domains and as such is the model from which all domains create their messages.

HL7 RIM Backbone

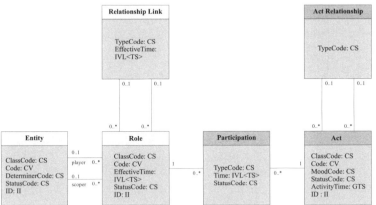

Figure 4 RIM's Core Concepts (Classes) and Attributes [15]

The RIM explicitly represents the connections that exist between the information carried in the fields of HL7 messages. It consists of a group of analysis patterns for

---

[20] http://www.openehr.org/specifications/spec_roadmap_2008.html.

[21] http://www.oceaninformatics.com

[22] http://www.hl7.org/about/about2.htm

messages and other components. It contains a mixture of variant and invariant ontological concepts and doesn't supply needed data structures. HL7 see their RIM as essential to their ongoing mission of increasing precision and reducing implementation costs. The RIM's core concepts as shown in figure 4 as a UML diagram needs to be read as - every happening is an:

- **Act** (Procedures, observations, medications, supply, registration, etc.),
- Acts are related through an **Act_relationship** (composition, preconditions, revisions, support, etc.),
- **Participation** defines the context for an Act (author, performer, subject, location, etc.),
- The participants are **Roles**, (patient, provider, practitioner, specimen, healthcare facility etc.)
- Roles are played by **Entities**, (persons, organizations, material, places, devices, etc.)

The RIM's core attributes as shown in figure 4 consist of six kinds that are:

1. type_cd (class_cd),
2. cd, (concept_descriptor)
3. time,
4. mood (determiner),
5. status,
6. id

These RIM concepts (classes) together with their attribute value sets are shown in figure 5

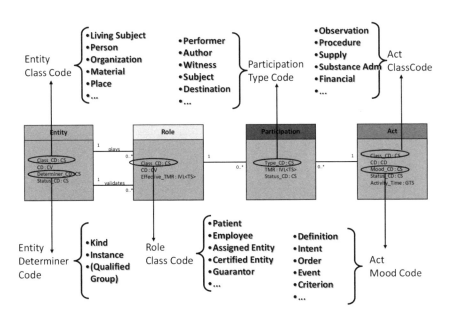

Figure 5 RIM's Classes and Attribute Value Sets

From the RIM, more detailed domain message information models (D-MIMs), as well as reference message information models (R-MIMs) and Hierarchical Message Descriptions (HMDs) —progressively refined knowledge models-cum-schemas - are developed to inform message design. Common Message Element Type (CMETs) are reusable RMIM fragments.

HL7's clinical context object workgroup (CCOW) has developed a context management standard that defines a protocol for securely "linking" applications so that they "tune" to the same context. This entails the coordination and synchronization of applications so that they are mutually aware of the set of common things - known as the context - that frame and constrain the user's interactions with applications. These standards specify technology-neutral architectures, component interfaces, and data definitions as well as an array of interoperable technology-specific mappings of these architectures, interfaces, and definitions.

HL7 has also released a clinical document architecture (CDA Release 2.0) standard that provides an exchange model for clinical documents (such as discharge summaries and progress notes). It is essentially a RMIM (Refined Message Information Model containing an arbitrary and ontologically inconsistent set of concepts at the *open*EHR Entry level. A CDA document is a defined and complete information object that can exist outside of a message and can include text, images, sounds and other multimedia content. CDA specifies the structure and semantics of clinical documents and can be sent inside an HL7 message as well as exist independently. The CDA derives its semantic content from the shared HL7 Reference Information Model (RIM) and uses the HL7 v.3 Data Types.

In addition to CDA, HL7 has developed data structure templates based on the HL7 RIM. This expresses the data content needed in a specific clinical or administrative context. This is a system for the representation of clinical document templates written in XML (SR XML). The union of standard information structures with standard vocabulary sets allows clinical information to be transmitted between health care applications in a way that maximises interoperability. These templates provide standard data structures based on the RIM that may be stored in a meta-data repository for multiple parties (internal and external) to interact with. The concept is based on the union of standard information structures with standard vocabulary sets. HL7 v.3 messages are based on building information structures derived from a standardised object information model. The linking of structures with vocabulary sets creates clinical templates.

4.6 Information Model Harmonisation Possibilities

Only two of the information models (CEN 13606 and *open*EHR) can be harmonised. The HL7 v3 RIM has a very different structure and is based on linking systems via messages. The latter is far more complex and takes a considerable amount of message standards development time. National HL7 affiliates influence the development of these general standards to ensure international needs can be met. They also develop implementation standards to suit their local national environment. HL7 v.2.x messages are now able to incorporate archetypes enabling a higher quality of clinical data transfer between systems. An Australian draft standard (Project No: 7355) for representing archetyped data in HL7 Version 2 closed for public comment on 29 July 2008 so is expected to be available in the very near future.

One could view the HL7 standards as being more appropriate for use during the transitional arrangements towards EHRs as the adoption of these messaging standards enable healthcare organisations to make better use of existing systems. However to realise the ideal EHR vision a different approach is required. Given the choice of EHR architectures and associated implementation issues, it is difficult to decide which one should be adopted as the key foundation for a national e-health strategy. The ISO 15498 Standard for Information and Documentation Records Management and the ISO 9000 quality standards also apply.

4.7 Data Types

In ISO/IEC 11404:2007 Information technology -- General-Purpose Datatypes (GPD), a shared document between ISO and HL7, a "datatype" is defined as:
- a set of distinct values, characterized by properties of those values, and by operations on those values.
- a data type consists of three main features: a value space, a set of properties, and a set of characterizing operations

This definition has also been adopted in the draft international standard ISO/DIS 21090 Health Informatics — Harmonized data types for information interchange that is now available for review by ISO members. Voting was completed September 2008.

4.8 Patient and Provider Unique Identifiers

The Standards Australia Health Informatics Committee IT-14 is in the process of updating their existing standards with input from the relevant HL7 and ISO TC215 standards development committee members. A specific Standard for Health Care Provider and Client Identification for clinical and administrative data management purposes (data structure and specification) promotes uniformly good practice in identifying individual providers and recording identifying data. Compliance with such a standard significantly assists in ensuring that records relating to each patient or individual provider will be associated with that individual or organisation and no other. This standard considers the issue of identification as well as the systems used to support identification. This draft notes that "without such a Standard, the unique identification of providers and health care clients will be jeopardized and there is a risk that different parties may develop inconsistent methods of identification". The ISO/CD TS 27527 for provider identification is also under development. Safeguards would need to ensure a high level of link accuracy, and for example, that there was no risk of an individual being issued with more than one Unique provider identifier (UPI) or of two individuals having the same UPI. This standard is necessary not only for the successful implementation of EHRs but also for the management of the health supply chain.

Developing a standard for Unique provider identifiers is particularly complex especially for organisational providers as a variety of healthcare facility characteristics exist such as ownership, management, types of services provided, geographical locations, funding arrangements, contractual arrangements with individual providers. Such characteristics may be classified into party/entity type, role type, fund type, service type, service insurance type, service delivery location etc. These identifiers need to enable providers to be classified into homogeneous groups from a statistical perspective in order to for example make relevant performance comparisons and for policy development/funding purposes. From a health supply chain perspective this needs to enable accurate delivery location, in some instances link to a specific patient as well enable on-line procurement and the appropriately management of all financial transactions.

4.9 Domain Knowledge Constraint Models (Archetypes, Templates)

These were introduced from a modeling perspective in Chapter 8 and discussed from a development perspective in the previous chapter. Heard [16] explains that :

"Archetypes are the fundamental shareable specifications of clinical information we need to provide quality health care, and have been formally accepted as a European standard in 2007 (CEN 13606 Part II) and now being considered by ISO. Each archetype represents a whole, discrete specification which is as inclusive as possible, always in terms of the *open*EHR reference model. The reference model itself guarantees that the key attributes for information in health records (such as who, when and where) are already taken care of and do not need to be addressed in each archetype. Further, the reference model has 5 different entry classes which provide the attributes and structures required for all the different sorts of information stored in a health record. Templates are a further means of building clinical models; these are composed of one or more archetypes and add further constraints required for the use of those archetypes in a particular setting".

The HL7 Patient Care committee is undertaking a project that specifically develops and maintains a set of Detailed Clinical Models (DCM), that are usable within the HL7 Clinical Statement, HL7 template specification, HL7 terminfo requirements, the CEN/IOS 13606 and OpenEHR archetype environment, and the Clinical template specification, among others [17]. This work primarily aims to fit with the HL7 Reference Information Model (RIM). It is argued that the content for DCMs and archetypes is the same but that this content is represented using different models. Ideally we'll find a way to enable this clinical content to be easily converted from one model to another so that we do not need to re-invent the wheel and duplicate such efforts.

It is necessary to establish a national Domain Knowledge Governance (DKG) process to achieve semantic interoperability. This is supported by the Australian National e-Health Transition Authority [2] who stated that 'undisciplined creation and application of archetypes threatens the goal of semantic interoperability'. To adequately support Domain Knowledge Governance, Information Technology support is required. DKG comprises:

"...all tasks related to establishing or influencing formal and informal organizational mechanisms and structures in order to systematically influence the building, dissemination, and maintaining of knowledge within and between domains" [18].

4.10 Can Standards Work Together (or Merge) to Produce EHRs?

Given the many standards already available and under development we need to ask how can we choose the right set of standards required to meet the desired purpose? The overview provided should have alerted you to the many variations encountered in standards produced to date. Each standard is developed to suit a specific purpose or schema, many have only one use. Beale [19] suggests we need a small topology to begin to understand the differences. He provided a number of message standards as examples and was able to identify variations in modeling, degree of interoperability, clinician engagement and economics all of which demonstrated that it was not possible to 'merge' these in any way.

Another group of messaging standards are developed for more generic purposes or schemas, so that these can carry a wide variety of content. Again he noted significant variations in modeling, degree of interoperability, clinician engagement and economics and provided examples. The third group were described as standards that define concrete generic schemas plus a formal way of defining content used for actual documents, XML for example. These had a higher degree of interoperability, improved clinician engagement and significant variations in economics such as implementation costs. These types of standard begin to be more useful for generating EHRs. Examples are:

- the EN13606-1 + EN13606-2 although adoption of this standard does not provide a direct basis for many useful clinical archetypes and no templates.
- HL7 CDAr2 +HL7 templates – these are schema specializations of the CDA main schema but have limited re-use capacity.
- openEHR RM XSD + archetypes + templates

The last group are standards that define a framework for defining reusable formal clinical content models that can be used with abstract generic schemas to be able to generate various concrete generic schemas such as message defs, XDs, Xforms, java code, DB schemas) and to generate concrete purpose-specific concrete schemas. This is the kind *open*EHR has been working on? It's important to understand the qualitative differences between these groups of standards as the economics such as implementation costs change over time and should not feature as the primary reason for choosing a particular ehealth strategy and associated sets of standards systems need to comply with in any nation.

5.   Integrating the HealthCare Enterprise (IHE) and Technical Interoperability

The Integrating Healthcare Enterprise (IHE)[23] began as an unincorporated organisation of many member organizations a few years ago and continues to grow. It is expected to be incorporated sometime in 2008. Health professionals and industry initiated IHE's establishment in response to the recognition that in the process of adopting any standard, gaps, options and room for conflicting interpretations are discovered. Experience has shown that no standard maps perfectly to the complex and ever-changing information domain of a healthcare enterprise. Filling the gap between standards and systems integration has, until now, required expensive, site-specific interface development. To close that gap a process for building a detailed framework for the implementation of standards was needed. IHE now provides that process via domain committees who develop and maintain the IHE Technical Frameworks (profiles) that spell out how specific systems can best be connected to others thus addressing interoperability in their respective clinical and operational areas of healthcare. Beale [19] refers to the IHE as a 'standard' for a transport system for other content developed by whatever means.   Technical communication protocols and standards were presented in chapter 5 on interoperability.

---

[23] http://www.ihe.net/

The ISO TC 215 has produced a Health informatics standard relevant to this topic. It is ISO/TR 18307:2001 Health informatics—Interoperability and compatibility in messaging and communication standards—Key characteristics.

6. Data Transmission Media

You also need to have some understanding of the transmission media infrastructures, or physical paths that may or may not be available in particular geographic locations. This is likely to have an impact on the adoption of EHRs or any other required data transmission. The available media such as telephone wires, satellites, fibre optic cables determine the speed, size limitations and possible distance of data transfer. The greater the bandwidth of a signal, the higher the achievable rate of data transfer. Optical fibre is the best possible guided media and minimises transmission impairments. Interference is a problem. It can occur with both the use of guided and unguided media such as wireless transmission, although it is a greater problem with the use of unguided media. Wireless technology has provided another dimension in addressing some of the limitations of the fixed network. Wireless LAN is a family of protocol from the IEEE standards (802.11), supporting transmission up to 11Mbps, which is much faster than broadband solutions like DSL and cable modems. Other technology like Bluetooth (also a wireless communication technology) is able to provide short range wireless networking to PDAs, mobile computers and even headsets using a frequency hopping scheme in the unlicensed 2.4 GHz ISM (Industrial-Scientific-Medical) band [20].

The telecommunications infrastructure is of paramount importance as it dictates the external connectivity capacity and associated costs for any healthcare organisation. In other words, software engineers have some work to do to enable effective communication between systems.

7. Record Ownership

Principles of data or information ownership begin to blur when applied to electronic records where, for example, any number of distributed databases are used to compile such records. In other words, data may be generated by any number of entities towards the compilation of a single record in which case the originator may well keep control of its own database even though it is linked electronically. This is the case with, for example, laboratory or diagnostic reports produced by private practices but submitted electronically to the entity requesting this service who then assumes responsibility for its inclusion into the patient's record. Medical staff need to determine the minimum data that needs to be made available to other healthcare providers. One can conclude that not only do we need standards to govern e-health record access but we also need appropriate legislation and governance processes to support a national e-health strategy.

8.   Risk Management (Enterprise View)

Risk management refers to loss of data, data corruption, inaccurate data processing, adoption of non evidence based protocols or practice guidelines in information and decision support systems that may lead to decisions with adverse consequences. EHRs need to be structured and managed in a manner that eliminates or at the very least minimises the opportunities for such events. This is especially critical when information is being extracted for use in decision support systems. There are no standards that meet this particular need and little work on this topic was apparent via web and literature searches other than the EHR certification protocols in use in the USA as mentioned previously.

9.   Conclusion

Developing health informatics standards is a complex and time-consuming process requiring ongoing international cooperation between teams of experts who collectively have the required expertise and knowledge as well as input from many stakeholders including researchers. It is about deciding how best to support national e-health strategy implementation to enable such strategies to be successful over time. There are many standards organisations working in this space. This chapter couldn't cover all of the work in progress, it's too extensive and constantly changing. The focus has been on the most significant standards development concepts associated with meeting national business requirements in a generic sense and EHRs in particular.

References

[1]   *European Union's e-health action plan 2004*
     http://ec.europa.eu/information_society/activities/health/policy/index_en.htm viewed June 2008
[2]   Australian Government Information Interoperability Framework – sharing information across bounderies, April 2006 Australian Government Information Management Office p.5 http://www.finance.gov.au/publications/agimo/docs/Information_Interoperability_Framework.pdf
[3]   Walker J, Pan E, Johnston D, Adler-Milstein J, Bates DW, Middleton B. The value of health vare information exchange and interoperability. Health Affairs [on line]. 2005 Jan 19; [cited 2008 Jan 2]. Available from: http://content.healthaffairs.org/cgi/content/full/hlthaff.w5.10/DC1
[4]   Elkin PL, Froehling D, Bauer BA, Wahner-Roedler D, Rosenbloom ST, Bailey K, et al. Aequus communis sententia: defining levels of interoperability. In: Kuhn K, Warren J, Leong TY, editors. Medinfo2007: conference proceedings. Amsterdam (NL): IOS Press; 2007. p.725.
[5]   Friedman TL. The world is flat: the globalised world in the twenty-first century. London (UK): Penguin Books; 2006.
[6]   Health Level Seven (HL7) 2003 Electronic Health Record Functional Model http://www.hl7.org/ehr/ cited June 2008
[7]   European Union final draft of the eHealth-INTEROP Report in response to EU Mandate/403-2007. available from: http://www.ehealth-interop.nen.nl/
[8]   Ringholm Whitepaper HL7 message examples http://www.ringholm.de/docs/04300_en.htm viewed November 2009
[9]   EU 1998/48/EC Information in the field of Technical Standards & Regulations Directive amending Directive and 98/34/EC1998/34/EC Information in the field of Technical Standards & Regulations Directive http://www.etsi.org/WebSite/AboutETSI/RoleinEurope/ECDirectives.aspx viewed November 2009
[10] Hayrinen K, Sarato K, Nykanen P 2008 Definition, structure, content, use and impacts of electronic health records: a review of the research literature. International Journal of Medical Informatics Vol.77 pp.291-304

[11] Lobach D F, and Detmer D E 2007 Research challenges for Electronic Health Records American Journal of Preventive Medicine Vol.32 (5S pp. S104-S111

[12] Garde S, Knaup P, Hovenga E, Heard S (2007): Towards Semantic Interoperability for Electronic Health Records: Domain Knowledge Governance for openEHR Archetypes. *Methods of Information in Medicine.* 46(3): 332-343.

[13] Beale T and Heard S 2007 An ontology based model of clinical information In: K.Kuhn, J.R Warren,

[14] Lowell Vizenor, Smith Barry, and Ceusters Werner. 2004. Foundation for the Electronic Health Record: An Ontological Analysis of the HL7's Reference Information Model. Unpublished, July 20. http://ontology.buffalo.edu/medo/HL7_2004.pdf

[15] Shafferman M – Past HL7 Chair, presentation slide presented at the Euromise conference, Prague 2004.

[16] Heard S April 2008 update of the *open*EHR wiki on health information models at http://www.openehr.org/wiki/dashboard.action cited May 2008.

[17] Goossen W 2008 Personal communication via email to the dcm@lists.detailedclinicalmodels.org list dated 2 May 2008.

[18] Garde, S, Heard, S & Hovenga, E 2005, 'Archetypes in Electronic Health Records: Making the case and showing the path for domain knowledge governance', HIC 2005: 13th Australian Health Informatics Conference, Melbourne, 31.07.2005–02.08.2005, eds. H Grain & M Wise, Brunswick East, Vic: Health Informatics Society of Australia.

[19] Beale T email communication to the openehr-clinical mailing list 6 September 2008

[20] Rao, S (ed.) 2002, IST-2000-25153 Review of Status of Early Relevant standard, IR6WINI Europe, *International Journal of Medical Informatics*, vol. 60, no. 3, pp. 281–301.

Review Questions

1. What is the relationship between standards and your national e-health strategy?
2. Describe and comment upon national and international standards development organizations and their standards development processes.
3. What would a suitable national Health Informatics standards roadmap look like in your country and what types of standards should it include?
4. Explain the benefits of the national adoption of Health Informatics standards

Health Informatics
E.J.S. Hovenga et al. (Eds.)
IOS Press, 2010
© *2010 The authors and IOS Press. All rights reserved.*
doi:10.3233/978-1-60750-476-4-156

12. Health Information Systems:- Requirements and Characteristics

Angelika SCHLOTZER[1], Assoc. Dip. Computing (CIAE), B App. Sc. (Computing)(CQU), Grad. Dip. Further Education (USQ)[a b], Maria MADSEN BS, BSc(Hons), GDAC, MB(IS), MACS PhD Candidate [b c]
[a]School of Computing, Bundaberg Campus, Queensland
[b] Central Queensland University, Australia
[c] School of Management and Information Systems, Director eHealth Education Pty Ltd

Abstract. This chapter gives an educational overview of:
- The purpose of health information systems (HIS).
- The characteristics of health information systems for the future.
- System interoperability as an essential feature in a modern HIS.
- Why user requirements must be established before an HIS is designed.
- How to transform a requirements specification into a request for tender.

Keywords. Information Systems, Health, Systems Analysis, Computer Communication Networks, User Requirements, Software Design, Health Facilities, Systems Theory, Data Management Systems, Database, Computer Security, Request for Tenders (RFT)

Introduction

The purpose of this chapter is to introduce key aspects of information systems design and development for health care. As such this chapter is not a comprehensive discourse on information systems development. Health Information Systems (HIS) have some unique requirements and problematic implementation issues. The implementation and adoption of electronic health records is both a unique requirement and a problem area. Another is the need to design or redesign systems to be interoperable with each other. Yet another, is how to ensure that HIS designed today will survive into the future through continued change to technology, legal requirements, and policies.

The chapter begins by emphasising the organization as a system and the importance of the clinical data in the system. Then we discuss database management systems including distributed systems and systems security. Next interoperability is examined from a health care perspective. Finally the process of requirements analysis and specification are discussed since it is more cost effective to get the design correct than to try to correct the system once it is operational.

---

[1] Corresponding author: a.schlotzer@cqu.edu.au

1.   The Systems View of an Organization

The systems view of an organization is the foundation of information systems theory. An open system accepts inputs from its environment and processes these inputs into outputs. The outputs and their results feed back into the system so that the system can continually improve its performance. An open system is also responsive to the environment in which it exists. In the case of health care organizations, the environment is a highly political one especially in countries where health care is publicly funded, Australia for example. Other external influences include standards, legislation, professional codes of practice, changing technology, and changing medical knowledge. A system can also be divided into subsystems. Sometimes these subsystems are logical division or grouping of processes, for example all payroll processes. Sometimes the subsystems are physically separate systems, for example a database management system. Thus the scope of an information system project can be large encompassing a whole of organization, for example an enterprise system, or it may be small encompassing only one limited subsystem, for example an electronic order entry system. In this chapter, the scope of the information systems we are discussing are enterprise wide. Thus a health information system, for our purposes, encompasses both the administrative information systems and the clinical information systems in a health care organization.

All information systems, including health information systems, are comprised of people, technology (eg. computers, networks, databases, input devices, output devices, and clinical equipment), and the organization (eg. policies, functions, goals, constraints, and existing resources). These three principle components contribute equally to the design of a successful information system. The way in which the technology of the system is connected and integrated constitutes the system's architecture. Blobel [1$^{pp.455-456}$] suggests that "future-proof" health information systems will need to be designed with the following characteristics:

- distribution;
- component-orientation (flexibility, scalability);
- separation of platform-independent and platform-specific modeling [i.e.] separation of logical and technological views (portability);
- specification of reference and domain models at meta-level (semantic interoperability);
- interoperability at service level based on concepts, contexts, and knowledge (user acceptance);
- enterprise view driven design (user acceptance); multi-tier architecture (user acceptance, performance, etc.);
- appropriate multi-media GUI (illiteracy);
- common terminology and ontology (semantic interoperability).

A health information system is successful if it does what it is supposed to do and people are willing and able to use it. What is a health information system supposed to do? A health information system needs to collect, store, protect, and deliver clinical data to those who need it for both primary and secondary uses. Modern health information systems should also implement electronic health records rather than continuing to rely on paper-based files. Therefore the clinical data is at the heart of the health information system.

2.   The Value in the System

Clinical data are a valuable and critical resource. All of the other technologies in a health care organization are there to ensure that clinical data are used appropriately to deliver safe and cost effective health care. Stead et al. [2] have summarised health care data as belonging to three overlapping dimensions. The dimensions based on data use are: Healthcare Provider, Personal Health, and Population Health. In the overlapping sections of these three sets of data they have grouped the data and information that must be shared across the sets. At the centre of this diagram are data that must be shared among all three sets including data for mandatory reporting.

Examples of content for the three dimensions and their overlap

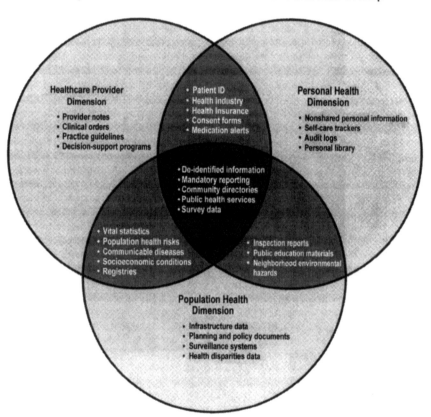

Figure 1 The Three Dimensions of Health Care Data [2 p. 114]

Figure 1 highlights how health care data are distributed across many different organizations, are used for many different purposes, and may exist in many places simultaneously. Managing the collection, storage, and use of these data is an important and complex task. There are many groups working on developing methods for improving the management of health care data. One example is the latest HL7 standard (version 3) which is based on an object model, the reference information model (RIM). The rim can be used to guide the development of new health information systems even though this was not its original purpose. Doing so would simplify the implementation of HL7 version 3 messaging for those systems. A different method, is the *open*EHR archetype approach which takes a higher-level view of health care data. While there are several different paradigms that can be used for data modeling and management, see chapter 8, the relational database remains the most widely implemented design and will be the focus of the discussions that follow.

3. Health Care Data Management

A database management system is a set of computer programs and files designed for the management (acquisition, organisation, storage, distribution, use, protection, archiving, and removal) of a data resource. Such a system is customarily purchased as a package with a number of options from one major software vendor. The features of these systems are discussed in the next section. The common acronym for database management system is DBMS. By taking a broad view of the organisation's information resources, future uses of information technology can be anticipated and accommodated without needing to replace or discard the existing investment in information systems. It has been observed that the data used by an organisation is relatively stable, whereas the processes that use this data, and the structure of the very organisation, is not. Separating the design of databases from that of the organisational units and structures that use the data gives a high degree of independence, stability, and value. Databases that have been designed with modern, well-developed concepts can be used to lever the effect of new technology and innovation, and not hold these effects back.

4. What is it About Database Management Systems That Make Them Important?

Database management systems are perhaps the primary mechanism for getting control of the organisation's information resource. By design, the data within a database can be shared, it has a logical, meaningful structure, and it can support the strategic and tactical goals of the organisation. Most, but not all, database management systems will exhibit all of the following features. A database management system consists of a set of data (database) stored on files, a data dictionary describing the format, structure, and location of the data stored, a user interface allowing interactive query and update to the database, a set of utility programs for monitoring what is happening on the database, re-organising the database, backing up and recovering the database, and an application program interface allowing programs written in one of many computer languages to access the database. Slightly less common features, yet becoming increasingly important in health information systems, include a system for managing concurrent use of the system by many people, security and access control features, see Chapter 13, and higher level languages suitable for developing entire applications. A system is not complete without the people involved with it. In the case of a database management system we usually see a database administrator, software developers, and end-users. A database management system rarely allows access to the data by any means other than its own software (they are proprietary systems). In many cases this software implements a security system restricting access to authorised use. By forcing programs to use the database management system software, data independence is achieved. Changes to the database may be made with only minimal changes required to application programs that use the data.

5. Distributed Databases

Most health care organisations are dispersed, occupying at least several buildings, and often having offices separated by hundreds of kilometres. The ability to share information quickly and easily across the organisation is important and essential. Mail systems, couriers, telephones and facsimile machines are all used to enable this dissemination. With computer networks, the computer-based information resources of the organisation can be easily on tap wherever needed. There may be a number of reasons why a database should be distributed. These reasons are usually based on cost, performance, or both. Compared with a centralised database, distributed systems offer the potential for greatly reduced communication charges, since the data resides closer to where it is actually used. Control of costs can be devolved, and local autonomy and accountability increased, with distributed databases. Response times for the more common transactions should improve considerably, since the bottleneck of the central computer has been removed. Parts of the network may be able to keep operating when the central site or network is malfunctioning. Some sites may be able to operate at different hours from others, they may not be constrained by the needs of others. Growth may be accommodated gradually, without the need for drastic spurts.

6. Health Information System Interoperability

Not only are health information systems within one organization often distributed geographically, from Fig. 1 above, it is clear that health care data must be shared across many unrelated information systems and that they will be used for many different purposes. One of the greatest barriers to the implementation of the electronic health record is the problem of how to share health care data across these disparate systems. In this section we present a brief overview of the interoperability as it relates to health care information.

Morris et al. [3] have investigated interoperability issues in military systems and have used the diagram in Fig. 2 to illustrate these issues at the different layers of interoperability from the technical to the political. They suggest that the *Knowledge/Awareness* layer is the transition layer where interoperability issues move from being technical issues to being organizational issues.

Fig. 2 highlights the fact that systems interoperability will not be achieved through technical solutions alone. Elkin et al. [4 [p. 725]] specify three types of interoperability, pragmatic, semantic, and syntactic that can be applied to the layers of Fig. 2.

1. Syntactic Interoperability   - Structural Interoperability
2. Semantic Interoperability   - Interoperability of a common and shared meaning
3. Pragmatic Interoperability   - Deals with external constraints on the system. Here we take to mean how easy is the type of interoperability to implement.

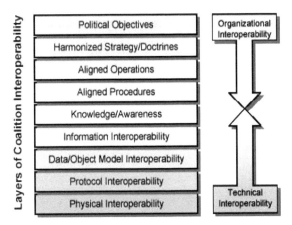

Figure 2 The Layers of Coalition Interoperability (from Tolk 2003 in [3 ^{p. 9}]

The lower three layers of Fig. 2 fit under the heading of *Syntactic* interoperability. The middle three layers of Fig. 2 fit under the heading of *Semantic* interoperability. And the top three layers of Fig. 2 fit under the *Pragmatic* interoperability heading. It is the semantic interoperability that has received the greatest attention in recent years in all information systems including health information systems because semantic interoperability is thought to be the key to knowledge sharing. Interoperability between systems using different database designs, different terminologies, and different infrastructures is difficult but not impossible. The most significant technology to aid interoperability in the last decade has been the HL7 messaging standards. HL7 has enabled health information systems that would otherwise be incompatible, to exchange clinical information with relative ease.

So we now know that a sound database design and semantic interoperability are two important requirements for future health information systems. But these are broad categories that tell us little about exactly what it is that is needed by the intended users of the system. These specific needs are yet to be discovered and will differ in certain respects from one organization to another even though the general requirements for all health information systems are the same.

7.   Discovering User Requirements

Information systems are built to be used by people to improve productivity, quality, efficiency, and effectiveness of their work and subsequently improve the outcomes for the organization. To build a successful information system it is therefore important that **what** the users do and **what** they need is understood. Information systems projects that follow the guidelines and recommendations of a recognised systems development methodology, such as performing requirements analysis and specification, and which have the support of one or more key managers within the organization who will sponsor the project are the most likely to succeed. It is critical to have such sponsorship otherwise the project is at risk of being under-resourced, prematurely terminated, or undermined in other ways.

There are a number of documents that result from the process of identifying and specifying requirements. The actual number of documents and the format in which they are generated depends on the discipline area involved, the guidelines/standards being used and the anticipated complexity of the new HIS. These standards or guidelines are not set in concrete. As HIS and other information systems become increasingly more complex, standards or guidelines are changed to adapt to these new levels of complexity[2]. The "Open Group Architecture Framework" [5] provides a comprehensive and detailed approach to systems development that is focused on requirements management. For our purposes, only the major pieces of documentation generated from a requirements analysis will be discussed based on information systems and information technology discipline guidelines.

7.1 Requirements Analysis

Once the decision has been made that an HIS is needed, the first step is to determine and document the requirements of the new system. Any errors or omissions made at this stage become very costly if they have to be fixed at a later stage. For example, Boehm and Basili [6] have identified that problems can be 100% more expensive to fix once a system has been implemented than if they had been found and corrected during the requirements or design stages. So it is well worthwhile to invest the time and resources needed to fully identify requirements.

Sharp, Rogers, and Preece [7 [p.474]] argue that there are two main aims in undertaking requirements activities. One aim is to understand as much as possible about the users, their work and the context of their work, so that the system can support them in achieving their goals; this we call "identifying needs". Building on this, our second aim is produce, from the needs identified, a set of stable requirements that form a sound basis to move forward into thinking about design.

This is also a good time to review workflow practices to determine whether any changes are needed. The resultant requirements will also form the basis on which "request for tender" documents are generated. More discussion on this follows later.

The sole focus of a requirements analysis is **what** the new system needs to do to fulfill the goals and needs of its stakeholders, not on how this will be accomplished. There are, however, constraints that do need to be considered; for example – the amount of funding available; reporting requirements; the organization's strategic objectives; and legislative requirements.

7.2 Stakeholders and Identifying Needs

It should by now be clear that all stakeholders must be involved in order to fully identify requirements. This includes everyone from top-level administrators to clinicians and technical staff. In some cases, it may also include external entities, for example, researchers. Each group of stakeholders has differing expectations, work functions and needs that the HIS is expected to address. For example, top-level administrators are generally interested in various reports that enable them to make management decisions. These are usually summaries that contain aggregated data such

---

[2] An example of this complexity can be found at the web site for The Open Group [http://www.opengroup.org/] which is an international consortium who envisage a global **Boundaryless Information Flow™**.

as how many patients presented with a communicable disease in the past quarter or statutory reports required by government. At the other end of the spectrum are the people at the "coalface", those clinicians who need to enter information applicable to an individual patient or update inventory and so on. These are significantly different perspectives of the system. Earlier systems were largely developed to meet top-level administrator needs, but dealt poorly (if at all) with the needs of other users. A stakeholder group that feels their needs are not being met by a system will circumvent it or possibly even undermine it.

There are a number of techniques that can be used to establish stakeholder needs. The major ones are interviews, focus groups, analysis of existing documents, observing users at work, questionnaires, use cases to visually illustrate a workflow practice and scenarios used to narrate workflow practices. Once this data has been collected, it is collated into the Needs Document (ND). This document is then analysed to group needs into categories and to identify overlapping needs. The output of this process is the Needs Analysis Document (NAD), which is reviewed with representatives of stakeholder groups for confirmation of accuracy. The NAD is written more concisely than the ND. Needs are stated in terms that can lead to verifiability in the completed system, but still in a natural language that non-technical users can understand. In addition, the needs are prioritised in case budget constraints lead to a situation where all of the needs cannot be implemented at this time. These needs become the user requirements in the formal Software Requirements Document.

7.3 Software Requirements Document

The Software Requirements Document (SRD) (also referred to as System or Software Requirements Specification (SRS)) consists of two major parts [8 p. 98]:

- User requirements: statements (including diagrams) in natural language of the services the system is expected to provide and any constraints under which it must operate.
- System requirements: a detailed set of precise, unambiguous statements about system services and constraints. These may be used as a contract between the system purchaser and the system developer.

Box 1 provides an example of User and System requirements specifications. Requirements tend to be classified as functional or non-functional. Functional requirements correspond to the user requirements; i.e. the services that the system should provide. Non-functional requirements are constraints under which the system will operate. Examples of a few of these include system response times, backup requirements, documentation standards, interoperability requirements (e.g. how this system will "communicate" with one or more legacy systems), privacy and confidentiality requirements, which user groups have access to which information and so on. How many and what type of non-functional requirements need to be included depends on the HIS to be developed. An example of a non-functional requirement might be: After five continuous minutes of keyboard inactivity, the system should blank the screen and lock the computer.

Box 1 Example User Requirement and System Requirements Specification

An example of a documented user requirement:
1.   The system must provide users with the ability to access and deal with basic client information in a timely manner.

A few of the corresponding set of System Requirements Specifications might be:

- Users should be able to add a new client record to the system interactively. This information consists of the client's name, address, contact details, date of birth, gender, marital status, next of kin, Medicare number and private health care provider (if any) details.
- Users should be able to update an existing client's record details interactively.
- Authorised users should be able to delete an existing client record.
- The system must respond to requests to add, update or delete a client record within a maximum of 10 seconds.

The software requirements document can be used as a basis for either the purchase of off-the-shelf systems software and hardware or for producing requests for tender for purpose built systems. The next section explains what is in a typical request for tender.

8.   Requests for Tender

As stated earlier, requirements form the basis on which request for tender (RFT) documents are prepared. Whether these requirements should be the user requirements or the system requirements specifications tends to be an area of debate. There are a number of factors that will influence the decision including the uniqueness of the system to be developed, whether system development will be outsourced or in-house, whether an off-the-shelf system is to be purchased, the criticality of system requirements and so on. For example, assume that the intention is to purchase existing software from a vendor. There could be a number of vendors who offer software that might satisfy the new system's requirements. If you talked with each of these vendors about your system needs, each one would praise their product as being the best solution; however, each product will have somewhat different functionality. To ensure that all vendors need to address all of the requirements of the new HIS without stifling potential innovative vendor solutions or adaptations, the user requirements would be included in the RFT. The content and format of RFT documents tend to vary, but the Pharmacy Guild of Australia's RFT document content sections provide a good example. These are outlined in Box 2. As you can see, the RFT document in this example is very detailed and can be adapted to suit most RFT needs.

Health information systems are complex systems and present the developer with some unique problems and requirements. Most important of these requirements are the management of clinical data for both primary and secondary uses. Blobel [1] identifies *portability, flexibility, user acceptance, semantic interoperability, performance, and scalability* as some of the key features required for "future-proof" health information systems. Performance and user acceptance are features that are unlikely to be met unless a full Requirements Specification is produced before a new system is purchased or a Request for Tender is released.

Conclusion

This chapter has described the characteristics of and why we need to adopt the use of information systems in the health industry. The need for system interoperability between health information systems was explained. Indeed it was demonstrated that system interoperability is an essential feature of successful Health Information System implementations. This is largely dependent upon having identified well developed user requirements to ensure that the systems adopted are designed to meet user needs. The chapter concluded with the presentation of how user requirements specifications can be transformed into requests for tender.

Box 2 Outline of Sections in a Request for Tender Summary

LODGEMENT OF TENDERS
        For hand delivery
        For postal delivery
COPIES REQUIRED
FAX TENDERS
LATE TENDERS
CONTACT OFFICER
PART A – CONDITIONS OF TENDER
        1. Invitation
        2. Enquiries by tenderers
        3. Lodgement of tenders
        4. Alterations, erasures, additional information or illegibility
        5. Ownership of tender documents
        6. Tender validity period
        7. Compliance
        8. Language, measurement and currency
        9. Tenderers to meet costs
        10. Tenderers to inform themselves
        11. Improper assistance and collusive tendering
        12. Affirmative action
        13. Acceptance of tenders
PART B – STATEMENT OF REQUIREMENT
        1. Background
        2. Research Requirements
        3. Management of the Project
        4. Reporting Requirement and Deliverables
        5. Costing the Evaluation
        6. Contracting the Evaluation
PART C – EVALUATION PROCESS AND RESPONSE FORMAT
        1. Evaluation Method
        2. Tender Evaluation Criteria and Information Required from Tenderers
        3. Compliance Criteria
        4. Evaluation Criteria
        5. Achieving the Requirement
        6. Tenderer's Capacity and Infrastructure
PART D – DRAFT CONDITIONS OF CONTRACT

References

[1]   Blobel, Bernd. 2007. Comparing approaches for advanced e-health security infrastructures. *International Journal of Medical Informatics* 76, no. 5-6: 454-459. http://www.sciencedirect.com.ezproxy.cqu.edu.au/science/article/B6T7S-4M7CMJS-1/2/9a636c5588b29f43261d1215ab74c4a6.

[2]   Stead, WW, BJ Kelly, and RM Kolodner. 2005. Achievable Steps Toward Building a National Health Information Infrastructure in the United States. *Journal of the American Medical Informatics Association* 12, no. 2: 113-120.

[3]   Morris, E, L Levine, C Meyers, and D Plakosh. 2004. *System of Systems Interoperability (SOSI): Final Report*. SEI Technical Report. Pittsburgh: Software Engineering Institute.

[4]   Elkin, Peter L, David Froehling, Brent A Bauer, et al. 2007. Aequus Communis Sententia: Defining Levels of Interoperability. In *Medinfo 2007*, ed. Klaus A. Kuhn, James R. Warren, and Tze-Yun Leong, Part 1:725-729. Brisbane: IOS Press.

[5]   The Open Group. 2008. The Open Group Architecture Framework Version 8.1.1. Organization. *The Open Group - Making Standards Work*. http://www.opengroup.org/architecture/togaf8-doc/arch/toc.html.

[6]   Boehm, B, and VR Basili. 2001. Software Defect Reduction Top 10 List. *IEEE Computer* 34, no. 1: 135-137.

[7]   Sharp, H, Y Rogers, and J Preece. 2007. *Interaction Design: Beyond human-computer interaction*. 2nd ed. Milton.

[8]   Sommerville, I. 2001. *Software Engineering*. 6th ed. Essex: Pearson Education Limited.

Review Questions

1. Explain why the clinical data is the most valuable asset in a health information system.
2. Examine the Request for Tender document outline, above, and briefly describe what might be found in the compliance section of an RFT for a new order entry system in your country.
3. Discuss performance improvements when clinical data are distributed across different areas (geographical or functional) of the organization for: a) a system that still uses paper-based records; and b) a system that has implemented a complete electronic health record.
4. Examine the features of a "future-proof" health information system as suggested by Blobel et al. (2007). Why is user acceptance found in this list? And who do you think are the users to whom the authors are referring?
5. Explain why requirements specifications are about "what" is required in the system and not "how" the system should be built?

Health Informatics
E.J.S. Hovenga et al. (Eds.)
IOS Press, 2010
doi:10.3233/978-1-60750-476-4-167

13.   Privacy, Security and Access with Sensitive Health Information

Peter CROLL[1] BSc (hons), PhD (Sheff), FACS, FBCS CITP, CEng,
Director, Better Life ICT, Brisbane, Qld Australia

Abstract. This chapter gives an educational overview of:

- Confidentiality issues and the challenges faced;
- The fundamental differences between privacy and security;
- The different access control mechanisms;
- The challenges of Internet security;
- How 'safety and quality' relate to all the above.

Keywords. Code of Ethics, Confidentiality, Privacy, Personal Information, Sensitive Information, Computer Security, Legislation& Jurisprudence, Professional Practice, Access and Evaluation, Risk Adjustment, Safety, Informed Consent

Introduction

In matters of health we can expect some degree of confidentiality when dealing with a healthcare provider. How much will depend on the circumstances and who we are dealing with at that time. Let us consider two extremes of the spectrum when dealing with issues of confidentiality.

On the one extreme where someone was discussing their mental state with a psychologist we would expect the highest level of confidentiality to apply. The patient has taken the psychologist in their confidence and expects whatever has been said to remain with them. The psychologist may wish to discuss aspects with his colleagues to gain a better insight to the case. The patient would reasonably assume that their psychologist would not personally identify them in such discussions unless they had given their specific permission to do so.

On the opposite extreme someone might be telling a person they don't know particularly well that they often suffer from migraines. They would not subsequently be too surprised if this person then mentioned this to others, especially if this occurred in a public place like a party or social gathering. These extreme examples highlight the two key issues associated with confidentiality:

    1. Who are you telling, and;
    2. What are you telling them?

There are assumptions made regarding confidentiality that are associated with the type of person and how sensitive the information is that you are revealing to them. A person's type might be determined by their profession which in turn might influence the sensitivity issues.

---

[1] Corresponding Author: peter@blict.com

With the medical profession the need to establish the highest ethical standards has been evident for over 2000 years. This can be traced back to the 'Hippocratic Oath' believed to originate from around the 4th Century BC most probably from Hippocrates, sometimes known as the father of medicine. It has been the tradition for physicians to take up the oath, although this is no longer obligatory, as a rite of passage for medical practitioners. Translated from the original Greek, the excerpt in the Oath relating to confidentiality reads: "Whatever, in connection with my professional service, or not in connection with it, I see or hear, in the life of men, which ought not to be spoken of abroad, I will not divulge, as reckoning that all such should be kept secret." [1]. Physicians would encapsulate these values by ensuring that discussion about an individual's conditions be confined within a practice or department for the primary purpose of helping the patient concerned. For secondary use of information that can be highly beneficial to the advancement of medical knowledge, normal practice would be to avoid identifying the individual concerned unless they had consented.

The more recent advancement of digital technology and e-health is providing a revolution in both medical know-how and healthcare provision. But with this advance the traditional boundaries are being breached. The concept of confining information in written form to a physical location, such as a surgery, is gradually disappearing. The remote and high speed access that today's digital technology brings presents new challenges and not only with healthcare providers but for governments, the ICT industries, lawyers and individuals alike.

Until the advent of the electronic computer and high speed communications confidentiality has been much easier to control. With spoken and written manual records it has been much easier to direct one's sensitive information to the right people. Judgements can be made about whom you trust and how much you tell them. This can limit the amount of sensitive information that is available in any one location. Hence, even if you find out that your general practitioner or local hospital is somewhat lax in its confidentiality you didn't necessarily worry about this being linked to a central medical record that could contain your psychiatric reports as well. With a given electronic record system this may not actually happen. The concern is that you have to trust systems that you may not be familiar with and people that are unknown to you. The reliance on third party support is widely adopted with today's IT systems. With the many media reports of privacy violations with electronic based information it is difficult to know who to trust and how to judge them. IT privacy and security issues are addressed later in this chapter since they are an essential component in the trust paradigm. If you don't trust the systems being employed you cannot be sure that confidentiality of your sensitive information will be adequately handled.

Figure 1 shows the basic relationship between Confidentiality, Trust and Privacy. This has been introduced to help simplify your understanding of these important aspects. Many of the texts that can be read on this subject area attempt to define each term. Unfortunately there is not much consistency in these definitions. In addition, although many definitions are factually correct, they can be hard to decipher as to their meaning in any practical sense with the handling of personal information. Hence the following diagram is used to identify the key concerns. Later in this chapter, the relationships are developed further to introduce security and safety.

Before we look at privacy and security, let us consider why it is now more challenging to be sure about confidentiality with IT systems:

1. The key issue of 'who are you telling' might have been extended beyond just your medical practitioner to include others who have access rights (including non-medical technical staff);
2. The key issue of 'what you are telling them' does not necessarily get handled any differently inside the computer system (except in the rare cases where different degrees of data sensitivity measures have been built in);
3. You have to place trust with systems that have third party support (including maintenance and backup);
4. IT security is a challenging topic for all concerned and it is not necessarily well understood by the medical professionals who are responsible for good governance measures to minimise the risks;
5. The media regularly reports on privacy violations with computer systems and it is difficult to judge what measures have been employed to protect your information from similar occurrences.

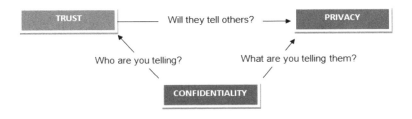

Figure 1. Confidentiality, trust and privacy mapping.

The key learning objective with this chapter is to appreciate what the critical criteria are for providing confidential IT systems used for health and to understand the best approach for achieving a trusted solution.

1. Trust with Health Information

The previous section looked at Confidentiality in the context of health information. We identified that there is a direct relationship with Trust. For the purpose of health information we have focused here on the human aspects of Trust. There is a lot of literature that now talks about 'Trusted Systems' in the context of computer systems that demonstrate high reliability, integrity and security measures [2] [3] [4] [5] [6] [7] [8]. These are important technical aspects and will be addressed later in this chapter. The reasoning for separating out the human from the technical aspects is because traditionally they are measured and handled in different ways. Attempting to use the same analysis techniques can result in widely differing results due to the types and range of users we find across the healthcare spectrum. When non-technical people are asked to gage their trust they generally give more weighting on perception rather than facts since IT systems, topics like reliability, security and integrity are all complex and technically demanding to comprehend. Technical people can be frustrated by these perceptions, as is evident in the electronic banking sector, but are now adopting measures to accommodate perceived fears [9].

The relationship developed between Confidentiality and Trust was "Who are you Telling". Note that the emphasis here is on 'Who' not 'What'. For the average member of the public the Trust they place on a computer system will depend mostly on who owns and operates it. People generally trust their Doctors and other qualified medical staff. They extend this trust to the services and equipment they employ in the doctor's practice. Only in the infrequent cases where the patient is knowledgeable about the computer systems being used and the manner that the medical staff use them can they make any informed judgement. In the absence of direct health IT knowledge, or any adverse prior experience of these IT systems failing, they rely heavily on their perception. Hence, from the view of the general public, Trust relates more with the people they deal with. This extends beyond the public since many medical staff are often just as poorly informed with the technical side of computing. Finding the truth requires this in-depth technical knowledge. Unlike other safety conscious industries, such as aviation, there is no mandatory investigation or central reporting facility when computers fail. It is therefore difficult to locate a trusted body of knowledge that can provide objective answers to the reliability and integrity of a given IT system.

2. Privacy with Health Information

Everyone is in agreement that Privacy is a high priority when dealing with Health Information. The response on how to deal with Privacy does get confused with the measures needed for IT Security. How they differ is explained through examples given below. Attaining absolute privacy is not particularly conducive with healthcare. If we adopt the definition of privacy as "*a person's right to be left alone*" then it would be obvious that they could not be left completely alone as healthcare requires some interaction with the person and knowledge of their condition.

The expression 'striking the right balance' is often used to describe how issues of privacy need to be weighed against benefit for the patients. This is particularly evident when health data is used for research purposes. The balance being struck here is the risk of privacy violation against the outcomes of for the good of the public. Looking at health data, even if the patients identifying information has been removed, this runs the risk that someone might be able to determine to whom that data belongs. This is particularly true when either the individual in question is known by the researcher or the individual has either unique or an unusual set of conditions making them easier to trace. So when data is used or presented there is always some privacy risk. Measures can be put in place to minimise these risks are discussed later in this chapter. The public good aspect refers to what positive outcomes can be derived from allowing health data to be used for research purposes. It may provide new valuable knowledge in population health studies or help identify an outbreak of an infectious disease. Too rigid a privacy policy will limit the effectiveness of health knowledge discovery while too loose a policy may result in an unacceptable number of privacy violations.

Finding the right balance for research can be ascertained by an ethics committee who will judge the risks and benefits. From an individual's perspective it is less clear how this is achieved. Many privacy advocates stress the need for individuals to have 'control' over their personal data. The law of most countries that have health privacy legislation usually allow for individuals to have the 'right' to determine the privacy of their data. Having the right and having control are not the same thing. Since, with IT systems, the patients rarely enter the data or own the computer systems. They have to give up their control to the medical staff involved. To further compound this, medical staff usually depend on third party support to determine the degree of control they actually have. That is, control is determined by the applications, the operating systems, the database systems, the policies and procedures of the organisation and IT or technical staff.

This emphasises the relationship between Trust (of the individuals involved) and Privacy as shown in Figure 1 as: "Will they tell others?" We have to trust that the individuals involved provide a supportive system that will minimise the risk of inappropriately disclosing personal information. The supportive system stretches well beyond the IT system and has to include implementation of those policies and procedures that make up good governance of your personal information. For example, when admitted to a hospital or medical clinic where you are asked to sign a consent form that included statements about who can see your personal data and for what purpose. Privacy policies and consent forms are varied in healthcare. Some act more to protect the individual others to protect the organisation from legal recourse. It is usually the latter that dominates.

3. How does Privacy Differ from Security?

To appreciate the difference between privacy and security consider an exhibition that is displaying valuable antiques. The display cabinets can be made of reinforced glass and well secured. The contents are intentionally visible for all to see but kept locked to prevent anyone from stealing them. Now with an IT system such stealing might involve using a removable storage device such as a memory stick or even an MPEG player to remove data. This could also be achieved remotely via the internet or other network connections. A range of security measures can be employed to prevent unauthorised copying of information, e.g., firewalls, smartcards or one of a number of password protected access control mechanisms [10]. A privacy violation might not involve copying and stealing data but simply viewing it as in the case of the exhibition display cabinets. To view private information either on a screen or because your account access rights permit it may well be improper. This is more likely to occur internally within an organisation due to the IT security measures put in place but need not be the case if the system is configured to allow remote viewing. One of the main problems facing organisations is determining what constitutes an unauthorised person viewing a record and how to handle this in a pragmatic manner. Because of the way contemporary systems are configured some people have wide ranging access rights. For example, in Australia we have seen this problem emerge with the Tax Office and the social service department Centrelink [11]. From a medical view point, personal data should only be viewable on a 'need-to-know' basis. That is, the individuals concerned should be part of a case file, or they have given consent permission to look at their information, or their life is in danger, or access has legal authority (the legal issues are covered in the next chapter).

Consent is a complex and often emotive issue. It is not always clear-cut that permission may have been granted for general access within a healthcare organisation and, furthermore, each organisation and even divisions within the same health authority often develop and use their own consent forms. The legal standing of these forms again is often unclear and one of the reasons why, for example, the Health Informatics

Society of Australia (HISA) has in a submission to the Australian Law Reform Commission [12] strongly recommended changes.

When it comes to health information you cannot talk about security without reference to privacy. Health information relates to individuals, either staff or patients and any security measures must try to protect the privacy of that individual. Also, it is not easy to segregate these issues within any electronic implementation since access control, cryptography and authentification are essential security mechanisms that also provide degrees of privacy protection.

The simplest way to differentiate these issues is to consider health Security as the mechanisms used to keep unauthorised people out and Privacy as the way that authorised people can only see information on a 'need-to-know' basis. The two issues for health security access mechanisms therefore are:

1.   *Restrict to only those authorised and trustworthy, and;*
2.   *Restrict to only those that need to know.*

Figure 2 shows these relationships with Trust and Privacy:

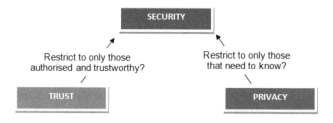

Figure 2. Security, Trust and Privacy Mapping.

4.   Access Control Mechanisms

Computer systems can employ a number of control mechanisms to provide privacy and security for personal and sensitive data. These originated as a means of limiting the damage that the inexperienced user might make on a system. That is access to certain files and programs and whether they could add, delete or modify them could be controlled to some degree at the discretion of the administrator (also known as the Superuser). This basic mechanism still forms part of the majority of today's computer operating systems and is referred to as a DAC (Discretionary Access Control) mechanism. Other more stringent methods have been employed such as MAC (Mandatory Access Control) mechanism that use specialised access control policies to mandate who can see and run all the objects that make up a system. Within the programs themselves RBAC (Role Based Access Control) mechanisms have been employed that specify who can do what based on the job function within an organisation. Note that this program protection mechanism is referred to as an 'application level' protection as opposed to 'systems level' protection. A systems level protection is much safer as any application level protection can be more easily bypassed by knowledgeable users or hackers. Whatever mechanism is employed no mechanism is 100% safe from misuse and the risks need to be determined and weighed up against the cost of protection. Furthermore, as security mechanisms are introduced then other factors such as ease of access and usability can be detrimentally affected.

5. Internet and Network Protection

The biggest challenge is to provide protection mechanisms that prevent unauthorised access from the network connections, particularly the global Internet. Allowing remote access can be highly beneficial to an organisation but that can allow for unauthorised anonymous users to hack their way into the system. The careful governance and auditing of accounts, use of strong passwords, restriction to specific machines and encryption of data using secret keys will reduce these risks significantly. With the Internet there are many occasions when this is not suited to the business model. Ingenious mechanisms such as PKI have been developed that allow for a compromise yet provide a fair degree of security. PKI stands for Public Key Infrastructure which is a method of using publicly available access keys together with trusted third party authorities to allow medium level security remote access for the general public across the internet. Public key certificates and the associated asymmetric cryptography is sophisticated and complex and hence often misunderstood. It is therefore frequently and inappropriately suggested as the best solution for many problems in healthcare internet security. It has a role to play like the many solutions that are commercially available but will not necessarily provide the degree of security and privacy that sensitive health information requires. The failing is not necessarily the mechanisms employed but how they are governed and more importantly how well protected the personal computers are that connect to the network. Ensuring good Internet protection will remain a challenging problem for the foreseeable future.

6. Safety and Quality

Since the publication of the alarming rates of safety in public hospitals the drive towards safety and quality has been intensified. The report 'To Err is Human...' showed that error rates and fatalities far exceeded any other industry including the automotive one [13]. Computerised systems were regarded as an essential tool to reduce errors, particularly in areas of medication management. For example, doctor's handwriting has always been notoriously difficult to read and the use of printed pharmaceutical prescriptions together with the ability to do some automatic checks on dosage, interactions etc. should dramatically reduce some of these errors. Compared with pen and paper computer systems are a more complex technology and can themselves fail in unsuspected and subtle ways. Any computer mechanism that is introduced to reduce harm should be assessed to see if it can itself cause harm. This is a non-trivial task as the level of understanding required to do a safety assessment on computer technology is very challenging. Awareness of these safety issues is very important especially when people's lives are at risk.

A safe system should be the central basis form which electronic healthcare systems are derived. As discussed above, security can have a detrimental effect on other quality factors such as usability and ease of access. These in turn can have a detriment effect on safety as there are many interdependencies in a given software design [14]. In this chapter we are focusing on Privacy, Security and Trust. For Privacy the concern is what harm can be caused by inappropriate access to your personal information. For security the concern is the harm that any modified or corrupted information (i.e. the data integrity) may have on safety. For Trust the concern is if the people you have entrusted your health with will do what is required to protection your information. These key issues can be stated as:

> Can what they know harm you;
> Can poor integrity harm you, and;
> Will the people you trust protect you?

Figure 3 completes the picture in terms of Privacy, Security, Confidentiality and Trust by placing Safety as the central issue.

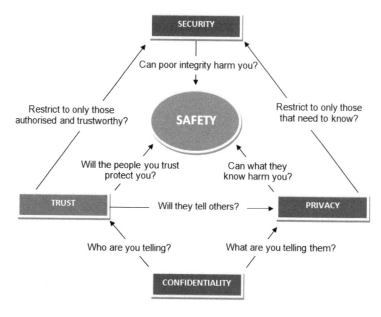

Figure 3. Safety at the Centre of the Privacy, Confidentiality, Security and Trust Mapping.

7.   Conclusions

Confidentiality is a fundamental requirement with health services. Its wider application with today's electronic computer systems requires adequate privacy policies and trust in the systems deployed. This is more challenging due to the common use of third party vendors to supply computer systems and the separation of control away from the medical practitioner who has built up your trust. Privacy and Security are often misunderstood terms that get used interchangeably. The computer implementations only add to this confusion by employing mechanisms that handle both through the same technology. The model produced in this chapter clearly identifies the complementary roles each has to perform for health information. Security mechanisms have been outlined that can provide a wide range of protection. These all come at a cost, not only financially but in terms of restricting other quality attributes such as usability and ease of access. Any quality health service should put the patient first and have the highest standards in terms of 'safety and quality'. It has been demonstrated that safety can be made the central attribute in a trustworthy system and the key issues that relate each property can be identified in an unambiguous manner.

References:

[1]   "Harvard Classics, Volume 38" Copyright 1910 by P.F. Collier and Son.
[2]   AS17799:2006 – Information Technology Security Techniques – Code of practice for information security management, Standards Australia.
[3]   Croll PR & Croll J, Privacy Compliance – Managing the Risks when Integrating Health Data, Health Informatics Conference Sydney, Aug. HIC 2006a.
[4]   Croll PR, Special Issue: Health Information Privacy and Security, electronic Journal of Health Informatics ww.eJHI.net, Vol 3, No 1 2008.
[5]   Jones, Safeguarding personal information, LEGISLATIVE COUNSEL'S DIGEST AB 1298, Bill introduced by Assembly Member Jones, State Legislation California, 2007.
[6]   Liu V, May L,Caelli W, Croll P Strengthening Legal Compliance for Privacy in Electronic Health Information Systems: A Review and Analysis, electronic Journal of Health Informatics, 2008; 3(1): e3.
[7]   Magnusson R, 'The changing legal and conceptual shape of health care privacy' 32 Journal of Law, Medicine & Ethics 680-691 2004.
[8]   PIA - Privacy Impact Assessment, Australian Government, Office of the Privacy Commissioner (www.privacy.gov.au), Aug 2006.
[9]   Croll, PR.& Morarji, H. Perceived Risk: Human Factors Affecting ICT of Critical Infrastructure. Proc. The Social Implications of Inf. Security Measures on Citizens and Business, pp. 213-222 2006b
[10]   Liu V, May L, Caelli W, Croll P, A Sustainable Approach to Security and Privacy in Health Information Systems, 18th Aus Conf. on Information Systems (ACIS'07), Dec 2007 , pp 225- 265.
[11]   ABC "Centrelink staff sacked for privacy breaches", news report ABC online, Wed, Aug 23, 2006.
[12]   ALRC   "Review of the Australian Privacy Law", Discussion paper 72, Australian Law Reform Commission (www.alrc.gov.au), Sept 2007.
[13]   Kohn LT, Corrigan JM, Donaldson M, eds. To Err Is Human: Building a Safer Health System. Committee on Quality of Health Care in America. Institute of Medicine; 2000.
[14]   Croll PR and Croll J, Investigating risk exposure in e-health systems . International Journal of Medical Informatics , Volume 76 , Issue 5 - 6 , Pages 460 – 465 2007

Review questions

1. What are the two key issues associated with confidentiality and how might they be explained in terms of health care applications?
2. Research into security standards that should be applied when implementing a health information system. Did you think they made adequate reference to privacy issues?
3. Explain how you might differentiate between the safety of a patient and the safety of a patient administration system?
4. What different types of access control systems are commonly used and which provide the best security?
5. Find out more about where PKI has been used in health applications. Do you think it provides good security and privacy for the applications proposed?
6. Non healthcare providers are now supporting electronic health record systems, e.g. Microsoft's health vault (www.healthvault.com). What security and privacy mechanisms do they provide and do you trust these sites – explain why or why not?

Health Informatics
E.J.S. Hovenga et al. (Eds.)
IOS Press, 2010
doi:10.3233/978-1-60750-476-4-176

14. Medico Legal Issues

Geraldine MACKENZIE[1], LLB, LLM, PhD[a], Hugh CARTER B.A., LL.B., LL.M.,
Barrister at Law[b]

[a]*Professor and Dean, Faculty of Law, Bond University, Gold Coast, Queensland,*
[b]*Lecturer, University of Southern Queensland, Springfield, Queensland, Australia*

Abstract. This chapter gives an educational overview of:

- An awareness of the legal issues involved in health informatics,
- The need for the privacy and security of the patient record
- The legal consequences of a breach of the security of the patient record.
- The concept of privacy law and what precautions ought to be taken to minimize legal liability for a breach of privacy and/or confidentiality

Keywords. Medical Informatics, Code of Ethics, Confidentiality, Privacy, Personal Information, Sensitive Information, Computer Security, Legislation& Jurisprudence, Professional Practice, Informed Consent

Introduction

It may be obvious that there is a need for privacy and confidentiality of the patient record, but the legal implications of a breach of either of these are not always considered and understood. Medical records are by their very nature intensely personal, and a patient must be able to have complete trust in the privacy and security of this information in order to provide it with confidence. Breaches can lead to serious consequences for a patient.

Because of a computer's increased capacity for storage, its enhanced ability to retrieve information quickly and the potential to network large numbers of computers, it is possible for a large number of people to have access to the patient record. Not only is there the possibility that this will result in the leakage of sensitive information, there is also the possibility that electronic records could be altered by unauthorised persons. Although this is also the case with paper records, the potential for harm where records are on paper is not so great. This chapter examines some legal issues in health informatics; in particular the privacy and confidentiality issues in the electronic storage of health records. [2]

1. The Right to Privacy

It is probably fair to say that members of the general public would be of the opinion that they had a right to privacy of their confidential health records. In general ethical terms, they do, but legally it is another matter. The "right to privacy" is somewhat of a misnomer. Generally speaking, there is no such thing as a legal right to privacy in

---

[1] Corresponding author: gmackenz@bond.edu.au
[2] All references in this chapter are to the law as applies in Australia.

Australia. There has been some recognition of such a limited right in, for example, the *Privacy Act* 1988 (Cth) which establishes rights in certain circumstances.

Most breaches of privacy will also be breaches of confidentiality, for which there are other legal remedies available. The *Privacy Act* was passed by the Commonwealth Government in response to the OECD Guidelines on the Protection of Privacy and Transborder Flows of Personal Data. Initially it applied only to "agencies" which are established under the Commonwealth, and therefore applied only to bodies such as Commonwealth hospitals, the Health Insurance Commission, and the like.

Central to the Act are the 11 Information Privacy Principles which are contained in section 14. They specify such things as the reasons for which information can be collected, how the information shall be stored, how access can be gained to the records, the use to which the records can be put, and the limits on disclosure of personal information. Principle 11 which is particularly relevant, states:

> "A record-keeper who has possession or control of a record that contains
> personal information shall not disclose the information to a person, body
> or agency, (other than the individual concerned) unless..."

A number of grounds upon which the information may be released are then stated, including: "(b) the individual concerned has consented to the disclosure".

The Act creates the office of Privacy Commissioner (s 19), who has the power to investigate complaints under the Act. If the Commissioner finds that a complaint is made out, he or she has the power to make various orders, including an order that the complainant be compensated for any loss or damage suffered. Because there had been concerns expressed that the Act was not broad enough in its jurisdiction, and there was a need for some sort of legislation to cover medical records more generally, ie, records held by State bodies and private bodies such as records held by a private GP, rather than just Commonwealth agencies, the *Privacy Amendment (Private Sector) Act (2000) (C'th)* was passed to resolve these problems. Taking effect in 2001 this legislation regulates the way in which organisations in the private sector can collect, use, keep and disclose personal information and gives individual people the right to find out what information is held by an organisation about them and a right to correct or add further information if the record is incorrect or incomplete. Some States, including New South Wales, the Australian Capital Territory and Victoria have passed privacy based legislation specifically related to health based information.[3] Further to the *Privacy Act*, it is also an offence under s 70 *Crimes Act* 1914 (Cth) for a Commonwealth Officer to disclose information they had a duty not to disclose.

2.   The Duty of Confidence

Breach of confidence in a minor matter concerning a patient may be bad enough, but when the breach, for example, reveals that the patient has HIV/AIDS, the consequences for that person can be catastrophic. A duty of confidence can arise in a number of different ways. It can arise by virtue of the ethics of a profession for example, the Australian   Medical   Association   Code   of   Ethics,   which   states:

---

[3] See *Health Records and Information Privacy Act* 2002 (NSW), *Health Records (Privacy and Access) Act* 1997 (ACT) and *Health Records Act* 2001 (Vic)

"In general, keep in confidence information derived from your patient, or
from a colleague regarding your patient, and divulge it only with the
patient's permission, except where a court demands".

There are also guidelines set down by the various health departments[4] These types
of guidelines can sometimes have a quasi-legal effect, as the courts have examined
them when determining whether a duty of confidentiality exists.[5] There are also statutes
in the different jurisdictions which create obligations for confidentiality of health
records[6] Furthermore, a duty to keep personal patient information confidential may be
an express or implied term of a contract which a patient may enter into with a health
provider.

The law also imposes duties in other situations where there is an obligation of
confidence arising from the circumstances in which the information was obtained. In
order to succeed in this type of legal action, the plaintiff (i.e., the person taking the
action), must show that the information has the necessary quality of confidence about it
in the sense that the preservation of its confidentiality or secrecy is of substantial
concern to the person taking the court action.[7] This would almost certainly be the case
in a doctor - patient relationship, and other health professional - patient relationships.
The second element is that the information must have been imparted in circumstances
importing an obligation of confidence; and thirdly that there must be a threatened or
actual unauthorised use or disclosure of that information to the detriment of the party
communicating it.[8]

3.   Negligence

Depending on the nature of the breach, the patient may be able to take other legal
action against the person responsible. This may be for example, because of the
negligence of the record holder in releasing confidential information. Taking such an
action can be very difficult, take a long time, and be very expensive. This can be a
deterrent in a lot of cases. According to the law of negligence, a health provider would
be liable if he or she owed a duty of care to a patient, that the duty of care was breached
by the health provider, and that damage resulted which was causally linked and not too
remote. As part of this test, the health provider would be liable if he or she failed to

---

[4]   See e.g., Health Commission of NSW Circulars No 82/369 and 84/82; Department of Health NSW
      (Hunter) *Policy for the Management of Acquired Immune Deficiency Syndrome and Hepatitis B*, 1 July
      1988; NSW Health Dept *Infection Control Policy for HIV, AIDS, and Associated Conditions* 1992,
      Queensland Privacy Guidelines for Hospitals, Department Standing Committee on Privacy and Health and
      Medical Records, April 1986; WA Health Department *Guidelines for Release/Access to Health Records
      1986*; SA Health Department *Guidelines Regarding the Release of Information*.
[5]   See e.g., the case of *W.* v. *Egdell* [1990] 1 Ch 359 where the UK Court of Appeal relied on the General
      Medical Council's *Advice on standards of professional conduct and of medical ethics* when determining
      whether a doctor had breached his duty of confidence.
[6]   See e.g., *Health Act* 1937 (Qld) s.49(1), *Health Services Act* 1991 (Qld) s.5.1, *Public Health Act* 1991
      (NSW), *Health Administration Act* 1982 (NSW), *Public and Environmental Health Act* 1987 (SA) s.42,
      South Australian Health Commission Act 1976 s.64, *Public Health Act* 1962 (Tas), *Health Act* 1958 (Vic),
      Health Services Act 1988 (Vic) s.141, *Health Act* 1911 (WA) s.314, *Health Services Act* 1990 (ACT),
      Health Services (Consequential Provisions) Act 1990 (ACT), *Notifiable Diseases Act* 1981 (NT).
[7]   *Moorgate Tobacco Co. Limited v Philip Morris Limited* (1984) 156 CLR 414, at p 438.
[8]   *Coco v A.N. Clark (Engineers) Ltd.* [1969] RPC 41, at p 47.

take the necessary steps to eliminate reasonably foreseeable and significant risks of injury to the plaintiff.

4. Avoiding Legal Action

The key to avoiding legal action, both for the sake of the patient, and in order to avoid being sued, is to ensure that proper precautions have been taken. This will include putting in place such things as: proper procedures for record keeping; adequate staff training on an ongoing basis; close and regular monitoring of these procedures, including adequate staff supervision; and review of these procedures making sure that they are sufficient. Taking these precautions will minimise the exposure to liability for the health professional. It is probably impossible to completely eliminate the risk.

5. What Security Measures Are Needed?

The question of what security measures have to be put in place to safeguard patient records is a difficult one to answer. There are no strict standards which apply generally to give guidance in this matter. Implicit in this issue though is the need to not only provide an appropriate level to cover all known risks, but also to have a level of security which is sufficient to minimize the risk of legal action.

What precautions must be taken depend on the concept of foreseeability of the breach. The courts have held that even though the risk may be unlikely to occur, it should still have been foreseen, provided that it is not far-fetched or fanciful.[9] This means that a record holder must take all reasonable steps to safeguard the security of the information. This involves taking proper security measures, such as password protection and not leaving files open on the screen when there is the possibility of access to them by unauthorised persons.

If a record holder takes all reasonable steps to provide proper security, and a breach of security still happens through an event which could not possibly have been foreseen, the record holder would probably not be negligent. This could be contrasted with the position where the record holder has not taken proper precautions, eg staff have not been properly trained, and a breach of security occurs. In these circumstances, the record holder probably would be negligent. Whether or not the record holder actually is negligent is a question which has to be answered in every case. The above examples are a guide only.

With advances in information technology it is now vital that organisations holding medical records take all necessary precautions in terms of information technology security measures, including the installation and regular updating of anti-virus and anti-spyware software, with the appropriate use of firewalls and other protective measures. Restricting access to medical records is the most critical factor. Medical records held in networked computers are particularly vulnerable. The potential for outside interference, e.g., by hackers, is real, and must be taken into account. It would be prudent therefore to seek advice from an appropriate IT professional in order to determine the security

---

[9] Council of the Shire of Wyong v Shirt (1980) 146 CLR 40, at p 48.

measures necessary. It must also not be forgotten that these will be subject to change as time passes, due to the changing nature of the computing industry. What is adequate protection today may not be so in one year's time, and almost certainly will not be adequate in five years' time. If no alterations are made to computer security measures to take account of the changes in information technology and changes in known risks, a person who has suffered harm by the release of the confidential information would have a far greater chance of establishing liability than would otherwise be the case.

6. Standards for Keeping Medical Records

There are no set standards which apply generally to the keeping of records, these issues are being addressed by a number of bodies. For example, the Royal Australian College of General Practitioners have in place a number of guidelines relating to information security[10] and confidentiality and privacy of health information.[11] Although the implementation of standards such as these is to be applauded, record holders adopting them are not automatically guaranteed immunity from legal action. There is still a need to be vigilant, and to note that information technology changes at such a rapid pace, that what is an appropriate standard now may not be so in the future. On the other hand, a failure to comply with these sorts of standards would leave a record holder vulnerable to legal claims should a breach of security occur.

7. When Can Confidential Information Be Disclosed?

There are exceptions to the rule that patient information must be kept confidential, and mandatory HIV/AIDS reporting is one of these. There are other times when access to the patient record is sought, e.g., for medical research, raising both ethical and legal issues. This has been discussed in a journal article [1]. In that article, he points out that disclosure of information in medical records for medical research without consent involves a breach of the duty of confidentiality. He then notes three exceptions to the general rule that confidential information cannot be disclosed:
   (1)   where the patient has consented to the disclosure;
   (2)   compulsion of law, where e.g., there is a compulsion to disclose information as part of judicial proceedings, or the mandatory reporting example given above; and
   (3)   where the disclosure would be in the public interest.
       An example of the third category occurred in the UK in the case of X v Y.[12] In that case information was supplied to a newspaper that two doctors were carrying on general practice despite having contracted AIDS. One of the issues in the case was whether it was in the public interest that the information be published. The court held that the public interest in preserving the confidentiality of medical records in identifying AIDS sufferers outweighed the public interest in publishing the

---

[10] See Criterion 4.2.2-Information Security unde the RACGP Standards for general practices

[11] See Criterion 4.2.1- Confidentiality and privacy of health information under the Racgp Standards for geeral practices

[12] X v Y [1988] 2 All ER 648.

information, and that this was necessary so that victims would not be deterred from seeking treatment.

A court in the United States has held that in certain situations there is a duty to disclose confidential information in order to warn others who may otherwise be at risk[13]. The cases of *BT v Oei* (1999) NSWSC 1082 and *PD v Dr Nicholas Harvey and another* (2003) NSWSC 487 in Australia have recently addressed this issue. In *BT v Oei* the court held that a doctor owed not only a duty to the patient as regards diagnosis and treatment of HIV, but also owed a duty to the patient's sexual partner. This duty to the patient's partner about testing and treatment., though, would be satisfied if the doctor appropriately advised and counselled the patient.

In *PD v Dr Nicholas Hervery and another* the court also came to the conclusion that a duty was owed by the doctor to the patient's partner, where the patient was HIV positive, but this still did not extend to breaching the duty of confidence owed to the patient by disclosing to the partner the patient's HIV status. The Doctor was still considered negligent though as he breached statutory reporting obligations owed to the Director General of Health who then could legitimately warn the patient's partner that she was at risk.

8. Access to Information

Contrasting with the situation previously where patients had limited (if any) access to their medical records, there is now much greater access available with the advent of Freedom of Information (FOI) legislation, although the record is still owned by the person who created it. Freedom of Information Acts are present in every Australian jurisdiction[14]. They operate to allow access to information held by certain specified public bodies and do not apply to private bodies, like private hospitals, or medical practitioners in private practice. In some jurisdictions, there is no need to rely on procedures under Freedom of Information legislation, as administrative access to records is possible. For example, the Queensland Health Department have since 1994 utilised a policy concerning *Administrative Access to Health Records*. This allows patients access free of charge to their medical records held by Queensland hospitals.

9. Conclusion

The electronic storage of patient records is now commonplace, both in relation to privately held records and records held by the public sector. This brings additional problems of privacy and security of the information stored in those records. With these problems comes the threat of legal liability to the record holder if confidentiality is breached. The only way to minimize legal liability and comply with duties of confidentiality is to be aware of the issues, and put in place appropriate mechanisms to

---

[13] See *Tarasoff v Regents of the University of California* 17 Cal 3d 425, 551 P 2d 334 (1976).

[14] Freedom of Information Act 1982 (Cth); Freedom of Information Act 1992 (Qld); Freedom of Information Act 1989 (NSW); Freedom of Information Act 1982 (Vic); Freedom of Information Act 1991 (SA); Freedom of Information Act 1989 (ACT); Freedom of Information Act 1991 (Tas) Freedom of Information Act 1992 (WA); Information Act 2002(NT)

address them. It is necessary in doing this to seek advice from computing / data protection professionals, and where appropriate, take precautionary legal advice. Not only should the legal issues be considered, but also the ethical and moral issues, because the information contained in the patient record is extremely sensitive and it is clearly the obligation of the record holder to safeguard that information. Only then will the health profession continue to maintain the confidence of the public that it presently enjoys.

References

[1] Thomson C J H, Records, Research and Access: What Interests Should Outweigh Privacy and Confidentiality? Some Australian Answers. Journal of Law and Medicine 1:95-108, 1993

Further Reading

1. O'Connor K, Emerging Information Privacy Issues in Health Care. *Proceedings of the Second National Health Informatics Conference* Melbourne, Australia: Health Informatics Society of Australia 21-25, 1994
2. Trindade F & Cane P The Law of Torts in Australia, 2nd edn. Oxford University Press, Melbourne 1993

Review Questions

1. Explain what legal issues are involved when adopting clinical information systems such as electronic health records.
2. Are healthcare providers able to ensure that legal patient information privacy principles are complied with, and how is that best achieved?
3. What are the legal consequences of non-compliance for individual health care providers in your country?
4. What precautions should healthcare enterprises take to minimize their legal liability for a breach of privacy and/or confidentiality?

Section 3

Supporting Clinical Practice

Health Informatics
E.J.S. Hovenga et al. (Eds.)
IOS Press, 2010
185
doi:10.3233/978-1-60750-476-4-185

15. Consumer Health Informatics

Jessica HO[1] DipPM, BN, RN, GradDipIT(software), MHlthSc, MACS, PhD candidate
Director of Interagency Information Policy Development (DIIPD), Australian Government Department of Defence, Canberra, Australia

Abstract. This chapter gives an educational overview of:
- The concept of consumer health informatics
- Technologies being used to empowered consumers today
- The impact of these new technologies on the health care delivery models

Keywords. Medical Informatics Applications, Caregivers, Health Promotion, Communication, Socioeconomic Factors, Personal Information, User Computer Interface, Information Management, Information Systems, Information Services, Internet

1. What is Consumer Health Informatics?

Consumer health informatics is no different to the other branches of informatics in healthcare other than it primarily represents the consumer interests and is about providing the consumer with the right tools, skills, support and knowledge to better manage their health care.

Gunther Eysenbach [1] defined consumer health informatics as,

"the branch of medical informatics that analyses consumers' needs for information; studies and implements methods of making information accessible to consumers; and models and integrates consumers' preferences into medical information systems."

Accordingly, the American Medical Informatics Association, Consumer Health Informatics Working Group [2] has defined consumer health informatics *as*

"a subspecialty of medical informatics which studies from a patient/consumer perspective the use of electronic information and communication to improve medical outcomes and the health care decision-making process."

Therefore, what differentiates consumer informatics from its parent discipline is not so much its technical substrata as the users it serves [3]. Medical informatics and nursing informatics professionals and their technical colleagues are accustomed to focusing on the needs of health care providers. It will take a different discipline and perspective to service the needs of consumers.

In a sense is consumer health informatics just technology hype? Individuals search for information regardless of the existence of technology such as the Internet. Any concerned individual will seek clarification and explanation not only from their own medical doctor but they also engage in conversation with their neighbours, social groups

---

[1] Corresponding author: jessicaho@grapevine.com.au

and friends alike. Technology advances have allowed these exchanges and information gathering to happen over the wire. This chapter highlights the differences when working with consumer health informatics.

2. Historical Context

The assumption that doctors (or nurses) know best when it comes to making health care decisions for their patient should no longer have a place in modern medicine. The doctor or nurses are or should be well informed about diagnostic, prognosis, treatment options and preventive strategies, but only the patient or consumer knows about his or her experience of illness, social circumstances, habits and behavior, attitudes to risk, values and preferences. Therefore both types of knowledge are needed to manage illness successfully, so both parties should be prepared to share information and make decisions jointly [4].

Consumerism, a market ideology of the 1980s, has infused health policy in many countries leading to consumers being more responsive and demanding towards their own health and well being. The problem with consumerism is that it encouraged consumers to make demands but failed to emphasise reciprocal responsibilities. The creation of static websites which dispersed health care information, health promotion and prevention directly to consumers such as Health*Insite*[2] using Web 1.0 technology filled this particular consumer demand. Consumers were confident with the information they obtained, especially when these sites subscribed to the Health On the Net (HON) code. The HON code approved subscribed medical and health websites based on its authoritiveness, complementary to the doctor-patient relationship, privacy, sources of published information, justifiability, transparency, financial disclosure and advertising policies.

Efficient and effective health care provision is a two way process, where the emphasis is on shared information, shared evaluation, shared decision making and shared responsibilities. The adoption of a Partnership concept is therefore a more effective policy platform for improving health outcomes which can be comfortably delivered through the Internet using Web 2.0 technology. This allows for more collaboration, content-rich and media-rich content and offers a user-friendly interface to promote social networking purposes.

According to Best [5], the characteristics of Web 2.0 are: rich user experience, user participation, dynamic content, metadata, web standards and scalability. Three further characteristics that Best did not mention about web 2.0 are: openness, freedom [6] and collective intelligence by way of user participation – all should be viewed as essential attributes of Web 2.0. Therefore, harnessing these new technologies may empower consumers and assist them in forming a truth partnership with their health care providers in achieving their desirable health outcomes.

However, a key ingredient to the trends cited above is a fresh openness towards consumer access to and contribution of, information. By contract the health care industry is moving more slowly towards providing consumers with online access to data and services, as evidenced by the Australian national electronic health records programs (i.e: National E-Health Transition Authority – www.nehta.gov.au).

---

[2] Health*Insite* is an Australian Government initiative, funded by the Department of Health and Ageing. It aims to improve the health of Australians by providing easy access to quality information about human health.

3. Empowering Consumers – the modus operandi of today's health care delivery

Today's consumers are seeking for ways to gain access to more information, manage their health outcomes and communicate with other like individuals. Consumers use a multitude of technology, devices, platforms and applications to enable the above objectives. The following describes the modus operandi of today's health care delivery from the consumer's perspective.

3.1 Personal Health Records (PHRs)

PHRs encompass a wide variety of applications that enable people to collect, view, manage, or share copies of their health information or transactions electronically. Although there are many variants, PHRs are based on the fundamental concept of facilitating an individual's access to and creation of personal health information in a usable computer application that the individual (or a designee) controls [7]. Some PHR models allow a range of information downloaded from clinical settings – electronic health records (summary), laboratory information systems, medication management systems and/or insurance details – into the PHR platforms where a consumer is able to independently decide about subsequent disclosure. Others require the consumer to enter their data electronically or download their data from a portable device into a portal which allowed them to electronically select the health care providers they wish to transmit the data to. Nevertheless, they all shared a few basic traits:

1. Highly useful – provide rapid utility and convenience by taking available data, making it digestible and providing immediate value to consumers
2. Easy to use – simple user interfaces
3. Free or Inexpensive – attracts high consumer usage

Technology companies such as Google and Microsoft see business opportunities [8] whereas Fortune 100 companies in their role as employers see efficiencies and cost savings when consumers can securely store, access, augment and share their own copy of electronic health information [9]. Notwithstanding, it is important to note that a PHR is not a substitution for the legal and professional obligation for recordkeeping by health care professionals and entities. In addition, PHR potentially carries a high risk where data will be out of sync with the health care provider EHR which may potentially be a health risk to the consumer. Synchronisation has to be performed regularly to allow the data to remain effective for consumers and health care professionals alike.

3.2 Internet Forum

An Internet Forum is a web application for holding discussions and posting user generated content, also commonly referred to as web forums, newsgroups, message boards, discussion boards, electronic discussion boards, discussion forums, bulletin boards or simply a forum [10]. They are regularly used by specific groups of people sharing specific common interests, for example a thread for a discussion could range from "How to breastfeed successfully" or "Should I administer Panadol to a one month old baby?" to "Where do I get birth control pills without my parents knowing?".

Internet Forum users may be anonymous, which allows the users freedom to ask specific questions regarding a topic. The comments and advice provided are usually from the general public rather than an authorised source of information. Users may also opt to share their medical history with the Internet Forum group. Some examples include the sharing of vodcast[3] of ultrasound images of in-vitro babies.

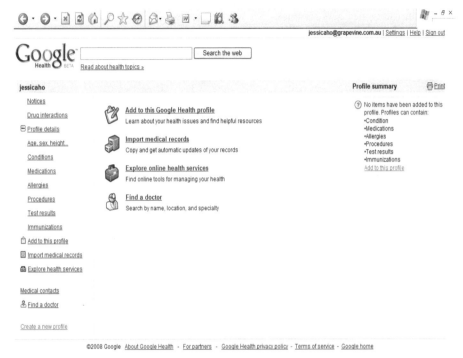

Figure 1: Example of the Free Personal Health Record System Offered by Google (https://www.google.com/health/html/about/index.html)

3.3 Wikis

A wiki (from the Hawaiian *wiki*, to hurry, swift) is a collaborative Web site whose content can be edited by anyone who has access to it [11]. Wiki can be used as a source for obtaining health information and knowledge, and also as a method of virtual collaboration, e.g., to share dialogue and information among health care consumers in caring for disabled children, or to allow health care consumers to engage in learning with each other, using wikis as a collaboration environment to construct their knowledge or to be part of a virtual community of practice.

Wiki features include easy editing, versioning capabilities and article discussions. Frequently, the consumer has to register to update a wiki. See an example of a depression wiki below, where consumers with depression can share their personal stories, and build a database of helpful information.

---

[3] Video podcast (sometimes shortened to vidcast or vodcast) is a term used for the online delivery of video on demand video clip content via Atom or RSS enclosures. The term is an evolution specialized for video, coming from the generally audio-based podcast and referring to the distribution of video where the RSS feed is used as a non-linear TV channel to which consumers can subscribe using a PC, TV, set-top box, media center or mobile multimedia device.

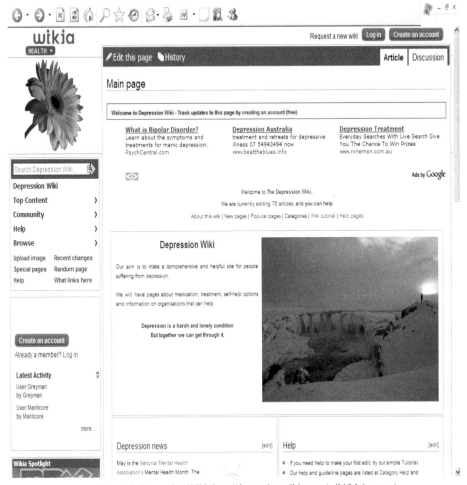

Figure 2: Depression Wiki (http://depression.wikia.com/wiki/Main_page)

3.4 Blogs

A blog (an abridgment of the term web log) is a website that contains dated entries in reverse chronological order (most recent first) about a particular topic [12]. Blog functions as an online journal and can be written by one person or a group of contributors. Each entry may contain commentary and links to other websites and images. Standard blogs include easy posting, archives of previous posts, and a standalone web page for each post to the blog with a unique URL. A blogger may post using text, videos (videoblog), photo (photoblog) to a potentially world wide audience on the Web. Consumer health related blog includes pregnancy diary, health products reviews, testing, managing autistic child diary, etc.

Blogs engage consumers with like interests in knowledge sharing, reflection and debate. They often attract large dedicated readerships who are interested in sharing their opinion and comment around a common topic within a community of practice.

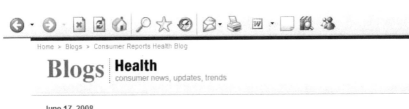

Home > Blogs > Consumer Reports Health Blog

Blogs | Health
consumer news, updates, trends

June 17, 2008

Looking for an excuse to barbecue this summer?

It's hard to know whether every suggested lifestyle change will really benefit my health. I'm more likely to pay attention if the reported news makes it very clear how the new study may or may not affect my future. So I paid attention to a recent study on how oily fish could protect against a common cause of blindness.

The study was a review of all the research on omega-3 fatty acids and age-related macular degeneration, a condition that affects the vision of about 5 in 100 Americans over the age of 60. AMD blurs the sharp central vision you need for activities such as reading, sewing, and driving, and can lead to blindness.

Researchers are especially interested in finding a way to prevent AMD, because although there are some treatments that can slow down vision loss, doctors have no way of restoring vision that's already been lost.

The new study found that eating at least two portions of oily fish a week reduced the risk of getting AMD by about a third.

Continue reading "Looking for an excuse to barbecue this summer?" »

🖨 Printable Version | Comments **(0)**
Posted to Natural health

June 03, 2008

Q&A: Pain relief from herbal products?

Are there any herbal products that help relieve pain and inflammation? —*L.H., Reading , Mass.*

Figure 3: Consumer Report Blog (http://blogs.consumerreports.org/health/2008/06/looking-for-an.html)

3.5 Virtual Coach, Avatars, SecondLife

An Avatars, is described as a computer user's representation of himself or herself, whether in the form of a three-dimensional model used in computer games, a two-dimensional icon (picture) used on Internet forums and other communities, or a text construct found on early systems (screen name)[13]. Avatars are commonly used in SecondLife, a game-like application where users are able to interact and re-enact some specific culture, event, activity and other concepts. SecondLife comprises of various diverse, user-driven subcultures. Users (referred to as Resident) in SecondLife engage in many activities, just as people do in real life, however unlike real life there is no biological need to seek food or shelter. Resident explores, interact and create new content. With the lack of pre-determined structure, the evolution of SecondLife society takes on to meet the wants and needs of its Residents. This virtual environment thrives on the interactions of real world individuals and their CGI residents or avatars. The avatars interact with people, businesses and organizations in a 3D environment. There are currently 7.5 million residents in Second Life.

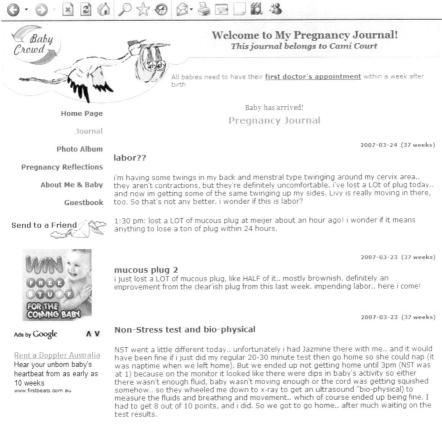

Figure 4: Pregnancy blog (www.babycrowd.com)

The Center for Connected Health in Boston is among those developing such a virtual health coach and studying its impact on users and professional staff alike. The aim of this program is to determine whether the Relaxation Response (RR), designed by the Benson-Henry Institute for Mind Body Medicine, can be successfully taught using the medium Second Life. Research in stress reduction treatment has revealed positive physical and mental benefits to patients.

Other examples include the commercially available EEG headband to allow a person to control a character walking around the SecondLife virtual world, all through raw brain power. Keio University in Japan is investigating its potential to be further customized for use by disabled individuals.

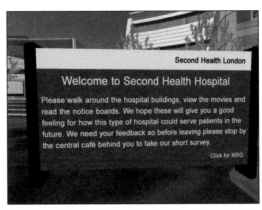

Figure 5: The Imperial College of London's Virtual Hospital (http://secondhealth.wordpress.com/)

Notwithstanding all the new disruptive technology described above, the most important and relevant sources of information for consumers are still the 'official' sites or portal which are supported by Governments directly or by the health care organizations. The diffusion of e-Health related patient empowerment tools is favored by the general actions promoting e-Health and information society (technology push), as well as specific consumer demands, in addition to benefits perceived by medical organizations, health care professional and Government (market pull). Simultaneously there is also resistance, originating from health care organizations, health care professionals and consumers with concerns such as the practical relative slow pace of adoption and day by day use of e-Health tools. Consumers will be more motivated to use e-Health systems that produce visible benefits and solving real actual needs.

4. Issues Associated With Consumer Health Informatics

As consumers, there are many inherent risks associated with using unverified and unidentifiable information and advice made available through the Internet or any new technology mediums. Consumer has to be able to distinguish what accurate advice is given by professionals, medical hypes and or purely commercial marketing from drug companies and/or individuals.

The potential for biased information that may have been developed by a person or organisation with a vested interest, may steers the consumers toward a certain type of treatment or medication. This could create an artificially high level of demand, which in the long run could cost society more if patients are taking medications that are harmful and not needed. The HON code mentioned previously, would be able to provide some assurance to consumers when access these information.

Access to networked computers and the cost of establishing and maintenance such as fees for Internet connection may also hinder accessibility. Other issues influencing access were physical barriers, such as those living in remote areas, and physical handicaps, hindering easy access to and use of computers. However, with the development of cheaper computer systems and Internet capable mobile phones for consumer and the gradual decline in connectivity prices, this trend may encourage consumer to use technology more often to manage their information and daily activities.

Other issues such as security and privacy are still a concern to consumers who may want to discuss sensitive health care issues, such as addiction and drug abuse. It may be a significant hindrance factor in major consumer informatics implementations if not addressed earlier.

5. Working with Consumer Health Informatics

An undeniably important aspect of healthcare is human interaction; caring and compassion to help patients navigate the inevitable difficulties associated with making the best possible use of our imperfect health systems. As technology and healthcare increasingly merge, it will be interesting to see how the social landscape evolves, and if we can achieve an appropriate balance of high tech and high touch in patient care.

As health professionals, the information we have traditionally been taught to impart to our patients are no longer your standard 1-minute advice as the patient is leaving the hospital: 'here is the list of your medications, don't get your bandage wet, some fact sheets about keeping your wound clean and come back and see us in 2 weeks'. Part of the new world is that patient/consumer will go out on to the Internet to seek their own Ix (Information Therapy). Ix describes the timely prescription and availability of evidence-based health information to meet individuals' specific needs and support sound decision-making.

We are able to engage with consumers more effectively to manage their care if we are able to improve our understanding and accessibility to Ix technologies. The average consumer's ability to access data and communicate electronically is proliferating exponentially and is transforming the culture of health care delivery. By providing consumers with direct access to networked data we essentially may have eliminated our professional gatekeeper role in managing their healthcare. The ability for consumers to shop for information and select their health care delivery modus operandi, although beneficial to insurers and payers, it may have eroded the way we have traditionally known health care service delivery. Health care providers have to ensure that they still remain relevant in the new world genre and be the central point coordinating the access to patient health care. Such a partnership is worth exploring as it will deliver the optimum health care results in managing illness successfully.

6. Conclusion

Consumer health informatics in an environment supported by health care providers and organizations will bring 'high expectations to healthcare relationships'. These expectations can improve the way the system interacts with the patient and the way care is delivered. It has the potential to transform the way health care is currently being delivered.

Many new technologies are developed with regard to empowering consumers in taking a more proactive approach to their health care. It is evident that consumers are also pushing the limit on how these technologies are used. However there are some aspects that lie beyond technology, which are part of the new social and relational context of the emerging more connected, more collaborative generation of consumer. The question that health care providers need to address is, "are we willing to embrace the new health care modus operandi" to ensure we remain in the centre of health care provisioning?

References

[1]   Eysenbach G. 2000 <u>Recent Advances: Consumer Health Informatics</u>. *BMJ;* v.320, pp 1713–16
[2]   American   Medical   Informatics   Association,   C.H.I.W.G.AMIA,   2008,
      <u>http://www.amia.org/mbrcenter/wg/chi/index.asp</u> cited on the 17 Jan 2008
[3]   Tetzlaff , L. 1997 "Consumer Informatics in Chronic Illness" *J Am Med Inform Assoc. 1997* Jul–Aug;
      4(4): 285–300. <u>http://www.pubmedcentral.nih.gov/articlerender.fcgi?artid=61246</u>
[4]   Coulter A. 1999 <u>Paternalism or partnership?</u> *BMJ*, v.319, pp 719-720 (18 September)
[5]   Best, D., 2006. Web 2.0 Next Big Thing or Next Big Internet Bubble? <u>http://page.mi.fu-</u>
      <u>berlin.de/best/uni/WIS/Web2.pdf</u>, cited 24/6/2008
[6]   Greenmeier, Larry and Gaudin, Sharon. <u>Amid The Rush To Web 2.0, Some Words Of Warning -- Web</u>
      <u>2.0 -- InformationWeek</u>. www.informationweek.com. cited on <u>2008-04-04</u>.
      <u>http://www.cnn.com/2008/TECH/02/21/google.records.ap/</u> cited on 24/6/2008
[7]   Markle Foundation, 2006 "Connecting for Health: Connecting Americans to their health care: a common
      framework for networked personal health information" <u>www.connectingforhealth.org</u> cited 3/12/2007.
[8]   CNN, 2008 "Google ventures into health records biz" Feb 21, 2008
[9]   Mandl, K 2008 "Tectonic Shifts in the health information economy" *New England Journal of Medicine,*
      vol.358, no.16, p1732-1737.
[10] Wikipedia, 2008a "Internet Forum" <u>http://en.wikipedia.org/wiki/Internet_forum</u> cited 24/6/2008.
[11] Wikipedia, 2008b "Wiki", <u>http://en.wikipedia.org/wiki/Wiki</u> cited on 24/6/2008.
[12] Wikipedia, 2008c "Blog" <u>http://en.wikipedia.org/wiki/Blog</u> cited on 24/6/2008.
[13] Wikipedia 2008d "Avatar" <u>http://en.wikipedia.org/wiki/Avatar_(virtual_reality)</u> cited on 24/6/2008.

Review Questions

1. Describe how you see consumers making use of their understanding about health informatics principles or consumer health informatics as a concept.
2. Make a list and describe the many technologies now available for consumers to use to support the management of their own helath and well being.
3. Explain what impact factors you see resulting from the widespread use of these technologies on current healthcare delivery models.

Health Informatics
E.J.S. Hovenga et al. (Eds.)
IOS Press, 2010
195
doi:10.3233/978-1-60750-476-4-195

16. Engaging Clinicians in Health Informatics Projects

Erika CABALLERO MUÑOZ[1] RN, RM[a], Carola M. HULLIN LUCAY COSSIO RN,
BN, Hons, PhD (Melb.Uni)[b]

[a]*High Risk Neonatal Nursing Specialist, Master in Instructional Design,*
Vice-President of Virtual Community of Child Health, Director of School of Nursing at
San Sebastian University, Santiago Chile
[b] *Co-Founder eHealth Systems, Santiago, Chile, Melbourne, Australia*

Abstract. This chapter gives an educational overview of:
- The importance of the engagement of clinicians within a health informatics project
- Strategies required for an effective involvement of clinicians throughout a change management process within a clinical context for the implementation of a health informatics project.
- The critical aspects for a successful implementation of a health informatics project that involves clinicians as end users
- Key factors during the administration of changes during the implementation of an informatics project for an information system in clinical practice

Keywords. Medical Informatics, Communication, Socioeconomic Factors, Computer Literacy, Information Systems, Health, Project Management, Change Management, Clinical Governance, Risk Management, Safety

Introduction

The effective involvement and engagement of clinicians within a Health informatics Project is essential for the safety of patients. Engaging clinicians is one of the success factors within the context where clinical health informatics projects are undertaken. In a Latino American context these types of projects are viewed as innovation penetration to their healthcare facilities and work practices. This is a significant factor associated with the delivery of healthcare services when there no clinical staff resources to spare, especially in developing countries where there is a heavy reliance on a public health system approach. It is important and critical to view the implementation of an information system as a means to educate all clinicians about the real benefits of using information and communication technologies to support daily work and how their trust regarding a health informatics project is critical for an appropriate implementation plan and deployment in their local clinical context to benefit patients.

One of the most relevant aspects of managing a Health informatics Project is the way clinical users change their practice especially given that new innovations are not usually positively welcomed. Sometimes such projects are viewed as an obstacle to providing

---

[1] Corresponding author: ecaballero@uss.cl

humanistic care to their patients. A health informatics project is expected to progress effectively following the engagement of clinicians since they will take ownership of the new technology for their workplace as a work tool based on evidence of cost effectiveness, quality of data and information. This especially reflects back to their organization's quality of services and their acceptance of these technologies to support their daily workflow.

This chapter aims to analyse some of those critical aspects that should include a health informatics Project in order to effectively engage clinicians' throughout all the stages of implementing an information system for clinical practice. The Latin-American context is viewed in detail based on these authors professional experience at the clinical and educational levels amongst healthcare professionals in Chile and Australia. It is argued that the incorporation of clinicians within any health informatics project, including not only in a project's implementation stages but also in the planning and designing stages.

1.   Health Informatics Projects

The introduction of a health information system needs to be carefully considered in order to acknowledge the right engagement of clinicians. Within a clinical context, this determines the success level of such a system implementation within any healthcare facility [1]. Also, the potential changes expected to have an impact upon the organization resulting from a clinical system implementation need to be considered at the level of risk factors for patient care delivery. Usually implementation of these systems requires a significant shift from the manner workflow was conducted before an information system is placed. This is where a leader of the project needs to engage all the healthcare professionals expected to use a new information system. At the same time, the manager and administrator of a health informatics project may not be the same as the actor viewed as the clinical leader who the users look up to for guidance throughout the implementation process. Consequently, the project manager is an important member of the team for engaging clinicians in an effective manner by providing realistic expectations from all involved with defined roles, especially where the clinical champion is viewed as a leader of their professional peers.

It is well recognised within clinical practice that the positive participation from the clinicians at the bedside will guarantee the right adoption and use of information systems for daily work duties so that an information system will not become an obstacle for patient care delivery. It is a challenge for all stakeholders involved within an organization to effectively implement a health information system since this means lots of changes of current work practice and to the way healthcare services are provided to their community.

Success of a health informatics project requires a strong leadership approach as a component of the strategies adopted for engaging all clinicians effectively. This enables the adoption of the most appropriate implementation strategies for managing change, specifically the manner risk management is handled. Not involving bedside care giving clinicians is known to have a negative impact on the organization's return of investment.

Ruiz & Molina [2] indicate some of the elements that need to be identified prior to the development of a large and complex information system (IS) in a clinical context. These include:

- The usual workflow procedures and practice
- The most essential information used in daily practice

- The profile of end users of the system
- The defined support team for before and after implementation of a system, viewed as a visible part of a health informatics project

The usual workflow procedures and practice dictate the specific information needs for the end users of an information system and how this will impact the clinical context where it will be implemented. The end users are viewed as part of a healthcare team that achieve effective work on a daily basis as collective decision makers for patient care delivery. In addition, this is viewed as one part of an integrative approach to join the clinical information system to administration requirements and management information systems.

At the same time, managing a project that ensures an appropriate engagement of clinicians, requires some steps to be taken in order to incorporate the processes needed by them as end users into the new information system, these include:

1) a plan of design,
2) plan of development,
3) plan of specific actions and
4) a change management approach for implementation.

This planning process needs to be confined to the defined scope of the project itself. This will indicate explicitly how far an information system is going to meet the clinical user needs and support current work processes. The success level of adoption and adaption of an information system to the daily routine work depends on the clarity of the above stages mentioned.

Scope management is viewed as ensuring the right processes are incorporated within a clinical information system development process. Phases of developing a well structured scope plan of actions may include:

a) scope planning,
b) definition of scope,
c) verification of scope and
d) controlling unexpected changes and potential risks.

Time management of a health informatics project ensures that all planned timelines are met. This requires:

a) action definition,
b) sequences of actions,
c) estimation of duration of each action,
d) development times and events,
e) time control by hours.

Cost management, allows the health informatics project to meet a prescribed budget that includes:

a) plan of resources available,
b) estimation of cost for each stage,
c) Cost control.

Quality Management of the health informatics project is required for satisfying all stakeholders involved in all events of the implementation stages. These steps are:

a) plan of quality measurement,
b) ensuring quality outputs of the clinical systems in terms of quality of data and information, and
c) control and monitoring systems for ensuring quality of services by using the information system.

Human resources management is critical for engaging the right clinicians at the right clinical context for implementing an information system for their practice. Stages that will be analysed in detail in this chapter that are required for an effective outcome involves:

- Organizational plan
- Approach definition to effectively involve human personnel and end users
- Definition of the development team

Communication management describes all the right processes required for ensuring the right time for each event, recollection, dissemination, storage, utilisation and re-utilisation of the information required for overall health informatics project. Some steps of this communication management are:

- Communication plan
- Information distribution among all stakeholders of the Project
- Productivity monthly reports to all interested parties
- Closure all the administration steps

Risk Management is the identification and analysis of the manner risks are handled within a health informatics project. This requires:

- Identification of potential risks
- Prioritisation of risks and its impact to the project
- Prevention measures to identified risks
- Quantification of risks
- Structured respond to risks
- Respond control approach to risks

Managing services during the implementation of a health informatics project requires a description of the processes that are required to be undertaken to ensure appropriate resources are allocated enabling these processes to be handled adequately during the implementation period. This includes the following actions:

- Services plan
- Requesting resources and services plan
- Providers selection plan
- Contracts administration
- Completion of contracts

This chapter emphasises some of these aspects mentioned previously in order to secure the right involvement of clinicians as end users of a clinical information system. These aspects are viewed as significant in clinical practice including the human resources management, especially during the design and development stages of a health informatics project. Refer to the chapter on project management for further details.

2. Clinicians and Executive Involvement In a Health Informatics Project

The involvement of clinicians within an implementation of a clinical information system is not an easy task for all stakeholders involved since the resistance from healthcare professional is real and hard to manage. The involvement of clinicians during the implementation stages is critical for the right identification of their information requirement according to a study about an implementation of an Electronic health record at a public healthcare facility conducted by Delany [1]. It was viewed as one of the most important success factors within their health informatics project

Another aspect viewed as important for successful implementation of a clinical information system is the right involvement and collaboration between executives from a healthcare facility and clinicians from the bedside level of patient care. Areas for collaboration are:

- the level of quality of data expected by all stakeholders from the newly information systems;
- discussion of definition of roles of each stakeholder within the health informatics project;
- the cost efficiency of the information system for the given organization; and
- the approaches to gain full executive support in order to empower clinicians throughout the health informatics project.

Regarding the Project administration team, the main factor recognised as critical for the success of a health informatics Project is the process to gain an indepth understanding and acknowledgement of the world of the end user, clinicians in this case. This understanding will allow the right channel of communication amongst all the stakeholders to the project. Usually, communication amongst clinicians already exists, therefore communication about the progress of the health information project must make use of these means.

The role of communicating the progress of a health informatics Project to all stakeholders is a significant process of educating how innovation can improve their daily work in their organization. In addition, it needs to provide incentives for self reflecting in their clinical practice as a learning strategy that ensures quality of care by using a new information system for their practice. The elements involved in this process include:

- to know the competencies required to perform a given informatics task in their practice, such as the right attitude, skills and knowledge,
- to identify the appropriate users requirements for the information system,
- to reflect the philosophical model of care provided by the end users based on health expectations and outcomes, for example in the case of a Latin-American expectation is to provide patient care as a person that is part of a given family, community and defined society.

It is important to remember to gain an understanding of the competencies required for using the information system during the process. This will dictate the requirements for developing the appropriate educational and training approach for achieving a successful implementation process. Also, the skills and knowledge provided to all end users will reflect the best strategies required to manage change and unexpected risks involved from the users' expectations from the information system.

The above point is viewed as critical among clinical practice, since it is well known amongst professional peers that resistance to change is well lived when new information systems are implemented to their daily practice, therefore, including this fact as a prevention of risk is important to the project manager and the administration team of a health informatics project.

The manner to gain an understanding of clinical data requirements is to involve the clinicians from the bed side into modelling their information needs for decision making, this will allow an active involvement in their own semantics to explicitly demonstrate their key requirements of data, information and knowledge for an information system. All the findings of the information modelling will provide the requirements for implementing an information system for their daily work, since the active collaboration from the clinicians as end users will provide the strategies that can be used for designing the system; the manner to test the system before going alive, and openly discuss with the users the expectations from the system to their daily work. This has been proven to effectively reduce the resistance to change among clinical practice and ensure active participation from all stakeholders during a health informatics project.

3.   Managing Change in Health Informatics Projects and Specific Strategies

The following section effectively analyses some of the successful strategies that work in clinical practice when implementing an information system for their daily work. All are directly related to the clinical requirements and organizational needs as a manner to evaluate the positive involvement of end users, in this case clinicians.

3.1 Administration and Management Strategies

Approaches to ensure the positive inclusion of clinicians into all the stages of developing an information system, requires the inclusion of different approaches in order to meet all stakeholders expectations. For example, from an administration and management perspective, the new information system needs to meet the organizational strategic directions as a healthcare facility, while for a clinical system, this needs to meet clinical outcomes following patient care delivery. The objective of a health informatics project needs to be explicitly reflective of daily work in order to achieve success. The integration of all systems into a health information system would be most effective. In practise each information system is developed in a progressive manner leaving enough space for fragmented systems within an organization. Also, the stakeholders that participate in the decision making for selecting an information system for clinical practice may not be the end users themselves. Clinical systems have only recently been viewed as significant for patient safety. Also the technology has recently achieved a maturity level to provide the right information to the right end users.

Some elements administrators and Project Managers need to be aware of include an understanding of having a correct system architecture for the overall requirements of the healthcare facility. In practice, the new system needs to be compliant with some type of standards enabling the technical requirements and clinical needs to be met. In addition, the understanding of the competencies required from their personnel in terms of training and education programs need to be carefully considered as a strategy to manage the change process the organization needs to go through. This strategy is significant from a management point of view since the training process will inform all end users about the organization's mission, vision and strategic direction as a healthcare facility. All these should be part of the implementation components of a health informatics project within a given context.

3.2 Organizational Analysis of Previous Learning Process and Change Management

An aspect that is viewed as fundamental for assessing the readiness of a health care facility for implementing an information system is the analysis of their workplace culture and their understanding of their own current organisational structure of decision making. This will determine the approach required to manage change and how to achieve the effective changes required to improve their daily work and health outcomes by using an information system, especially at the bedside level.

The results of an analysis of their workplace culture is a significant factor to know before implementing an information system in order to achieve a successful acceptance level from the end users. The approach to gain an understanding of their workplace culture includes an analysis of their daily routine, seek the frequent work symbols of information they use on regular basis, search for their work local myths and their clinical ideology for providing healthcare to their patients. Some techniques to achieve this understanding are a) conducting focus groups amongst all the stakeholders, especially within clinical groups of healthcare professionals and b) the creation of users group amongst clinical practice specialties. In clinical practice, the group of end users are viewed differently from a clinical model of care and the experts that implement the information system as a health informatics project.

A strategic factor to include for achieving a successful implementation process is to ensure the manager of the health informatics project is directly involved in training development and educational approaches to involve all the stakeholders. This factor will provide the necessary opportunities for the administration and management team of the information system to gain an understanding of the real requirements from the end users for using the new innovation to their daily work. Techniques to achieve this include: tutorial delivery, local assessment information needs, end users group meetings on request in order to empower clinicians and facilitate positive participation for decision making during the health informatics project.

Working with all the stakeholders of a health informatics project requires lots of time management and resources, but when clinicians feel part of this process they are prepared to change all the daily routines to meet the expectation of health outcomes. This involves real commitment from all the stakeholders that will be impacted by the information system implementation.

Within a health informatics project a change agent will be identified, some of those clinicians are positive for the overall aim, while others will find this most challenging. An aspect for any implementation process is the handling of the negative change agent within a clinical context. Some strategies that may work to handle this situation are, the involvement of all stakeholders and especially the resistant end users to inform them about the decision making process for implementing an information system for daily practice. The most transparent the communication process is kept the less anxiety level will be experienced by end users that refuse to change their daily practice. This is a well known factor among nurses who are over fifty years old, especially in the aging population of healthcare professionals that is part of this generation within a health system. It is a significant factor to include when planning a major change of clinical practice by implementing an information system, this will avoid the risk of duplicating data, production of clinical errors and generation of wrong information from healthcare delivery.

This organizational analysis in the context where the information system will be implemented will provide and determine the level of risk involved in actively engaging clinicians for achieving success in the overall health informatics project. Some factors to include in the risk management planning include: possible clinical scenarios and potential obstacles to achieve data entry from the end user, the way clinicians are expected to change their current workflow, specially in their daily work and how this correlated with current needs for patient care delivery.

3.3 Evaluation Strategies

The evaluation of information system is a key element for a health informatics project within a clinical context due to the impact to healthcare delivery. Some evaluation strategies used in clinical practice for this reason include the seeking of information from the end users regarding their expectations from an information system's impact on their daily routine. This can be done as a survey using a semi structured approach or a more structured questionnaire measuring their information needs. Another strategy is to conduct focus group discussions before and after the design and development of an information system. This approach is very useful when creating the model of information for the system. In depth interviews of end users working in a given clinical context is another strategy. These are very productive for specialised clinical systems for example emergency medicine, intensive care units and/or aged care areas. All these evaluation strategies and approaches can be strengthened by documenting all the processes required for the development of an information system and by including effective real observations of the clinical tasks associated with the daily work.

The evaluation strategies within a health informatics project start before the information system is designed and keeps going during and after the implementation process in the clinical context by engaging clinicians as a factor for achieving success.

4.   Five Key Success Factors for Managing a Health Informatics Project for Positively Engaging Clinicians

In order to achieve success in managing a health informatics project by engaging clinicians, five key success factors have been identified as useful in clinical practice. An information system development cycle includes many approaches for technical involvement, however, the focus here is to actively view the information systems from an user-centred design and development perspective, which in this case focuses on active clinicians taking care of patients.

4.1   Well Defined Objectives and Scope of the Project

The definition of the objective and scope of the project will dictate directly the success level of the implementation of an information system in clinical practice. This key factor will clearly communicate to all stakeholders of a health informatics project the expectations and limitations of a clinical system for the daily work. Factors that need to be considered are: a) clear objective development by engaging the end users, b) creation of real clinical benefits by using an information system at the local level, c) development of self assessment queries to all stakeholders for identifying the appropriate scope of the project such as:

- What are the real improvements expected from clinical practice by using an information system?
- What is the end user profile who is expected to enter the data to the newly developed information system in the clinical context?
- What is the scope of the project and which clinical context is expected to use it?

Once the scope of the project is well defined by engaging all clinicians, this will clearly provide all the competencies required for all end users and project the appropriate requirements of resources for the manager to carry all actions required for training and education

4.2 Planning and Defining Procedures for a Health Informatics Project.

This Key factor is crucial for understanding exactly all the tasks and procedures required for a well defined health informatics project. This includes activities such as:

   a) plan of actions to achieve a return of the investment for the organization,
   b) plan of actions to achieve clinical outcomes explicit to the organization and/ or specific area of clinical practice,
   c) plan of actions to achieve empowerment of all clinicians involved in the health informatics project.

All these procedures require a well documented process that clearly defines the stakeholder who will carry out the specific action to achieve the overall aim of the health informatics project. This approach will provide the right strategies for all stakeholders to achieve positive results and ensure communication among clinicians are included during all the steps required for a successful implementation process.

One of the approaches used at the clinical level to achieve an effective plan of actions within a health informatics project is called Work Breakdown Structures –WBS, which consists of the decomposition of the project tasks into small stages or parts. This process includes:

- definition of key aspects to follow,
- estimation of specific times required to complete each stage and activities to achieve results,
- definition of activities that depend on external factors of the projects to prevent failures during implementation stages,
- provision of alternative decision making processes in case of budget constraints in order to complete successfully all the programmed actions.

It is critical to carefully consider the external factors of a health informatics project since this will dictate some of the timeframe required to prevent resistance from the end users. A technique that is useful at the clinical level includes a working chart with expected times for carrying out each activity within the project; this will allow a clear communication process among all the involved clinicians and stakeholders.

To achieve all of the above requires critical, effective and transparent communication approaches among all the stakeholders. That is it needs to be a regular practice among clinicians making daily decisions for patient care. In addition, a plan of adoption of the new information systems into clinical practice can effectively demonstrate the real benefits for clinical practice relative to the time expected from them to get involved. This is viewed by clinicians as a way to prevent harm to patients and prevent health issues with all the stakeholders within a health informatics project. As previously mentioned within this chapter, it is a focal point for clinicians that all clinical systems at the bedside aims to support the provision of care to patients, as a person who belongs to a family, community and defined society. From an implementation point of view, three aspects have been identified as relevant to consider within a health informatics projects, including:

- Technical functionalities - computational, as telecommunication tools, involving directly health modelling techniques that reflect clinical tasks. Vidal [3] clearly indicates that an effective technological development needs to efficiently include all the functionality specifications that a healthcare provider requires for their daily work , especially clinicians at the bedside in a healthcare facility. To achieve this, the adoption of standards for the definition of data, information such as classification approaches and terminologies need to follow health concepts effectively.

- Skilled personnel for administering and managing a health informatics Project, involving the health informatics competencies. This will provide the right skills to manage, plan, direct, control and motivate all the stakeholders involved in a health informatics project. The authors of this chapter are extremely aware that this type of personnel does not exist in Latin-American yet, however, in the last couple of years a strong need has developed for this type of workers within a health system.
- Change agent identification within a health informatics project involving the right clinicians and executives within an organization, that have the right skills to engage effectively all the decision makers at the right timeframe and right context. This is critical to maintain a positive engagement from all clinicians who do not necessarily understand the technology as a hardware tool but they are experts handling the data, information and knowledge require for patient care delivery.

4.3   Follow up and Reporting Processes

This key factor for success is related directly with the manner by which a health informatics project is monitored regarding the aim of the information system before implementation and how this was achieved in real time. It is important to actively report on a regular basis before, during and after the implementation of the information system. This factor is critical for engaging clinicians and keeping them informed in an explicit manner. A calendar indicating all the actions taken within the project and expressing the changes will provide the right channel of communication amongst the entire project team members. Late variations must be documented as well in order to maintain trust in the project from all team members and clinicians who are expected to use the information systems on daily basis. As a final point for this key factor, it is critical to have a well defined committee from the health care facility that can effectively monitor the project in an objective and proactive manner. This will ensure clarity among all stakeholder and a well structured approach to provide accountability for all tasks involved in a health informatics project.

4.4 Change Management

Change Management is the most important key factor for success within a health informatics project because any type of information technology introduced to clinical practice will impact how patient care delivery is performed. It is well known in clinical practice that changes occur within any health informatics project, however, the most important ones considered when engaging clinicians are the ones that impact directly on the safety of patients. Nurses will not touch the new information systems if they think that the new information system will reduce the hours they have available to directly interact with their patients. They may not verbally express their lack of satisfaction with the system, but they would not actively interact with the information system as part of their daily workflow.

An approach to manage changes in the clinical context is to ensure to have a well identified clinical leader among the healthcare professionals' team. The leader will provide strong direction to achieve the right changes in the clinical context by providing the right manner of decision making that ensures patient safety.

Change in clinical practice, is not an easy task since patient care delivery is complex in nature. However, if clinicians are involved from the early stages of designing an information system as a user-centred project, it is most likely that clinicians will change the appropriate elements to achieve success in the implementation process. Some identified factors amongst clinicians that prevent a successful implementation include, a lack of training in health informatics, a lack of understanding of computational needs for collecting data, a lack of clear engagement of end users at the clinical context due to different semantics between experts developing the systems and healthcare professionals providing healthcare.

4.5 Risk Management

This last key factor for achieving a successful health informatics project is one that can very easily impact negatively to the overall aim of an information system. Consequently, it is important to always incorporate a risk management plan to achieve effectively positive results. Identified risks are related directly to end user' past experiences with change and associated with information and communication technologies in their workplace. Consequently, the meeting of training needs is a well recognised risk of failure or success for an implementation of information system for clinical practice. This requires a well planned approach to prevent identified risks and leave some space for unexpected risk that a project can experience due to external factors.

The risk analysis for managing a health informatics project is essential as a manner to ensure the right resources are allocated appropriately for all stakeholders involved. This is very significant when engaging senior clinicians such as medical specialists nurses' consultants, expert healthcare professionals who are extremely busy in their clinical areas. In addition, this will ensure the time and space for all clinicians to include their code of professional ethics for the protection of their patients.

A scale that has been used in projects include a grading of potential risks such as (1) potential risk, (2) possible risk and (3) probably to happen, at the same time, the time can be defined as the level of impact to the project, high impact (3), medium impact (2) and low impact (1). This scale can be used as a numerical table by multiplying both results of the identified risk and measure the possibility to happen and assess the level of impact to the health informatics project. The results of using this scale will determine the level of failure by not controlling the risk involve in implementing an information system for clinical practice [3].

Finally, risk management as a key factor for success of a health informatics project is the manner that tasks are defined as potential danger for the implementation of an information system for clinical practice that has carefully considered contextual and professional factors such as physical constraints, logistics requirements, administration and the legal framework for ensuring the clinical areas are safe and optimum to handle a major change of behaviour for daily practice.

5. Conclusion

This chapter has described, in some detail, how clinicians can effectively be engaged before, during and after a health informatics project. The authors conclude that all the success factors, perspectives and approaches shared with the readers can be effectively applied to paper or digital system projects. All the elements viewed as critical for obtaining positive results were strongly based on clinical experience and real cases of implementing clinical systems for improving healthcare delivery. In addition, emphasis was given on the importance of engaging the right stakeholders to their part of the overall project.

Our argument has strongly focussed in the importance of engaging the clinicians not only for implementing an information system for their practice, but also to ensure the end users are actively involved in the design, development and deployment of an information system that is expected to generate some changes in their daily routine. This chapter has shared real techniques in-depth by describing how to handle the five key success factors in a health informatics project. As a background requirement for the overall strategy for engaging clinicians, education was viewed at all times as the most significant aspect that must be included during all the steps of implementing an information system to support clinical practice. Furthermore, the philosophy of caring for people must i positively consider how clinicians provide care models on their daily workplace, including the way transparent communication occurred during all project related activities and have as a focal motive to care for the patient as a person that is part of a family, community and well defined society.

References

[1]   Delany R (2005) Editorial: Success in Health Care - Making IT Work. Health Care and Informatics Review Online™ 7(1); June 2004. On line en
      http://hcro.enigma.co.nz/website/index.cfm?fuseaction=editorialdisplay&issueID=52
[2]   Ruiz González Francisco, Molina Tejedor Miguel Angel. Gestión de Recursos Humanos en Proyectos Informáticos. Universidad de Castilla-La Mancha. Escuela Superior de Informática, Planificación y Gestión de Sistemas de Información. Ciudad Real, 15 de Mayo del 2000.
[3]   Vidal Ledo María. Información, tecnologías y ética en la salud. Rev. Cubana de Informática en Médica. 5(3) ISSN: 1684-185. Online at
      http://www.cecam.sld.cu/pages/rcim/revista_9/articulos_htm/eticaensalud.htm

Review Questions

1. Explain the importance of engaging clinicians prior to and during the implementation of Health informatics projects.
2. What strategies need to be adopted to effectively involve clinicians throughout change management processes adopted?
3. List and describe the critical aspects for effective and successful system implementations in clinical settings.

Health Informatics
E.J.S. Hovenga et al. (Eds.)
IOS Press, 2010
doi:10.3233/978-1-60750-476-4-207

17. Physiological Monitoring

Mohanraj K. KARUNANITHI[1] PhD
*Research Team Leader, The Australian E-Health Research Centre, ICT Centre, CSIRO,
Brisbane, Qld, Australia*

Abstract. This chapter gives an educational overview of:
- the evolution of commercial physiological monitoring over the years
- the importance of physiological monitoring in an electronic health record (EHR)
- issues to be addressed to enable an integrated EHR
- benefits and future perspectives of physiological monitoring and its relevance to an EHR for patient care

Keywords. Medical Informatics Applications, Telemedicine, Computer Systems, Data Collection, Personal Information, Decision Support Systems – Clinical, Physiology, Medical Record Systems-Computerised, Monitoring, Standard

Introduction

Physiological monitoring is defined as a method of tracking continuously, in real-time, the vital signs of a patient, accomplished by bedside technologies in a clinical setting [1]. The purpose of physiological monitoring in clinical practice is to detect changes in the vital physiological parameters from the normal (healthy) range of values in the event of illness or disease. Subsequently, interpretations of these values are used to provide appropriate clinical management such as medication, electrolyte/blood replacement fluid administration, and diet to return and maintain physiological parameters to their normal range of values.

Reportings of physiological monitoring date back to the ancient Greek physician, Herophilos, a physician of Alexandria (ca. 460-377BC) who emphasised the importance of heart rate, from the radial artery pulse and a water clock, to assess patients with fever [2]. One of the first inventions of physiological monitoring device was the electrocardiograph (ECG) in 1887 by Willem Einthoven, which led to cardiac monitoring [3]. Even at this time, Einthoven realised the relevance of distance monitoring by trialling the ECG monitoring from his laboratory, connected by cables, to a patient in a hospital over a distance of 1.5km [2].

Although the importance of physiological data in diagnosing and treating disease began with the inclusion of the four vital signs: temperature, pulse rate or heart rate (HR), respiratory rate and blood pressure (BP) on patient charts, and the first instrumental recording of these signs, before 1900, its application in clinical practice did not begin till later in the 1940s. The vast revolution in technology since then, particularly the recent developments in the microelectronics in biosensor, microprocessor power and display technology in the last few decades, physiological monitoring has expanded to include

---

[1] Corresponding author: Mohan.karunanithi@csiro.au

other measures such as electrocardiography (ECG), electromyography, phonocardiography, non-invasive blood pressure, thermodilution cardiac output, blood gases (pO_2 and pCO_2), and blood pH.

The application of physiological monitoring has been predominantly in the acute care settings such as intensive care units and operating theatres. Many of these monitoring procedures are performed with complex bedside monitors that are capable of monitoring and displaying traces/waveforms of vital signs simultaneously. In recent years, these monitors are being integrated into clinical information system (CIS) and/or hospital information system (HIS) to become part of an integrated component of patients' health record. Moreover, there have been initiatives to migrate this into a centralised electronic health record. Aside from acute care, there have been also initiatives and developments in physiological monitoring focussed at the management of chronic diseases, in particular due to the ageing population. With the prevalence of chronic diseases and its burden on the healthcare system, there has been increasing developments in technology to provide remote physiological monitoring capabilities for patients to be cared from homes or the community.

This chapter will explore the evolution of commercial physiological monitoring over the years to its present state of integration to CIS and HIS in the acute care setting. The chapter will also discuss the importance of physiological monitoring in an electronic health record (EHR) and the issues to be addressed to enable an integrated EHR. Furthermore, the chapter will look at the benefits and future perspectives of physiological monitoring and its relevance to an EHR for patient care in both acute care and remote care settings. The fact that physiological monitoring has components of sensor/medical devices and bedside monitor to view the signals, the terms used through out the document would be sensor(s) and patient monitor(s). Both components together will be termed as a physiological monitor(s).

1. Evolution of the Commercial Physiological Monitors

A recent review on the commercial production of physiological monitors demonstrated the technical evolution of physiology monitors over the last 5 decades [4]. The first reported use of physiological monitor, called the cardiotachoscope, had the fundamental attributes of current patient monitors such as a cathode ray tube (CRT) to view ECG, a heart rate (HR) indicator, alarms for high and low HR thresholds, and a connection to a conventional electrocardiograph for printouts. This was later referred to as electrocardioscopes or cardioscopes and was first commercially produced for use in operating rooms by Cambridge Instrument company, in 1954. This monitor included a small round cathode ray tube CRT display and analog indicators. In 1956, Electrodyne produced a cardioscope mounted on top of a large pacemaker and introduced these as physiologic monitors into clinical setting, not specific to operating room use only.

In 1960s, intended functions and configuration features of physiological monitoring systems were similar to what is available in modern systems. Although numerous physiological parameters were technically available, such as ECG, encephalogram (EEG) or the recording brain activity, invasive BP, and temperatures, monitors were restricted to standard measurement of ECG. Modular pre-amplifiers were made available from vendors to cater for various combinations of patients and parameters. By mid 1960's, prominent vendors such as Sanborn (later Hewlett Packard) offered equipment in modular pieces for central monitoring of alarm conditions for HR indication, temperature, pacing, tape memory, etc. Sanborn also offered a numeric readout accessory module for blood pressures, temperatures, and HR. EEG monitoring became a common use during this decade for assessing the depth of anaesthesia during surgery.

There was also the development of monitoring all bedside monitors centrally from one location. Due to the lack of display technology to view waveforms simultaneously, at the time, central monitoring was performed with a star pattern cabling to a separate switching box that enabled monitoring of one bed at a time. From 1966 and onwards, vendors began to incorporate monitors with a larger and rectangular CRT which unlike the round CRT was better able to display multiple waveforms. The Hewlett Packard Model 7803A "Monitorscope" released in 1968 was one such example, in which featured a horizontal line progressing at the bottom of the screen with the HR as a bar graph.

In the 1970s, the impact of digital electronics and eventually microprocessors made significant improvements to the capability of physiological monitors in the presentation of the signals and real-time processing of arrhythmia and also addressing patient safety. The introduction of memory monitors incorporated analogue to digital converters and small memories to briefly store several seconds of incoming data, enabled non-fade persistent display of waveforms. First of these monitors was introduced by Electrodyne in the Computa View patient monitoring system. With the introduction of microprocessors in the mid 1970s, vendors such as Spacelabs, HP, and Philips began integrating HR information on the CRT display as a numeric value. Arrhythmia analysis of ECG signals was introduced but relied upon connection to an ancillary computer. Hence, vendors such as Mennen-Greatbatch and American Optical produced arrhythmia computers that would learn normal ECGs which is fairly standard with the modern physiological monitoring systems. During this period, General electric and Mennen-Greatbatch began incorporating isolated ECG inputs for patient electrical safety.

In the 1980s, there were significant developments in patient monitoring technology. These included more modular monitoring systems, arrhythmia analysis at each bedside, color displays in monitors, and monitors becoming computerized and networked. The modularity moved allowed a "hot-swappable" feature which meant actual parameter measured can be adjusted from one patient to the next. This meant that not all bedside monitors required the loading of all parameters but only those specific to each patient's requirement of monitoring. The HP Merlin system introduced in 1989 was an example of such modular system.

In 1983, Burdick introduced their Color-Trend monitor which featured the colour screen with different parameters displayed with unique colours. In the early 1980s, Nihon Kohdon and Spacelab introduced bedside monitors with arrhythmia analysis incorporated. Subsequently, this became a centrally coordinated feature of the central monitoring station from vendors such as General Electric, Becton Dickenson, and Vigilant arrhythmia.

Unlike the previous decade(s), where monitoring systems of different departments of a hospital such as emergency department, intensive care unit and operating room (s) would tend to have different makes and models of bedside monitors, a more standardized approach came into practice with the introduction of transport monitors. Transport monitors featured parameter modules that were transferrable between the bedside monitors of the same vendor. This meant that the same parameter module could remain with the patient independently of where the patient is transferred within the hospital and yet maintain the storage of their information and trended data. Examples of such monitors are Spacelabs PC Express (1990) and PC Scout (1994). Another standardized approach was to establish vendor specific monitoring network connections at many bedside locations, thus enabling network-compatible monitors to be connected on the monitoring network, at whichever location of the hospital the patients is transferred to. Unlike the transport monitors, this approached allowed the entire monitor to travel with the patient and be connected in their next hospital location of care. Examples of this type of monitor include the Spacelabs Quicknet Interface (1994) and the Siemens "Pick and Go" system (1996).

Another type of monitor such as the Spacelabs flexport (1990) was able to connect to other types of critical equipment at the bedside such as ventilators, pulse oximeters, and infusion pumps. This provided the capability of transmitting new data and alarms. The challenge for monitors was to be able to maintain the integrity of the different information of the equipment being relayed over the network. This triggered developments of monitors such as the Spacelabs UCW (1996) and the HP Viridia system (1997) to run standard Windows operating systems to interface with hospital information systems.

Another advanced feature in monitoring device was also the move from the bulky CRT display monitors to the monochrome flat and thin LCD displays in monitors. This enabled designs of a more compact bedside monitors such as the Siemens SC 9000 of the late 1990s.

2. Physiologic Monitoring in the 21st Century

Physiological monitoring systems have continually incorporated operating systems and network connectivity and highly software driven. Today's physiological monitoring systems have now become scalable to the type of patient across the continuum of care from emergency department through to the operating system and intensive care unit, as part of a health care enterprise solution.

To enable the ease of integration of physiological monitoring within the health care enterprise, the hardware technology has also shifted towards a PC model with built-in connectivity. Hence, the function of physiological monitors has changed from just a display unit to that of an integrated information management tool. Vendors have, therefore, risen up to this challenge by integrating information standards in their systems architecture at all levels of product design which directly impacts scalability and post-implementation support, as well as the ability for monitors to interface with clinical information systems.

Continuous monitoring of vital signs of less-critical patients and those at the end stage of recovery such as rehabilitation, who needs to ambulate, was enabled by telemetry or wireless systems of physiological monitoring. Although both are of wireless modes, telemetry system consisted of a vital signs transmitter that is attached to the patient sending signals over a radio-frequency (RF) through antenna subsystems, fixed within the infrastructure of a care unit. These antennas communicate the digitized data from the transmitter to a set of receivers connected to the nurse's central monitor workstation. Unlike the hardwire and telemetry systems with installations of permanent connections and antenna network at specific locations, the wireless system of monitoring has the advantage of being non-station specific and less costly on the overheads of healthcare institutions. The wireless configuration makes monitoring devices non-station specific and enable continuity in the monitoring being available outside the care unit and in overflow areas such as hallways, bathrooms, or during transfers between care units.

The wireless system approaches uses spread spectrum and cellular as communication protocols within transmitter/receiver pair on every patient monitors and central monitors. Although medical telemetry system has been used since the 1970s, its uptake was limited by the infrastructure cost of implementation, the narrow bandwidth limiting the number of patients' monitors being monitored at a time, and its availability to only ECG monitors. With the start of digital TV within the same RF band as the medical telemetry system, a designated RF band for wireless medical telemetry service (WMTS) was created in 2000,which has been developing since then [5]. The only thing that's going for WMTS is that the designated RF spectrum is protected for medical telemetry. However, there are still numerous flaws with WMTS that affects medical telemetry systems such as interference from hair dryers, fluorescent lights, and co-channel digital TV broadcasters.

At the same time WMTS was designated, the IEEE approved the first standards for wireless networking, which included 802.11 (also known as 802.11FH or frequency hopping), 802.11a and 802.11b. With the existence of both WMTS and the new IEEE 802.11x standards, major medical device vendors evaluated both options but differed in their wireless standards for physiological monitors. Welch Allyn chose to go with 802.11 standards. GE launched Apex Pro 5-lead ECG, non-invasive BP and pulse oximeter monitor using WMTS, while using 802.11 for their patient monitors. Spacelabs, Datascope and others ran their telemetry on WMTS, putting 802.11 in their wireless medical devices. Philips was the only exception, who decided on their patient monitoring devices (telemetry, patient monitors, defibrillators) to be on WMTS. The more recent Philips Intellivue telemetry system uses a smart-frequency hopping technology with WMTS protocol in their patient monitors and central monitors, which can co-exist in a wireless 802.11 network. The advantage of having monitoring devices on separate wireless infrastructure is the elimination of a single point of failure, such that if telemetry, was lost wireless system medical devices would continue to operate. Overall, 802.11 standard has proven to be more reliable and safe than WMTS and hence, has become the defacto standard.

3. Physiological Monitoring Interface to Clinical Information Systems

Clinical information system (CIS) is a system that interoperates with bedside monitors, bedside peripheral devices, and hospital information systems (HIS) in providing an integrated clinical information charting and data management support system in a local area network configuration [6]. Among other bedside devices such as ventilators, infusion pumps, etc., that connect to the CIS, physiological monitors are considered to be high-end bedside medical devices capable of monitoring all of the vital signs simultaneously in real-time with the capability of adjusting the number of parameters according to the patient acuity. Typically monitoring system network runs at 10 megabits/second with network utilization in the range of 25-30% of total bandwidth. As much as physiological monitors need to interface with CIS to receive vital signs and track trends, they also need to be in the same network with HIS to create or relate to patient medical record with important identifiers and billing purposes.

Although the physiological monitors are able to connect to the same enterprise network as the CIS and HIS, they often reside on the private network due to the bandwidth requirement and uptime guarantee. This is often overcome by routing HIS patient identifier data to the physiological monitor using dedicated gateways.

4. Developments of Physiological Monitoring Technology for Remote Monitoring

Recent advances in electronics with biosensors on microchips have led physiological monitoring technology to become integrated in wearable devices. This integration has been in the form of clothing, watches and jewellery. Similarly, advances in communication technology have led to these sensors being able to transfer data wirelessly. Using the oxygen saturation sensors that have been long used in finger based pulse oximeters [7], ring sensors are being investigated for vital signs such as arterial pulse pressure, heart rate and activity using plethysmography [8] [9] and pulse transit time techniques, in major universities. More recently, another similar innovative health monitoring wristwatch technology was introduced by Chubb Telehealth Products, but with a built-in Bluetooth wireless capability.

The traditional clinical practice of arterial BP measurement with cuff inflation around the brachial artery has been applied to developments of ambulatory blood pressure monitors using oscillometric technique by major vendors of BP monitors [10] [11]. The reliability and accuracy of BP measurement from such device depends on the wearer keeping the monitored arm immobile while the cuff inflates [12].

Of the vital signs, BP remains as one of the critical measures for the elderly for most chronic diseases, particularly with regard to the medications they are managed with. Reactions to medications can be different in each individual. Therefore, the availability of continuous ambulatory BP could effectively detect missed medications and abnormal fluctuations in BP. There is an ambulatory arterial BP measurement device that provides continuous BP that works on the volume clamp technique, called Portapres [13] developed by Finapres medical systems. Its application for everyday use remains questionable as it encumbers both a finger and a wrist and requires a battery pack to be worn around the waist.

A more practical approach to wearable monitoring technology has been explored to integrate sensors in clothing items on the basis that clothing is a daily part of life and the body is close to the signal source. Moreover, the approach of using the upper body as the area for sensing vital signs aligns with the region of vital organs and the current practice of medical assessments/examinations performed by clinicians.
Some initiatives in this field have been the Lifeshirt by Vivometrics [14] and Smartshirt by Sensetex [15]. Lifeshirt has been very comprehensive in the numerous physiological measurements it can provide, but its integrated sensors, requiring a cumbersome recorder and peripheral attachment to be carried around, deviate from an ambulatory use for a daily wear, especially for elderly patients. The smart textile approach of Smartshirt, uses innovative nanotechnology to weave optical fibres into the fabric to communicate with sensors and data collection, also embedded within the fabric.

Unlike the Lifeshirt, it is a fairly new technology with only limited measurements to ECG, respiratory rate and heart rate. Because of its recent introduction, it is at the testing phase and therefore, its potential application among the elderly remains to be seen. Smart textiles has become one of the thriving areas of application for nanotechnology research for the purpose of fitness and health monitoring [16] [17] and remains to be explored for durability in wash and wear.

5. Integration of Physiological Monitoring in Remote Monitoring Capabilities

Utilization of patient information monitored by the wearable physiological monitoring devices can provide two purposes: (i) enable clinician or other members of the multidisciplinary care team to assess and advise or attend to the patient in need of care; (ii) inform the patient or his/her relatives of his/her health status and progress. In most cases full utilization of such wearable monitoring technology in elderly patients would be in the assessment by the multidisciplinary care team to address to their care. To enable such information flow to the care team, the physiological monitoring technology needs to be integrated to an environment of remote monitoring capability such as in the infrastructure of telecare.

Telehealth is a component of the broader infrastructure of telecare that utilises physiological monitoring technologies by specifically focusing on home/community monitoring via remote monitoring technologies of patient vital signs to conduct clinical process. Some of the telehealth systems include: Chubb Telehealth Products, Tunstall Telecom [18], Docobo [19] and Philips medical system [20].

A brief description of these telehealth systems are outlined below. Chubb and Tunstall [21] telehealth systems have clinical telemonitors that provide individuals the capacity to monitor their own vital signs at home with supplied BP cuff, pulse oximetry and weighing scales. These data are transmitted over a telephone or internet connection to a database server where they can be accessed remotely by a clinician. Docobo telehealth system [19], like that of the Chubb, connects to a web based home monitoring service, known as "doc@home, for sending information from external sensors and monitors to the clinicians.

The Doboco telehealth system has a bluetooth wireless enabled Medical Device Directive approved handheld unit (called the Health Hub). The Philips Medical System has a TV based telecare platform, called Motiva [22], where a patient with chronic diseases receives a set top box to deliver the multimedia care experience and a wireless vital signs device. The patient data is made available to the medical care provider through a broadband connection for review and generate patient care plans. Another successful implementation of a telehealth system used in United States has been the Health Buddy system [23], for remote monitoring of vital signs via monitoring technologies, of advanced chronically ill patients at home.

In review of the above telehealth systems, there is a large disconnect between these systems and the integration to wearable monitoring technologies, instead they are mainly connected to home monitoring stations. That is patients have to interact with monitoring technologies that are not ambulatory but tethered to a computer eg. a BP cuff monitor). This may be one reason why most telehealth systems are confined to one type of care setting, such as residential care or home, or to a general practitioner/medical centre via a call centre, and not integrated into a healthcare service, where continuum of patient care can be monitored from the time of first admission in the hospital, to independent living at home and/or residential care. One model of approach for an integrating healthcare service infrastructure would be to have a centralised telehealth system that will network all physiological monitoring systems and the different healthcare settings (hospital, medical centre, home, residential care) of a region or locality, as described in a recent review on monitoring technology for the elderly patient [24]. This telehealth model would be feasible under a standardised interoperable monitoring, data management and communication technology environment. This would then make it feasible for the patients to adopt a wearable monitoring technology that is interfaced to a telehealth system, from the time of their commencement of episodic care in a hospital, through to their journey to a community care setting. The community care would include interaction with a community health centre providing remote monitoring services and guidance to patients in either homes or residential care settings. The adoption of such a model would not only enable a uniform streamlined approach in the care practice, in which care planning can be structured and followed with one system, but also allow patients to adapt to such a system at the early stage of care. Thus the patient's early introduction to the wearable monitoring technology during episodic care can act as a trial for the patient in a controlled environment with close monitoring by clinical staff, before they wish to adopt it subsequently, for their ongoing care at home. This will not only enable a smoother transition of care but also enable continuous patient assessment by any member of the multidisciplinary care team having accessibility to patient's monitored information from the one system or centralised server.

6.   Physiological Monitoring and EHR

Electronic Health Record (EHR) defined by the Health Information Network for Australia [25$^{p.Xv}$] report in Australia, is:

> "… an electronic, longitudinal collection of personal health information, usually based on the individual, entered or accepted by healthcare providers, which can be distributed over a number of sites or aggregated at a particular source. The information is organised primarily to support continuing, efficient and quality healthcare. The record is under the control of the consumer and is stored and transmitted securely."

The core data that initiates a patient's health information in an EHR is that from physiological monitoring of vital signs for his or her medical condition, whether it is from a general practitioner or the hospital as their first clinical assessment/examination. Physiological monitoring data again becomes a vital part of the longitudinal collection of health information gathered before, during and after diagnostic procedures (eg. medical imaging), interventional procedures, therapeutic (including medication) management, during patients' continuum of care.

7.   Issues of Physiological Monitoring and EHR

At the point of care, interpretation of physiological data from monitoring is critical, particularly in operating rooms and ICU. One of the common problems of physiological monitoring is signal artifacts that are displayed on patient monitors [26]. The sources of artifacts on ECG signals are electro surgical knife interferences, power line, movement artefacts during surgery. In invasive blood pressure measurements, artifacts are caused by pressure line occlusion, medication injection and movement of pressure tubing. Artifacts in pulse oximetry (oxygen saturation) signals are caused by movements and ambient light interference. Similarly other physiological signals such as non invasive BP, capnography (CO_2 levels in expired breath) and temperature measurements are also affected by artifacts. These artifacts can lead to wrong interpretation and false alarms especially at the crucial time of surgical intervention or emergency situation in the ICU. These data can also become inadvertently propagated into data recorded in the clinical database and subsequently migrated into an EHR, which are used for assessments, reporting, and retrospective analysis. To overcome problems of artifacts, engineering measures that need to be addressed would be two fold (1) improving the design of biomedical senses to be less tolerant of artifacts; (2) improving signal processing that enable better detection and filtering of artifacts.

Together with artifacts, interpretation of multiple physiological waveforms, alphanumeric values and alerts can become overwhelming to the clinical staff, as an additional task to managing the bedside monitoring interfaces and physiological sensors, and also normal routine of patient care. This will become more unmanageable with increasing workload that healthcare workers are currently facing to meet the increasing trend in nursing shortages and the population ageing. To overcome some of these problems, developments of clinical decision support system needs to adopt more complex intelligent signal processing techniques such as neural networks and fuzzy logic for higher level automated decisions. Although clinical decision support systems (CSSD) are prevalent in existing CIS, these models could be extended to fusion of data from different bedside monitors, medication management systems, pathology results to assist in therapeutic management such as the regulation of hypotensive drug infusion flowrate with variation in BP measurements.

Unlike the evolving standards of DICOM for diagnostic radiology images, data format of various physiological signals is still widely open for interoperability standards. Several generic formats for medical sensor data have been proposed such as the Japanese favoured protocol, MFER for medical waveform Format Encoding Rules and SCP ECG for Standard Communications Protocol ECG. Recently, openXDF was proposed as an open standard for digital storage and data exchange of time series physiological signals and annotations [27]. This data format for physiological signals is more likely to appeal to technology providers because it is compatible with the standard web 2.0 programming language for structured data, XML (Extensible Markup Language).

At the connectivity end of physiological monitors, like other bedside monitors, there is still an issue with interoperability between devices and clinical information systems. The same interoperability issue exists between other clinical information systems in the HIS architecture such as messaging information between ancillary systems such as that from pathology, pharmacy, medication management, emergency departments. While HL7 is becoming an accepted interface standard between clinical information systems and HIS, not all vendors of physiological monitors have conformed to it. Even if interfaces were standardised for physiological monitors, integrating physiological data into an EHR would still remain problematic as most HIS interfaces are proprietary. When a HIS does conform to an interface standard, there again many standards exist, such as HL7v2.x, HL7v3 CDA, CEN ENV 13606 EHRExtract, openEHR Archetypes, that prevents interoperability (refer chapter 11). Hence, creating an integrated EHR to share between disparate EHR repositories from healthcare institutions remains to be addressed.

Current shifts in healthcare to remotely monitor physiological signals in an ambulatory setting poses many challenges in adopting these physiological data in an integrated EHR, as part of a longitudinal health record. Firstly, wireless wearable physiological monitoring devices would need to ensure transmission of data over the wireless network has a wide coverage and reliability (and security), even at times of failure in networks. As a result, quality of monitoring should not be compromised in any emergency situation of alerts. Secondly, the streamed data format needs to be standardised and interoperable with the database system at the centralised server where data is transmitted, for access to various members of the multidisciplinary team. Thirdly, the communication protocol would need to be interoperable with other EHR repositories from hospital HIS and other allied health services which a patient may attend for his care.

An initiative to enable an interoperable architecture for an integrated healthcare with remote monitoring capabilities and connectivity to a HIS is being addressed in a European Union funded project, called Saphire [28]. The Saphire project is developing an intelligent healthcare monitoring and decision support system on a platform to integrate the wireless medical sensor with HIS.

To address some of the interoperability problems of proprietary data formats of wireless physiological monitoring devices, four layers of processing is undertaken. Firstly, it goes through the networking layer of Bluetooth and TCP/IP stacks for streaming the data. Secondly, it passes through sensor driver layer for communication protocol to determine the data structure. Thirdly, the data point layer is used to determine if a sensor driver is needed. Fourthly, the virtual device layer determines if another physiological parameter needs to be processed from one or more of the sensor data through algorithm(s). These data from the virtual device layer is then stored in a database and exposed as semantically enriched web service, which is used by CDSS.

Similarly, the EHR records are also exposed as semantically enriched web services. This enables data exchange between EHR and sensor data through semantic interoperability. Sharing of EHRs between healthcare institutions was enabled by Integrating the Healthcare Enterprise (IHE) cross-enterprise document sharing (XDS) architecture. With local repositories of EHR registered to an XDS registry along with a set of metadata, relevant EHR documents can be accessed and discovered from wherever they are stored. For CDSS to exploit data stored from EHR, EHR documents represented as HL7 CDA documents are published to the XDS registry through their metadata.

8.   Benefits of Physiological Monitoring and EHR

Benefits of physiological monitoring spans across many points of patient care from the early detection of medical symptoms to determination of further diagnostic procedures to therapeutic care such as medication management to tracking the progress of therapeutic management to the collation of patient health records in a EHR. This breadth and depth of physiological monitoring applied in patient care and everyday life as one ages, demonstrates the importance of accessibility such data in an EHR form, so that quality of care can be improved. Similarly, subset of EHR information in the form of personal health record becomes important for the emphasis made on self-management in remote monitoring care models.

The availability of physiological monitoring in an EHR form availability at any point of care anytime, whether in acute care setting or remote monitoring from the community or homes, has the following benefits:-
   (i)   Reduction in medication errors
   (ii) Reduction in healthcare costs by reducing unnecessary hospital and emergency department visits.
   (iii) Increase in the efficiency of services provided by directing clinicians to more serious cases of patient care.
   (iv) Increased access to care in rural and remote locations and patients living at home.
   (v)   Remote monitoring of vital signs and feedback provides a sense of security and empowerment towards self management to patients.

9. Future Perspective of Physiological Monitoring

As much as technological evolution in physiological monitoring owes to the advances in visual representation through improved display technology, so would the future of physiological monitoring advance towards a dynamic representation of real-time processed diagnostic medical images. This is certain with the rapid advances in the micro-processing power being able to transform clinical practice of offline medical image processing in diagnosis to be available in real-time. With the evolving standards of DICOM in the interoperability of diagnostic images for exchange, store, view, and retrieval integration of clinical and archiving systems for diagnostic images will become seamless. However, physiological monitoring in remote monitoring will remain with streaming from wireless medical devices due to bandwidth limitation in communication technologies. The integration of both medical images and physiological signal data will become more prevalent on the EHR as interoperability and standards become established. Clinical decision support systems will utilise this enriched, integrated EHR and real-time physiological monitoring to provide higher level automated decisions of disease severity, assist therapeutic management, clinical states and functional status. Networks for communication between clinical systems and EHR repositories between health care institutions will lean towards a single high- speed wireless Internet platform. This will enable clinicians with readily accessible for of real time physiological monitoring with integrated EHR for review, decision making and actions. PHR will also become more enriched with integrated EHR data and better visual representation for their medical condition for self management.

References

[1]   Subramanium S. Physiologic Monitoring and Clinical Information Systems. *Clinical Engineering Handbook*. MA, California, UK: Elsevier Academic Press; 2004:456-463.
[2]   Geddes LA. Perspectives in physiological Engineering. *Medical Instrumentation.* 1976;10(2):91-97.
[3]   Gorges M, Staggers N. Evaluations of physiological monitoring displays: A systematic review. *J Clin Monit Comput.* 2007;22:45-66.
[4]   Engineering staff of Femtosim Clinical Inc. Fifty Years of Physiologic Monitors Available at: http://www.femtosimclinical.com/History%20of%20Physiologic%20Monitors.htm. Accessed 8 May 2008.
[5]   Medical Connectivity. An Assessment of Wireless Medical Telemetry System (WMTS). Available at: http://medicalconnectivity.com/2008/04/27/an-assessment-of-wireless-medical-telemetry-system-wmts/. Accessed 21 May 2008.
[6]   Dyro JF, Poppers PJ. Improving Patient Care Through Integrated Computing. *Int J Clin Monit Comput.* 1986;3(3):217-218.
[7]   Nellcor Pulse Oximetry Sensors. Available at: http://www.nellcor.com/prod/list.aspx?S1=POX&S2=SEN. Accessed 25 October 2006.
[8]   Asada HH, Shaltis P, Reisner A et al. Mobile monitoring with wearable photoplethysmographic biosensors: Technical and clinical aspects of aring sensor for ambulatory, telemetric, continuous health monitoring in the field, in the hospital, and in the home. *IEEE Engineering in Medicine and Biology Magazine.* 2003;May/June::28-40.
[9]   Clarke M JR, Bratan T et al. Providing remote patient monitoring services in residential care homes. Healthcare Computing: Developments in primary care. 2004:114-122.
[10] Omron Healthcare. Available at: http://www.jadavey.com.au/default.htm. Accessed 22 October 2006.
[11] Welch Allyn. Available at: http://www.welchallyn.com/medical/products/catalog/country.asp Accessed 20 May 2008.
[12] McGrath BP. Ambulatory blood pressure monitoring. . *Med J Aust.* 2002;176(12):588-592.

[13] Portapres. Available at: http://www.finapres.com/customers/portapres.php. Accessed 20 October 2006.

[14] Vivo-metrics. Life-shirt. Available at: http://www.vivometrics.com/site/system.htm. Accessed 20 May 2008.

[15] Sensetex. Smartshirt. Available at: http://www.sensatex.com/smartshirt.html. Accessed 21 May 2008.

[16] Muhlsteff J SR, Schmidt M, Perkuhn M, Reiter H, lauter J, et al. Wearable approach for continuous ECG – and activity patient monitoring. International Conference of the IEEE Engineering in Medicine and Biology Science (EMBEC) San Francisco, USA (20. Wearable approach for continuous ECG – and activity patient monitoring. International Conference of the IEEE *Engineering in Medicine and Biology Science (EMBEC)* 2004.

[17] Paradiso R. Wearable health care system for vital signs monitoring. *Proc. IEEE Conference Information Technology in Applications in Biomedicine.* 2003:283-286.

[18] Tunstall. Available at: http://www.tunstall.co.uk/ Accessed 18 May 2008.

[19] Docobo. Available at: http://www.docobo.co.uk/ Accessed 20 May 2008.

[21] Chubb. Telehealth Products.

[22] Philips Medical System. Available at: http://www.medical.philips.com/us/products/telemonitoring/products/motiva/. Accessed 20 May 2008.

[23] Health Hero Network. Health Buddy. Accessed 21 May 2008.

[24] Karunanithi M. Monitoring Technology for the Elderly Patient. *Expert Rev Med Devices.* 2007;4(2):267-277.

[25] Commonwealth of Australia, A Health Information Network for Australia, Canberra 2000

[26] Takla G, Petre JH, Doyle J, Horibe M, Gopakumaran B. The Problem of Artifacts in Patient Monitor Data During Surgery: A Clinical and Methodological review. *Anesth Analg.* 2006;103:1196-1204.

[27] OpenXT Consortium. Open Exchange Data Format. Available at: http://www.openxdf.org/.

[28] Saphire Intelligent Healthcare Monitoring System. Available at: http://www.srdc.metu.edu.tr/webpage/projects/saphire/. Accessed 20 May 2008.

Review Questions

1. Describe the evolution of commercial physiological monitoring over the years and the associated impacts on e-health strategy implementations.

2. How can the importance of physiological monitoring data's inclusion in EHRs best be accommodated?

3. What are the issues that need to be addressed for successful EHR implementation?

4. What variations in physiological monitoring devices are we likely to have to accommodate in the future?

Health Informatics
E.J.S. Hovenga et al. (Eds.)
IOS Press, 2010
doi:10.3233/978-1-60750-476-4-219

18. Image Management and Communication

Liam CAFFERY[1] BInfoTech, Dip App Sc (Diag Rad)[a], Lawrence SIM PhD[b]
[a]Centre for Online Health, University of Queensland, and the Royal Children's Hospital, Brisbane, Australia
[b]Scientific Advisor - Radiology Support Services, Clinical and Statewide Services, Queensland Health, Australia

Abstract. This chapter gives an educational overview of:

- various digital imaging technologies, systems and standards
- key components of a Picture Archiving and Communication Systems (PACS)
- advantages of a digital medical imaging service over a film-based service
- standards used in PACS
- how PACS integrates with an image-enabled electronic health record
- future trends in digital imaging

Keywords. Medical Informatics Applications, Data Collection, Medical Records-Computerised, Radiology, Computer Systems, Documentation, User Computer Interface, Risk Management, Systems Integration, Clinical Governance, Multimedia, Image Management

Introduction

The development of technologies for digital acquisition of medical images has changed the way medical imaging departments manage their data and information. As the popularity of digital imaging systems has increased, so has the need for systems that will store, retrieve and distribute medical images and facilitate review of medical images in digital form. These systems are known as Picture Archiving and Communication Systems (PACS).

This chapter will examine the various technologies, systems and standards that facilitate these tasks that are known collectively as image management. After completing this chapter the reader will be able to describe the key components of a PACS, list advantages of a digital medical imaging service over a film-based service, describe in broad detail the standards used in PACS, describe how PACS integrates with an image-enabled electronic health record and identify future trends in digital imaging

1. Image Management

Traditional medical image management techniques were based around the production of images printed onto sheets of film. A patient's films were placed in a packet and stored in a file room (Figure 1). A patient's imaging packet was retrieved manually and physically distributed to their treating clinician. Films were reviewed by placing the film

---

[1] Corresponding Author: lcaffery@coh.uq.edu.au

on a light box to illuminate the image. The viewing of images in this manner is referred to as *hard-copy* review.

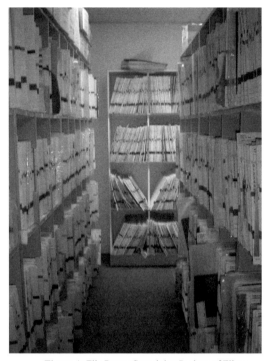

Figure 1: File Room Containing Packets of Films.

A PACS is a computer system — both hardware and software — used for the storage, distribution and review of medical images. A PACS is made up of many components — including a database, an image archive and one or more computerised review stations. All the components of a PACS are connected by a data network. PACS is a necessary infrastructure for digital image management.

PACS allow a hospital to operate a filmless imaging service where medical images are acquired in a digital format, stored digitally in an archive and retrieved and viewed using software running on a computer. The viewing of images on a computer monitor is often referred to as *soft-copy* review.

The concept of digital image management arose with the need to manipulate digital medical images following the invention of the computed tomography (CT) scanner — the first modality to produce images in a digital format [1]. The development of CT was also the catalyst for the development of the Digital Image Communication in Medicine (DICOM) standard [2]— a set of rules governing the formatting of images and the exchange of images between the modality, archive and the review stations.

2.   Advantages of PACS

Digital image management provides a number of advantages over traditional film-based image management. These include:-

- Instantaneous access to images as soon as they are acquired.
- The elimination of manual storage and retrieval of images on film because a patient's complete radiological history is online.
- A reduction in lost films.
- The ability for more than one person to view the same image simultaneously at different locations.
- The elimination of image processing and image processing chemicals from the workplace.

Evaluation of PACS has shown an improvement in the quality and productivity of radiological services based on a number of metrics such as a turn-around-time, patient waiting times and decreased length of hospital stays [3] [4] [5] [6] whilst at the same time delivering substantial cost-reduction for the service [3] [6] [7]. In addition to the quantifiable cost-savings, many authors point out intangible benefits of PACS and digital imaging that cannot be easily costed. These include a reduction in a clinician's time spent looking for lost films and less repeat examinations [4] 6] [8]. PACS is also credited with improving the productivity of both radiologists and radiographers [9] [10]. Diagnosis also improves due to a higher proportion of examinations being reported by a radiologist [4] and the ability to digitally manipulate an image — for example, changing the brightness and contrast [4].

3. Image Acquisition

A modern hospital will produce medical images from a number of sources — predominantly from the radiology or medical imaging department. Medical imaging uses X-rays, ultrasound waves, radio-isotopes and magnetic fields to produce images of the human body, skeleton system, arterial system, soft-tissue structures and organs for the purposes of disease diagnosis and to monitor the progress of treatments.

The medical imaging departments may have a number of modalities including computed tomography (CT), magnetic resonance imaging (MRI), ultrasound (US), angiography and nuclear medicine (NM). By their very nature these modalities produce digital images i.e. an image produced as a result digital data acquisition and processing by computer algorithms.

Plain X-rays — for example, a chest X-ray — are traditionally acquired in an analogue format using a film-screen combination and chemical processing to produce a film-based image. To acquire a digital plain X-rays — an imaging plate or receptor has replaced the film-screen combination. This is referred to as computed radiography (CR) or direct radiography (DR) depending upon image receptor [11] [12].

Other departments within a hospital will also produce digital medical images. In their simplest form these are digital photographs of parts of the human body. Some examples include endoscopic or colonoscopic images from the gastroenterology department — for example, digital photographs of ulcers, polyps or tumours in the gastrointestinal tract. Further examples of non-radiological imaging include retinal images used in ophthalmology (Figure 2), laryngoscope images of the larynx, otoscopic images of the ear, colposcopic images of the cervix and digital photographs of skin lesions for dermatology. These types of non-radiological images are known collectively as visible-light objects.

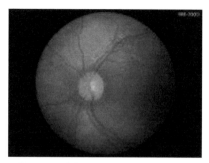

Figure 2: Visible Light Object of a Retina.

3.1 Archiving

An archive in a PACS is a repository of medical images. The function of the archive is to not only store images but also allow the retrieval of images for clinical use.

3.2 The digital image

A digital image is formed from a number of rows and columns of data elements referred to as an image matrix. The individual elements of the image matrix are known as pixels (which is an abbreviation of *picture elements*). Each pixel is one homogenous shade of grey in a greyscale image or one homogenous colour in a colour image. A digital image also has depth which allows structures of different contrast to be displayed. Image depth is the number of shades of grey that each pixel can represent in a greyscale image or the number of colours each pixel can represent in a colour image. If a pixel can represent any one of 256 (2^8) different shades of grey, the image is said to be an 8-bit or 1-byte (8 bits = 1byte) image. Typical digital medical image depth is in the ranges of 12 to 16 bits.

3.3 Compression

A digital image is stored as a file. The file size of an image is the product of the number of rows, columns and depth of an image and can be determined as follows:

Image Size (in bytes) = Rows x Columns x Number of bytes/pixel

This formula gives an uncompressed file size. To reduce storage requirements compression algorithms are used. Reducing the individual file sizes reduces the archive storage space needed (which in turn, reduces the cost of storage). File compression also reduces the transmission time across a network, say from an image archive to a review station. There are many different techniques and file formats for image compression. The joint photographic expert group (JPEG)[13] has defined the JPG and JPG2000 compressed file formats which are commonly used in image compression techniques for medical images.

Compression can either be lossy or lossless. Lossless compression means the decompressed file is an exact replica — pixel for pixel — of the original file whereas, using a lossy compression algorithm means the decompressed file may vary from the original file's pixel values. At high levels of compression an image may display obvious visual differences from the original. At low levels of compression a lossy compression algorithm may result in an image that is visually indistinguishable from the original.

The amount of compression applied to an image is referred to by a ratio of the original file size to compressed file size. Typical values of compression ratios for lossless compression of DICOM images using JPEG techniques are in the range of 2:1 to 2.5:1. Lossy compression techniques can yield a much higher and often user selectable compression ratio.

The major concern with lossy compression is that subtle abnormalities might be lost in a compressed images and this may lessen the ability to diagnosis from the image. Hence, most PACS will archive images in a lossless format. There is considerable debate to what extent medical images can be compressed using lossy compression algorithms without the loss of diagnostic information [14]. Until clear policies are established by the various professional organisations with regard to the use of image compression and agreed standards are developed it is probable that PACS archives will continue to use lossless compression of images. Table 1 contains typical image metrics and storage requirements for different modalities.

Imaging Modality	Rows	Columns	Bit depth (bytes per pixel)	Uncompressed image size (MB)	Typical number of images per examination	Uncompressed study size (MB)	Compressed study size (MB)
CT	512	512	2	0.5	200	105	48
MRI	512	512	2	0.5	300	157	71
Angiography	1024	1024	2	2.1	30	63	29
Digital mammography	4096	4096	2	33.6	4	134	61
Computed radiography	2048	2048	2	8.4	2	17	8
Ultrasound	576	768	1	0.4	30	13	6
Nuclear Medicine	860	1076	1	0.9	3	3	1

Table 1: Image Metrics for Different Medical Imaging Modalities. Calculated Compression Assumes a Compression Ratio of 2.2:1

3.4 Archiving Strategy

The purpose of archiving is two-fold — clinical and legislative. Review of previous imaging stored in an archive is an integral part of diagnosis and treatment of a patient [15]. Medical images are used during a course of treatment which may extend from a number of hours to a number of years. This is referred to as the period of clinical usefulness for an image. The period of clinical usefulness is variable and influenced by such factors as the age of the patient and the disease or injury suffered.

An archive will need to store images for the period of time mandated by legislation. Under legislation medical images (and all medical records) need to be retained for a minimum period of time. The *Queensland Health (Clinical Records) Retention and Disposal Schedule* [16] of the state's health department specifies a minimum retention period for medical images of five years.

3.5 Archiving Architecture

Typically a PACS archive is made up of a number of tiers (or levels) of storage. The use of a multi-tiered approach to archiving is a balance between cost, reliability and speed of retrieval. The first-tier, stores images for the period of clinical usefulness on high quality, high reliability hard disk drives (often called spinning disk) to facilitate the rapid retrieval and viewing of images. At the end of the period of clinical usefulness, images may be migrated to more cost-effective storage mediums to meet legislative retention requirements — for example, digital versatile disk (DVD), compact disk (CD), magnetic tape and more recently on lower cost disk arrays. This is called the second-tier archive.

4.   Disaster Recovery

A third-tier approach to archiving is sometimes used for disaster recovery. Disaster recovery is used to mitigate risks such as fire and natural disasters by having a copy of the archive located in a different geographic location to the primary archive. This is called off-site storage.

4.1 Storage Devices

4.1.1 Disk Devices

PACS archives use an industry standard technique called redundant array of independent disks (RAID) to ensure the reliability of storage. RAID groups multiple hard-disks, say six disks, into an array. When data is stored, it is replicated to a number of disks in the array. If one physical disk fails, the data can be recovered from other disks hence, the term redundant. Multiple arrays make up an archive. (Figure 3)

The use of spinning disks can be either direct-attached or networked. Direct-attached storage (DAS) is physically connected to a host server. The operating system of the host server controls the input and output to the storage array. Networked storage does not have a host server. It has its own network address, allowing multiple servers in a PACS to share the same storage area. This architecture is useful in a busy PACS environment as a number of servers can load-share the tasks of image file input and output. Depending on the particular technical arrangement, network storage is known by the terms network attached storage (NAS) or storage-area network (SAN). Any of the "spinning disk" architecture is referred to as on-line storage.

4.1.2 Removable Media

The second-tier of storage in a PACS archive often uses removable media housed in a jukebox. This type of storage architecture is referred to as near-line storage. The most common formats are DVD with a capacity of around 4.5 GB per disk or one the magnetic tape formats. Magnetic tape media use half-inch magnetic tape — similar to video-tape — wrapped around a spindle and stored inside a cartridge for physical protection. Two categories of magnetic tape are Digital Linear Tape (DLT), with a capacity of up to 40GB per tape and Linear Tape-Open (LTO) with a capacity of up to 800 GB per tape (Figure 4).

A jukebox (Figure 5) can have hundreds of storage slots for removable media, and one or more drives for reading/writing images to the media. Whilst the media is housed in the jukebox it is available for retrieval by a clinician using a review station. Media can physically be removed from the jukebox. When removed it is referred to as off-line. The media can be returned to the jukebox in the event of a clinician needing to review an image stored on the off-line media.

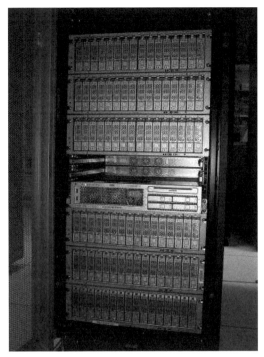

Figure 3: Arrays of Hard-Disk Drives in RAID Configuration Used as a PACS Archive.

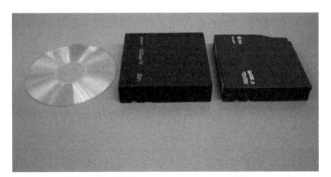

Figure 4: DV D (left), DLT Cartridge (middle) and LTO Cartridge(right).

As the cost of spinning disk arrays has fallen it has become feasible for PACS vendors to offer non- removable media in the form of spinning disk arrays for near-line storage. These near-line disk array systems are usually configured as RAID devices using lower specification disks which are considerably less expensive than the higher quality first-tier arrays.

Archiving strategy, terminology and devices are summarised in Table 2.

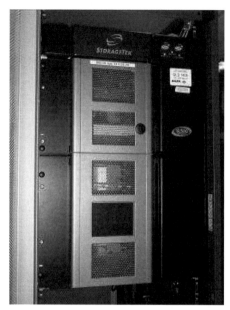

Figure 5: A LTO jukebox. This jukebox can house 50 LTO tapes.

Tier	Terminology	Options	Role
1	Online	High speed RAID device for example, NAS, SAN or DAS	Facilitate the rapid retrieval of images during the period of clinical usefulness
2	Near-line	Removable media jukebox for example, DVD, DLT or LTO jukebox or RAID device (typically slower and cheaper than Tier 1)	Minimizes the cost of storage whilst maintaining the ability to i) store and retrieve images for occasional clinical need and ii) store images for period of time required image retention legislation.
3	Disaster recovery or Offsite	RAID device or removable media jukebox	A redundant image archive housed in a separate geographical location used to mitigate the risk fire or other disaster.

Table 2: A Description of the Terminology, Options and Role of a PACS Archive

5.   Communication and Networking

The individual devices that make up a PACS are connected by an industry standard data network e.g. Ethernet in either a local area network (LAN) or wide area network (WAN) topology. Network performance is a very important consideration for PACS operation. Medical image studies are large — for example, a single CT study may contain 50 MB of data (Table 1). Good connectivity and clinically acceptable data transmission rates are requirements for an effective PACS service. What constitutes "acceptable" for data transmission rates will depend upon the particular circumstances. It may be acceptable to wait 5 minutes for the transfer of a CT scan from another hospital but images "on demand" will be required for the surgeon in operating theatres. For a service where productivity depends upon the rate at which images can be viewed (i.e. radiology) any noticeable delay in image transmission (from archive to viewing station) is undesirable. Reliability is another consideration for medical information transmission and this introduces considerations of redundancy, resilience and security.

Continuous streaming technologies are already part of wide area PACS implementations. Streaming is a web-based technology that refers to the continuous sending of portions of data from source (e.g. archive) to client (e.g. review station) rather than sending all the data first and viewing only after the data transmission is completed [17]. Streaming enhances the efficient use of available bandwidth by PACS applications. The development of streaming technologies has facilitated greater use of web techniques in PACS applications.

6. Review Stations

Medical imaging studies are undertaken for clinical purposes and as such the images produced must be reviewed by clinicians. Images will usually be seen by a radiologist, who will produce a documented report on the findings in the imaging study. This process is called *primary diagnosis*. The radiologist's report and images will be used by patient's treating doctor to aid the management of the patient. When the treating doctor reviews the images and report it is called *clinical review*.

To a clinical user the review station or workstation they use to review images stored on a PACS is the most visible component of the PACS and the only part of the PACS they may ever interact with [18]. A review station is typically a personal computer (PC) which runs image viewing software (Figure 6). The software allows searching of the image archive and display of a patient's images. The PC is coupled with a monitor or monitors appropriate for reviewing medical images [19].

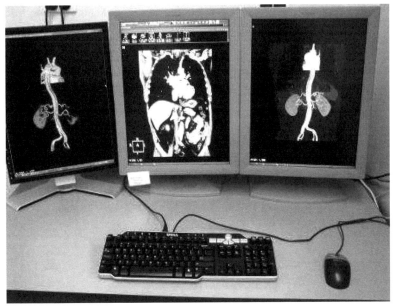

Figure 6: A PC-Based Diagnostic Review Station Using a 3 Monitor Configuration.

There are two main types of review stations — diagnostic and clinical review stations. The monitor and display (video) card specifications are the principal difference between a diagnostic and clinical review station. The monitor may be a standard PC monitor, as is often used in clinical review stations or a high- resolution, high-brightness, greyscale monitor purpose-built for primary diagnosis.

Review station software can be implemented either as a web-browser system or in a client/server architecture — where dedicated image viewing software is installed on the PC. Using a web-browser system means viewing software does not need to be installed manually on a clinician's PC. The clinician uses a standard web-browser — for example Microsoft's Internet Explorer — to search the archive and display images. This architecture allows ease of access and is often a more economical solution for review stations than client/server. Web-browser systems also lift the geographical restrictions of workplace. Radiologist reporting from external sites is reality now in many sectors. This has the potential to provide radiological interpretations remotely, delivering quality clinical imaging services regardless of geography.

7. Digital Image Communication

An international standard called digital imaging and communication in medicine (DICOM) was developed to allow medical images to be sent from modality to archive to review station regardless of the manufacturer of the device. The DICOM standard has facilitated the growth in PACS-based image management.

The DICOM standard was developed as a joint initiative of the American College of Radiology (ACR) and the National Electrical Manufacturers Association [2]. The first version of the standard was released in 1983 and has subsequently undergone a number of iterations. The current version is version 3.0; however, DICOM is now considered a version-less standard. Instead of releasing new versions, the existing version is updated or corrected each year with new supplements added to the standard when necessary and outdated sections retired. At the time of writing the DICOM Standard consists of 17 Parts and 137 Supplements.

DICOM defines a file format for medical images. A single DICOM file is made up of two parts. The first part is called the header and contains text based information such as the patient's demographics and study information. The second part is the actual image pixel data. DICOM supports different images compression techniques — for example, JPEG.

A DICOM service class is set of rules governing what actions can be performed on a DICOM object (file) — for example storing or retrieving the file from an archive or printing the file. A service object pair (SOP) is a combination of the DICOM object and service class — for example, store a CT image. The presentation context of a DICOM transaction is the combination of SOP and transfer syntax — for example, store a CT image using JPEG compression. Before two DICOM compliant devices can exchange an image they must first establish an association. This process involves agreeing on a presentation context. Once the association has been established the image can be transferred.

DICOM Part 14 defines a greyscale standard display function (GSDF) to facilitate the consistent display of images on review station monitors.

DICOM has also defined methods for web-browser application to query, retrieve and view a DICOM image. Web access to DICOM objects (WADO) methods are used by web-based review station or electronic health records (EHR) portals. WADO methods typically use streaming technology for fast access.

Vendors of medical imaging modalities and PACS devices issue a DICOM conformance statement listing the DICOM objects, services classes and transfer syntaxes their device supports. DICOM conformance does not guarantee connectivity between two devices. Interoperability is tested during regular multi-vendor events called connectathons that are facilitated and managed by a body called Integrating the Healthcare Enterprise (IHE) [20]. IHE has been enthusiastically embraced by the PACS industry and has rapidly spread beyond the realm of radiology. It is now a major consideration for all health related software development. IHE oversee the connectathons and issue integration statements for vendors who prove interoperability (refer chapter 11).

8. Interoperability Feeder Systems

A PACS is not a stand-alone system and is often connected to other information systems within a hospital. A PACS will normally communicate with the hospital information system (HIS) and all patient registrations, admissions and discharges will flow from the HIS to the PACS. This allows updates to a patient's information; say a change of name in the HIS to be replicated in the PACS, ensuring consistency of patient information and a reduction in manual data entry.

The PACS will also communicate with the radiology information system (RIS). The RIS is used to schedule radiological examinations and record the radiologist's report on an image. Having this information flow to the PACS means the images and radiologist's report can be viewed side-by-side during clinical review (Figure 7).

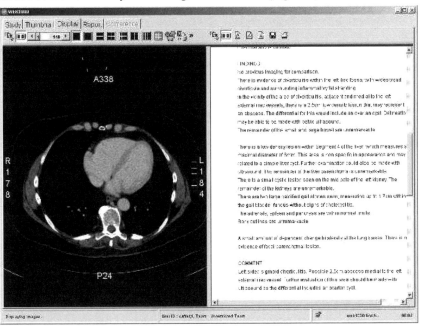

Figure 7: Screenshot From a Web-Based Review Station Displaying Both the Image and Associated Radiologist's Report.

9.   PACS and the Electronic Health Record

PACS can also be integrated into an image-enabled EHR as demonstrated schematically in Figure 8. Cross enterprise document sharing (XDS) and cross enterprise document sharing for imaging (XDS-i) are the primary architectures for achieving PACS/EHR integration. XDS architecture involves the creation of a persistent radiology objects — for example, a radiologist report with embedded images. This object is stored in a central clinical data repository (along with objects from other clinical information systems) and viewable from a portal — often a web-browser. Typically key images that demonstrate an abnormality are selected for embedding in the report. To allow access to the full image set, a second technique — where hyperlinks to images stored on PACS, are included in a radiologist's report. Selecting the hyperlink enables users of the EHR portal to retrieve and view images stored in a PACS using WADO.

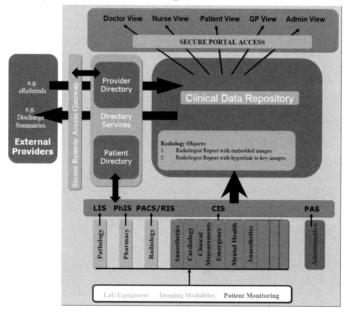

Figure 8: Schematic Representation of the Relationship Between Clinical Information Systems (including PACS), EHR Clinical Data Repository and Portal Access for Viewing Objects.

10. Teleradiology

Teleradiology is the umbrella term for the transfer of medical images over a network from one geographic location to another [21]. A teleradiology system may use a local area network (LAN) to transfers images within a hospital campus or a wide area network (WAN) to transfer images between hospitals. The Internet can be used to transfer images internationally.

Teleradiology has two distinct purposes. The first is to provide a primary diagnosis, reporting service where a radiologist reports images acquired in multiple sites, thus achieving economies of scale. The second is to provide expert medical opinion. Medical specialists tend to congregate in large, metropolitan tertiary hospitals and their expertise can be sought by doctors working in rural and remote areas. For example, a neurosurgeon can review the CT scans of a head injury patient via teleradiology, and advise the local doctor on treatment or recommend transfer to the tertiary site. A study from Hong Kong has shown that employing teleradiological support of a neurosurgical service reduced unwarranted patient transfers by around 20% and reduced complications — such as hypoxia — occurring during transfer by around 25% [22].

In Singapore, the use of teleradiology has been considered in order to address difficulties in providing radiological services – in particular a shortage of radiologists [23]. The expected benefits of teleradiology for Singapore include:

- Ready availability of radiological interpretation services.
- Access to subspecialty radiological input.
- Out of hours radiology service and consultation.
- Enhanced education and information sharing.
- Increased availability of radiological resources.
- Possible healthcare cost reduction.

Teleradiology systems utilize the DICOM standard to transfer images. Teleradiology can be implemented in a number of architectures — for example, commercial-off-the-shelf teleradiology systems are available for purchase from numerous vendors or alternatively a hospital can use its PACS to implement teleradiology.

A number of architectures can be used when using PACS to implement teleradiology.

- Remote modality: The same way a local modality — such as a CT scanner — can be connected to a PACS, a remote modality can be connected via a WAN. This allows images that are produced at a remote site, perhaps a rural centre, to be archived and reviewed at a tertiary hospital.
- Remote review station: A review station can be connected to a PACS over a WAN. This architecture is often used by on-call clinicians, where a review station is installed in the clinician's home.
- PACS to PACS image transfer: Disparate PACS system can transfer images from one site's archive to another. This architecture is often employed when a patient's care is transferred from one facility to another.

11. Future Trends

11.1 Multi-Slice CT and the Digital Data Explosion

Traditional CT scanners used a linear detector to produce a single cross-sectional image of the body during each rotation of the X-ray tube. CT scanners now use multiple detector rows which allow the simultaneous acquisition of multiple slices for each X-ray tube rotation. 64-slice per acquisition is common place and 256-slice (and greater) is now emerging.

Multi-slice CT allows the rapid acquisition of numerous images. These axial images are typically processed into three-dimensional (3D) images which improve the visualisation of anatomy. (Figure 9 and 10) 3D imaging is also known as volumetric imaging. Volumetric imaging of the arterial system is non-invasive and has supplemented (and in some cases replaced) a range of traditional angiographic procedures — where the artery is punctured to allow the introduction of contrast media via a catheter.

The consequence of multi-slice CT is an increase in the number of images produced and the resultant need to store and display these images. This is called the digital data explosion. See the case study below for an example of the effect of the digital data explosion.

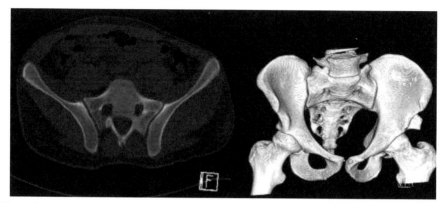

Figure 9 : Numerous Axial Slices Acquired During CT Scanning (left) are Processed into 3D Images (right).

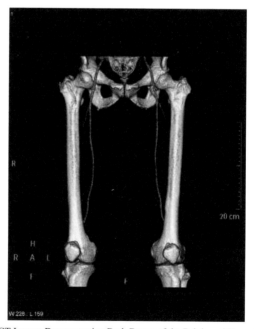

Figure 10 : Volumetric CT Images Demonstrating Both Bones of the Pelvis and Upper Legs and Arteries.

11.2 Globalisation

The increasing bandwidth and decreasing cost of the Internet has made possible the advent of nighthawking. Nighthawking is a teleradiology service that takes advantages of different world time zones to provide after-hours radiological cover. Kalyanpur,

Weinberg et al [24] describe a service where after-hours CT scans acquired in the United States of America (USA) are transmitted — via the Internet — to a radiologist working in India — where it is day time. The CT scan is reported by the Indian radiologist and the report is transmitted back to the referring doctor in the USA. The turn-around-time for this process was 40 minutes. Teleradiology is a global growth industry with services presently offered by numerous commercial operators.

11.3 Image Fusion

Image fusion (in a medical imaging context) refers to the overlay and registration of images from two or more modalities in order to gain the benefits of both modalities. Typically, image data from computed tomography (CT), magnetic resonance imaging (MRI), single-photon computed tomography (SPECT), and positron-emission tomography (PET) are superimposed pixel by pixel to generate a combined (or fused) image.

In the early days of image fusion, MRI scans were fused with CT scans to take advantage of the improved soft tissue contrast of the MRI. With the development of advanced nuclear medicine technologies, it is now common to create fusion images from SPECT or PET super-imposed on CT or MRI scans [25]. This fusion combines the functional or physiological image characteristics from nuclear medicine imaging with the detailed anatomical information from radiological images.

Image fusion was originally performed on at least two sets of images taken on different machines at different times, using specialized software. This is not a simple process as the sets of images to be fused will have dimensional differences due to a variety of factors including differences in body position, image scaling techniques, and slice thicknesses.

More recently, specialized scanners have been developed to acquire the required sets of images close in time and without needing to move the patient. The PET/CT scanner [26] is a good example of such a combined scanner. An example of a fused PET/CT image is shown in Figure 11.

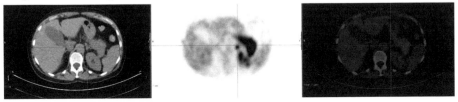

Figure 11: CT Image of Abdomen (left), PET Image of Abdomen (middle) and Resultant Fused Image of Abdomen (right)

12. A Case-Study: The QPACS project

The QPACS project installed PACS and RIS into the Royal Brisbane and Women's Hospital (RBWH), Royal Children's Hospital (RCH) and the Princess Alexandra Hospital (PAH) in Brisbane, Australia between April 1999 and March 2001. The QPACS project coincided with the re-building of both the RBWH and the PAH. During the planning for these facilities, decisions were made that when each hospital moved into their new facility; they would offer a filmless radiology service. A combined tender process selected the Agfa-Gevaert group as the prime vendor for these PACS projects.

The RBWH and RCH are on the same campus and single PACS installation serviced both hospitals. A separate PACS was installed at PAH. The QPACS project was completed in 2001 when all QPACS hospitals officially moved from PACS Project mode to a PACS operational mode, and since this date both hospitals have been filmless. Since 2001 all hospitals have experienced an approximate 10% compound growth in the number of studies performed annually (Figure 12) however, the number of images has grown exponentially (Figure 13) predominantly due to multi-slice CT and the resultant digital data explosion.

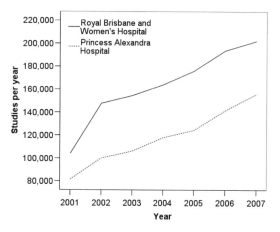

Figure 12: Number of Studies Performed at the Royal Brisbane and Women's Hospital and Princess Alexandra Hospitals since Installation of PACS.

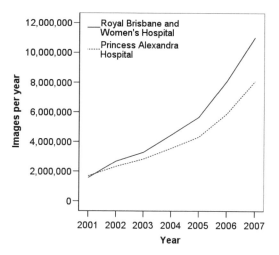

Figure 13: The Number of Images Produced per Year at the Royal Brisbane and Women's Hospital and Princess Alexandra Hospital.

12.1 Archiving

The original installation in 2001 used three-tier archive architecture. Online storage was provided by 200GB of direct-attached RAID arrays, near-line storage used a DLT jukebox with 400 tape capacity and offsite disaster recover was a second DLT jukebox.

In addition, both sites installed web servers for hospital-wide image delivery - with approximately 200 GB of disk storage operating in *first in first out* storage. Very soon after these systems went live it became evident that the web storage space was unable to effectively cope with the clinical work requirements. This was generating multiple requests for retrievals from the tape archive to the web and consuming system resources with resulting poor performance. The web cache sizes at both sites were upgraded to 1TB and the result was much improved performance for the clinical users. This in turn led to a much improved level of acceptance of the *filmless* system for managing medical images.

The initial 200GB online storage at RBWH was upgraded to 4TB in 2003, and upgraded again in 2006 to 10 TB. At PAH the initial 200GB online storage was upgraded to 4TB in 2003.

In 2007, the storage architecture at both sites was changed. This decision was made due to the obsolescence of the DLT media. A three-tier architecture with the in-situ direct-attached RAID storage is still employed. A further 25 TB of SATA arrays are now used for near-line storage, and a LTO jukebox is used for offsite disaster recovery at both sites.

12.2 Viewing Stations and Monitors

Both hospitals have around 50 diagnostic review stations with high brightness, high resolution monochrome monitors. These workstations are installed in a client/server architecture in dedicated areas with control of ambient light in a majority of instances. These diagnostic review stations are installed mainly in the radiology departments of the respective hospitals, however some are installed in the intensive care unit (ICU), intensive care nursery (ICN), emergency department and orthopaedic departments.

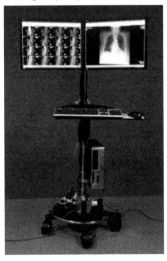

Figure 14: Mid-Tier Clinical Review Stations Developed at Princess Alexandra Hospital for Operating Theatre Use.

In addition, to the diagnostic review stations each hospital utilises a web-server for the distribution of clinical review images. Any hospital PC can access the web-server and view images (with appropriate authentication) from within the hospital intranet. A number of clinical departments requested improved viewing platforms over the standard PC screen. A number of high quality colour LCD panels were acquired. The typical specification for these devices was 20" screen, 2MP display, 250 cdm^2 luminance (or better) and incorporating calibration software for automatic DICOM Part 14 GSDF conformance. The monitors were connected in pairs to a standard PC via a high quality dual output video card and used to run the web based enterprise delivery application. The acceptance by the respective clinical areas of these "mid tier" clinical review stations was overwhelmingly positive. (Figure 14)

13. Conclusion

PACS is a digital image management system used by medical imaging services. It has largely replaced traditional film-based image management and is proven to reduce the cost of running an imaging service. PACS also improves productivity of staff and reduces the number of lost images.

PACS requires images to be acquired in a digital format. These images are stored in an archive. Before being stored they are compressed to save storage costs and facilitate the faster transmission across a network. PACS typically use lossless compression algorithms. Most PACS will use a multi-tier approach to archiving as a balance between cost, reliability and performance. There are numerous storage devices that can be used as an archive — for example, RAID arrays of hard-disk drives and magnetic tape jukeboxes. Review stations run software that allow the searching and retrieval of images from the archive. Once retrieved, images are *soft-copy* reviewed on a computer monitor. Review station software may be run in a client/server architecture or as a web-browser application. Web-browser applications take advantage of streaming technology for the fast delivery of images to the review client.

DICOM was developed to standardise both the format and transfer of medical images from one imaging device to another regardless of the device's manufacturer. IHE oversee connectathons where different manufacturers test their compliance to the DICOM standard.

PACS / EHR interoperability can be achieved in a number of ways. The first is where a radiologist's report contains embedded images and the second where the report contains hyperlinks to images stored on the PACS archive. An EHR portal — typically a web-browser application — allows an end user to search a clinical repository for these reports, and view them with along side information from other clinical information systems.

Digital imaging has made the possible the development of a number of advanced imaging techniques. Multi-slice CT has allowed the rapid acquisition of large numbers of CT slices. These slices are processed into 3D images. This is known as volumetric imaging. The increasing bandwidth and decreasing cost of the Internet has made possible the inter-continental teleradiological transfer of images. Another advanced technique is fusion of images. Fusion combines the functional or physiological image characteristics from a nuclear medicine image with the detailed anatomical information from a radiological image. The resultant fused image has both the physiological and anatomical image characteristics in a single image.

References

[1]   Hounsfield GN. Computerized transverse axial scanning (tomography): Part I. Description of system. 1973. *Br J Radiol* 1995;68(815):H166-72.

[2]   National Electrical Manufacturers Association *DICOM Home Page.* See http://medical.nema.org/ (cited May 2008)

[3]   Nitrosi A, Borasi G, Nicoli F, Modigliani G, Botti A, Bertolini M, et al. A filmless radiology department in a full digital regional hospital: quantitative evaluation of the increased quality and efficiency. *J Digit Imaging* 2007;20(2):140-8.

[4]   van de Wetering R, Batenburg R, Versendaal J, Lederman R, Firth L. A balanced evaluation perspective: picture archiving and communication system impacts on hospital workflow. *J Digit Imaging* 2006;19 Suppl 1:10-7.

[5]   Watkins J, Weatherburn G, Bryan S. The impact of a picture archiving and communication system (PACS) upon an intensive care unit. *Eur J Radiol* 2000;34(1):3-8.

[6]   Crowe B, Sim L, Manthey K, Stuckey S, Whitter V. Clinical and productivity gains from introduction of PACS at major teachning hospitals in Australia. *Int J CARS* 2006;1(Supp 1):94-95.

[7]   Fang YC, Yang MC, Hsueh YS. Financial assessment of a picture archiving and communication system implemented all at once. *J Digit Imaging* 2006;19 Suppl 1:44-51.

[8]   Weatherburn G, Bryan S, Cousins C (2000) A comparison of the time required by radiologists for the preparation of clinico-radiological meetings when film and PACS are used, *European Radiology*, vol 10, pp 1006-1009

[9]   Canadian Association of Radiologists *PACS Position Paper.* See http://www.car.ca/Files/media_PACS.pdf (cited May 2008)

[10] Mackinnon A, Billington R, Adam E, Dundas D, Patel U. Picture archiving and communication systems lead to sustained improvements in reporting times and productivity: results of a 5-year audit *Clinical Radiology Jul;63(7):796-804. Epub 2008 Mar 25*

[11] Cowen AR, Workman A, Price JS. Physical aspects of photostimulable phosphor computed radiography. *Br J Radiol* 1993;66(784):332-45.

[12] Yaffe MJ, Rowlands JA. X-ray detectors for digital radiography. *Phys Med Biol* 1997;42(1):1-39.

[13] Joint photographics expert group *The JPEG committee home page.* See http://www.jpeg.org/ (cited June 2008)

[14] DICOM Working Group 4 *Update on the CAR evaluation of Irreversible Compression for Medical Images.* See http://medical.nema.org/Dicom/minutes/WG-04/2007/2007-02-21/Irreversible_Compression_of_Medical_Images.ppt (cited June 2008)

[15] Mun SK, Goeringer LT. An image management and communications (IMAC) system for radiology. *Med Prog Technol* 1992;18(3):165-79.

[16] Queensland Government *Queensland Health (Clinical Records) Retention and Disposal Schedule: QDAN 546 v.3.* See http://www.archives.qld.gov.au/downloads/QDAN00546V3.pdf (cited May 2008)

[17] Pohjonen H. Web-based PACS for all users. *EuroPACS 2006.* Trondheim, Norway, 2006.

[18] Li M, Wilson D, Wong M, Xthona A. The evolution of display technologies in PACS applications. *Comput Med Imaging Graph* 2003;27(2-3):175-84.

[19] Andriole KP. Display monitors for digital medical imaging. *J Am Coll Radiol* 2005;2(6):543-6.

[20] IHE *Integrating the Healthcare Enterprise.* See http://www.ihe.net/ (cited May 2008)

[21] Caffery L, Coulthard A. Telemedicine and Neuroradiology. In: Wootton R, Patterson V, editors. *Teleneurology*: The Royal Society of Medicine Press Limited, 2005.

[22] Poon WS, Goh KY. The impact of teleradiology on the inter-hospital transfer of neurosurgical patients and their outcome. *Hong Kong Med J* 1998;4(3):293-295.

[23] Cheng LT, Ng SE. Teleradiology in Singapore--taking stock and looking ahead. *Ann Acad Med Singapore* 2006;35(8):552-6.

[24] Kalyanpur A, Weinberg J, Neklesa V, Brink JA, Forman HP. Emergency radiology coverage: technical and clinical feasibility of an international teleradiology model. *Emerg Radiol* 2003;10(3):115-8.

[25] Wiest PW, Hartshorne MF. Image Fusion. *Appl Radiol* 2001;30(4):9-16.

[26] Townsend DW, Beyer T. A combined PET/CT scanner: the path to true image fusion. *Br J Radiol* 2002;75 Spec No:S24-30.

Further reading

1. The PACSnet website (http://www.pacsnet.org.uk/) is run by United Kingdom's National Health Service (NHS) Centre for Evidence-based Purchasing. The Education section of this web-site contains a *Beginner's guide to PACS* and a comprehensive *Glossary* of PACS and terms. (cited June 2008)
2. *PACS and Imaging Informatics: Basic Principles and Applications* authored by H.K. Huang and published by John Wiley and Sons is a comprehensive text on PACS, related standards and imaging informatics.
3. Paskins Z, Rai A. The impact of Picture Archiving and Communication Systems (PACS) implementation in rheumatology. *Rheumatology (Oxford)* 2006;45(3):354-5.

Review Questions

1. Identify and describe various digital imaging technologies, systems and standards.
2. What are the key components of a Picture Archiving and Communication Systems (PACS) ?
3. Explain the advantages of adopting a digital imaging service over a film based service.
4. What standards are used in PACS?
5. Describe how PACS integrates with an image-enabled electronic health record.
6. What are the future trends in digital imaging?

Health Informatics
E.J.S. Hovenga et al. (Eds.)
IOS Press, 2010
doi:10.3233/978-1-60750-476-4-239

19. Telehealth and Remote Access

Anthony MAEDER[1] PhD FIEAust

Professor in Health Informatics, School of Computing & Mathematics, University of Western Sydney, Australia

Abstract. This chapter gives an educational overview of:
- concepts concerning the nature and usage of Telehealth systems in some common clinical settings
- the expected structure of typical interactive (synchronous) and non-interactive (asynchronous) Telehealth scenarios
- various characteristics of human usage and physical infrastructure pertaining to typical Telehealth systems

Keywords. Telemedicine, Computer Communication Networks, Medical Informatics, Data Collection, Referral and Consultation, Health Facilities, Caregivers, Quality of Healthcare, Software

Introduction

In current times a major issue for health care has become rapidly increasing costs, coupled with reduced workforce capacity and increased consumer demand. Also, the health care sector has acknowledged the importance of widespread incorporation of safety and quality methods in health care practices. Various changes in the way health care is delivered are becoming adopted partially in response to the above two drivers:
- Health agencies are moving towards *more localised* (i.e. decentralised) models for point-of-care delivery which allow more *individualised, patient-centric care* and ease pressure on hospitals through promotion of *community and home care.*
- Requirements for *mobility of patients, carers, health workers and clinicians* to attend provider locations places an unnecessary *travel burden* on the mobile party and leads to *avoidable time wastage* and associated distress.
- Capacity to *systematise elements of care* addresses variations in safety and quality of *service and decisions* due to lack of *patient-specific detailed information* and different levels of *experience and training in care team members.*

Telehealth (or "health care at a distance") has been promoted as a means of enabling some of these changes, as well as providing related system wide efficiency gains and access equity. This has led to the establishment of numerous Telehealth programs locally in hospital groups or geographical/political regions, such as the National Health Service in Britain, Infoway in Canada and several States in the USA. Telehealth is seen as applicable to developing countries, where large distributed populations are serviced by minimal health care systems, as well as for developed countries, where complex and expensive differentiated health care systems are already in place. However, its

---

[1] Corresponding Author: a.maeder@uws.edu.au

widespread uptake has been slower than expected, due mainly to the challenges of balancing human factors with technical aspects, as well as some frequent bureaucratic and economic impediments. This area of Health Informatics relies on careful blending of human control and interaction with the enabling computer software and equipment, to be effective. This section will provide a broad background to Telehealth, including some key terms and concepts.

1. What is Telehealth?

Telehealth is a term widely used to denote health care delivery activities in which the parties involved may be *located separately in place and/or time.* Information and communications technologies are used to bridge these two gaps in appropriate ways. For example, a patient interacting with a clinician in real time by videoconferencing for a consultation about a health condition (i.e. teleconsultation), or a patient whose vital signs are being monitored over a computer-based network to track their health status and alert a carer if danger levels are reached (i.e. telemonitoring), are both examples of Telehealth. Similar closely related terms such as Telemedicine and Telecare are often used interchangeably with Telehealth, although technically they may have narrower meanings within their own specialist domains.

The *World Health Organisation (WHO)* [1[p.1]]) refers to the concept of Telemedicine (health) as:

> "delivery of health care services, where distance is a critical factor, by health care professionals using information and communications technologies for the exchange of valid information for diagnosis, treatment and prevention of disease and injuries, research and evaluation, and for the continuing education of health care providers, all in the interest of advancing the health of individuals and their communities".

The *International Organization for Standardization* [2] defines Telehealth as

> "use of telecommunication techniques for the purpose of providing telemedicine, medical education, and health education over a distance", as distinct from Telemedicine as "use of advanced telecommunication technologies to exchange health information and provide health care services across geographic, time, social and cultural barriers".

Based on these definitions, we observe that Telehealth processes consist of several essential components:

- a health care **delivery** activity which is part of the process of caring for a patient, such as consultation, examination, diagnosis, monitoring, or carrying out a procedure;
- two or more **parties** who are cooperating in the health care delivery activity: a party may be a human, such as a patient or clinician, or may be an automated system such as a decision support system;
- separate **location** in place and/or time, such as the patient in a different building or town from the clinician, or the clinician reviewing a series of patient sessions some period after they have been captured;
- a **communications** system such as a telecommunications link or a computer network, which can be used to move or store the associated electronic information;

2. Special Instances of Telehealth

Teleconsultation is seen as the most longstanding, widespread and generally understood deployment for Telehealth, and so it is natural that it should have developed some diversity and specialisation. The application of Telehealth in many different clinical areas has led to diversification of the techniques involved, and to differences in how the basic elements of a Telehealth activity are applied. Consequently these areas have adopted labels for their type of Telehealth, such as telepsychiatry, telepediatrics etc. For example, a teleconsultation conducted with a psychiatric patient might be one-on-one with the clinician, and might require a full body view of the patient so that body language signs can be read. On the other hand, a teleconsultation with a child patient might require other participants (such as parent or nurse) and might need to include means of engaging the child in the interaction (such as an attractive setting or interface). In some situations, the Telehealth environment can be simple (such as webcam-to-webcam discussions between clinicians) while in others it can be very complex, aggregating or integrating multiple channels and devices together (e.g. tele-intensive-care systems which incorporate video feeds of the patient, nurse and various clinicians, medical device outputs, and images such as histology samples or X-ray films).

There are also some clinical areas in which Telehealth activities differ quite considerably from a consultation setting, such as those not conducted in real time (e.g. teleopthalmology, teledermatology) and those which involve multiple parties and special equipment (e.g. tele-intensive-care and tele-surgery). We might consider these rather as *tele-investigation* or *tele-collaboration* activities. For example, in teleopthalmology, images or videos of the eye captured with a specialised fundus camera may be submitted to a central repository from which clinicians download a set of images assigned to them for further study and their recommendation on how to deal with the patient. In tele-surgery, joint access to intra-operative monitoring by cameras and other instruments or medical devices, and shareable control over use of the surgical instruments may be provided for clinicians within the operating theatre and at another remote site. It is reasonable to expect that there will be further proliferation of such special instances of Telehealth as well as their associated distinctive terms in the future, especially as other clinical areas adopt Telehealth methodology and solutions.

The WHO and ISO definitions referred to previously also included *health education* within their scope, because historically many interactive Telehealth systems have been used for this purpose at times when they are not occupied by clinical users. For example, videoconferencing networks in state hospital systems can typically be used for administrative and educational sessions (including netmeetings or broadcasts) for as much (if not more) time as on direct health care activities. While education is an important and legitimate purpose to which Telehealth technology can be applied, it should perhaps not be regarded as an intrinsic Telehealth activity. In the same way, electronic searching for health information (by a patient, carer or practitioner) in order to be informed about a health condition or treatment, could not be said to be a mainstream activity of Telehealth. As online learning and other aspects of education conducted remotely over computer and telecommunications networks are fundamentally similar to other types of electronic education, and distinguished here only by having health care content, we will not consider them further in this chapter.

Another area in Health Informatics which is sometimes described as Telehealth is the *transfer and access of various types of health data* from computer systems for human usage. For example, systems for distributed access to image data for human viewing and interpretation (such as teleradiology, telepathology, teledermatology) are commonly included as part of Telehealth, on the basis that they permit human-computer interaction to occur between the clinician and the database. If these actions are being considered as part of an overall health care activity involving caring for a patient, and the matters under consideration cover the whole health care process and not just the data access issues, then this view is philosophically defensible. However, the recent emergence of widespread use of unified data storage repositories (such as PACS) and integrated multiple database systems (such as data warehouses) has led this area of need to be well served now by conventional Health Informatics solutions, whether locally within a hospital or between separate locations. This distinction applies even more so to conventional health data flows such as messaging or patient record retrieval. So the basic technical solutions used for distributed storage and access to health data should not themselves be seen as fundamentally Telehealth.

3.   Why is Telehealth Useful?

Telehealth offers a range of diverse benefits (including human and economic) for patients, health professionals, and health systems. It allows the provision of health care to proceed when patients and clinicians are separated by distance, at a level comparable with that achieved in a normal face-to-face session. This allows both patients and clinicians to use their time more efficiently, and helps patients in distant locations avoid the time, effort and expense of travelling to the location of the clinician. This form of benefit can be evaluated using simple economic models and so has been widely reported in research literature. The *improved access to and use of resources*, be they human or physical, remains the most significant factor which is used to propose or justify the introduction of new Telehealth interventions.

Another avenue for benefit occurs when a patient is being looked after by one or more carers. Telehealth provides the means *to allow carers to make contact with the patient when required*, without needing to remain with the patient or visit the patient as often. This is especially useful when there is a choice of clinicians, perhaps at different sites, and any one can be chosen to respond depending on suitability or availability. An extension of this idea is the use of telemonitoring of patients who are in a lengthy period of treatment or recovery, using sensors worn by the patient or fitted to the physical environment surrounding the patient. This monitoring task can be performed by a computer program which alerts the patient or a carer if the situation appears abnormal or threatening, and supplies routine summaries at other times. An alert can be achieved by an alarm being activated to attract attention by the patient or carer, or by making contact with and giving advice to the patient through the monitoring computer system or from a medical telephone (or video) call centre. This concept has been extended to use the same methods to help people maintain wellness by measuring and feeding back information about their activities of exercise or even daily living. Various trials have established the effectiveness of Telehealth in improving patient satisfaction with health care and their increased participation or compliance in health care processes.

Telehealth also permits *flexibility when multiple clinicians or carers are involved*, as it will enable multi-party consultations and case discussions to occur with minimal disruption of the parties' other work. This in turn brings benefits of improvements to the knowledge and practice of individuals in the care team, as they can be advised or coached by more experienced professionals sited remotely. This model can also be applied to situations where clinicians must work together closely and instantaneously in a team to deal with an acute or trauma situation (such as emergency or intensive care), although they are in different locations from each other. Ultimately, clinicians aspire to achieving greater safety and quality of care through use of Telehealth rather than any alternative method, but this claim has not been validated in medical literature to any significant extent.

4. Fundamental Telehealth Concepts

Telehealth is fundamentally a means for undertaking of clinical tasks, so we should first be able to identify the associated *stages of activity* at which different Telehealth interventions are possible:

- Patient data gathering by observations and devices (including images and test results)
- Patient data transfer (communication) between health personnel and/or computer systems
- Patient data aggregation and summarisation to exclude redundant details
- Higher level information extraction from data for use in supporting clinical decisions
- Interaction and feedback between health parties on clinical decision matters
- Extraction of clinical evidence from patient data and support of population and longitudinal studies.

These stages can be further characterised according to the conventional Information Systems concepts of *input, process, and output*. For example, observations made by the consulting clinician during a telepsychiatry teleconsultation session may constitute an input activity; investigating longterm correlation of patient behaviour patterns with medication dosage levels via a multi-party expert conference may be seen as a process activity, and discussion of the care approach needed for the patient with other members of the care team may be seen as an output activity.

Next we should consider how to characterise the various *modes of action or interaction* which occur between the various potential parties in a Teleheath situation:

- Patient Self-care (e.g. wellness programs) where there is solely patient-computer interaction and the computer software provides advice and information;
- Carer-Patient and Clinician-Patient (e.g. telehomecare) where there is some Telehealth based patient-computer (or patient-clinician-computer) information gathering aspect, and some Telehealth based interaction between one or more health care professionals and the patient.
- Clinician-Carer and Clinician-Clinician (e.g. care planning) where the Telehealth interactions are between health care personnel for the purpose of managing the delivery of health care services to the patient.

These three options can be labelled as *patient-specific, patient-clinician, and clinician-specific*. It is also possible that a device or a computer could take the place of one of the parties in the above options, serving as an "agent" or surrogate for human presence, or even that two devices might communicate directly with each other on behalf of a patient, carer or clinician (e.g. active monitoring of patients). However, at some point the process must be grounded in a human interaction of one of these types.

The most basic and obvious distinguishing features of any Telehealth activity are the *technical factors*: that is, the details of structure or operation of the Telehealth enabling technology. These are not necessarily identifiable with any explicit Health aspects. Some of these factors are:

- Timing: whether the Telehealth interaction takes place in real-time (synchronous, such as teleconsultation) or separated (i.e. delayed) in time (asynchronous, such as telepathology – sometimes called "store-and-forward")
- Medium: how the interaction is conveyed, such as by voice, video, tactile device, physiological signals
- Mechanism: which type of capture and presentation (display) devices are used for the interation, such as a videoconferencing unit, webcam, PDA, wearable sensors
- Channel: which telecommunications means is employed to deliver the interaction, such as broadband, network, wireless, store-and-forward
- Properties: how the performance criteria for the interaction are specified, such as reliability, affordability, quality-of-service, error rates and recovery
- Human: how the user related aspects of the system are specified, such as user interface, realism, useability, acceptability.

A vast body of technical knowledge exists for all of these areas, and specifics are best addressed by the appropriate technical specialists such as electronics engineers or medical technicians. This is a domain in which Telehealth must fall back on the more general foundations of the Health Informatics operational environment in which it exists.

5. How Telehealth Works

Telehealth most frequently replaces human-to-human health care processes with human-to-computer-to-human processes. Therefore we need to understand both the computer based elements, and the human based elements, to make a sensible appraisal of a given Telehealth situation. Refer also to chapter 25 where associated issues from legislative and policy development perspectives are discussed. This section describes how these different elements work, and provides brief walkthroughs of two different scenarios for how they would be used in practice.

5.1 Computer Systems and Peripheral Components

The mechanisms and channels for Telehealth operations are usually of limited choice for the user, as they are often provided as hardwired infrastructure within the particular health services unit and cannot be modified. Generally the physical *front end nodes* of a Telehealth system are a number of computer based units which provide interface functionality for interaction purposes, often through plug-in peripheral devices. Some examples are:

- Commercial teleconferencing units (e.g. Polycom) or videoconferencing units (e.g. Tandberg) which operate in turnkey mode;
- Desktop or laptop computers using microphones and/or webcams, connecting to an in-house network or via web based services (e.g. Skype) which require local configuration of standard software;
- Computer controlled or hand held cameras for acquiring patient images
- Wearable or user operated tabletop physiological monitoring devices.

These units are connected by a *communications network* such as a broadband web or internet environment, or a dedicated (closed) wired or wireless network. They are subject to special *control software*, which is often provides different layers of sophistication for the scope of control (e.g. systems administrator, session manager, individual user). Typical control software would offer a range of functions, possibly including:

- Register users for access to the Telehealth system, indicating their access rights or allowed user roles;
- Regulate access to the system by authenticating users at time of access;
- Configure a Telehealth session, by initialising connection of all users and allowing dynamic connections or disconnections during the session;
- Allow adjustment of operating parameters (e.g. sound volume or picture clarity) locally, remotely or globally during a session;
- Enable or disable recording of the session or capture of other information (e.g. snapshots or button presses) interactively by users during the session;
- Retrieve and replay past sessions, and apply some analytical tools to summarise sessions or find occurrences of interest in those sessions;
- Provide access to stored patient data, external clinical reference information, and decision support tools;
- Maintain usage logs and provide summaries and statistical breakdowns of system and session utilization characteristics;
- Perform hardware and software resets including peripheral device setup and calibration operations.

The control software for a Telehealth system can thus be quite complicated in its full scope of functionality. Nevertheless, most clinical users do not need to know how to make use of any more than a small fraction of this functionality and will usually rely on Telehealth system coordinators and other technical or clinical services support personnel to supply any additional knowledge at the time of need.

5.2 Human Involvement

The human is an essential component of any Telehealth process at some point. Due to the remote nature of the users (or agents) it is important that appropriate *procedural and behavioural protocols* be adopted, in much the same way as one makes allowances when interacting with people of different cultures who might not understand nuances or colloquialisms, or when expressing oneself in e-mail when unintended meanings can be read into words without other cues. Often some of the additional information we gather during real human encounters (e.g facial expressions and body language) is not as obvious during a Telehealth session, and this can lead to misunderstandings and distractions. To achieve a smoothly flowing and productive interactive Telehealth session, a number of good practice matters should be observed:

- All participants should be aware of who is involved in the session (usually this is achieved by "round the table" introductions at the start);
- All participants should be connected appropriately to allow them to participate fully (e.g. to hear/see others clearly throughout the session and to be able to make clear inputs themselves);
- One of the participants should play the role of the session moderator (controller) who will progress the session according to a session plan (agenda) which is made clear to all participants near the start of the session;
- The session moderator should intervene if the session is not going to plan, or if participants stray from best practice behaviour, and should bring the session to conclusion when the business is finished or the time period has expired;

- If some participants are not as visible (e.g. if connected by voice only) or not as vocal in personality as others, the moderator should ensure they are invited to participate as often as the other participants;
- Each participant should try to participate in a natural way, but have regard for efficiency of the session (i.e. avoid long rambling conversation, or interrupting when others are delivering);
- Sensitivity is needed by all participants to behave politely and inclusively, and not to take advantage of the fact that the other person is in another place and cannot fight back!

Some of these aspects are illustrated in the scenarios described below.

5.3 Teleconsultation Scenario

Patient A at town X has been scheduled for a pre-surgery Telehealth session with the scheduled anaesthetist B at the hospital in city Y a few days before an operation. A is assisted in the session by nurse C at town X, who gives A a preparatory briefing and then sits in on the session with the available patient notes. B initiates and manages the session, by calling up the state health department videoconference unit in the town X clinic: both A and C can appear comfortably on the same screen as they are sitting next to each other. B introduces himself and checks the patients name and date of birth verbally, and asks A if he can hear and see B well enough. He discusses the anaesthetising process with A, then asks about A's previous history of anaesthesia and allergies. He asks about breathing issues and asks A to show his open mouth close up to the camera so that he can get an idea of any difficulties with teeth or throat abnormalities. C assists A with this process having done it before with other patients, as A cannot see himself in the picture-in-picture while in that pose. B also asks A to undertake a spirometer test to obtain lung capacity and breathing performance estimates. C administers this test and reports the results to A and B. B asks C to confirm from the records whether there is any other relevant patient history and medication information he might take into account. B asks A whether he has any questions about the anaesthetic procedure, or the Telehealth session. B ends the session by thanking both A and C for their participation and making a positive comment about the upcoming operation.

5.4 Telemonitoring Scenario

Patient P has recently suffered a mild heart attack. She is sent home after a short hospitalisation period, with a telemonitoring device which she must wear during the day when she is active and mobile. The device logs several vital signs and motion information continuously, and transmits aggregate data back to the base unit at the hospital by wireless every hour. Her case nurse Q has given her a briefing on how the device works in general, and ensured that it is working and she can fit it comfortably and securely herself. Q is responsible for making daily phone calls to P to check on her health and to give her feedback on how she is progressing according to the care plan developed on her discharge. She has established a convenient time of day (late afternoon, before dinner) with P for this event. She makes the phone call and begins with a general conversational introduction showing some interest in P's personal life. She checks that P is sitting comfortably and ready for some health discussion. She then asks P is there has been anything abnormal with her behaviour or feelings in the past day. She reviews the results of the downloaded data which has been passed through an analysis program which checks for physiological aberrations, provides a classification of all P's mobility activities in the past day, and compares vital signs and gait from those activities with similar activities in previous days. Q is able to congratulate P for keeping to her prescribed amount of walking activity, and tell her that her heart signals show she is responding better than was expected by this time. Q asks P if she would like to increase or vary her mobility activity regime at once, or wait for her next weekly review point at which the care plan would normally be modified. Q reassures P that if the data shows it has been too much, then P would be advised to return to the previous regime at once. Q asks if P has any other questions and reminds her that she can call the clinic at any time if she has concerns. Q then ends the session on a personal note of looking forward to the next day's call.

6. Characteristics of Telehealth Systems

Telehealth systems are quite diverse in their nature and so it is helpful to be able to classify them according to their detailed characteristics. This allows specification and selection of systems to be carried out in an informed way, and provides a means for systems to be compared and evaluated technically. It also allows the identification of elements in Telehealth systems which may need to be subject to systems development decisions, such as adoption of standards, interoperability or modularity considerations. This section discusses several such types of characteristics according to an overall classification structure or "taxonomy" into which they fit and within which some shared understanding and discourse can occur between people with different expertise and interests.

6.1 A Taxonomy for Telehealth

A simple and natural way to divide up the space of Telehealth is to recognise that there are two considerably different "applicability" or "discourse" domains which have fundamentally different views of what constitutes the characteristics of interest in a Telehealth system [3]:

- the "Tele" (or data) domain includes technical scientific and engineering characteristics (e.g. information or equipment related aspects, including software, telecommuncations, human factors);
- the "Health" (or usage) domain includes clinical or applications aligned characteristics (e.g. health care processes and systems).

If there is ambiguity about which domain is more appropriate, one should consider whether the item of interest is specific and unique to the health care environment, in which case the "Health" domain might be deemed more appropriate for it. For example, the choice of a videoconferencing configuration which will provide acceptable quality for human conversational interaction may be associated with the "Tele" domain, while the controls on image resolution and lighting/colour settings to allow remote clinical decision making for wound care may be associated with the "Health" domain.

From these two primary domains, we next derive major subsets associated with functional differences corresponding to the time sequenced nature of tasks in both of the domains. In the "Tele" domain, the functions deal with stages in the handling of data during a Telehealth process, while in the "Health" domain, they deal with stages of severity and complexity of intervention in the treatment of patients. Each of these functional stages is then broken down further into components and sets of standards or standardisable tasks can then be described for this level. Table 1 below provides a map of the existing and potential standards space using this taxonomy: we will not discuss the individual specific standards further as that is a highly specialised topic. In addition to understanding the landscape of Telehealth according to this taxonomy, we also need to consider aspects of performance and useability which make a Telehealth system "fit for purpose" in given operational circumstances. These aspects will be discussed in the sections following.

Table 1 Map of the Existing and Potential Standards Relative to Functions and Their Components

DOMAIN	*FUNCTION*	*COMPONENT*
Tele (Data)	Capture	Physical Characteristics e.g. colour, measurements Device Types e.g. audio, image, video, sensors
	Storage	Compression e.g. JPEG, MPEG Content e.g. regions of interest, physiological signals
	Transmission	Coding e.g. protocols, packets, errors
	Processing	Transforms e.g. scaling, noise
	Quality	Display e.g. screen properties Observer e.g. subjective opinion
Health (Usage)	Assessment	Clinical guidelines Screening/consultation Telepresence/robotics
	Diagnosis	Reporting guidelines Remote testing and imaging Decision making and expert consultation
	Treatment	Prescribing and medication Formulation of care plans
	Management	Execution and modification of care plans Coordination of multiple carers
	Monitoring	Recording from medical devices Messaging / terminology Analysis of data, images, signals Carer-patient e-mail/web usage

7. Physical Performance Properties

As with any computer or telecommunications system, there are many physical characteristics in a Telehealth situation which are determined by selection or configuration choices. It is widely variable which of these can be adjusted by users, or even by system administrators, since many Telehealth systems are set up in a fixed mode of operation (or at least with very few choices allowed). This type of *pre-configured* or "turn-key" behaviour is often preferred because it is easiest for users (i.e. the threshold of training and familiarity required before use is low) and also easiest for administrators (i.e. the number and variety of user queries to be handled is low). The expedience of having a system which can simply be switched on and expected to work with few if any further keystrokes is very attractive, especially in time-critical settings such as health care.

Nevertheless, some thought must be put into the choice of these characteristics at the time of acquisition or installation of the Telehealth system, so it is appropriate to mention a few of the most important ones. The three essential physical components in an end-to-end Telehealth system are:

- interaction acquisition/presentation front end;

- telecommunications coding and transfer channel;
- computing engine (including related data access).

These can be seen as separate subsystems, and in each case there is a vast body of scientific and engineering knowledge associated with understanding them. That is well beyond the scope of this text, but we will give an overview of some fundamental aspects which may provide helpful context when making use of Telehealth systems.

Of these, the *computing engine* is the least specific to explain because it is usually customised to be vendor- or application-specific. The computing functionality needed to support a person-to-person conversational videoconferencing session is quite well standardised and can be achieved with the use of embedded off-the-shelf hardware or publicly-available software libraries, with minimal additional computational overhead or further sophistication necessary. On the other hand, tele-surgery or tele-examination procedures using particular medical instruments and requiring a degree of feedback to the user with fail safes on allowed manipulations, would require highly specific software which could not reasonably be fully pre-specified and so must rely on the decisions of the product vendor. Between these extreme cases is the possibility of blending access to other information technology resources within the Telehealth session: for example, allowing the clinician to inspect electronic medical records, or to review past Telehealth sessions, while the current session is in progress. While these functions could be provided by a separate information system independent of the Telehealth system, there are some applications where the need is sufficiently frequent that it makes sense to integrate them (e.g. when monitoring changes in the condition of a wound over time by inspecting an image sequence).

By contrast, the *telecommunications* aspects of a Telehealth system are highly standardised and often amount to little more than a choice between common market products. The choice of channel types (e.g. PSTN, ISDN, ADSL, Broadband, Ethernet) and the physical connection medium (e.g. copper, coaxial cable, optical fibre, wireless, microwave) is highly technical and details should be sought outside of this text if necessary. The choice of communications protocol (i.e. the way in which the data being communicated is coded for transfer) relies to a large extent on those other choices, as access to the channel seldom comes without locked-in service provision arrangements. For example, certain telephone service delivery channels are appropriate to support video teleconsultations, because the associated communications protocols necessary for their normal task of interactive voice traffic ensure only minor time delays. This characteristic would also permit a realistic impression of motion to be achieved in video communication, and the channels can also incorporate real-time error correction and recovery which is necessary when coded video transmission fails. On the other hand, packet data delivery channels are generally not as useful for video teleconsultations, as they may allow prolonged delays in transmission, and may require substantial retransmissions to recover from serious errors.

Some elementary properties of the chosen communication system or the particular configuration will be of primary interest to Telehealth system users. The *speed* of communication refers to the amount of information transferred per unit time, usually expressed as Kilo-bits per second (Kbps) or Mega-bits per second (Mbps). This can be misleading because often much more information is transferred than just raw data: there is an overhead for the transfer protocol that "wraps" the data with coding information and supports error recovery, as well as for channel control purposes. Also, there may be many separate communications in progress simultaneously over a channel, with sharing (or multiplexing) of the available channel capacity between them, which can result in a much slower speed being achieved than the channel would appear to support. Generally channel characteristics are therefore specified instead as *bandwidth*, which determines the maximum speed possible, when all such overhead effects are taken into account. A major influence on achieving a good share of the bandwidth is the amount of *noise* or variation in the raw data values that occurs due to manipulations of the data (e.g. transforming electrical signals to digital values), requiring time and compute expense to be invested in reducing or smoothing the noise. In addition, *errors* may occur involving loss or corruption of information in the communication protocol during transmission. Error recovery may be achieved by use of redundant extra information to allow reconstruction of the original, or else errors may simply be concealed by post processing of the faulty decoded information. The various parameters that can be controlled to have an impact on noise and errors are termed "quality of service". It is usually accepted that video teleconsultation requires channel bandwidths of at least several 100s of Kbps to cater for all these different factors. While the user may benefit by being aware of these technical concepts and may readily identify disadvantages in a Telehealth system due to them, it is unlikely that any of them would be easily user configurable at the start of a session!

Finally, the human-computer *interaction* properties at the front end in a Telehealth system depend very strongly on the type of data that is being acquired or presented. Conversational *audio* data requires comparatively little bandwith (around 10 Kbps) for good quality delivery, but more may be required for subtle information with higher frequency components such as speech abnormalities, and stethoscope or heartbeat sounds. If simple *physiological signals* (eg temperature, pulse oximetry) from the patient are being transmitted continuously from sensors or medical devices, it is realistic to expect that at least another voice channel of bandwidth would be necessary for carrying this information, usually in a compressed form. When *images* are transferred, careful consideration must be given to spatial resolution (the number of pixels or individual points of digital information needed to represent the picture) and intensity resolution (the amount of information per pixel, specifying brightness or colour at that point). Generally, images of several 100,000s of pixels are necessary to allow sharp visual presentation on a computer display screen at sizes that are most natural for human viewers. This is achievable with many of the digital cameras of today in the consumer market, but not with lower end phonecams or webcams. Human vision cannot easily distinguish more than about 100 intensity shades in monochrome images, but can see many 100s of colour variations, so typically these images are represented with 8 or 24 bits of information per pixel respectively. Medical imaging modalities usually operate at the higher end of this range, with digital image resolutions of several Megabytes of pixels and up to 16 bits per pixel in monochrome. Multislice and multimodal imaging (such as MRI and 3D-CT) typically provide images of lower resolution than this but as sets of many 10s of images. When dealing with colour images, it is important to cater for the effect of the colour of the illumination as this may affect skin tones, lesion appearance etc. When communicating with *video*, many of these image characteristics are retained but there is an additional load of transmitting many images (or "frames") per second to provide motion (and lip synch for conversation), so that several Mbps of bandwidth is really needed for smooth, realistic presentation.

8. Human Useability Properties

Human factors in design is an extensive area of study, which has many lessons to offer Telehealth. Useability in this context refers to how easily and effectively the user can apply the system to achieve known objectives. As Telehealth sessions are often substituting for human-to-human interaction activities, the degree to which they accurately mimic real presence is a key aspect of their useability. The *quality* of the presented information, be it audio, image or video, can be represented by numerous quantitative measures but ultimately it is the *subjective* opinion of the user which matters most. Our sensory systems are surprisingly tolerant of some aberrations and not of others, so there must often be some tuning or balancing of competing presentation aspects in a system. For example, the human visual system is highly sensitive to the rate of display of frames for perceiving motion, with any rate less than about 15 frames per second giving a *flicker* or jitter impression.   Similarly, a time *lag* between an action and the presentation of the action to the user of more than a few 100s of milliseconds can be very disruptive. On the other hand, compromising audio quality and picture resolution can be more easily accepted by most users.

Another set of useability factors is concerned with operational matters for the Telehealth system as a whole. The *reliability* of the system refers to how often failures occur that cause interruption or termination of sessions, often measured as *availability* or up-time when the system could potentially be used. Load on the system is measured by *utilization* which is the fraction of availability that is actually made use of by user sessions. Most Telehealth units will *schedule* usage so that it is spread throughout the periods of availability, and try to prevent *saturation* or bottleneck conditions. The system must also achieve *robustness* in its operation, to ensure that system failures cannot be easily provoked, and *resilience* so that users cannot easily misuse it so as to cause failures of the applications software.   The provision of a Telehealth coordinator or system administrator is essential in overseeing these aspects and in matching up human expectations with system capabilities and configuration.

9. Standards and Interoperability

As with many areas in Health Informatics, standards are critical to the existence and advancement of Telehealth. We can distinguish standards in the Tele domain, which are usually generic (i.e. apply in many areas beyond Telehealth) and of a technical (i.e. scientific or engineering) nature, from those in the Health domain, which are more specific in their direct association with clinical areas or processes. We shall briefly consider some examples from these two classes.

Telehealth could not easily make use of existing telecommunications infrastructure for activities like teleconsultation and tele-investigation, if that infrastructure were not constructed according to international standards for equipment, wiring, electrical characteristics, data and control signals, protocols and presentation, most of which are controlled through the International Organisation for Standardisation (ISO) (see chapter 11). Of these, the most tangible impacts on the user come from the coding and presentation of data which can cause perceptible changes for users. For example, single images are coded by a group of standards developed by the Joint Photographic Experts Group (JPEG) committee[4], as mentioned in the previous chapter, and high quality video is coded by those developed by the Moving Picture Experts Group (MPEG) committee[5], both convened under the auspices of the ISO [6].

The adoption of these standards allows guaranteed interoperability of different devices and systems which adhere to them, in the same way that Health Messaging standards (such as HL7 and IHE) allow exchanges of information between data entities. Standards such as JPEG and MPEG have been subject to a considerable amount of debate and trials, and while they may contain tradeoffs the choices will have been very well informed. If visual artifacts or degradations are seen by the viewer when using these standards, it can be assumed that these are hard limitations of the way the Telehealth system has been set up (e.g. with bandwidth limitations) than some unexplained quirk of the software. Consequently there is usually less value in trying to reconfigure coding and transmission applications software to improve useability, than in seeking an upgrade of the system to improve performance or a revision of the system architecture to make better use of the applications.

In the Health domain, standardisation follows a different model. Rather than adopting an overarching standardization process (and organisation), standards specific to certain clinical areas tend to be developed and adopted by the related professional bodies or government agencies. For example, the international medical image format standard used in radiology, DICOM, was developed the American College of Radiology (ACR) and the National Electrical Manufacturers Association (NEMA) also mentioned in the previous chapter [7]. In this environment, emerging standards are often promulgated as "clinical guidelines" or "best practice procedures". The lack of a formal standardisation mechanism in many such cases, and the reluctance to adopt changes to fixed clinical practice without conclusive clinical evidence of its efficacy, has led to this area moving comparatively slowly. In such circumstances, it is essential to share knowledge and exemplars, including case studies or success/failure anecdotes to help drive the acceptance of these putative standards further.

10. Future Developments in Telehealth

As noted above, Telehealth has been seen as a promising area of e-Health but it has not yet achieved widespread adoption. There are many reasons for this, from achieving cost benefit on appropriate scales, to dealing with human resistance to change. Some of the more immediate future areas for development in Telehealth below will contribute to overcoming some of these barriers and boosting uptake.

10.1 Universal Connectivity

The expectation that our future world will provide an environment of mobile and ubiquitous computing, allowing access to information systems for everyone, anywhere, anytime and with unlimited bandwidth and computational resources, will overcome one of the greatest limitations with current Telehealth systems. The expense and complexity of operating dedicated channels of high integrity and availability, as required by the critical nature of some Telehealth services (especially *synchronous* situations like teleconsultation or tele-surgery), would be negated in such a universal environment. One of the major problems to be solved for this to happen is that flexible, seamless transitions must occur between different forms of telecommunications channels, communications protocols, data representations, and information input/output devices, so that the user still obtains acceptable (indeed best case) performance when moving from a higher bandwidth richer presentation situation to a more constrained one (or vice versa). This concept is termed "scalability" and it will require considerable progress in the convergence (or harmonization) of currently highly disparate standards, or at least the introduction of a meta-standard that defines dialogue and negotiation between services running on those different standards. In the *asynchronous* arena, universal connectivity will also benefit Telehealth, as it will enable easier collection of physiological signals and behavioural data for patient monitoring without the need for explicitly instrumenting the patient's living environment. The health care system will then be better positioned to offer individualised care responding to actual patient disposition and progress, and to move the patient treatment focus further away from hospital- or clinic-based care.

10.2 Privacy and Security

The legal and social sensitivities which require careful adherence to privacy and security principles when dealing with Health Data have been covered elsewhere in this text. Telehealth is an area which holds greater risks than many, due to the difficulty of controlling access to the transfer and presentation components of sessions. Telecommunications across public networks, or over long distances with multiple hops between intermediate systems, are more prone to snooping and interception. Concealed presence or covert eves dropping by additional parties at the remote end controlled by a carer or clinician, of which patients would be unaware, can constitute a violation of their rights. Recording or summarizing of teleconsultation sessions (e.g. on CD) can lead to personal information being available outside of the normal controlled confines of the health service information system. Handling of patient monitoring data by proprietary systems not bound by universal standards can result in potentially catastrophic changes or losses in that data. There is much to be done to establish some principles initially and eventually some standards to address these issues.

10.3 Realism and Intelligence

An aspect of teleconsultation systems which is often criticised is the lack of realism, which detracts from the effectiveness of the session as compared with true human presence. A similar limitation affects tele-investigation and tele-collaboration situations, where clinicians feel restricted in the range of actions or interactions they can perform naturally. The greater the number of participants in a joint group interactive session, the harder it is to achieve a realistic (and controlled) session. These conditions can be improved with greater bandwidth, as well as more sophisticated functionality including some built-in adaptation or "learning" by Telehealth systems so that they actively predict or extrapolate from the past behaviour of session participants. A further enhancement along these lines would be the automatic extraction of information from Telehealth sessions, to provide automatic summarisation and capture of factual information from a session as part of the patient record. This could in turn feed into some clinical decision support system which assisted the clinician with achieving the objectives of the session, such as making a diagnosis or revising a care plan. Ultimately this may lead us to the "computer-as-doctor" situation where Telehealth includes in its gamut the provision of automated health care services.

References

[1]   World Health Organisation, Department Essential Health Technologies, "Information technology in support of health care", http://www.who.int/eht/en/InformationTech.pdf   no date, cited 6 October 2008
[2]   ISO/TR16056:2004 International Standards Organisation, Technical Report "Interoperability of telehealth systems and networks", ISO TC 215, Geneva 2004.
[3]   SA TR 2961:2007 Standards Australia, Technical Report "Telehealth standards scoping study", SA IT-14-12, Sydney 2007
[4]   Joint Photographic Experts Group (JPEG), http://www.jpeg.org/
[5]   Moving Picture Experts Group (MPEG), http://www.chiariglione.org/mpeg/
[6]   International Organisation for Standardization (ISO), http://www.iso.org/iso/home.htm
[7]   National Electrical Manufacturers Association, Digital Imaging and Communications in Medicine *DICOM Home Page.*See http://medical.nema.org/ (cited May 2008)

Further Reading

Journals:

1.   Royal Society of Medicine Press, *Journal of Telemedicine and Tele-care,* 1995-
2.   Mary Ann Liebert Publishers, *Telemedicine and e-Health,* 1995-
3.   Hindawi Publishing Corporation, *International Journal of Telemedicine and Applications,* 2008-

Books:
1.   Darkins AW & Cary MA, *Telemedicine and Telehealth: Principles, Policies, Performance and Pitfalls,* Springer, 2000.
2.   Norris AC, *Essentials of Telemedicine and Telecare,* John Wiley & Sons, 2001.
3.   Wootton R, Craig J & Patterson V (eds), *Introduction to Telemedicine*, RSM Press, 2006 (2nd ed).
4.   Wootton R; Dimmick S, Kvedar J (eds), *Home Telehealth: Connecting Care Within the Community,* RSM Press 2006.

Review Questions.

1.   Describe the primary concepts concerning the nature and usage of Telehealth systems in some common clinical settings.
2.   Explain some expected structures associated with typical interactive (synchronous) and non-interactive (asynchronous) Telehealth scenarios.
3.   What are the characteristics of human usage and physical infrastructures pertaining to typical Telehealth systems?

Health Informatics
E.J.S. Hovenga et al. (Eds.)
IOS Press, 2010
doi:10.3233/978-1-60750-476-4-255

255

20. Primary Care Informatics and Integrated Care

Siaw-Teng LIAW[1] MBBS, PhD DipObst, GrDipPHC, FRACGP, FACHI [a], Douglas I. R. BOYLE PhD, FACHI[b]

[a]*Director, SSWAHS General Practice Unit, Professor of General Practice Faculty of Medicine, The University of New South Wales, Australia*
[b]*Senior Research Fellow (Health Informatics), University of Melbourne, School of Rural Health, Shepparton, Victoria, Australia*

Abstract. This chapter gives an educational overview of:
- The biopsychosocial model of primary health care and longitudinal relationships;
- Management of undifferentiated problems and chronic illness within the clinical relationship;
- Patient–centred care in the context of health promotion, early detection and effective care of patients with chronic illness;
- Inter-professional networks, connectedness, connectivity and interoperability;
- Record linkage and health information sharing/exchange for clinical, audit, quality assurance, professional development and research purposes.

Keywords. Primary Healthcare, Computer Communication Networks, documentation, Healthcare Quality, Medical Informatics Applications, Electronic Prescribing, Referral and Consultation, Health Promotion, Quality Control, Communication, Interoperability, Risk Adjustment, Safety, Health Care Systems, Decision Support Systems-Clinical, User Computer Interface

Introduction

This chapter will examine connectivity across clinical professions and disciplines from the perspective of general practice and primary care. The context is safety and quality of acute and chronic disease management across the continuum of care. The scope will include clinical practice, safety and quality audit, evaluation and research, community health, management and policy dimensions. The focus will be patient-centred primary and chronic care, reflecting the biopsychosocial model and longitudinal relationships between patients and professionals, where patients present with unstructured and undifferentiated problems to specially trained primary care professionals. The unique features of family and general practice (FP/GP) in office based community settings and the discipline of dealing with all ages, sexes, and health conditions over the lifetime of a patient and his/her family require unique models of the cognition and decision-making thinking, leading to unique issues in health and medical informatics in general practice and primary care. Various perspectives matched to the diverse needs of primary care

---

[1] Corresponding Author: siaw@unsw.edu.au

health professionals, managers, policy makers and ICT systems and services vendors will be discussed. Where indicated, international relevance and harmonisation will also be examined.

1.   The Australian Health System

The Australian health system is underpinned by the universality of Medicare Australia, Pharmaceutical Benefits Scheme (PBS) and public hospital care. The PBS and Medicare Australia subsidise medicines and health services respectively. In addition, there is a cap on individual annual expenditure on medicines and health services after which the citizen receives PBS and Medicare services free. The Repatriation PBS (RPBS) provides veterans with free medicines. Medicines included in the PBS may be prescribed in three categories: (1) unrestricted, (2) restricted to specific conditions, or (3) require an authority to prescribe. An authority to prescribe is requested over the phone with a trained clerical person, a time-consuming process seen as a cost containment strategy with an inappropriate clerical role for doctors [1]. The recent streamlined authority codes scheme [2] allowed doctors to prescribe a list of (cheaper) drugs, using a drug group number available online, bypassing the phone approval process.

The majority of Australian general practitioners/family physicians (GP/FP) use computers to prescribe and print scripts [3]. This has been promoted by the Australian government through Practice Incentives Payments (PIP) for using information and communication technologies (ICT) to prescribe and do business using the Internet-based Medicare Online[2] and EFTPOS-based Medicare Easyclaim[3], and subsidies to use ICT infrastructure like Broadband for Health (BFH). The National E-Health Transition Authority (NEHTA)[4] was established to develop required interoperability standards for health information sharing and a national electronic health record system, HealthConnect [4] which has a medicines component (MediConnect). With increasing evidence supporting the cost-effectiveness of computerised decision support Kawamoto et al [5]. proposed strategies to promote a national eHealth and decision support program [6] and the emphases of the 2008 Australian National Health and Hospitals Reform Commission (NHHRC)[5], the future is likely to involve eCommerce, ePrescribing and decision support systems.

As prescribers and gatekeepers to the Australian health system, GP/FP are key determinants of health care and medicines utilisation volumes and patterns. The domains of general/family practice are first contact care, longitudinality, coordination of care, comprehensiveness and patient-doctor relationship [7]. This is consistent internationally as family medicine in the USA identified a New Model of Practice characterised by a patient-centred team approach; elimination of barriers to access; advanced information systems, including an electronic health record; redesigned, more functional offices; a focus on quality and outcomes; and enhanced practice finance [8]. These attributes form a framework for the examination of how medicines and health services are used [9].

The 2008 Australian National Health and Hospitals Reform Commission emphasised the following for the Australian Health System:

---

[2] http://www.medicareaustralia.gov.au/provider/business/online/medicare-online.shtml
[3] http://www.medicareaustralia.gov.au/provider/medicare/claiming/easyclaim/index.shtml
[4] www.nehta.gov.au
[5] www.nhhrc.org.au

- integrated and coordinated care across all aspects of the health sector and between primary care and hospital services, acute and aged care services and rural and metropolitan health services;
- a greater focus on prevention, healthy lifestyle and early intervention in chronic illness; improving rural and indigenous health services and outcomes; and
- a well qualified and sustainable health workforce into the future.

Optimal primary care is information-enhanced and evidence-based [10]. It is comprehensive, longitudinal and patient-centred, usually delivered as integrated care by inter-professional teams. A key component of integrated care is continuity, which has three dimensions [11]:

1. Informational continuity—the use of information on past events and personal circumstances to make current care appropriate for each individual;
2. Management continuity—a consistent and coherent approach to the management of a health condition that is responsive to a patient's changing needs; and
3. Relational continuity—an ongoing therapeutic relationship between a patient and one or more providers.

Australian GP/FP conducted more than 100 million consultations in 2006-7, managing about 1.50 problems per encounter [12]. This increase of 5.4 million consultations from 1999-2000, with a significant increase in longer consultations, reflects an ageing population with increasing chronic disease, such as diabetes, cancer, cardiovascular disease and mental ill health. Also increased are referral rates to medical specialists, especially cardiologists, and psychologists, podiatrists and dietitians; and imaging and laboratory investigations. Overall GP/FP prescribed 83.3 prescriptions per 100 encounters in 2006-7, down from 94 in 1999-2000. At least one medicine was prescribed, supplied or advised to obtain over the counter for over half the problems managed by GP/FP [12]. Extrapolating to the 103 million GP/FP encounters claimed from Medicare in 2006-7, it is estimated that Australian GP/FP prescribed more than 85 million medicines (82%); supplied 9.1 million medicines directly to the patient (8.8%); and recommended medicines for OTC purchase on 9.6 million occasions (9.2%). This represents half of PBS-subsidised pharmaceuticals and one-fifth of OTC purchases.

From the safety perspective, an estimated 16% of hospitalised patients suffer an adverse event, with 50% of these events being preventable [13]. About 10.4% of the 17.5 million people who make 95 million visits to their GP/FP annually will experience an adverse drug event (ADE); about 1 million ADE being moderate or severe and 138,000 requiring hospitalisation [14]. Half (56%) of preventable ADEs occur during drug ordering and 4% at dispensing [15].

Health services and quality use of medicines (QUM) research requires data collection and monitoring systems, linking drug utilisation, health services and clinical information, to examine cost-effectiveness, safety, quality, and appropriate prescribing of medicines, including those used off-label and outside PBS-approved indication ("*leakage*"). The main sources of information about Australian prescribing activities are the Australian Statistics on Medicines (ASM) [16] and BEACH (Bettering the Evaluation And Care of Health) reports, "General practice activity in Australia" [17]. The ASM dataset does not include a large proportion of public hospital drug use, over the counter purchases (except for S3 Recordable medicines) or the supply of highly specialised drugs to outpatients through public hospitals under Section 100 of the National Health Act 1953. These national data sets are insufficient to further understanding of QUM beyond prescribing rates; information is incomplete on some classes of drugs, characteristics of the patients or indications for their use. In contrast, the more comprehensive patient-level information from the electronic prescribing packages of participating GP/FP enabled an assessment of the appropriateness of therapy [18].

There must be universal benchmarks in defining and measuring appropriate use of health services and medicines, in relation to health outcomes. In addition to developing performance indicators, especially with regular reporting requirements, there is a need for resources to develop the data collection, linkage and aggregation systems as part of routine practice in this next generation health system. This is especially important if there is a need to collect patient-level data, including linked data, to measure the continuum of a person's health service needs and utilisation patterns over time. A comprehensive understanding of the health statistics require an appreciation of the biopsychosocial model of primary health care and longitudinal relationships, the reality of managing unstructured problems and uncertainty within the clinical relationship, and providing patient–centred care in the context of health promotion, prevention, early treatment, and rehabilitation.

2.   The Place of Informatics

The unique features of family and general practice (FP/GP) in office based community settings and the discipline of dealing with all ages, sexes, and health conditions over the lifetime of a patient and his/her family require unique models of the cognition and decision-making thinking, leading to unique issues in health and medical informatics in general practice and primary care. Research is urgently needed to verify the models of thinking that physicians use during patient care encounters and the associated nomenclatures and classifications which support them. User interfaces need to be optimized for accuracy and speed. Standards for medical records computing in general and family practice need testing and validation [19].

To this end, an appropriate definition of primary care informatics [20] is

"… the scientific study of data, information and knowledge, and how they can be modelled, processed or harnessed to promote health and develop patient-centred primary medical care. Its methods reflect the biopsychosocial model of primary healthcare and the longitudinal relationships between patients and professionals. Its context is one in which patients present with unstructured problems to specially trained primary care professionals who adopt a heuristic approach to decision making within the consultation".

As part of health system reform, the NHHRC[6] has highlighted a number of challenges with the fragmented Australian health care system, especially in relation to preventive strategies and a reformed chronic disease management system, that require primary care and informatics solutions that are ethical, secure and protect personal privacy. These include:

- "…fragmented responsibilities between Commonwealth and state governments and poor communication and sharing of information between hospital maternity care and primary and community care hinders effective provision of services…" (Challenge 3);
- "…With many different programs and services with different rules and

---

[6] www.nhhrc.gov.au

funded in different ways, there is little ability for service continuity, responsiveness in planning and implementing local models of integrated care, or use of new communication technologies that are focused on the needs of people in their local communities..." (Challenge 4).

- "...In the longer term, preventive strategies and a reformed chronic disease management system with improved management of care and information across the many interfaces of care will reduce demand on public hospitals and allow better access to elective surgery..." (Challenge 6).
- "...Improvements need to tackle systemic, communication and information management issues including better patient identification, handover and decision support..." (Challenge 8).
- "...It is imperative to implement a robust and standards-compliant information management system that enables individuals to authorise access to their vital health details across all health care environments including hospitals, GPs and other health professionals, where they choose to do so, in an agreed privacy regime..." (Challenge 11).

These challenges and their solutions require an understanding of informatics tools such as record linkage and health information sharing/exchange for clinical decision support, audit, quality assurance, professional development and research purposes. Patient safety and the quality of care can be improved in a number of ways:

1. Making health and medical knowledge available to the clinician and patient when it is needed at point of care;
2. Information sharing and prompting about duplications e.g. tests ordered because investigations carried out by the GP are not available to the hospital consultant, leading to greater cost-efficiencies in health services; and
3. Prompting to reduce potential errors in use of medicines e.g. wrong drug for diagnosis, drug-drug interaction, and out of range values or activities in managing health problems e.g. diabetes protocols.

As part of routine health care, a range of biomedical, clinical and community health research data is collected on the patient in a number of settings from laboratories to bedside to general practice consulting rooms. To maximise the utility of these information and personalise health care, the information need to be linked to specific individuals. However, significant quality, ethical, legal and social issues are associated with record linkage, de-identification and re-identification, information sharing and central information repositories.

Routinely collected electronic health care data, aggregated into large databases, is being used for audit, quality improvement, health service planning, epidemiological study and research. However, studies in primary care have demonstrated that gaps exist about how to find relevant data, select appropriate research methods and ensure that the correct inferences are drawn [21]. Routinely collected primary care data could contribute more to the process of health improvement; however, those working with these data need to understand fully the complexity of the context within which data entry takes place [22]. Metadata are important. Explicit statements are needed to explain the source, context of recording, validity check and processing method of any routinely collected data used in research [23]. Presentation of data about mortality in practice populations can enable practices and teams to reflect on their clinical policies, leading to improved quality of care and patient safety [24]. At the enterprise level, this type of information has demonstrated that Kaiser Permanente achieved better performance, measured as prompt and appropriate diagnosis and treatment, at roughly the same cost as the NHS because of integration throughout the system, efficient management of hospital use and greater investment in information technology [25].

The opportunities for health practice and research are:

- Growing volumes of routinely recorded data, especially for the growing number of patients with chronic disease and complex interactions between disease and drugs;
- Improved and improving data quality [26] and standardisation;
- Technological progress enabling large datasets to be processed;
- The potential to link clinical data with other data including genetic databases; and
- An established body of know-how within the international health informatics community.

However, there are challenges, including:

- Growing complexity and pace of change in medicine and technology with almost 500K new publications in Medline every year;
- Research methods for analysing and interpreting data in large datasets are limited;
- Integrating systems where there is often no reliable unique identifier and between health (person-based records) and social care (care-based records e.g. child protection);
- Informed consent and achieving appropriate levels of information security and privacy; and
- Legal and social issues related to health care policy, financing and professional practice.

In terms of technology diffusion, the drivers for adoption of informatics and electronic decision support (EDS) tools in eHealth, eResearch and eLearning include:

- Private and secure information exchange;
- Accurate patient identification to underpin epidemiological research and post-marketing surveillance;
- Accurate disease detection (sentinel) and surveillance;
- Safe and accurate clinical decision support systems for patient and provider;
- Personalised use of evidence from the literature and patient records to guide individual management e.g. "*virtual n-of-1 clinical trial*";
- Staff/workforce capacity and capability;
- Organisational / Administrative drivers;
- Population / public health drivers;
- Community / Sociocultural drivers; and
- Legislative / policy / political drivers.

The efforts of the Australian government in the last decade has led to almost universal electronic script-printing in general practice [3]. The Australian approach has been to build the national infrastructure, provide a supportive environment and develop interoperability standards to encourage the computer industry to build a national shared EHR and standards-based eHealth systems. In developing a 'person-centred' system, many countries are starting to focus on the personal health record (PHR), as part of the EHR strategy. A national eHealth implementation agency is being mooted to complement the National E-Health Transition Authority (NEHTA), whose role was to develop the required standards. The National Health and Hospitals Reform Commission has emphasised eHealth and has KPIs for "improving and connecting information to support high quality care". Despite demonstrated benefits from well-designed information management and decision support systems, in both electronic and non-electronic formats, across a wide range of health care environments [27], there is still not acceptable levels of safety and quality in the health care in Australia [28], USA [29] and the rest of the world [30].

A well designed and managed health information exchange and network, with good standard operating procedures supported by education and training, is a fundamental requirement for safe and accurate information-enhanced health care, improve continuity of care and prevent identity theft or leakage. This health information exchange is also essential for conducting quality multi-centre practice-based clinical and health services research and evaluation, health informatics and clinical decision support research and epidemiological and community health research.

3. Ethical and Secure Information Sharing in Integrated Care

A health information exchange (HIE) mobilises healthcare information electronically across organizations within a region or community, linking the personal information of a single individual held on different databases, while maintaining the relevance and meaning of the information being exchanged. HIE facilitates access to and retrieval of clinical data to provide more timely, efficient, effective, equitable, patient-centered care. In most countries that have embarked on this path, the planned architecture of a national HIE is logically a network of regional HIE. In the USA, Regional Health Information Organizations (RHIO) are geographically-defined entities which, using a range of business and financing models, develop and manage a set of contractual conventions and terms, arrange for the means of electronic exchange of information, and develop and maintain HIE standards [31]. The UK NHS has also divided the country into several regional HIE.

The University of Melbourne Collaborative Network and Data Using IT (CONDUIT) research and development program aims to develop such a HIE for clinical, audit and research purposes[7]. CONDUIT has developed a set of utilities, called GRHANITE™, to achieve this HIE by accurately and efficaciously linking data from multiple sources without needing or using any identifying information or third-party key holders. GRHANITE™ moves and manipulates information across the Internet, using state-of-the-art encryption and comprehensive security programming techniques to overcome longstanding confidentiality and security issues associated with health information sharing. Personal identifiers are removed before any movement of data. The system also manages consent and retrospective withdrawal of consent. GRHANITE™ ensures that the identity of an individual can be established only by authorized users at sites that originate the patient data.

With GRHANITE™ installed in all participating organisations in a collaborative Internet-based network, the patient, provider and site will be identifiable in a very secure and confidential manner, as long as consent is valid and the system is connected to the Internet. Outside of the source system, all information about the patients and providers are encrypted and not re-identifiable as illustrated by Figure 1.

The GRHANITE™ record linkage methodology builds on current techniques of privacy-preserving data linkage programs [32] [33] [34] [35]. The efficacy of the GRHANITE™ techniques have been statistically ascertained through a comparison with an industry standard probabilistic record linkage technology (from Sun Microsystems) linking 45,000 records from 10 different data sources. An extensive in-house test, using a

---

[7] www.conduit.unimelb.edu.au

database of 850,000 individuals in Victoria and the 2006 Australian Census [36] have further confirmed the efficacy and accuracy of the GRHANITE™ Statistical Linkage Keys methodology. GRHANITE™ uses the security inherent in its implementation to achieve a middle ground between absolute anonymity and pragmatic de-identified record linkage. Details of the specific techniques employed were reported at the HIC2008 Conference, Melbourne 2008.

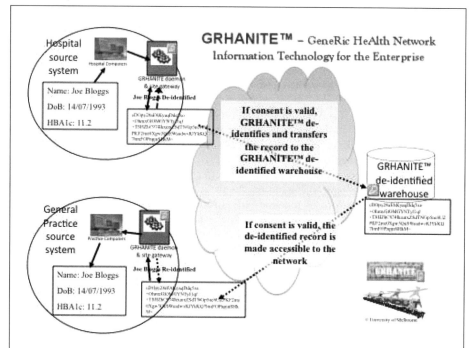

SCENARIO: Joe Bloggs attends a hospital service. If consent is not withdrawn or has been waived, GRHANITE™ automatically de-identifies Joe's personal and clinical information and transfers them to the GRHANITE™ de-identified data warehouse, making them available to the network. Joe's GP can download Joe's de-identified information and GRHANITE™ can decrypt the information for clinical purposes within the practice. Decryption can only occur in the source system. All information outside of the health service is stored or manipulated encrypted.

Figure 1. Ethical and Secure Information Sharing with GRHANITE™

GRHANITE™ is currently being used for:
1. **health surveillance** in the Australian Collaboration for Chlamydia Enhanced Sentinel Surveillance (ACCESS) project, with waiver of consent. This involves 68 sites across Australia (30 general practices, 30 laboratories and 8 family planning centres). This is done in collaboration with the Burnet Institute[8].
2. **audit, epidemiology and governance reporting** in CONDUIT Phase 1, where non-identifiable patient information is being extracted and aggregated from GP information systems (Medical Director and Practix) in rural Victoria, using an opt-out consent model. This is in partnership with Divisions of General Practice.

---

[8] www.burnet.edu.au

3. **clinical information sharing** in CONDUIT Phase 2, where GP information systems in Phase 1 are to be linked to a hospital-based diabetes care clinic with re-identification of the patient in the health service which provided the information; consent is opt-out. This is in partnership with BioGrid Australia[9] , health services and Divisions of General Practice.

4. **other inter-sectoral uses:** There are numerous other potential uses of GRHANITE™ in all professional domains e.g. education, law and banking. Post-marketing surveillance of pharmaceuticals is an obvious domain being explored.

Record linkage oversight processes are simplified with security, record linkage and consent mechanisms being part of one package, with no need for humans to be in the loop routinely. The approach adopted enables information sharing with minimal risk of patient identity exposure en-route or during storage, allowing data to flow among systems without ever exposing identity. Just as important, it does not "lock in" any vendor or service/support contracts. It makes central registers possible without risking patient identity exposure or theft and overcomes reservations by health authorities about identifiable data leaving their organization for record linkage purposes.

4. Information Sharing to Improve Chronic Disease Management

The commonly used software applications in Australia collect information that are common to most patient groups and used by most providers, including:

- alerts and allergy information
- laboratory data
- diagnostic images
- other investigative data e.g. consult notes
- medication management and orders
- lifestyle issues questionnaires
- vital signs and statistics eg. Height, weight, blood pressure
- referrals to other providers and support systems
- patient plans and goals
- outcome measures

However, the capture, storage and retrieval of such information are not always convenient, organized or meaningful to the practitioner or the practice in primary care. The potential to share information is also not being realized to support patient-focused communication between health care providers (HCP), enable HCP to be informed of key factors and indicators that mark the progress of the stages in a disease, and assist coordination of care by sharing information and supporting workflow.

Apart from a small number of pilot regional projects e.g. the HealthConnect[10] pilot projects and lack of long-term prospects[11], there are currently no formal regional health information exchanges or networks in Australia[12]. Point to point email is still a minority practice. Multiple paper copies of health care records are kept at different locations and no one record contains all the information. There are linkages to pathology and imaging

---

[9] www.biogrid.org.au

[10] www.health.gov.au/healthconnect

[11] www.australianit.news.com.au/story/0,24897,16727512-15306,00.html

[12] www.health.gov.au/internet/main/publishing.nsf/Content/eHealth)

laboratories for reports, but little else. Relevant information from laboratories may become lost in the large volume of laboratory test results that are returned or generated daily. Key health record information is not available at all locations where patients with chronic conditions are managed. As a result, timely and appropriate communication between clinicians, caregivers, and patients is inhibited.

The chronic care model (CCM) envisages a system in which informed, activated patients interact with prepared, proactive practice teams. It consists of 6 interrelated components [37]:

1. *Community resources and policies* refers to the mobilisation of community resources to meet patient needs, encouraging patients to participate in community programs, health care organizations forming partnerships with community-based organizations, and advocating for improved patient care;

2. *Health system organisation* refers to the support for the creation of organisations and systems that promote safe, high-quality care, comprehensive health system change/reform, provision of incentives to improve quality of care, and systems to coordinate care across organizations;

3. *Self-management* refers to support for activities that empower and prepare patients to manage their health care, enhance patients' central role in care and treatment and improve self-management support strategies, including assessment, goal setting, action planning, problem solving, and follow-up;

4. *Delivery system design* refers to ensuring delivery of effective and efficient clinical care and self-management support, promoting roles definition among the clinical care team, an internal and external communication strategy and service delivery between the team members and clients, and regular follow-up;

5. *Decision support* increases the capacity of the clinical team to promote care that is consistent with scientific evidence and patient preferences, reflect treatment guidelines, improve information sharing with patients, based on proven methods of provider education and integrate specialist expertise and primary care; and

6. *Clinical information systems* to facilitate effective care, use data to monitor the performance of the care system, provide reminders to providers and patients, facilitate case planning and provide information necessary for coordinating care among patients and their providers.

The goal of chronic care or disease management is to address the illness with maximum effectiveness and efficiency, regardless of the treatment setting. The various components of the CCM can improve the care of patients with chronic illness. The value of the CCM is reflected in the literature, especially in that related to the care of people living with diabetes. A systematic review of 39 studies of diabetes care programs that applied at least one component of the CCM found that the intervention improved at least one process or outcome measure in 32 of the 39 studies. Studies focusing on specific chronic conditions - congestive heart failure, asthma, and diabetes - demonstrated that CCM interventions resulted in reduced health care costs and reduced use of health care services. No specific element of the CCM was found to be critical for effectiveness. However, 19 of 20 interventions using a self-management component improved a process or outcome measure in diabetes [37].

In another CCM-related study [38], the *Allies Against Asthma* coalitions collaboratively identified and addressed problems related to system fragmentation and to improve coordination of care. Each coalition developed a variety of interventions related to its specific needs and assets, stakeholders, stage of coalition formation, and the dynamic structure of its community. Despite common barriers in forming alliances with busy providers and their staff, organizing administrative structures among inter-institutional cultures, enhancing patient and/or family involvement, interacting with multiple insurers, and contending with health system inertia, the coalitions demonstrated the ability to produce coordinated improvements to existing systems of care [36]. Common success factors for disease management include understanding the course of the disease, targeting the patients most likely to benefit from intervention, increasing patient compliance through education and behavior change strategies, providing full care continuity, and evaluating outcomes.

Software tools to support chronic care across the continuum of care are key levers to enable the full realization of the cost-benefits of a shared electronic health record [39]. The shared EHR and chronic care information systems (CCIS) are usually focused on:

1. Enhanced provider and consumer communication, through an online portal or as automated messaging (fax, e-mail, HL7, etc.), to facilitate electronic referrals between care providers;
2. Electronic order entry and result messaging across the continuum of care;
3. A single longitudinal EHR for each client for all programs and services;
4. Standard chronic illness care plans, with the CCIS as the integration point for cross-continuum care plan development and administration; and
5. Enhanced communication and information sharing for individuals, health care providers, researchers and the system as a whole.

Secure on-line access to their personal electronic health records, using personal identifiers, will enable patient access to their personal health information and a broader base of general information on health issues. With the click of a mouse, individuals with chronic illness can access relevant information to allow them to play a more direct role in managing their own health.

Clinicians would have access to patient records at the point of a clinical encounter as well as clinical decision support tools to facilitate evidence-based practice. The EHR and CCIS would help manage the massive amounts of complex health information, ensure access to complete and accurate information about patients' health and health care histories, and improve clinicians' ability to access the latest information, select the best course of action, and use evidence to guide their decisions.

Researchers, planners and policymakers concerned with chronic diseases would have access to aggregate data compiled through the EHR system. These data, extracted generically for health research purposes may be *non-identifiable* or *re-identifiable*. Re-identifiable health information allows certain illnesses or health-related factors to be tracked over time, monitoring and measuring patient outcomes in the management and treatment of chronic illnesses; it will also allow data mining to generate hypotheses and ask pertinent research questions. Privacy-preserving technologies [32] [33] [35] and organisational protocols are essential to ensure that the privacy of individuals can be effectively protected to allow re-identification. The CONDUIT and GRHANITE™ utility is a useful approach with generic application.

5. Conclusion

To achieve meaningful reform within the universality of Medicare, PBS and public hospital care, it is essential that resources and information are shared among people and information systems. Interpersonal sharing requires connectedness, connectivity and semantic standards; sharing among information systems requires interoperability (technical, syntactic and semantic) standards. Optimal information sharing and exchange requires informed consumers and providers; accurate, secure and confidential identification of patient, provider and location; accurate and standardised information; robust and secure information systems; and well-grounded standard operating procedures and governance protocols.

Information exchange and sharing is complex, especially in the real world of disparate legacy systems and lack of implemented interoperability standards. HIE needs interfacing and aggregating mechanisms that circumvent the current lack of standardisation and provide an affordable migration path for data from legacy systems into newer technologies as they become available. This requires a secure and ethical environment for informed consent, patient identification, data encryption, extraction, linkage, aggregation and exchange within an Internet-based service oriented architecture. The solution must also be low-cost, open-source, modular, re-configurable and adaptable.

Supportive nationally-coordinated government policies and strategies which transcend jurisdictional and partisan politics, good transport and communication infrastructure, an adequately-funded and well-trained workforce and ongoing training and support programs are essential to maintain the safety and quality of the health system.

A cultural change in health services and government to emphasise capacity building, education, training and support - including specific training in eHealth and informatics tools - is key to recruiting and retaining a high-quality workforce. A quantum shift is required to move from the current very small scale and fragmented approaches to a nationally coordinated health research, education and informatics capacity building program in Australia.

The Australian College of Health Informatics[13] and the Australian Coalition for eHealth[14] has argued for a national eHealth strategy and work plan with a solid business case and credible funding over a realistic timeframe. This has since been taken up by the Australian Health Information Council (AHIC)[15] although AHIC was discontinued as from June 2008. Apart from coordinated investments in standards-based interoperable ICT and clinical systems, there must also be a systematic and coordinated capacity building program to ensure adequately skilled resources are available to support the implementation of the eHealth work plan.

A transparent and performance assessment approach to implementation is essential, with open access for public review and comment. The milestones and review points over the planned timeframe must enable appropriate and timely corrective action or fine tuning of the strategy as required following appropriate ongoing consultation involving key stakeholders, consumers and clinicians. A change management and communication strategy is critical. An evaluation research plan to monitor and measure performance outcomes achieved against specified objectives must be in place. In addition to clinical performance indicators, there is also a need to develop quality indicators for the data collection, linkage and aggregation systems to collect patient-level data, to enable the measurement of the continuum of a person's health service needs and utilisation patterns over time and across the health system.

If sufficiently funded and resourced, the implementation of a national eHealth program will require at least a decade to complete. But it may never be completed successfully without a health and health informatics workforce with the range of

---

[13] http://www.achi.org.au

[14] http://www.ceh.net.au/

[15] http://www.health.gov.au/internet/main/publishing.nsf/Content/ehealth-futuredirections

competencies and knowledge described. As Roy Romanow, Chief Commissioner of the Commission into the Future of Health in Canada emphasises,

> "Some might wonder why a chapter on information would figure so prominently and be placed at the beginning of a report on the future of Canada's health care system. The answer is that leading-edge information, technology assessment and research are essential foundations for all of the reforms outlined in subsequent chapters of this report" [40]

References

[1] Liaw, ST, C Pearce, P Chondros, B McGrath, L Piggford, and K Jones. 2003. Doctors' perceptions and attitudes to prescribing within the authority prescribing system. Med J Aust 178:203-206.
[2] Medicare Australia. 2008. Streamlined authority process, 2007 12 17 2007 [cited 18 Jan 2008 2008]. Available from http://www.medicareaustralia.gov.au/provider/pbs/doctor/streamlined-authority-process.shtml.
[3] Liaw, ST, and R Tomlins, eds. 2005. Chapter 12. Developments in information systems. Edited by C. D. o. H. F. Services. Vol. May 2005, General Practice in Australia 2004. Canberra: Aust Gov Publishing Services
[4] Health Insurance Commission, Australia. 2008. MediConnect. Medicare Australia 2008 [cited 22 Jan 2008 2008]. Available from http://www.medicareaustralia.gov.au/provider/patients/mediconnect.shtml.
[5] Kawamoto, K, CA Houlihan, EA Balas, and DF Lobach. 2005. Improving clinical practice using clinical decision support systems: a systematic review of trials to identify features critical to success. BMJ 330 (7494):765-.
[6] National Electronic Decision Support Taskforce. 2002. Report to Health Ministers: Electronic Decision support in Australia. Canberra: National Health Information Management Advisory Council.
[7] Buetow, SA. 1995. What do general practitioners and their patients want from general practice and are they receiving it - a framework. Social Science & Medicine 40 (2):213-221.
[8] Martin, JC, RF Avant, MA Bowman, JR Bucholtz, JR Dickinson, KL Evans, LA Green, DE Henley, WA Jones, SC Matheny, JE Nevin, SL Panther, JC Puffer, RG Roberts, DV Rodgers, RA Sherwood, KC Stange, CW Weber, and Future of Family Medicine Project Leadership Committee. 2004. The Future of Family Medicine: a collaborative project of the family medicine community. Ann Fam Med 2 (Suppl 1):S3-32.
[9] Anastasio, GD, MP Dutro, and LS Parent. 1986. Applying family medicine concepts to prescribing. Family Medicine 18 (5):259.
[10] Davidoff, F, B Haynes, D Sackett, and R Smith. 1995. Evidence based medicine. BMJ 310:1085-1086.
[11] Haggerty, JL, RJ Reid, GK Freeman, BH Starfield, CE Adair, and R McKendry. 2003. Continuity of care: a multidisciplinary review. BMJ 327 (22 Nov 2003):1219-1221.
[12] Britt, H, GC Miller, J Charles, C Bayram, Y Pan, J Henderson, L Valenti, J O'Halloran, C Harrison, and S Fahridin. 2008. General practice activity in Australia 2006–07. In General practice series no. 21; AIHW cat. no. GEP 21. Canberra: Australian Institute of Health and Welfare.
[13] Wilson, RM, and MB Van Der Weyden. 2005. The safety of Australian healthcare: 10 years after QAHCS. MJA 182 (6):260-261.
[14] Miller, GC, HC Britt, and L Valenti. 2006. Adverse drug events in general practice patients in Australia. MJA 184 (7):321-324.
[15] Leape, LL, DW Bates, DJ Cullen, J Cooper, HJ Demonaco, T Gallivan, R Hallisey, J Ives, N Laird, G Laffel, and et al. 1995. Systems analysis of adverse drug events. ADE Prevention Study Group. JAMA 274 (1):35-43.
[16] Commonwealth Department of Health and Aged Care (in conjunction with PBAC DUSC). 2005. Australian Statistics on Medicines 2004-5. AGPS, Canberra.
[17] Britt, H, GC Miller, J Charles, Y Pan, L Valenti, J Henderson, C Bayram, J O'Halloran, and S Knox. 2007. General practice activity in Australia 2005–06. In General practice series no. 19. AIHW cat. no. GEP 19. Canberra: Australian Institute of Health and Welfare.
[18] Robertson, J., D. Henry, T. Dobbins, A. Sprogis, R. Terry, and M. Ireland. 1999. Prescribing patterns in general practice. A comparison of two data sources. Australian Family Physician 28 (11):1186-90.
[19] Bernstein RM, Hollingsworth GR, Viner G. Evaluation of controlled medical terminologies for use in primary care electronic records. Discussion paper prepared for the American Medical Informatics Association Primary Care Working Group Conference, 1995 Nov 1; New Orleans.

[20] de Lusignan The National Health Service and the internet *J R Soc Med 2003*;**96**:490-493 doi:10.1258/jrsm.96.10.490
[21] de Lusignan, S, and C van Weel. 2006. The use of routinely collected computer data for research in primary care: opportunities and challenges. Family Practice 23 (2):253-263.
[22] de Lusignan, S, N Hague, J van Vlymen, and P Kumarapeli. 2006. Routinely-collected general practice data are complex, but with systematic processing can be used for quality improvement and research. Inform Prim Care 14 (1):59-66.
[23] de Lusignan, S, JF Metsemakers, P Houwink, V Gunnarsdottir, and J. van der Lei. 2006. Routinely collected general practice data: goldmines for research? A report of the European Federation for Medical Informatics Primary Care Informatics Working Group (EFMI PCIWG) from MIE2006, Maastricht, The Netherlands. Inform Prim Care 14 (3):203-209.
[24] Sullivan, E, R Baker, D Jones, H Blackledge, A Rashid, A Farooqi, and J Allen. 2007. Primary healthcare teams' views on using mortality data to review clinical policies. Qual Saf Health Care 16 (5):359-362.
[25] Feachem, RGA., NK Sekhri, KL White, J Dixon, DM Berwick, and AC Enthoven. 2002. Getting more for their dollar: a comparison of the NHS with California's Kaiser Permanente Commentary: Funding is not the only factor Commentary: Same price, better care Commentary: Competition made them do it. BMJ 324 (7330):135-143.
[26] Soto, CM, KP Kleinman, and SR Simon. 2002. Quality and correlates of medical record documentation in the ambulatory care setting. BMC Health Serv Res 2 (1).
[27] Kohn, LT, JM Corrigan, and MS Donaldson. 2000. To err is human: building a safer health system. Washington, D.C.: National Academy Press.
[28] Barraclough, BH. 2001. Safety and quality in Australian healthcare: making progress. The newly formed Australian Council for Safety and Quality in Health Care has ambitious plans. MJA 174:616-617.
[29] Leape, LL, and DM Berwick. 2005. Five Years After To Err Is Human What Have We Learned? JAMA 293:2384-2390.
[30] World Health Organization. 2008. The launch of the World Alliance for Patient Safety. "Please do me no harm." 2004 [cited Feb 2008 2008]. Available from www.who.int/patientsafety/launch/en/.
[31] Adler-Milstein, J, AP McAfee, DW Bates, and AK Jha. 2008. The State Of Regional Health Information Organizations: Current Activities And Financing. Health Affairs 27 (1):w60-69.
[32] Agrawal, D, and CC Agrawal. 2001. On the design and quantification of privacy preserving data mining algorithms. Paper read at 20th ACM SAGACT-SIGMOD-SIGART Symposium on Principles of Database Systems, at Santa Barbara, California.
[33] Agrawal, D, and R Srikant. 2000. Privacy-preserving data mining. Paper read at ACM SIGMOD Conference on Management of Data, June 2000, at Dallas, Texas.
[34] Churches, T , and P Christen. 2004. Some methods for blindfolded record linkage. BMC Med Inform Decis Making 4 (9).
[35] O'Keefe, C, M Yung, L Gu, and R Baxter. 2004. Privacy-preserving Data Linkage Protocols. In Workshop on Privacy in the Electronic Society '04; . Washington, DC, USA.
[36] Australian Bureau of Statistics. 2006 Census. Australian Bureau of Statistics 2008 [cited 28 Feb 2008. Available from www.abs.gov.au.
[37] Bodenheimer, T, EH Wagner, and K Grumbach. 2002. Improving primary care for patients with chronic illness. The Chronic Care Model Part 1 JAMA 288 (14):1775-1779.
[38] Bodenheimer, T, EH Wagner, and K Grumbach. 2002. Improving Primary Care for Patients with chronic Illness: The Chronic Care Model, Part 2. JAMA 288 (15):1909–1914.
[39] Rosenthal, MP, FD Butterfoss, LJ Doctor, LA Gilmore, JW Krieger, JR Meurer, and I Vega. 2006. The Coalition Process at Work: Building Care Coordination Models to Control Chronic Disease. Health Promot Pract 7 (2_suppl):117S-126.
[40] Romanow, R. 2002. Building on Values: The Future of Health Care in Canada. In Final Report. Ottawa: Commission on the Future of Health Care in Canada.

Review Questions

- What is the importance of Inter-professional networks, connectedness, connectivity and interoperability in primary care settings relative to the adoption of Patient–centred care in the context of health promotion, early detection and effective care of patients with a chronic illness?

taken to make sure that the right medication, right dose, right patient, right time, and right route is selected each and every time. It is the failure of any one of these that makes medication errors one of the leading causes of adverse reactions in all parts of the health systems all over the world [3] [4]. Many of the processes used in hospitals around the world are still paper based, which leads to problems of poor legibility, lack of standardisation of drug dosing and frequency nomenclature and hence the risk of more errors appearing. There are many examples of adverse events occurring based on the incorrect interpretation of an illegible prescription on a paper based medication chart or paper prescription. Errors occur due to dispensing the wrong medication or giving the wrong amount of a medication.

As modern medicine advances, medications and medication regimes are becoming more complex. Clinicians have to try to remember large numbers of complex interactions, not only drug to drug interactions, but also drug to disease interactions. The potential for errors to occur in a busy and stressful hospital or private clinic becomes even more likely. When patients are moving from one health service to another, where different clinicians are making changes to medication regimes, it is extremely important that those changes are adequately communicated between clinical settings.

2. Benefits of Electronic Medication Management

For the last 30 years, the practice of health informatics has promised to revolutionise healthcare by automating many parts of the health care environment. There have been many advances in health informatics and technology in that time span, however the vision of a world where health information is available across the whole continuum of care has not yet been realised. For various reasons, medication management is seen as a process that lends itself well to computerisation and is seen as providing a number of benefits. These benefits come under the following broad headings:

2.1 Reduced Medication Errors and Adverse Events

Most of the literature about the benefits of electronic medication management concentrates on this aspect. The use of electronic medication management systems should reduce the number of medication errors in all three of the areas of prescribing, dispensing and administration.

In the prescribing area this is by improving legibility and standardising the ways in which medication can be ordered as well as providing decision support at the point of prescribing to warn of such things as allergies, drug to drug interactions, drug to disease interactions, dosing guidelines etc.

In the area of dispensing of medication, legibility and standardisation of dosing nomenclature is paramount, especially in a community pharmacy, where the pharmacist may not have direct access to the clinician.

At the point of administering the medication, it can help to make sure that the drug is given to the right person, at the right time and that the dose is correct.

In all these areas, an electronic system makes it easier to see who did what and when so that a more complete record is kept about medication. There have been many studies done looking at the reduction in adverse events due to the use of CPOE and some of these have demonstrated reduction of adverse events by more than 50% and up to 80% [5]. This does seem to be dependent on the system used and where and how it has been implemented, as there have been cases, where introduction of a computerised system has actually seemed to increase patient mortalities [6].

2.2   Reduced Cost to the Health System

Reducing the number of adverse events caused by medication errors, will lead to a reduced cost burden on the health system and significant savings. This is estimated at up to one billion US dollars per year in the US alone [7]. Other areas where cost savings will occur is in better utilisation of medication.

2.3   Reduced Variance in Clinical Usage of Medication

As new medications become available and new treatments arise at a more and more rapid pace, it is becoming increasingly difficult for clinicians to keep up. Medication usage varies widely across the continuum of care and what one clinician uses for a particular problem may vary widely from another. This is often based on experience and comfort rather than national or international best practice.

Electronic systems can provide clinicians with best practice guidelines at the point of prescribing. This can lead to improved outcomes for patients and reduced costs for the health system.

2.4   Better Utilisation of Medications – Matching Indication to Drug

Electronic guidelines can improve utilisation of scarce resources in medication. A good example here is antibiotic usage, where the overuse and inappropriate use of these drugs has lead to increasing antibiotic resistance and increasing costs to the health system in treating with more expensive drugs for longer periods of time. Electronic systems can reduce antibiotic resistance, by promoting more appropriate use of the right antibiotic for the right indication.

2.5   Reduced Workload for Staff in Medication Management

A well designed and implemented medication management system should enable improvements in efficiency to enable better utilisation of time for other patient care. There have been some spectacular failures in implementing these systems, where change management hasn't been properly managed, and the systems themselves haven't been designed with clinician workflow in mind. If a clinician finds that using a system is more difficult or slower than their normal processes, without providing any other benefits, they will be reluctant to adopt it [8].

What are the requirements for an electronic medication management system, to enable it to provide the benefits as out lined above? This question is often asked by technicians and clinicians in one part of a health system, without giving much thought to the requirements of the whole continuum of care. What this means, is that a system that works in a particular vertical of the health services market i.e. a hospital, is not necessarily going to be able to share information with other parts of the health sphere such as family practice clinicians. Utilising standards and making sure that the data collected is able to be computed on is a very important part of enabling best use of a medication management approach.

3.   Prescribing

Prescribing software or CPOE is increasingly used in different parts of the world. In some parts of the world, it is the family physicians who have taken the lead in this area. In particular, in places like Denmark, Australia and the United Kingdom, the vast majority of primary care physicians use clinical applications to prescribe medications. Most of these systems still print out a prescription that is taken by hand to the pharmacy where it is dispensed. In this instance, the clinician has an accurate and detailed electronic record of the patient's medications and it is very fast and easy to add a new drug or re-prescribe an old one. In Denmark, clinicians can send a prescription electronically to the pharmacy and have it dispensed there with feedback that the medication has actually been dispensed.

There are a number of components that are essential in a CPOE system to enable the full benefits to be realised, especially for medication management across the health services continuum. These are:

- A unique patient identifier
- A common drug nomenclature or coding system
- A common format for describing a medication order that is useable for computation
- A common format for recording clinical information that is useable for computation
- A unique provider identifier and the ability to digitally sign an order

A **unique patient identifier** is a requisite building block for many parts of the health informatics environment and is worthy of a chapter in its own right. No attempt will be made here to define or describe it, save to say that to be able to identify who is the subject of a prescription is essential in all the parts of the medication management process. Chapter 11 has referred to this standard.

A **common drug nomenclature or coding system** is an important requirement for medication prescribing. At the point of prescribing, the clinician needs to be able to be presented with a current list of medications, the available strengths and forms of the drugs and pack sizes. This reduces the chance of making simple mistakes like misspelling the name or choosing a strength that is not available. Many of the commercial drug data lists will provide complete prescribing information that a clinician can look up at the point of prescribing for such information as indications, contraindications, interactions, side effects and dosing information.

More importantly, a common coding system for medications enables a computer system to recognise which drug has been prescribed and to enable decision support based on this information. When prescriptions are moved from one health service to another and one information system to another, a common coding system will enable these systems to recognise which drugs have been prescribed. This is very difficult to do from the drug name alone as the spelling and details may differ. For instance, one prescriber may use a generic drug name while another uses the brand name for the drug. Computer systems cannot easily recognise that these are the same thing without an identifier that uniquely matches the two. The ISO TC215 committee is working on resolving this issue.

A **common format for describing a medication order that is useable for computation** is very important when sharing information between computer systems or for decision support. A good example of the kind of information that needs to be recorded in this way is the timing of medication. Clinicians record the timing of medication in every medication that they prescribe. This can become very complex as it needs to cover such things as dose frequency, specific timing, dose duration, event related timing i.e. before meals, treatment duration, and changes based on triggers and outcomes. It is relatively easy for clinicians to record this on paper as there is an established short hand for these things although even that varies from place to place and clinician to clinician. However, to record this in a way that computers can utilise for accurately scheduling administration or for decision support is much more difficult. To enable this kind of data recording, the data must be accurately modelled using models that are computable. One such clinical modelling and electronic health record solution is called *open*EHR[2] and uses models called archetypes which are mathematically based models of clinical concepts as described in chapters 9 and 10.

When prescriptions are shared across different health services such as from a clinician to a community pharmacy, or from a hospital to a family physician, the ability for computer systems to reliably understand what the prescription means will enable clinicians to have a better knowledge of what medications the patient is currently taking and be warned about what the possible consequences of taking the particular medication might be. Having a common way of describing the prescription and also the processes that have occurred to that prescription i.e. dispensed, administered, ceased, etc., enable feedback loops to be implemented so that prescribing clinicians will be able to know whether a medication has been dispensed and where.

A **common format for recording clinical information that is useable for computation** is very important when decision support is required. A more detailed discussion of medication decision support is detailed below, however if a computer system is going to use data to inform a clinician about possible issues such as allergies or interactions, the underlying data needs to be in a format that is reliably computable. For decision support, if the data that the computer system is using for presenting possible issues to the clinician is not reliably computable, then the system may either present an issue that is not real or fail to present an issue that is real. In either case, the decision support is worse than none at all.

The unique provider identifier and the ability to digitally sign an order is also important so that an accurate and medico-legally binding record is maintained about who prescribed something. This is as protective for the clinician as it is for the patient, as it makes it much more difficult for someone to forge a prescription. Most digital signatures should utilise a public key infrastructure (PKI) process so that a signature can be verified by anyone using the clinician's public key as previously described in chapter 13.

4.   Dispensing

The commonest systems for medication management in hospitals today are those systems used by pharmacies to manage stock control and enable administrators to manage growing medication budgets. These systems have often grown to include clinical features for managing medication. Pharmacists provide a very important secondary mechanism for checking the suitability of drug indication, dosing and administration. In a hospital environment, the dispensing of a medication is often bound by rules relating to indication, cost and best practice. An electronic medication management system can make this process much more useable in a complex environment.

---

[2] http://www.openehr.org/

A completely electronic medication management system which worked across health system boundaries involves the ability for pharmacies to receive prescriptions electronically. This requires a common data format so that the pharmacy information system can accurately record what was dispensed and provide feedback to the clinician. In many countries, where a patient can visit any pharmacy of their choosing, a central repository of prescriptions will need to be developed so that when a patient arrives at a pharmacy, the pharmacist can access their prescription and dispense it. This process requires that the patient can be accurately identified both in the repository and by the pharmacist.

5. Administration

In the home or community, administration is usually carried out by the patient or the patient's carer. This is almost always a manual process, however with the advent of technologies such as Google health and home monitoring for blood pressure and other signs, it will soon be possible to record administration of medications at home. This is likely to be useful for the elderly and those that have carers so that information about what and how much medication is given can be known.

In the hospital situation, administration of medication, usually by nursing staff, is a major task that occurs at regular intervals during the day and night and more often for people undergoing intensive treatment. The application of information technology to this task, if the right software and hardware is used, can improve the process so that dose calculation and other possible errors are less likely and so that the task is more efficient. Information technology can make getting the correct patient right using barcode scanning or RFID tag scanning. Once the patient is identified, a medication management system should be able to say exactly what the drugs are that are required at that time, the dosage and the route of administration. The system should enable the accurate recording of what was given and when and by who – with a digital signature for the giver.

In general, the technology needed for hospital administration rounds, needs to be useable at the bedside. This means that hardware either needs to be mobile using hardened mobile and wireless equipment or needs to be at every bedside. Administration can be taken a step further and there are now systems that actually manage the physical medication and only release the right drug for the right person. These electronic storage cabinets are linked to prescribing, dispensing and administration software and are an attempt to completely close the loop so as to reduce administration errors as much as possible.

6. Decision Support and Medication Management

Medication management systems have the potential to be much more than just systems that make a doctors handwriting legible. As previously stated, modern medicine is changing at a great rate and it is difficult for any clinician to keep up with the changes and/or remember all the possible side effects or interactions for a particular drug. Indeed drugs are often not given in isolation and interact not only with other drugs, but foods and environmental things as well as disease processes. A good information system will be able to provide information to a clinician at the point of care, that is timely, accurate and most importantly, based on the individual who they are dealing with.

Decision support, whether in medication management or any other domain in health, is only as good as the information that it has to make decisions on. If that information is not accurate or not computable, then even the most sophisticated decision support algorithm will be of no value. Information needs to be in a format that is reliably computable and that reliably maintains the semantics or meaning of that information. To truly realise the power of decision support, clinical information must be available in forms such as *open*EHR which allow for complex clinical information to be captured with full semantics intact. When data is captured like this it will enable decision support and safety checks at many more points of the medication chain.

Decision support in medication management systems can cover a number of different areas and are most useful to the clinician at the point of prescribing.

- **Allergy warnings** – A good prescribing tool will warn a user, if the medication has one or more components that a patient may be allergic to. This should be able to be class based so that a person who is allergic to penicillins will get a warning about drugs that contain amoxicillin for instance.
- **Duplicate therapy checking** – making sure that the same thing isn't prescribed twice
- **Drug to drug warnings** – The prescribing software should be able to compare drugs already prescribed with the drugs that this person is already taking and warn of any potential interactions. This process needs to strike a balance between warning about too many things and not enough. If a clinician is bombarded with too many warnings, then it is possible that they will start to ignore warnings or take less notice. This requires the system to content on drug to drug interactions that is current and kept up to date.
- **Drug to disease warnings** – This process is more complicated as the data about diseases needs to be captured in such a way that the system can understand what a disease is. This also needs to have content about the interactions which is current and up to date. A number of commercial data providers can provide this kind of content. This kind of decision support can also support drug to pregnancy and drug to elite athlete warnings.
- **Dosing information** – A good system will enable users to calculate correct dosage for a medication based on factors such as the age, weight and sex of the patient. More complex systems can also take into account such things as renal function, however again this is dependent on the system being able to reliably access this data.
- **Care pathways and complex dosing regimens** – A good system should enable the prescribing of complex regimens and make it easy to comply with complex care pathways such as chemotherapy.

In summary for us to realise the benefits of electronic medication management we need to ensure that the flow of information concerning medicinal products locally, nationally and internationally is supported by standard unambiguous drug codes, as the more specificity with which a drug concept is entered into a computer for processing, the more specific the clinical information will be received in return. This is assisted by the adoption of standard clinical knowledge models (archetypes) so that the semantics of the clinical data remains in tact at all times throughout the electronic medication management process.

References

[1] Institute of Medicine (2000). To Err Is Human: Building a Safer Health System (2000). The National Academies Press.

[2] ISO/TR25257:2008 **Error! Reference source not found.** – final ballot draft version 2.2, ISO TC215, Geneva

[3] Phillips J, Beam S, Brinker A, Holquist C, Honig P, Lee LY, Pamer C., Retrospective Analysis of Mortalities Associated With Medication Errors - Am J Health-Syst Pharm 58(19):1835-1841, 2001. © 2001 American Society of Health-System Pharmacists

[4] Lazarou J, Pomeranz B H, Corey P N, Incidence of Adverse Drug Reactions in Hospitalized Patients: A Meta-analysis of Prospective Studies JAMA, Apr 1998; 279: 1200 - 1205.

[5] Bates D W, Leape L L, Cullen D J, Laird N, Petersen L A, Teich J M, Burdick E, Hickey M, Kleefield S, Shea B, Vander Vliet M, Seger D L, (1998). "Effect of Computerized Physician Order Entry and a Team Intervention on Prevention of Serious Medication Errors" (abstract). JAMA 280: 1311–1316. http://jama.ama-assn.org/cgi/content/abstract/280/15/1311

[6] Han YY, Carcillo J A, Venkataraman S T, Clark R S B, Watson R S, Nguyen T C, Bayir H, Orr R A (2005). "Unexpected Increased Mortality After Implementation of a Commercially Sold Computerized Physician Order Entry System". Pediatrics 116:No 6 pp1506–1512. doi:10.1542/peds.2005-1287 http://pediatrics.aappublications.org/cgi/content/abstract/116/6/1506

[7] RAND Healthcare: Health Information Technology: Can HIT Lower Costs and Improve Quality? http://www.rand.org/pubs/research_briefs/RB9136/index1.html

[8] Connolly, Ceci. "Cedars-Sinai Doctors Cling to Pen and Paper", The Washington Post, 2005-03-21. http://www.washingtonpost.com/wp-dyn/articles/A52384-2005Mar20.html

Review Questions

1. How can information technology best be used for medication management?
2. Where is the adoption of electronic medication most useful and what are its benefits?
3. What is required to implement these systems beyond the application requirements

Health Informatics
E.J.S. Hovenga et al. (Eds.)
IOS Press, 2010
© 2010 The authors and IOS Press. All rights reserved.
doi:10.3233/978-1-60750-476-4-278

22. Clinical Decision Support Foundations

Malcolm PRADHAN[1], MBBS, PhD[a], Siaw Teng LIAW MBBS, PhD DipObst, GrDipPHC, FRACGP, FACHI [b]

[a]*VP Research & Software, Alcidion Corporation, Adjunct Professor, Health Informatics, University of South Australia*
[b]*Director, SSWAHS General Practice Unit, Professor of General Practice Faculty of Medicine, The University of New South Wales, Australia*

Abstract. This chapter gives an educational overview of:
- The elements of a clinical decision;
- The elements of decision making: prior probability, evidence (likelihood), posterior probability, actions, utility (value);
- A framework for decision making, and support, encompassing validity, utility, importance and certainty; and
- The required elements of a clinical decision support system.
- The role of knowledge management in the construction and maintenance of clinical decision support.

Keywords. Decision Support Systems-Clinical, Medical Informatics Applications, Evidence Based Practice, Practice Guidelines, Knowledge, Data Management Systems, Quality of Healthcare, Professional Practice, Risk Adjustment, Safety, Software Design, Terminology

Introduction

Clinical Decision Support Systems (CDSS) have been an active area of research since the earliest days of health informatics [1] [2] [3], but despite this early interest there is very little computer-aided clinical decision support in routine use in the health care system today. What is the reason for this disparity between research and implementation? Could it be that the importance of CDSS were overstated, that health care does not need decision support, or that health care is simply too complex for computers to be of assistance? The determinants of the slow adoption of CDSS are more complex, requiring an optimal balance of a number of factors (otherwise the sections on CDSS would be significantly shorter).

1. The Need for CDSS

Why does health care urgently need clinical decision support? The progress of health care to improve our lives and increase survival have been significant, but evidence over the

---

[1] Corresponding Author: mp@alcidion.com.au

last 15 years has demonstrated clearly that problems in the effective delivery of health care results in patient harm, inefficient work practices, and unnecessary costs. For example:

- In Australia an estimated 12,000 to 14,000 people die in hospitals every year due to preventable errors (Wilson et al. 1995). Proportionate figures have been observed in the USA [4] [5].
- It has been estimated that up to 16% of hospitalised Australians will suffer an adverse event: 50% of these events will be preventable and 10% of these preventable events will lead to permanent disability or death [6].
- It is also estimated that about 10.4% of the 17.5 million Australians who make 95 million visits to their General Practitioner (GP) or Family Practitioner (FP) annually experience an adverse drug event (ADE): these ADEs are not trivial, with about 1 million being moderate or severe and 138,000 requiring hospitalisation [7].
- Up to 40% of results ordered in hospitals are never read by medical staff [8] [9] in hospitals with computerised pathology systems.
- Problems with managing high risk medications, such as Warfarin and Aminoglycosides result in significant patient complications such as bleeding, renal impairment and lengthy hospital stays.
- Approximately 40% of patients who are treated for myocardial infarction are not discharged on the appropriate medications [10] [11].

These systemic problems in health care are well recognised by government bodies and significant national level reports have been published in response in numerous countries [5] [4] [12]. The possibility that clinicians can inadvertently harm patients – *iatrogenesis* - has been long recognised; over 2000 years ago Hipprocrates created an oath for healers that included "never do harm" and was aware of the dangers of medications.

It is important to note that these high rates of error are in an industry with highly dedicated staff who work very hard to improve patient outcomes. How can a health care with highly skilled, dedicated staff have higher rates of error than any other industry? It is widely recognised by national agencies that problems in western health care are predominantly due to underlying problems in the way health care is delivered. Some error-promoting practices include:

- Memory-based: The delivery of health care relies on an individual's memory with little support from computers and other tools;
- Inefficient work practices: almost 60% of clinician time is spent in non-clinical, manual, administrative tasks, in addition there are high rates of interruptions [13] [14];
- Cognitive limitations: There are well recognised cognitive biases and limitations to the way individuals handle complex decision making problems [15]; and
- Lack of system-wide mechanisms to catch and prevent errors from causing patient harm [16].

In other industries high error rates and waste could not be so tolerated; such inefficiency would result in significant financial losses and a company that didn't invest in improving its performance would not be in business for long. However, health care in the public sector is not driven by normal competitive forces, since demand is high and resources are limited. In the private sector it could be observed that suboptimal performance results in more business rather than less. A key problem for health care is that it does not routinely measure its benefits, either in dollars or quality of life, so calculating cost-benefits for process improvement investments is very difficult to do. In the absence of outcome measures that reflect the primary goal of improving patient outcomes, other more easily measured targets become of the focus of the business, for example costs. Because health care does not routinely measure its benefits, administrative success is viewed as running a health care organisation within a budget rather than maximising benefit and minimising harm across the population of patients under care.

In the Australian health care context there is little incentive to invest in process improvements; for example, in contrast to a bank, a hospital board will not get removed if the preventable error rate in their institution is high. Litigation is also not often a significant driver for improvement in Australia as most public hospitals do not pay directly for their insurance and often the payouts are relatively low because punitive damages are not strongly weighed in damage calculations.

The lack of financial and organisational drivers for safety and process improvement has resulted in traditionally low rates of investments in health care compared to other information industries [17]. In recent years the investment in health care information technology (IT) has increased, predominantly in data systems, such as patient administration systems, booking systems, electronic results viewing and prescribing. Except for interaction checking during medication prescribing, there is very little interactive decision support for clinical staff.

The current status of health care is that clinician must deal with complex business processes, increasingly complex patients, more treatment choices and ever increasing evidence published in the literature with few IT tools to support them. Clearly there are many opportunities for health care to benefit from CDSS.

2.   Understanding Decision Making

Before discussing CDSS it is useful to define the elements of decision-making. Before reading on you may ask yourself if you can answer the following questions:
  1.   What is a decision?
  2.   What is a good decision?

While dictionaries commonly define a decision as "a conclusion reached after consideration" [18], we will define a decision more specifically as "an irreversible allocation of resources". In this context, thinking about giving up smoking as a new year's resolution is not a decision, it is an idea or consideration. A decision requires a commitment of resources such as throwing away all your cigarettes, buying patches and using them.

The definition of a *good* decision is often misunderstood, particularly in the legal system. Here are two scenarios, consider if the decisions are good ones:

  Scenario 1: A patient on a ward has a migraine and you prescribe aspirin. You realise after the patient has taken the aspirin that the patient has a low platelet count, and that the addition of the aspirin has dramatically increased their chance of bleeding. However, the patient does not bleed, and their headache goes away.

  Scenario 2: A patient has had significant blood loss, they meet the criteria for transfusion and you commence the treatment. Later that evening the patient suffers shock due to the transfusion and is admitted to the intensive care unit.

A good decision maximises the chance of a good outcome, it cannot guarantee a good outcome. This is an important concept because it separates the quality of the decision from the outcome, which means we can make a good decision based on the best information we have at the time and the quality of the decision does not change later when we have more information. In the first scenario a bad decision resulted in a good outcome, and in the second a good decision resulted in a bad outcome.

Making a decision has several steps and we will define the elements of decision making so we can use these concepts when comparing different approaches to CDSS. Let us assume a doctor is asked to assess if a patient has pneumonia and decide if the patient requires intravenous antibiotics. Before the patient is even seen the doctor will have an understanding of how likely the patient has pneumonia based on the age of the patient, where they live (at home or aged care facility), and perhaps the time of year. This estimate of baseline probability of pneumonia is the prior probability. A probability is a measure of how likely an event is to occur and is between 0 (no possibility of occurring) to 1.0 (certain to occur). Let's say the doctor estimates the probability at a 0.05 or 5% chance of pneumonia.

If we had a database with enough clinical data and outcome data then we could use it to determine the prior probability, but often we don't. When speaking to expert clinicians it is sometimes easier to acquire this probability by allowing them to think in population terms. The question "If you saw 100 people with these features how many of them will have pneumonia?" is easier to consider than "What is the probability of this patient having pneumonia?"

Back to our hypothetical patient: the patient has a cough and a fever, and is short of breath. This combination of findings has a certain likelihood of being present in pneumonia; based on the positive findings the doctor updates the probability of pneumonia to 35% (Figure 1). The likelihood depends on the sensitivity and specificity of the findings [19]. These data can also be gathered from the published evidence, from data analysis, or from expert opinion if necessary.

Probability of Disease

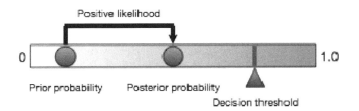

Figure 1. Updating the Probability of Disease.

In sequential information gathering the posterior probability becomes the new prior probability considering a new piece of information, such as the patient's white cell count, the posterior probability becomes the new prior probability, and the likelihood of the new information result in an increased new posterior probability if positive, or a reduced posterior probability if negative.

Should the doctor commence treatment? Is 35% enough certainty? Probability alone is not enough to guide decision making, we also need to understand the benefits and problems of each action. In this case we would need to consider the situations shown in Table 1.

Table 1. Potential Outcomes of Actions.

	Treat (Rx+)	**Don't Treat (Rx-)**
Disease Positive (D+)	Treatment when disease present, side effects may occur but disease is treated.	Disease is not treated and may worsen.
Disease Negative (D-)	Treatment is given, the patient is at risk of side effects for no benefit.	The patient is not at risk of side effects and no effects of disease.

Utility theory is the study of preferences or desirability of outcomes [20]. Each of the combination of outcomes in Table 1 can be assigned a value that corresponds to their relative desirability. While we would obviously like to have no disease and no treatment (D-, Rx-), this may not be possible. If the treatment is perceived as having few side effects and the cost of the treatment is low (e.g. paracetamol or herbal remedies) then treating the disease is considered as having little downside and people will often take medications at low probability of disease. However, if the treatment has significant side effects or is expensive (e.g. chemotherapy) then we want to be sure that it is warranted and will undergo invasive tests to confirm the diagnosis. The probability of disease at which we act is the decision threshold, and it is based on our preferences over each potential outcome.

It is important to note that utility is based on the preferences of the decision maker. Who is the decision maker in a clinical context? In theory the patient is the decision maker, who may seek advice from the doctor or, in most cases, delegate their decision to the doctor. However, the patient's preferences should determine the actions taken. The measure of utility of treatment benefits and side effects can be used to calculate a decision threshold. When the probability of disease is above the decision threshold the doctor should treat, otherwise the doctor should not treat or they should seek more information.

This description of decision-making is called normative because it highlights how decisions should be made, but in reality decisions are rarely made in this way. Experts do not formally manipulate probabilities in their mind; in fact, our minds are not designed to handle subtle changes in probability based on new information. Experts use prior knowledge and experience to make judgements about how likely problems are and do this very efficiently. However, when using or building CDSS we need to keep in mind how decisions are made so we can understand the assumptions that have gone into building the CDSS, and which problems can be assisted with the implementation of the CDSS.

To illustrate how CDSS may use these elements of decision making consider a simple CDSS that incorporates a logistic regression model found in the published literature to determine who is eligible for advanced chemotherapy. The logistic regression model uses histopathological features to determine the metastatic spread of breast cancer based on a sample from one or more sampled "sentinel lymph nodes" [21]. The model updates the prior probability based on each feature observed for a patient, such as the type of cells present, the degree of invasion into the sentinel nodes and the size of the primary tumour. The regression model then outputs a patient specific posterior probability of metastatic spread that can be used to determine further treatment such as chemotherapy and radiotherapy.

In an ideal setting we would try to understand the preferences of the patient by describing the side effects of the chemotherapy, and the potential extension of life. By using trade-offs between potential options we can quantify their preferences and use the probability obtained from the model to assist them identifying the best option. However, in our busy health care system we usually do not have the time (or skills) to ascertain each patient's preferences [22]. To make decision making practical clinicians often assume a population preference or sometimes a number of preference models. The assumed preferences will then define decision thresholds. If the probability of survival is low and side effects significant then no action (palliation) would be recommended; if the probability of survival is high (above the treatment threshold) then chemotherapy would be recommended; if the probability of survival is in between or particularly uncertain then a decision may be made for further tests (test threshold) to reduce the uncertainty in the decision [23] [24]. Decision models can also be used to calculate the expected value of information (EVOI), which is how much effort we should spend on seeking new information. If preferences are known then a CDSS with this capability can dynamically generate the most effective investigation strategy based on what is known about the patient and the diagnoses under consideration.

In clinical medicine there is much discussion about "best evidence" which determines the likelihood of treatment benefits. However, patient preferences will determine at what level of evidence we should act or seek more information. Unfortunately, clinicians often incorporate their own preferences into decision-making, for example the risk of being sued or occasionally financial gain. Therefore, the output from a normative CDSS may not be well received by clinical users if it is not "flexible" in its ability to be customised to local practice patterns.

3. Clinical Decision Making

Clinical decision-making ranges in scope from a narrow "make a diagnosis" in some specialty areas to "make a diagnostic formulation with a problem list" in general practice and family medicine, where the emphasis is on patient-centred comprehensive care within a biopsychosocial model. In a diagnostic formulation, the diagnosis is seen as part of a comprehensive problem list. Most clinical disciplines fall somewhere in between. Having made a diagnostic formulation, the clinician then makes management and medication decisions, taking into account the patient's age, gender, ethnicity, pregnancy and breast-feeding status; the safety, efficacy and cost of the therapy; drug indications, contraindications, interactions and allergies; care plans and review and assessment regimes.

Clinical decisions can be difficult for a number of reasons: there is significant uncertainty, potential actions have significant or costly outcomes, there are numerous options to remember and consider, or the time available to act may be limited. In health care many of these factors are present at once.

We have been considering each decision as a single item but organising the management for a patient involves creating a plan, or a series of linked decisions. The challenge is to update the plan if the state of the patient changes sufficiently. Errors in health care often occur because people forget to follow up plans when other patients demand their time. The literature demonstrates that CDSS are not as effective in assisting with diagnoses as they are in reminders and alerts [25].

Clinicians often use pattern recognition of signs and symptoms and heuristics to make assessments and diagnostic decisions - 'educated guesswork' to solve problems in uncertain situations. In heuristic problem solving, a difficult question is often answered by substituting an answer to an easier one [26]. On the other hand, evidence-based practice promotes computation-based reasoning over impression formation and intuitive judgements.

The dual-system model of cognition distinguishes between intuitive judgement, which is quick and associative, from the slower reasoning according to rules [27]. Intuitive judgment sits between the automatic parallel operations of perception and the controlled serial operations of reasoning; the representations on which intuitive judgments operate retain some features of perceptions in that they are concrete and specific, and they carry causal propensities and an affective charge [28]. As clinical expertise develops with the acquisition of knowledge and competencies, complex cognitive operations migrate from rules-based reasoning to intuitive judgement. Novice interns generally use the serial processing of computational reasoning to make a diagnosis or choose a therapy, compared to the almost instant intuitive judgement of expert experienced specialist clinicians. For these experts, pattern matching and heuristics has replaced conscious systematic serial processing.

The migration from explicit methods of decision making to implicit or intuitive methods has been termed by Johnson [29] as the "paradox of expertise"; the paradox being that as people gain expertise they are less able to explain the explicit steps taken to reach their decisions. This can be a problem for descriptive decision making methods, such as rules, that rely on experts to describe how they have solved a problem. In comparison, normative methods like decision models use evidence to achieve expert performance without mimicking each step an expert says they carry out.

Judgments of probability or frequency are often influenced by what is similar (representativeness), comes easily to mind (availability), and comes first (anchoring) [30]. However, intuitive heuristics often violate the conjunction rule, where the probability of the conjunction P(A&B) cannot exceed the probabilities of its constituents P(A) and P(B), resulting in large and systematic biases [30] [31]. For example, a conjunction may appear to be more representative than one of its constituents, and instances of a specific category can be easier to imagine or to retrieve than instances of a more inclusive category; the result is that this combination will make a conjunction appear more probable than one of its constituents. Systematic violations of the conjunction rule have been observed in the judgments of the lay and professional communities in a variety of contexts, including estimation of word frequency, personality judgment, medical prognosis, decision under risk, suspicion of criminal acts, and political forecasting. Semantics used to phrase the conjunction appear to be more important in violations than the format of the frequency or probability [32]. Research to improve our understanding of the semantics and cognitive processes involved is important. In the clinical context, errors of intuitive judgment raise two questions: "What features of intuitive judgment created the error?" and "Why was the error not detected and corrected by reasoning?"

In formal decision analysis, a diagnostic decision is made using likelihood functions associated with specific signs and symptoms. In the formal decision making process, a likelihood function of a positive or negative sign or symptom or test value will modify the prior or baseline probability. The reference values for these probabilities are usually derived from large scale prevalence studies in the relevant clinical settings and domains. For instance, the reference values for general practice and family medicine decisions can be calculated from large scale community prevalence programs like the Dutch Transition Project [33]. This is a "best of breed" example of a large and reliable database with a thesaurus standardising the structured data collected. This ongoing network research project started in the mid-80's, with data coded and collected from episodes of care in daily practice by family doctors in the Netherlands, Japan, Poland, Malta and Serbia. The data on patients' presenting complaints and doctors' interventions and diagnostic labels allows research into diagnosis in family medicine. The positive and negative likelihood ratios of a symptom against a diagnosis with an episode of care can be calculated for each pair of presenting symptom and diagnostic label. The Transition Project used its data to develop predictor weights to support diagnostic decisions. Table 2 demonstrates the calculations of predictive statistics to support ear pain as a predictor of otitis media in children aged 0-4 years in the Netherlands. Ear pain increases the probability of a diagnosis of otitis media in new episodes of care in young children more than its absence excludes this diagnosis.

Table 2. Example of Characteristics of a Predictor: Ear Pain as Predictor of Otitis Media.

Episode:	Otitis media	Row %	Other	Row %	Total
With ear pain	995	59.4	680	40.6	1675
With other reasons for encounter	840	8.5	9054	91.5	9894
Total:	1835	15.9	9734	84.1	11569
Sensitivity 0.54	LR +: 7.76	LR- : 0.49	PV+ : 0.59	Odds ratio: 15.77	Pretest Odds: 0.19
Specificity 0.93	95% CI: 7.14-8.44	95% CI: 0.47-0.52	PV- : 0.92	95% CI: 13.98-17.79	Posttest Odds: 1.47
NOTE: LR+:positive likelihood ratio; LR-: negative likelihood ratio; PV: predictive value; CI: confidence intervals. Source: WONCA Informatics Working Party CDSS Task Group					

Clinical inertia describes the failure to manage a chronic condition aggressively enough to bring it under control. When clinicians asserted that the BP was "usually well controlled", objective evidence frequently suggested otherwise [34]. Approximately 50% of diabetic patients presenting with a substantially elevated triage blood pressure did not receive treatment change at the visit; this was mainly due to clinical uncertainty about the true blood pressure value [35]. On the same note, clinicians are often unaware of their prescribing errors, reporting their lack of awareness of the potential clinical situation leading to 44% of the clinically significant ADEs that were identified by an alert system [36]. Clinical decision makers are more likely to accept recommended guidelines if they had completed residency more recently, rated evidence from randomised control trials as more important, were more concerned with harms of action, and were more likely to have a favourable opinion of alternative therapies to mainstream therapy [37].

4. Shared Decision Making

Patients with newly diagnosed prostate cancer value their current and future health states differently from their clinicians [38], highlighting the need for shared decision making with patients. Shared clinical decisions are based on 2 fundamental characteristics – importance and certainty. Importance reflects a combination of objective and subjective factors; certainty is present if one intervention is superior and absent if two or more interventions are approximately equal [39]. It has been proposed that for major important decisions that have low certainty, patients should be encouraged to be the primary decision makers, with physician assistance as needed [39]. It is recognised that patient engagement and participation depends more on the building of relationships than on making decisions [40]. Patient preferences for participation in decision making cannot be reliably judged based on patient communication behaviours during routine visits. Engaging patients in a discussion of preferences for decision making may be the best way to determine the role each wants to play in any given decision [41].

The emergence of multidisciplinary teams and inter-professional practice has highlighted the importance and desirability of shared decision making among the health care team. There are relatively few studies in the literature on the factors that influence, and how they are used in, case manager resource allocation decisions. Reported studies often lack conceptual clarity, theoretical frameworks and are not situated within the clinical decision-making literature [42]. The current reality is that medical practitioners, nurses, allied health practitioners and administrators still each see quality from their own perspective, which might or might not be similar to that of the patient. It has been recommended that the patient's perspective be assumed wherever possible to minimise ambiguity in issues of healthcare quality [43].

It is important that the health care team incorporates the patient's preferences to determine the best course of action. If the preferences of health care members are strongly incorporated then this can lead to defensive testing and treatment behaviour [44].

5.   Building Blocks of a CDSS

A fundamental question in building a CDSS is whether to develop a dedicated CDSS or write purpose built software that implements decision support algorithms. This dedicated approach has been commonly taken because the market for dedicated CDSS has been quite specialised. If a clinical unit wants to solve a particular problem, for example the head of the unit wants to implement a Warfarin dosing algorithm so all patients are dosed according to best practice, then it may be perceived as easier to hire a programmer to implement the algorithm using the locally available infrastructure such as an intranet than for the unit to procure an enterprise CDSS.

The local ad hoc approach to implementing decision support results in several significant problems. First, the ad hoc approach results in core business functions for the hospital being implemented chaotically in different parts of the infrastructure. How can an organisation know which algorithm or business logic is implemented in the database as SQL queries, in middle layer objects, in web page code, or in client applications? Furthermore, it is impossible to know when any of these critical algorithms require updating in the face of new evidence. For example, if a new improved Warfarin algorithm becomes available: who will know where it has been implemented and by whom throughout the enterprise? A similar problem can occur if the name or range of a pathology test or any data item in the hospital system changes. How can a manager tell which decision support modules are affected by the change? If a programmer leaves the organisation they often take with them critical information about what logic is implemented where, in what language, and the dependencies between modules. Another significant problem with the ad hoc approach is that it is hard, if not impossible, for an organisation to impose standards for testing and verification.

For these reasons, the ad hoc approach to implementing decision support has been discredited. In some institutions home grown decision support tools have been removed because of the risk of keeping them up to date. The alternative to the ad hoc approach is the dedicated CDSS.

An enterprise CDSS should comprise the following components:

- A clinical terminology and ontology that determine what the CDSS can reason with [45];
- A knowledge representation that can access clinical data in a coded form [46];
- Links into the hospital IT systems and other clinical data systems that trigger events within the CDSS; events can be based on data or user request;
- A maintainable knowledge representation that is linked to the ontology system; and
- A decision support engine that applies decision support algorithms against the knowledge base.

Commonly, a rule-based CDSS will be implemented in the following way:

- Knowledge engineers or informaticians work with clinical and business stakeholders to plan the decision support required to solve a problem;
- The knowledge engineer uses an editor to browse what information is available in the system (via the ontology), they map items in the ontology to data items that can be used in the construction of business rules;
- The business rules are stored in the knowledge management system with links to the terms used from the ontology, and the events that trigger the execution of the rule;
- As data flows into the CDSS via HL7 or other formats the decision support engine checks if any rules are associated with the event;
- Data items from the clinical data systems are mapped against terms in the CDSS and the rule is executed; and
- Any outputs from the rules are written to a database and can be used in other rules or in client applications e.g. alerting systems.

Rules can be relatively simple single propositions (a collection of if/then statements), or they may be implemented as cascades of rules with complex dependencies between them. Other problem solving methods can also be used such as statistical models (e.g. regression models, multivariate Gaussian models), or uncertainty management algorithms such as Bayesian networks [47].

As a problem becomes more complex and requires more sophisticated approaches the complexity of the decision support algorithms can become a barrier to implementation. For example, maintaining large rule sets has caused significant problems in maintaining consistency in the knowledge base and the time to compute rules grows rapidly [48]. Efficient algorithms have been developed to improve the efficiency of decision support algorithms such as the Rete algorithm for rules [49], or clique tree propagation for Bayesian networks [50], but the implementation of these algorithms is complicated, although numerous commercial and open source implementations exist. The complexity of decision support algorithms has made fuzzy logic an attractive method because it is relatively easy to implement and is effective for simple decision problems. Unfortunately it is not easy to map evidence based care or patient preference models to fuzzy systems; therefore its use in health care is limited [51].

As with any modelling task, parsimony is a goal. In other words it is best to use the simplest method to solve the problem at hand. In many instances, rules suffice in alerting and reminder tasks. However, rules are very inconsistent when dealing with uncertainty [52] [53] [54], where statistical methods are preferable. These methods include parametric statistical models and Bayesian models. Because probability and statistics is the language of evidence-based medicine, it is easier to translate evidence into statistical models for decision support. Other methods of building decision support models may include data analysis and gather data from expert opinion [55].

5.1 Data Integration

To avoid data re-entry and to keep up with the status of activity within a health care organisation an enterprise CDSS must integrate with the administration systems. In a hospital these include laboratory feeds, patient administration, radiology, emergency department information systems, and others. These data feeds are usually in a variation of HL7 [56], although smaller hospitals may require other forms of integration such as database access. In GP clinics integration is often more difficult because some brands of GP desktop software do not allow real-time access to the GP data.

Even if the data systems are easily integrated there is often a step to map the data items and values into a form that can be used by the CDSS. This can mean the mapping of codes used to identify data elements, and the verification of value types and ranges.

Unfortunately most data systems do not allow writing data back into the systems, which means that the output of a CDSS are often not easily integrated into core data systems. Some integrated clinical information system vendors in both the community and hospital prevent meaningful data integration as way of creating a competitive edge in the market place, so customers will be locked in the integrated solution rather than being able to choose best-of-breed systems that can be integrated as a unified system. With the advent of health care protocols, internet protocols and modern computing power data Integration is no longer a technical barrier rather than it is a political/strategic barrier.

Interoperability is often not a major factor in purchasing decisions in the health care sector because the purchasing decisions in IT are made to support administrative functions with little consideration to supporting clinical functions. There are therefore good reasons why error rates in health care are so high, and clinical tasks require so much manual effort.

5.2 Governance and Verification

A CDSS must support governance structures within health care organisations. An example of such a structure is a hospital guideline committee that ensures all guidelines and decision support meet the minimum criteria for evidence and compliance with best practice. Once approved, decision support can be implemented. However, it must be tested rigorously before implementation into the live or production environment where patient care is affected. A CDSS knowledge management system must support the fact that content can only be moved into production when governance approval has been given and the appropriate testing has been carried out. Testing may comprise unit tests for all key functions, as well as scenarios to test the behaviour of decision support in common and unusual situations (so called *edge conditions*).

The ability of CDSS to respond in a consistent way when faced with edge conditions, or in the face of inconsistent data is called "*graceful degradation*". This concept implies that decision support is built with the ability to know when it can be reliably applied, or if its advice may have a greater deal of uncertainty due to an unusual combination of inputs. The degree to which this kind of rigour is applied depends on the consequences of the decision support recommendations. Systems that do not degrade gracefully can output unexpected recommendations if their assumptions are not directly met and cause patient harm.

5.3 Clinical Workflow Integration

The greatest challenge to the widespread use of CDSS, after health care bureaucracy, is workflow integration. The combination of high workload and fewer health care workers means that there is little time to spare for using computers unless they are assisting with tasks that reduce workload. Often, computerisation in health care is seen as something that slows people down because they sometimes have to maintain electronic and paper records, or simply due to the bad design of clinical IT user interfaces (UIs).

There is an expression that says: "Buying a new phone doesn't guarantee you better conversations". Similarly, installing IT in health care doesn't guarantee you will improve safety, quality and efficiency. An extensive analysis of investments in technology over the last 30 years have shown that many investments fail to realise a return on investment [17]. The ability to realise technology benefits in health care can be even more challenging due to patient complexity, workflow complexity, workforce restrictions, and high degrees of uncertainty. Technology interventions must be clearly focussed on addressing change management of staff to new workflows, making sure that each stakeholder receives some workflow wins from using the system, and ensuring that the technology is robust and reduces errors. Ongoing evaluation post-implementation is also important to monitor sustained benefits in safety and efficiency.

Due to the relatively small penetration of CDSS in health care we are yet to see methods and standards that assist implementers to understand the implications of CDSS in modifying clinical behaviour and the consequences for patient safety. For example, in the late 1980's, articles appeared in the medical literature highlighting the increase in error rate due to computerised systems for results reporting because laboratory staff ceased manual alerting methods such as calling duty doctors on the telephone for abnormal results [57]. Even today there is no widespread decision support to address the concern raised over 20 years ago.

Another challenge for CDSS is the quality of the information that is presented, and how it is presented. Poorly designed CDSS can cause errors, due to two main factors. The first is that IT systems are often used to implement standardisation of practice, however a standard policy may not be suitable for all patients [58]. Junior clinicians in particular will follow the standardised practice to reduce their personal risk if a bad outcome follows a divergent decision. Second, the implementation of the decision support may not protect adequately against user errors [59].

The unexpected consequences of broadly applied guidelines are problems of process and governance, where new initiatives have not been verified against the target population. The user interface and decision support quality problem requires further work to (a) build standards such as visual semantics that clearly communicate risk and errors in clinical UIs, and (b) develop implementations of best practice guidelines that reduce the risk of error due to interface design.

Improved health care IT and decision support implementations will enable health care organisations to reduce variation in practice and potentially improve clinical outcomes, but the risks of unexpected errors will remain while health care does not routinely monitor clinical outcomes and error rates in real time to ensure that interventions improve patient outcomes and are sustainable.

5.4 Knowledge Management

Software development methodology has evolved quite rapidly in a relatively short period of time as IT projects become bigger and more expensive. It is well understood that about 70% of a software's cost over its lifespan will be incurred after the first release due to maintenance, bug fixes and change requests. If we consider CDSS content to be similar to software, then we can expect more effort to be spent on maintenance and update because of the progress of medical science. Therefore, managing CDSS content is vitally important to maintaining CDSS reliability and cost effectiveness.

5.5 Creating Evidence Based CDSS Content

When creating a decision support system we are creating a model of the problem domain and using some problem solving method to reason about the model. Different decision making methods represent the domain in different ways: rules see the world as chains of "if/then" structures linked by the parameters they use and assert; neural networks represent domains as links between neural nodes, the strength of which is defined by their activation parameters; Bayesian networks link nodes defined by probability relationships; decision models use probability and add utility nodes to represent explicitly the preferences for decision making; regression models express a model as an additive relationship between weighted parameters; and so on.

A model is by definition a simplification of the world we are trying to reason about. It is a statement of the scope of the decision support system: what are the parameters we are using to drive the CDSS? what the relative importance of the parameters. To be more precise, a model is a representation of the problem domain that expresses which parameters are independent of each other, which are dependent, and the strength of the dependencies. Just to make matters interesting when a CDSS is running and we are observing information new dependencies can be created or existing dependencies removed.

The knowledge management tools used to create, edit, test and deploy models in CDSS have a role to assist us in understanding the decision support models. Some representations are naturally expressed graphically, such as neural networks and Bayesian networks, while the underlying assumptions of rules may require some effort to understand.

5.6 Terminology

Building CDSS content is a process of mapping parameters gathered in health care to model parameters in the decision support model, executing the knowledge content represented by the model, and then integrating the output of the CDSS into the clinical workflow. Data sources may be lab systems, other IT systems, or data entered by clinical staff. The mapping of data into the model parameters relies on standards of terminology and ontology of the data in IT systems and electronic health records. IT systems have a huge variation in the way they represent information and the ontology and terminology issues are not often understood during IT purchasing decisions because the requirement for IT systems is usually to present data on screen rather than present data to a CDSS for automated processing.

An appropriate classification for symptoms, processes and diagnoses is essential to describe the events and knowledge within a profession or discipline. A clinical terminology may be conceptualized as comprising reference, interface and aggregating terminologies [60]. These terminologies are not formal entities on their own, but are formal transformations of one another, reflecting three overlapping functional dimensions of a terminology spectrum. The reference terminology is "an all-encompassing superset representation that either links to every other interface or reporting terminology or supports most of the useful interface or analytic functions within its own structure". The interface terminology, comprising preferred terms and synonyms, may be part or independent of but mapped to corresponding concepts in the reference terminology. Similarly, classifications or aggregating terminologies are separate and parallel terminology structures, related to reference terminology concepts by maps.

The International Classification for Primary Care (ICPC), generally accepted as the most appropriate classification for general practice and family medicine, is a related classification of the World Health Organisation - Family of International Classifications[2] [61]. The ICPC proposes a data model of episodes of care and, because it allows unique classification of concepts, has been used for diagnostic and therapeutic decision support [62]. However, because it does not capture data at a sufficient level of detail for clinical care, it has been mapped to International Classification of Diseases 10th edition (ICD10) [63] to allow a greater level of detail and specificity in coding clinical information. In many situations, even ICD 10 is not specific enough.

SNOMED-CT, the Systematized Nomenclature of Medicine-Clinical Terms, has been selected as a reference terminology in the United States of America and Australia, because it has more unique health concepts than ICD10. A large nomenclature such as the SNOMED-CT includes terms that can describe almost any symptom or diagnostic finding. Such specificity or granularity allows the building of decision support tools for very specific situations. However, the more terms there are for the clinician to choose, the lower is the reliability in coding: different doctors will choose different terms to describe the same condition, and even the same doctor can choose different terms at different times.

In many cases a CDSS may wish to reason about concepts rather than only about individual terms. For example, a decision support system may wish to know if a patient has had a history of ischaemic heart disease (IHD), and not specifically an anterior myocardial infarction, or any other numerous manifestations of IHD. An ontology is a formal relationship between terms, or concepts, that facilitates reasoning about the domain. In an ontology, individual terms are often assigned categories (or classes), and formal relationships between concepts and categories often defined in logic statements Therefore, "myocardial infarction" may belong to a category of IHD, and IHD would have a relationship called "disease-of-organ" that links to the concept "heart".

The effort required to construct ontologies for complex domains such as health care is immense. To make matters worse, the same domain can be represented by multiple, incompatible ontologies so efforts may not be reusable. A pragmatic approach is to construct ontology as needed for decision support reasoning with well-defined relationships and category definitions (Refer Chapter 9).

5.7 Machine Learning

Building decision support systems is a specialised and can be a difficult, multi-disciplinary task that involves integrating knowledge from experts and evidence from the

----

[2] http://www.who.int/classifications/en/

literature. Often the published literature doesn't provide all the data that is required to populate a model, so other data sources are often required such as clinical databases and research databases.

To avoid the manual work required to build CDSS models researchers have looked towards learning models from data. Examples include parametric statistical models such as regression models and their variants, neural networks, association rule learning, and Bayesian network models. Decision support models usually comprise two basic components (a) a structure or how parameters in the model are related, and (b) the values attached to the parameters. Machine learning can be used to learn both structure and parameter strengths, such as training a neural network, or just learn parameters as is the case in regression modelling. In model building the structure of a model plays an important role. First, learning structure requires a lot of data, where as learning parameters in a given structure is considerably less data intensive [64]. Second, the performance of a model with a structure that accurately reflects the problem domain is more robust to variations in parameters [65. In health care we often have some understanding of the underlying structure of problems regarding diseases, physiology, drug actions, and so on. This structure can be used to create models without having to learn everything from data.

There are two broad types of machine learning, supervised and unsupervised. Supervised learning is usually conducted in an episodic manner where data is analysed, new models constructed, tested, verified and then put into production. Unsupervised learning allows computer algorithms to update themselves as they work on new data. Unsupervised learning is generally not an option in health care where it is very easy for machine learning algorithms to create models that make sense mathematically but are an inaccurate representation of the problem. In a practical sense machine learning still requires expertise from researchers working in a multidisciplinary team; it is another tool in the arsenal of decision support development.

5.8 Managing Knowledge Management in CDSS

If the majority of effort in CDSS is to maintaining the quality and currency of the knowledge, then a CDSS should have the following facilities for knowledge management:

1. Tools to support full lifecycle development of content such as version control, rollback, auditing of changes, restriction of deployment to production.
2. Extensive support for testing during development including unit testing (function testing), system testing, and user acceptance testing before deployment into the production environment.
3. Restrict the output of decision support to key areas of the electronic health record that cannot override clinician-entered data and is clearly differentiated from it.

6.   Conclusions

This chapter has brought together numerous concepts in informatics including evidence-based health care, probability, psychology, terminology, ontology, human factors, workflow and a variety of computer science and IT concepts. While implementing a simple set of rules is a straightforward task, implementing more complex and system wide decision support is considerably more involved. Implementing CDSS relies on a strong multidisciplinary team and CDSS tools that support the robust implementation, testing and maintenance of knowledge. In the next chapter we will review where CDSS have been used, and which areas have been shown to be effective in improving health care.

References

[1] de Dombal, F. T., Hartley, J. R., & Sleeman, D. H. (1969). A computer-assisted system for learning clinical diagnosis. *Lancet, 1*(7586), 145-8.
[2] Pople, HE, Myers, JD, & Miller, RA (1975). DIALOG: A model of diagnostic logic for internal medicine. In *Proceedings of the fourth international joint conference on artificial intelligence.* (pp. 848-55). Cambridge, Massachusetts: MIT Artificial Intelligence Laboratory Publications.
[3] Shortliffe, E. H., Axline, S. G., Buchanan, B. G., Merigan, T. C., & Cohen, S. N. (1973). An artificial intelligence program to advise physicians regarding antimicrobial therapy. *Computers and Biomedical Research, An International Journal, 6*(6), 544-60.
[4] Kohn, L. T., Corrigan, J. M., & Donaldson, M. S. (2000). *To err is human: Building a safer health system.* Washington, D.C.: National Academy Press.
[5] CMO (2000). *Organization with a memory.* NHS, Department of Health.
[6] Wilson, R. M., & Van Der Weyden, M. B. (2005). The safety of australian healthcare: 10 years after QAHCS. *The Medical Journal of Australia, 182*(6), 260-1.
[7] Miller, G. C., Britth, H. C., & Valenti, L. (2006). Adverse drug events in general practice patients in Australia. *The Medical Journal of Australia, 184*(7), 321-4.
[8] Fordyce, J., Blank, F. S., Pekow, P., Smithline, H. A., Ritter, G., Gehlbach, S., et al. (2003). Errors in a busy emergency department. *Ann Emerg Med, 42*(3), 324-33.
[9] Kilpatrick, E. S., & Holding, S. (2001). Use of computer terminals on wards to access emergency test results: A retrospective audit. *BMJ (Clinical Research Ed.), 322*(7294), 1101-3.
[10] Mitra, S., Findley, K., Frohnapple, D., & Mehta, J. L. (2002). Trends in long-term management of survivors of acute myocardial infarction by cardiologists in a government university-affiliated teaching hospital. *Clin Cardiol, 25*(1), 16-8.
[11] Simpson, E., Beck, C., Richard, H., Eisenberg, M. J., & Pilote, L. (2003). Drug prescriptions after acute myocardial infarction: Dosage, compliance, and persistence. *Am Heart J, 145*(3), 438-44.
[12] Wilson, R. M., Runciman, W. B., Gibberd, R. W., Harrison, B. T., Newby, L., & Hamilton, J. D. (1995). The quality in australian health care study. *Medical Journal of Australia, 163*(9), 458-71.
[13] Chisholm, C. D., Collison, E. K., Nelson, D. R., & Cordell, W. H. (2000). Emergency department workplace interruptions: Are emergency physicians "interrupt-driven" and "multitasking"?. *Academic Emergency Medicine : Official Journal of the Society for Academic Emergency Medicine, 7*(11), 1239-43.
[14] Westbrook, J. I., Ampt, A., Kearney, L., & Rob, M. I. (2008). All in a day's work: An observational study to quantify how and with whom doctors on hospital wards spend their time. *The Medical Journal of Australia, 188*(9), 506-9.
[15] Tversky, A., & Kahneman, D. (1974). Judgment under uncertainty: Heuristics and biases. *Science (New York, N.Y.), 185*(4157), 1124-1131.
[16] Reason, J. (1991). *Human error.* New York, NY: Cambridge University Press.
[17] Landauer (1996). *The trouble with computers.* The MIT Press.
[18] *The New Oxford American Dictionary.* (2001). *The new oxford american dictionary.* USA: Oxford University Press.
[19] Sox, Blatt, MA, Higgins, & Marton, KI (1988). *Medical decision making.* Butterworth-Heinemann.
[20] von Winterfeldt, & Edwards,W (1986). *Decision analysis and behavioral research.* Cambridge University Press.
[21] Farshid, G., Pradhan, M., Kollias, J., & Gill, P. G. (2004). A decision aid for predicting non-sentinel node involvement in women with breast cancer and at least one positive sentinel node. *Breast (Edinburgh, Scotland), 13*(6), 494-501.
[22] Richardson, G., & Manca, A. (2004). Calculation of quality adjusted life years in the published literature: A review of methodology and transparency. *Health Economics, 13*(12), 1203-10.
[23] Pauker, S. G., & Kassirer, J. P. (1980). The threshold approach to clinical decision making. *The New England Journal of Medicine, 302*(20), 1109-17.
[24] Pauker, S. G., & Kassirer, J. P. (1981). Clinical decision analysis by personal computer. *Archives of Internal Medicine, 141*(13), 1831-7.

[25] Hunt, D. L., Haynes, R. B., Hanna, S. E., & Smith, K. (1998). Effects of computer-based clinical decision support systems on physician performance and patient outcomes: A systematic review. *JAMA : the Journal of the American Medical Association*, *280*(15), 1339-46.

[26] Kahneman, D; Frederick S (2002). "Representativeness Revisited: Attribute Substitution in Intuitive Judgment". in Thomas Gilovich, Dale Griffin, Daniel Kahneman. *Heuristics and Biases: The Psychology of Intuitive Judgment*. Cambridge: Cambridge University Press. pp.49–81.

[27] Gilbert, D. 1999. What the mind's not. in Chaiken, S. and Trope, Y. 1999. *Dual-Process Theories in Social Psychology*. Guilford Press. New York. pp. 3-11.

[28] Kahneman, D, & Frederick,S (2002). Representativeness revisited: Attribute substitution in intuitive judgment. In Gilovich, T (Ed.), *Heuristics of intuitive judgment: Extensions and applications.* New York, NY: Cambridge University Press.

[29] Johnson,PE (1983). What kind of expert should a system be?. *Journal of Medicine and Philosophy*, (8), 77–97.

[30] Tversky, A, & Kahneman,D (1983). Extensional versus intuitive reasoning: The conjunction fallacy in probability judgment. *Psychological Review*, (90), 293-315.

[31] Kahneman, D, & Tversky,A (1996). On the reality of cognitive illusions. *Psychological Review*, (103), 582-591.

[32] Mellers,B, Hertwig,R, & Kahneman,D (2001). Do frequency representations eliminate conjunction effects? An exercise in adversarial collaboration. *Psychological Science*, (12), 269-275.

[33] Okkes, I. M., Oskam, S. K., & Lamberts, H. (2002). The probability of specific diagnoses for patients presenting with common symptoms to dutch family physicians. *The Journal of Family Practice*, *51*(1), 31-6.

[34] Rose, A. J., Shimada, S. L., Rothendler, J. A., Reisman, J. I., Glassman, P. A., Berlowitz, D. R., et al. (2008). The accuracy of clinician perceptions of "usual" blood pressure control. *Journal of General Internal Medicine : Official Journal of the Society for Research and Education in Primary Care Internal Medicine*, *23*(2), 180-3.

[35] Kerr, E. A., Zikmund-Fisher, B. J., Klamerus, M. L., Subramanian, U., Hogan, M. M., & Hofer, T. P. (2008). The role of clinical uncertainty in treatment decisions for diabetic patients with uncontrolled blood pressure. *Annals of Internal Medicine*, *148*(10), 717-27.

[36] Raschke, R. A., Gollihare, B., Wunderlich, T. A., Guidry, J. R., Leibowitz, A. I., Peirce, J. C., et al. (1998). A computer alert system to prevent injury from adverse drug events: Development and evaluation in a community teaching hospital. *JAMA : the Journal of the American Medical Association*, *280*(15), 1317-20.

[37] Power, M. L., Baron, J., & Schulkin, J. (2008). Factors associated with obstetrician-gynecologists' response to the women's health initiative trial of combined hormone therapy. *Medical Decision Making : An International Journal of the Society for Medical Decision Making*, *28*(3), 411-8.

[38] Elstein, A. S., Chapman, G. B., Chmiel, J. S., Knight, S. J., Chan, C., Nadler, R. B., et al. (2004). Agreement between prostate cancer patients and their clinicians about utilities and attribute importance. *Health Expectations : An International Journal of Public Participation in Health Care and Health Policy*, *7*(2), 115-25.

[39] Whitney, S. N. (2003). A new model of medical decisions: Exploring the limits of shared decision making. *Medical Decision Making : An International Journal of the Society for Medical Decision Making*, *23*(4), 275-80.

[40] Rotar-Pavlic, D., Svab, I., & Wetzels, R. (2008). How do older patients and their gps evaluate shared decision-making in healthcare?. *BMC Geriatrics*, *8*, 9.

[41] Hudak, P. L., Frankel, R. M., Braddock, C., Nisenbaum, R., Luca, P., McKeever, C., et al. (2008). Do patients' communication behaviors provide insight into their preferences for participation in decision making?. *Medical Decision Making : An International Journal of the Society for Medical Decision Making*, *28*(3), 385-93.

[42] Fraser, K. D., & Estabrooks, C. (2008). What factors influence case managers' resource allocation decisions? A systematic review of the literature. *Medical Decision Making : An International Journal of the Society for Medical Decision Making*, *28*(3), 394-410.

[43] Gottlieb,J (2006). Analyzing quality data. In Chaiken, S (Ed.), *The quality solution: The stakeholder's guide to improving health care.* Boston, MA: Jones and Bartlett Publishers.

[44] Owens, D. K. (1998). Defensive diagnostic testing--a case of stolen utility?. *Medical Decision Making : An International Journal of the Society for Medical Decision Making*, *18*(1), 33-4.

[45] Kumar, A., Ciccarese, P., Smith, B., & Piazza, M. (2004). Context-Based task ontologies for clinical guidelines. *Studies in Health Technology and Informatics*, *102*, 81-94.

[46] Bleeker, S. E., Derksen-Lubsen, G., van Ginneken, A. M., van der Lei, J., & Moll, H. A. (2006). Structured data entry for narrative data in a broad specialty: Patient history and physical examination in pediatrics. *BMC Med Inform Decis Mak*, *6*, 29.

[47] Cowell, RG, Dawid, AP, Lauritzen, SL, & Spiegelhalter,DJ (2007). *Probabilistic networks and expert systems.* Springer.

[48] Stefik,M (1995). *Introduction to knowledge systems.* Morgan Kaufmann.

[49] Forgy,C (1982). Rete: A fast algorithm for the many pattern/many object pattern match problem. *Artificial Intelligence*, (19), 17-37.

[50] Lauritzen, SL, & Lauritzen,DJ (1998). Local computations with probabilities on graphical structures and their application to expert systems. *Journal of the Royal Statistical Society. Series B*, (2), 157-224.

[51] Cheeseman, P (1986). Probabilistic vs. Fuzzy reasoning. In Kanal, LN, & Lemmer, JF (Eds.), *Uncertainty in artificial intelligence.* New York, N.Y.: Elsevier Science Publishers.

[52] Heckerman, DE, & Horvitz, EJ (1987). On the expressiveness of rule-based systems for reasoning under uncertainty. In *Proceedings of the sixth national conference on artificial intelligence.* Palo Alto, Calif.: Morgan Kaufmann.

[53] Horvitz, EJ, & Heckerman,DE (1986). The inconsistent use of measures of certainty in AI research. In Kanal,LN, & Lemmer, JF (Eds.), *Uncertainty in artificial intelligence.* New York, N.Y.: Elsevier Science Publishers.

[54] Pearl, J (1988). *Probabilistic reasoning in intelligent systems: Networks of plausible inference.* San Francisco, CA, USA: Morgan Kaufmann Publishers Inc.

[55] Heckerman, D (1985). *A tutorial on learning with bayesian networks* [http://research.microsoft.com/research/pubs/view.aspx?msr_tr_id=MSR-TR-95-06]. Microsoft Research.

[56] *Health Level 7.* (2008). [http://www.hl7.org]. Health Level Seven Inc.

[57] Bradshaw, K. E., Gardner, R. M., & Pryor, T. A. (1989). Development of a computerized laboratory alerting system. *Computers and Biomedical Research, An International Journal*, 22(6), 575-87.

[58] Eslami, S., Abu-Hanna, A., de Keizer, N. F., & de Jonge, E. (2006). Errors associated with applying decision support by suggesting default doses for aminoglycosides. *Drug Safety : An International Journal of Medical Toxicology and Drug Experience*, 29(9), 803-9.

[59] Koppel, R., Metlay, J. P., Cohen, A., Abaluck, B., Localio, A. R., Kimmel, S. E., et al. (2005). Role of computerized physician order entry systems in facilitating medication errors. *JAMA : the Journal of the American Medical Association*, 293(10), 1197-203.

[60] Liaw, S, Grain,H, & Pearce,C (2002). *An approach to terminology standards for electronic health records: Background and conceptual framework.* Canberra: Commonwealth Department of Health and Ageing.

[61] Maddern,R, Sykes,C, & Ustun,T (2007). *World health organization family of international classifications: Definition, scope and purpose..* Geneva: World Health Organization.

[62] Okkes, I, Sk, O, van Boven, K, & Lamberts, H (2005). *Episodes of care in dutch family practice. Epidemiological data based on the routine use of the international classification of primary care (ICPC) in the transition project of the academic medical center/university of amsterdam (1985-2003).* University of Amsterdam.

[63] WHO (n.d.). *International statistical classification of diseases and related health problems (10th revision).* Geneva: World Health Organization.

[64] Gaines,BR (1989). An ounce of knowledge is worth a ton of data: Quantitative studies of the trade-off between expertise and data based on statistically well-founded empirical induction. In *Proceedings of the sixth international workshop on machine learning.* New York, N.Y.: Morgan Kaufmann Publishers Inc.

[65] Pradhan, M., Henrion, M., Provan, G., Del Favero, B., & Huang, K. (1996). The sensitivity of belief networks to imprecise probabilities: An experimental investigation. *Artificial Intelligence*, 85(1-2), 363-397.

Review Questions

1. Describe the elements of a decision making process.
2. What are the building blocks for and required elements of a clinical decision support system?
3. Discuss knowledge management relative to decision support systems.
4. What role does knowledge management play relative to the construction and maintenance of clinical decision support systems?

Health Informatics
E.J.S. Hovenga et al. (Eds.)
IOS Press, 2010
doi:10.3233/978-1-60750-476-4-296

23. Clinical Decision Support Implementations

Siaw Teng LIAW[1] MBBS, PhD DipObst, GrDipPHC, FRACGP, FACHI [a], Malcolm PRADHAN, MBBS, PhD[b]

[a]*Director, SSWAHS General Practice Unit, Professor of General Practice Faculty of Medicine, The University of New South Wales, Australia*
[b]*VP Research & Software, Alcidion Corporation, Adjunct Professor, Health Informatics, University of South Australia*

Abstract. This chapter gives an educational overview of:
- Evidence for the benefits of CDSS;
- Categories of CDSS including user and workflow requirements;
- A framework for the implementation of CDSS, including human factors and the problem of free text;
- a framework for the evaluation of CDSS.

Keywords. Decision Support Systems-Clinical, Medical Informatics Applications, Knowledge, Statistics, Evidence Based Practice, Practice Guidelines, Clinical Trials, Risk Management, Safety

Introduction

This chapter is the second of two on clinical decision support across the continuum of care from primary care/family medicine to hospital medicine. The first chapter dealt with the need for, rationale and foundations of clinical decision-making and clinical decision support systems (CDSS). This second chapter deals with CDSS applications in practice and the important principles underpinning implementation within the context of integrated care, including hospital- and community-based care.

1. Categories of Decision Support

The term "decision support" is used widely to market products that range from online text books to sophisticated inference engines. The term decision support is also used in the area of business intelligence (BI) in which data warehouses collate and present summarised information via reports and "drill down" queries that allow users to explore detailed views of the data.

In previous systematic reviews decision support has been defined as a "system designed to aid directly in clinical decision making, in which characteristics of individual patients are used to generate patient-specific assessments or recommendations that are

---

[1] Corresponding Author: siaw@unsw.edu.au

presented to clinicians for consideration" [1] [2]. A similar definition has been proposed by Wyatt and Spiegelhalter [3]: "active knowledge systems which use two or more items of patient data to generate case-specific advice." This definition implies that the CDSS synthesises new information from observations.

The key notions for CDSS in the definition are encapsulated in the following phrase: *patient specific assessment and recommendations*. A CDSS must be able to synthesise a patient-specific assessment, and customise its output taking into account patient context. Other contexts, such as user expertise, organisational goals, local practice should ideally also be considered. However, presenting a generic guideline document or a historical chart of previous laboratory results does not constitute a CDSS, although they may assist with decision making in general.

The preceding definitions of CDSS based on patient-specific assessment and recommendations summarise the current use of CDSS but they do not quite capture emerging applications where CDSS monitor populations of patients to identify optimal use of resources to manage risk. For example, when managing resources in community-based chronic disease management, or in managing patient flow in hospital through optimal discharge a CDSS may dynamically customise the resources allocated for managing categories of patients based on the current population characteristics, resource availability and best evidence. From concepts introduced in the previous chapter we can more precisely describe this variation of CDSS as maximising expected utility across a patient population rather than optimising the utility myopically for each patient hoping it will work best for all patients (sometimes called "trickle-down" utility maximisation).

A useful categorisation of CDSS should communicate the way in which the CDSS is to be used, and the sophistication of the system to inform implementers on how to test and verify the system, and how the system will be integrated into the clinical workflow. Sim and Berlin introduce a categorisation based on 24 axes [4] to accurately describe CDSS; we present a simpler categorisation of CDSS based on 5 categories that are designed to guide the reader on how to approach the implementation and evaluation of CDSS:

1. **Context**: What is the clinical setting e.g. General Practice, outpatient, inpatient, community? Who are the decision makers; whose utility are we maximising? How is the system to be integrated into the workflow? Is the system *passive* (awaiting users to invoke it) or *active* (automatically triggered by events)?

2. **Output**: How complex is the output from the system? Is the system *open-loop* (recommends actions to the clinician) or *close-loop* (directly implements a decision e.g. calibration of a ventilator)? Is it an alert, or is it a complete care plan? What is the time frame that the recommendation is valid? How will outputs be integrated into the workflow?

3. **Reasoning**: What is the *inference strategy* (e.g. Rules, statistical, neural network, etc.)? Does it incorporate evidence? Can it incorporate qualitative data or expertise? How can the system be tested across a large set of tests? How do you know the tests cover all the CDSS implementation? How is it maintained?

4. **Robustness**: What assumptions does the system make on data completeness (does it handle missing data)? How does the system respond to errors within data items? Does the system recognise cases which have contradictory information or that the system was not designed to handle (so called "graceful degradation")?

5. **Auditability**: Does the system keep track of all inference and recommendations made? Can a recommendation be tracked back to the original data that triggered it? Does the CDSS monitor its own outputs?

2.   The Evidence for CDSS

The previous chapter on the Foundations of CDSS highlighted the high rate of preventable deaths every year in Western Health Systems. A study of people in contact with the health care system in the United States revealed that just over half (54.9%) received recommended care [5]. Lomas and colleagues [6] documented a 5 year gap between the publication of guidelines and changes in routine practice in numerous Western health care systems. Obviously there is a potentially large role for CDSS to improve the quality of care and to narrow the gap between research and clinical practice. This section looks at the evidence for CDSS interventions.

The most common form of CDSS in primary care is interaction checking during prescribing. The act of providing decision support at the point of care, as clinicians enter data for ordering medications or laboratory tests and results, is commonly called computerised physician order entry (CPOE). CPOE has been shown in some cases to improve dramatically patient safety by reducing preventable prescribing errors and improved compliance to guidelines [7] [8]. However, in other settings such outpatient care [9] pathology ordering [10], the benefits are not as easy to evaluate and the study quality much more variable.

Other common forms of CDSS include reminders for missed appointments and preventative care (e.g. immunisations for children, PAP smears for women), reminders attached to the patient's electronic health record (EHR) for emerging risks such as renal function, specialised dosing algorithms for high risk medications (e.g. Warfarin, Aminoglycosides), reminders for improving compliance to best practice guidelines and care plans, customisation of care plans for patients. Despite the early historical interest in diagnostic systems, the majority of successful CDSS implementations are in a critiquing role that monitor for specific patient risks.

In the last 15 years numerous meta-analyses and systematic reviews have been conducted that demonstrate clearly the benefits of CDSS in clinical practice (Table 1). There is little doubt that a well-implemented CDSS will improve patient safety, compliance with best practice guidelines, compliance with best practice medication management, and can reduce the length of stay in hospital. There are two important caveats to this picture: while physician productivity and compliance has been demonstrated, very few evaluations of CDSS have included the measurement of patient outcomes, and many have not been able to demonstrate improvements in this area. Also, not all implementations of CDSS succeed in their goals [11], and systems may fail to be accepted by their target users. More recent studies have shown that poorly implemented information technology can promote new types of preventable error [12]. Table 1 summarizes recent systematic reviews on CDSS interventions.

The reviews in Table 1 represent over 200 randomized controlled trails, with the preponderance of evidence indicating the benefits of CDSS. Examples of specific intervention types [1] are summarized in Table 2.

Table 2 demonstrates that certain areas of CDSS applications are more successful than others, but success is not guaranteed.

Some consistent patterns on benefits have emerged from the CDSS literature:
1. Clinical alerts and reminders have the capacity to change behaviour and improve drug dosing and management;
2. Reminders and alerts have shown to be effective in reducing preventable error;
3. Physician order drug entry is effective in reducing prescription error and dosing errors;

4. The combination of physician order entry and CDSS has been shown to reduce serious drug-related errors by 55%;
5. CDSS is effective in improving compliance with clinical guidelines; and
6. CDSS have been shown to reduce length of stay and inpatient costs.

Table 1. A Summary of Systematic Reviews on the Effectiveness of CDSS to Improve Patient Care. The Number of Randomized Controlled Trials (#RCTs) Analysed in Each Study is Listed

Subject	Year	#RCTs	Comments
Computerized reminders and feedback in medications management [13]	2003	26	Reminders more effective than feedback
Computerized advice on drug dosage prescribing [7]	2008	23	Faster therapeutic level, lower toxicity, shorter length of stay.
Computer for clinical information and reminders [14]	1996	98	Successful interventions in reminders, patient education, treatment planning.
Clinical decision support systems [11]	2005	100	Benefits in drug dosing, preventative care, alerting. No significant benefit in diagnosis.
Clinical decision support and physician drug order entry for medication safety [15]	2003	12	Both order entry and stand-alone decision support improved drug safety.
Physician order entry provided with decision support [8]	2003	11	Integrated decision support is a critical feature of order entry.
CDSS in ambulatory care for practice guidelines and reminders [16]	2008	17	Thirteen of 17 (76%) studies shown to have positive effect for reminders and guidelines.

Table 2. Detailed Results and Patient Numbers for Selected Intervention Types

Intervention type	# Patients	# RCTs	# Positive	% Positive
Drug dosing	1113	15	10	67%
Reminders	38453	19	14	74%
Disease management	51908	26	19	73%
Diagnosis	-	5	1	20%

The extensive research in CDSS interventions also reveals areas to be aware of when designing and implementing CDSS systems:

- Feedback and reminder systems are most effective when presented close to decision making;
- Poor human interfaces can reduce the use of a system;
- Clinician acceptance of systems is reduced if required to enter redundant data;
- In an inpatient setting prevention advice is less effective as clinicians are more concerned with immediate problems;
- Systems require careful planning and the ability to be modified after deployment since physician behaviour may not match initial specification; and

- CDSS evaluations have failed to show a significant role in diagnostic tasks, however in well chosen, specialized tasks CDSS have been effective, for example [17]

The literature of the role of CDSS in nursing is less well developed and the quality of studies in the area are not of high standard. This is in part due to the more complex intervention required for CDSS in nursing tasks and the lack of defined outcome measures [18]. It is clear that further work is required to understand the best role for CDSS in nursing.

The most successful CDSS have been simple rule-based systems that draw attention to data and facts e.g., drug-drug interaction or abnormal values that the user already knows but may have forgotten at the moment of decision or have been to busy to check. Critiquing CDSS (71%) were more successful than consultative CDSS (47%). Provision of CDSS improves prescribing practices and treatment outcomes of patients with acute illnesses but appeared to be less effective in primary care [19].

Integration of CDSS with clinical information systems decreased selected types of medication errors throughout the medication-use process in a health care system and improved therapeutic drug monitoring in patients with renal insufficiency and in patients receiving drugs with narrow therapeutic ranges through the use of CDSS alerts [20]. Using an EHR to assess medication use in the elderly may reduce the use of psychoactive medications and falls in a community-dwelling elderly population [21] and an EHR-derived registry in an integrated delivery system can improve diabetes care [22].

Physicians generally have relatively positive attitudes towards CDSS. However, there is a novelty effect that needs to be maintained. Clinicians will use an online evidence retrieval system in routine practice; however, usage rates drop significantly after initial introduction of the system [23]. Their main expectations are flexibility, individuality and reliability of the system [24] to bring relevant information to the right person at the right time and the right place; highlight out of range or abnormal values; checking the patient's EHR for allergies or drug-drug/drug-disease interactions; and make recommendations based on patient factors. CDSS for prescribing are usually well received because they support a routine and important task, automate script generation especially for repeat scripts, and transmit scripts electronically to a pharmacy. User-friendly CDSS protocols and interfaces are important [25].

In his systematic review of computerised clinical decision support systems, [2] reported that automatic provision of decision support as part of clinician workflow, provision of recommendations rather than just assessments, and provision of decision support at the time and location of decision-making were predictors of success along with periodic performance feedback, sharing recommendations with patients, and requesting documentation of reasons for not following recommendations [2]. Clinician (and other stakeholders) involvement is critical for good system design and successful implementation in both specialist and general practice [26] [27].

Because external incentives are strong drivers of adoption, policies requiring reporting of chronic care measurements and rewarding improvement as well as financial incentives for use of specific information technology tools are likely to accelerate adoption of order entry with decision support [28].

A systematic assessment of end-users' perceptions of Veterans Health Administration Computerised Clinical Reminder system suggests that they need to be developed and implemented with a continual focus on improvement based on end-user feedback and better integration into the primary care clinic workflow/workload [29]. Unexpectedly, providing periodic performance feedback, sharing recommendations with patients, and requesting documentation of reasons did not lead to compliance with recommendations.

The most important predictors of success is an efficient infrastructure and infrastructure to promote the ubiquitous computing across the whole healthcare continuum: interoperable electronic records, electronic prescribing, clinical decision support, CDSS, workflow-based systems as well as a secure technical infrastructure. However, while the potential of ubiquitous computing to enhance effectiveness of health services delivery and organisation is great, it is also a great societal challenge [30]. It requires a comprehensive intersectoral and interprofessional approach to be successful. CDSS for earlier diagnoses and interventions, which can also optimise process of care or administration, can further improve the quality of care while reducing its costs [31]. Cost-effectiveness of interventions may be more easily measured and monitored with a CDSS in place [32].

3. The Secret to Successful CDSS Implementation

It is said that the key to selling real-estate can be summarised in 3 simple rules: Location, location, location. Similarly, the key to implementing a CDSS *successfully* also depends on 3 simple rules: workflow, workflow, and change management. Thus — at least on paper — implementing a CDSS is slightly more complex than selling real-estate. The basic concept for a successful CDSS is relatively simple: if it saves the clinician time then they will use it. Clinical users value time savings over other potential benefits such as improving the quality of care [33]. Achieving time savings in the clinical workflow is far from simple because it relies on the tight integration between a CDSS and the clinical workflow with no redundant data entry.

In the previous section we summarised the high quality evidence for the use of CPOE systems with integrated CDSS. Along with the demonstrated improvements in clinical practice CPOE systems have also been demonstrated to yield cost savings to the institution [34] [35]. Despite these well-documented benefits, the uptake of CPOE in US hospitals is around 10% [36]. In contrast, the uptake of CPOE for medications in General Practice is almost 90% [37]. The core reason for the disparity in uptake is workflow. In an ambulatory setting the doctor is at a desk and patients come to them. In a hospital the doctor moves between patients, often across wards, often carrying medical notes. There is significantly more complexity of integrating CPOE into the hospital workflows; computers on wheels (COWs) and bedside computers improve the workflow but maintaining a purely electronic drug chart without moving to a complete EHR presents change management and technology infrastructure barriers that spoil the cost/benefit equation for CPOE implementation [38].

Based on their extensive experience in implementing CDSS, Bates and colleagues [39] created a set of "Ten Commandments for Effective Clinical Decision Support". In summary they are:

1. Speed is everything. The software should be highly responsive.
2. Anticipate needs and deliver in real time. Don't keep clinicians waiting for data.
3. Fit into the user's workflow. Passive systems are not utilized as much as active systems.
4. Little things can make a big difference. Usability is important.
5. Recognise physicians will strongly resist stopping. Rather than asking physicians not to act, offer an alternative.

6. Changing direction is easier than stopping. Changing system defaults will reinforce recommended practice.
7. Simple interventions work best. Complex guidelines are harder to implement and change-manage.
8. Ask for additional information only when you really need it. Minimise data entry.
9. Monitor impact, get feedback, and respond.
10. Manage and maintain your knowledge-based systems.

We propose five additional user requirements that are important in the development and use of CDSS:

1. CDSS are flexible and allow different levels of entry (and exit) for the clinician, depending on experience and information seeking styles.
2. CDSS are interoperable.
3. CDSS data model supports encounters and episodes of care within a continuity of care framework.
4. CDSS must promote collaborative and shared decisions between clinicians and patients and among health professionals in the multidisciplinary health team; outputs of the system should be sensitive to the health literacy of the recipients.
5. CDSS must facilitate and support communication and interaction between the clinician and the system to promote knowledge exchange and an ongoing dialogue among the community of users.

Other factors in the implementation of a CDSS will include data integration, and stakeholder analysis for each participant in the project. Stakeholder analysis is an assessment for each member of staff involved in the intervention of the additional workload and the potential workflow wins that will occur. We have occasionally found that professional groups are sensitive to increases in workload if this benefits another professional group without realising benefits to their group.

It is important for a successful CDSS implementation to have opinion leaders in each of the stakeholder groups so each group understands the strategic importance of the initiatives. An opinion leader is person within a professional group whose opinions are highly regarded and will influence others in the group to participate in the project.

In an extensive analysis of 71 CDSS Kawamoto and colleagues [2] analysed features that may determine the success of implementation, many of the features chosen are in the "Ten Commandments" for CDSS. The authors found the following CDSS features to be statistically significant in improving the success rate of implementations (absolute rate improvements are shown, please refer to source for confidence intervals):

- Integration with the order entry system (37% higher rate of success)
- Computer based reminders (26% higher rate of success)
- Automatic decision support as part of the workflow (75% success compared to 0% for passive systems)
- Provision at time and location of decision making (48% higher rate of success)
- Request reason for not following recommendations (41% higher rate of success)
- Provision of recommendation, not just assessment (35% higher rate of success)

Factors that were not statistically significant but had some potential influence include: minimal clinical data entry, justification of evidence, and output of clinician and patient information. Factors that were not significant included: local involvement in development, noting agreement of recommendations, promotion of action rather than inaction, periodic feedback to CDSS implementers and CDSS accompanied by conventional education. It should be noted that this study required significant interpretation of reported trials and the details of how each factor was implemented in each study may differ significantly.

Some important features of CDSS were not documented in evaluations and could not therefore be compared by Kawamoto and colleagues[2]. These features comprise: Speed of the system, time savings, clear user interface, accuracy of recommendations, system development process, alignment of the CDSS to the organisational priorities, involvement of opinion leaders.

4.   The Problem of Unstructured Data Entry

With today's computing power and networked architectures the challenges in CDSS implementation are no longer hardware related but rather driven by workflow limitations. A significant challenge in realising benefits of CDSS is the presentation of structured data. For a CDSS to understand patient context and clinical intent, data from a structured EHR must be presented to the CDSS coded in a standardised terminology. Clinical users are used to expressing their thoughts (and uncertainties) in free text, whether it be on paper or typed into a text box on screen.

Free text is not a reliable way of driving CDSS. Consider the task of entering the concepts that a patient has "chest pain that does not radiate to the arm". The concept "chest pain" can be written in free text as "substernal pain" or "pain located in the chest." Translating these grammatical variations is error prone, even before considering spelling errors; in the latter case we have to estimate the proximity of the word "pain" to the concept "chest". Negation is another complexity that can have many variations in free text, so "does not radiate to the arm" could also be written as "left arm radiation is not present". There is also the nontrivial matter of disambiguating the word "radiation". Much progress has been made in natural language processing but the potential for errors in CDSS recommendations outweighs the potential convenience to the end user. Precision relies on important terms to be coded on data entry.

Clinical users are not used to entering coded terms via list selection, tags or text completion. But not all information needs to be coded, only the information required to drive the CDSS and any concepts required for research and evaluation. It is no surprise then to see that CDSS implementations have focussed on areas that require minimal user data entry or capture data such as medications that are easier to look up in a drug list rather than as part of a sentence structure.

In Australia the National E-Health Transition Authority (NEHTA)[2] is charged with developing interoperability standards to support a national EHR. Unfortunately many Australian national and State health IT implementations have in the past and today still use free text fields to avoid the complexity and potential workforce problems related to structured data entry. To make matters worse, many of the large health IT vendors chosen by State-based health agencies do not follow NEHTA's interoperability guidelines for communication between their data systems and external systems, such as CDSS. Health IT vendors' disregard for interoperability are usually part of a strategy to force out competitors, rather than for any technical reason.

---

[2] www.nehta.gov.au

5. Human Factors in CDSS Implementations

It has been recognised that the implementation of technology could cause new types of error [40] [41]. In 2005, a landmark paper was published that showed that the implementation of a clinical information system (CIS) and CPOE was related to an increase in mortality rate in a paediatric intensive care unit [42]. Further analysis of the tragic findings revealed a complex combination of factors that lead to a general break down in the function of the intensive care unit [43]. In this case contributing factors included: a lack of preparation for a hospital-wide CPOE implementation that occurred over a 6 day period; a change in the way drugs were ordered, stored and administered in the unit; a reduction in direct communication between staff members; a reduction in the time spent at the bedside; an increase in time required to enter common orders such as stabilization orders due to a deficient user interface, so a task that took seconds per medication before the CPOE took 1-2 minutes per medication afterwards; further reductions in productivity due to network bandwidth problems.

It is reassuring that studies in the similar environments before and since had not resulted in adverse outcomes [44] [45] [46]. On the contrary, CDSS implementations had demonstrated rapid improvements in patient safety and quality. However, the fact that technology diffusion was associated with an increase in mortality has caused researchers to look more closely at the workflow and social changes within an organisation brought by technology implementations.

There is now a focus on understanding the impact of system implementation and software usability on patient safety, through the impact these factors have on changing the behaviour and workflows of staff in health care [47] [48] [49]. This will hopefully yield some standards and implementation guidelines to maximise the benefits of CIS and CDSS implementations and minimise the risks.

The challenging task of improving the usability and workflow integration of CIS and CDSS is not assisted by the side effects of IT centralisation and procurement processes that exist in large organisations. Purchasing a CIS and CDSS is a complex process: the users of the system (clinicians) are not the purchasers of the system and do not set the standards for the implementation. Instead, the purchasers are the administration staff and standards set by the IT staff. In addition to this separation of responsibilities is the persistent challenge of creating an IT specification that embodies goals of usability and workflow integration. The specification document, a core part of the procurement process, is sometimes followed by a software demonstration. It is extremely difficult, if not impossible, to understand the full implications of an expansive computer system on every day tasks and workflows within a complex and often chaotic health care environment.

The role of a CDSS is to make patient-specific assessments and recommendations, and then convince the clinical user to act in the best way. Furthermore, the role of a CDSS is to sort through the myriad pieces of data that bombard clinical staff to ensure that important information is attended to in a timely manner to maximise benefits to the patients under the care of the clinicians. Therefore usability, workflow integration and the communication between the CDSS and clinicians are at the core of CDSS implementations. Currently it is common for the selection and purchasing process for CIS and CDSS to overlook considerations of human factor integration, risk management and usability because these have traditionally not been the criteria for IT procurement.

Along with improved standards it is clear that IT implementations in health care must go through a process of validation and measurement before being allowed operate "live" with real patients. It will be resource intensive to construct a realistic acceptance-testing environment that incorporates measurements on productivity, usability, errors, and workflow implications but these initiatives must be put into place to minimise the risk of adverse and unintended consequences of IT implementations in health care.

6. Evaluation of CDSS

The field of evaluation in health informatics is complex because an informatics intervention has multiple dimensions, such as:

1. IT System: Is the system usable? Is it fast?
2. Workflow: Does the system integrate into the workflow?
3. Data integration: Does the system integrate with data systems?
4. Productivity: Does the system improve clinical performance?
5. Outcomes: Does the system improve patient outcome?

When evaluating a new drug a study is constructed to randomise patients to between the new drug and a placebo or current therapy. Ideally both the clinician and patient do not know which drug is being received. The delivery of the new drug does not require a change in workflow or the installation of new IT systems, and usually the health care organisation is paid for running the trial. In contrast to a drug trial, health informatics interventions cannot be easily randomised for the clinician or patient, nor can they be easily isolated from organisational factors and change management issues. CDSS evaluations also have a problem with defining a "gold standard" for comparison, because experts often do not agree with the detail of each other's recommendations.

Observational studies or before/after studies are therefore more common in health informatics. Another challenge for health informatics evaluations is the problem of outcome measure. Health care does not routinely measure the outcomes of its activity in a way that can be evaluated. Therefore, collecting patient outcome data is expensive for all interventions. Because the evaluation of health informatics interventions covers so many dimensions across clinical personnel, organisation and management, data collection is often complex and more expensive than non-informatics interventions. Therefore CDSS evaluations require specific methodologies to be successful.

Evaluation methodology should be appropriate to the evaluation question or objectives. It can be formative to examine the processes and to determine if the "product" is ready for implementation in the field, or summative to examine if the ready "product" can achieve the outcomes envisaged e.g. improved management of asthma or improved health outcomes in asthmatics. Unrealistic expectations and premature summative evaluation of products that are not ready for larger scale implementation have been the weakness of many CDSS evaluations[50] [28].

The methods used should be comprehensive. This usually means a multi-method approach with complementary observational, qualitative and quantitative data collection to triangulate and validate the dataset. The methods would include log analyses of the use, snapshot surveys of the wider user groups and observational studies of the patterns of use. As an example, in the evaluation of an online health information resource [51], six data collection strategies were used:

1. An up-to-date and comprehensive literature review;
2. An initial series of focus group discussions and individual interviews with a purposive sample of doctors, nurses, and allied health professionals in metropolitan and rural hospitals (2001-early 2002). Discussions focused on EBP

in the workplace, factors such as the computer and online information resources influencing decision-making, and the CHC. Focus group questions were of a more general nature, while the interviews explored the practices of individual practitioners;

3. A paper-based '*Clinical Practice and Information Needs Survey*' of a purposive sample of hospital clinicians, to capture the perceptions of clinical users and non-users prior to a scheduled state-wide promotion of the resource. It examined current work practices, computer competencies, general information access issues and awareness of the resource;

4. A second round of focus groups and interviews in 1 metropolitan, 2 regional and 1 rural hospital. Three groups were targeted, with a focus on younger and older users and medium to high users. Questions focused on the extent, type and ease of use of the resource, and any changes in relation to resources or environment.

5. An online survey of clinicians who used the resource, which addressed self-assessed computer competencies, training provided, resource design and usability, extent and ease of use of the resource functionalities.

6. An observational study of the ways in which a purposive sample of clinicians access and use the resource in a metropolitan and a regional hospital.

Complex interventions such as CDSS require a multidimensional matrix to describe the impact on process, impact and outcomes measures, which must be appropriate. As an example, the dimensions adopted for the evaluation of the MediConnect internet-based electronic medication record [52] were:

1. system (technical): includes data integrity, security and timeliness
2. data quality: includes medication and demographic information
3. privacy and confidentiality: includes suppression and informed consent
4. access to information: includes technical and people aspects
5. workflow and support: includes technical and people aspects
6. education and support: includes training resources/programs for trainers/support officers, as well as community engagement
7. communication strategy: includes delivery media and community engagement
8. participation: includes event log, reasons for participation, nonparticipation and withdrawal
9. satisfaction with MediConnect: suppression, opt-in/opt-out, Medicare number/unique ID, penalties, training and support, access and incentives
10. cost-structure: direct and indirect costs.
11. outcome measures: drug–drug interactions, drug–disease interactions and hospital admission related to therapeutic misadventure.

Other relevant questions include: what is the optimal level and type of computer support required by GPs, a heterogenous group, at different levels of experience, operating in very different social, professional and educational contexts? It also depends on whether the CDSS is designed to be opportunistic/consultative or reflective/critiquing.

7. Conclusions

We have described how CDSS have been used in the past decades and what types of CDSS implementations have shown to improve clinical outcomes. We have presented a set of categories to use when considering the implementation and evaluation of CDSS. Because of the early adoption of IT systems in health care in the United States, many of the evaluations have been published in hospital settings, and many of them from the US. However, the fundamental concepts of CDSS and issues associated with the development and implementation of CDSS are very similar in other environment internationally and in ambulatory settings. A difference is that the EU and Australia had a strong GP/FP and primary sector compared to the USA, where most of the CDSS work has been hospital-based; in fact most of the innovative USA work has been done in 4 benchmark institutions.

The robustness of a diagnostic CDSS is enhanced by the use of objective data such as laboratory investigations as compared to the use of clinical symptoms and signs. There is a phenomenon of "waning specificity", where the likelihood of false positives increases in the course of a consultation as the diagnostic scope narrows. The additional interactive "learning", where the application asks specific questions of the clinician and suggests further testing in the form of specific questions or investigations, is a valuable enhancement consistent with accepted CDSS benchmarks [53]. The limitations and limited implementations have as much to do with the need for comprehensive and accurate electronic health records (EHR) as the safety and quality of the CDSS themselves.

The safety and effectiveness of therapeutic decision support systems have been well reported in the literature. One phenomenon is "alert fatigue", which means that many important drug interactions may be missed because of desensitisation resulting from too many clinically irrelevant alerts, which also intrude on workflow [54]. There is a need for a classification of drug interactions, so that only significant ones should appear. CPOE with integrated CDSS can decrease adverse events but can also cause errors such as fragmented display of medication orders, pharmacy inventory display of drug doses that were confused with recommended dosages, and ignored renewal orders for antibiotic therapy when notices were placed in the paper chart and not in the computer [55]. Nevertheless, the benefits overweigh the potential errors.

CDSS have clear benefit in managing reminders and alerts for disease management. This well documented benefit of CDSS could be realized if integrated with cancer and other risk factor screening programs that are rigorous, robust and useful. However, they need to be embedded in EHR to maximise the leverage on the use of computers. These programs can effectively promote patient participation in their own health care proactively. However, successful communication with the patient is pivotal in this approach; this requires time, skills and resources.

The effects of CDSS on patient outcomes have been insufficiently studied [11]; this systematic review found 52 studies of addressed patient outcomes, of which only 7 (13%) found a significant benefit. We have described the challenges of measuring patient outcome improvements in health informatics and CDSS evaluations in particular. These challenges must be overcome to demonstrate benefits to patient outcomes in CDSS evaluations.

There are significant opportunities for improving the safety of general practice computer systems. Priorities include improving the knowledge base for clinical decision support, paying greater attention to human ergonomics in system design, improved staff training and the introduction of new regulations mandating system suppliers to satisfy essential safety requirements [56]. While promising, CDSS require careful development and implementation within a comprehensive conceptual framework of intrinsic and extrinsic determinants of prescribing behaviour. Many questions remain: How "hard" are diagnoses made on clinical grounds alone? Are predictors evaluated using multivariate methods? Where do errors in decisions mostly occur? What are the types of errors and what are the significant ones? Is a universal and generic CDSS possible, supportable and sustainable? What is the cost effectiveness of CDSS?

Significant errors continue to occur despite demonstrated benefits from well-designed information management and clinical decision support systems across a wide range of health care environments [57]. Five years on very little has changed [58]. The situation is similar in Australia [59] and the rest of the world [60]. The need for successful CDSS implementations remains.

References

[1]   Hunt, D. L., Haynes, R. B., Hanna, S. E., & Smith, K. (1998). Effects of computer-based clinical decision support systems on physician performance and patient outcomes: A systematic review. *JAMA : the Journal of the American Medical Association, 280*(15), 1339-46.

[2]   Kawamoto, K., Houlihan, C. A., Balas, E. A., & Lobach, D. F. (2005). Improving clinical practice using clinical decision support systems: A systematic review of trials to identify features critical to success. *BMJ (Clinical Research Ed.), 330*(7494), 765.

[3]   Wyatt, J., & Spiegelhalter, D. (1991). Field trials of medical decision-aids: Potential problems and solutions. *Proceedings / the ... Annual Symposium on Computer Application [Sic] in Medical Care. Symposium on Computer Applications in Medical Care*, 3-7.

[4]   Sim, I., & Berlin, A. (2003). A framework for classifying decision support systems. *AMIA ... Annual Symposium Proceedings / AMIA Symposium. AMIA Symposium*, 599-603.

[5]   McGlynn, E. A., Asch, S. M., Adams, J., Keesey, J., Hicks, J., DeCristofaro, A., et al. (2003). The quality of health care delivered to adults in the united states. *The New England Journal of Medicine, 348*(26), 2635-45.

[6]   Lomas, J., Sisk, J. E., & Stocking, B. (1993). From evidence to practice in the united states, the united kingdom, and canada. *The Milbank Quarterly, 71*(3), 405-10.

[7]   Durieux, P., Trinquart, L., Colombet, I., Niès, J., Walton, R., Rajeswaran, A., et al. (2008). Computerized advice on drug dosage to improve prescribing practice. *Cochrane Database of Systematic Reviews (Online)*, (3), CD002894.

[8]   Kawamoto, K., & Lobach, D. F. (2003). Clinical decision support provided within physician order entry systems: A systematic review of features effective for changing clinician behavior. *AMIA ... Annual Symposium Proceedings / AMIA Symposium. AMIA Symposium*, 361-5.

[9]   Eslami, S., Abu-Hanna, A., & de Keizer, N. F. (2007). Evaluation of outpatient computerized physician medication order entry systems: A systematic review. *Journal of the American Medical Informatics Association : JAMIA, 14*(4), 400-6.

[10] Georgiou, A., Williamson, M., Westbrook, J. I., & Ray, S. (2007). The impact of computerised physician order entry systems on pathology services: A systematic review. *International Journal of Medical Informatics, 76*(7), 514-29.

[11] Garg, A. X., Adhikari, N. K., McDonald, H., Rosas-Arellano, M. P., Devereaux, P. J., Beyene, J., et al. (2005). Effects of computerized clinical decision support systems on practitioner performance and patient outcomes: A systematic review. *JAMA : the Journal of the American Medical Association, 293*(10), 1223-38.

[12] Koppel R, Metlay J.P, Cohen A, Abaluck B, et al Role of Computerized Physician Order Entry Systems in Facilitating Medication Errors *JAMA*. 2005;293:1197-1203.

[13] Bennett, J. W., & Glasziou, P. P. (2003). Computerised reminders and feedback in medication management: A systematic review of randomised controlled trials. *The Medical Journal of Australia, 178*(5), 217-22.

[14] Balas, E. A., Austin, S. M., Mitchell, J. A., Ewigman, B. G., Bopp, K. D., & Brown, G. D. (1996). The clinical value of computerized information services. A review of 98 randomized clinical trials. *Archives of Family Medicine, 5*(5), 271-8.

[15] Kaushal, R., Shojania, K. G., & Bates, D. W. (2003). Effects of computerized physician order entry and clinical decision support systems on medication safety: A systematic review. *Archives of Internal Medicine, 163*(12), 1409-16.

[16] Bryan, C., & Boren, S. A. (2008). The use and effectiveness of electronic clinical decision support tools in the ambulatory/primary care setting: A systematic review of the literature. *Informatics in Primary Care, 16*(2), 79-91.

[17] Durieux, P., Nizard, R., Ravaud, P., Mounier, N., & Lepage, E. (2000). A clinical decision support system for prevention of venous thromboembolism: Effect on physician behavior. *JAMA : the Journal of the American Medical Association, 283*(21), 2816-21.

[18] Randell, R., Mitchell, N., Dowding, D., Cullum, N., & Thompson, C. (2007). Effects of computerized decision support systems on nursing performance and patient outcomes: A systematic review. *Journal of Health Services Research & Policy, 12*(4), 242-9.

[19] Sintchenko, V., Magrabi, F., & Tipper, S. (2007). Are we measuring the right end-points? Variables that affect the impact of computerised decision support on patient outcomes: A systematic review. *Medical Informatics and the Internet in Medicine, 32*(3), 225-40.

[20] Mahoney, C. D., Berard-Collins, C. M., Coleman, R., Amaral, J. F., & Cotter, C. M. (2007). Effects of an integrated clinical information system on medication safety in a multi-hospital setting. *American Journal of Health-System Pharmacy : AJHP : Official Journal of the American Society of Health-System Pharmacists, 64*(18), 1969-77.

[21] Weber, V., White, A., & McIlvried, R. (2008). An electronic medical record (EMR)-based intervention to reduce polypharmacy and falls in an ambulatory rural elderly population. *Journal of General Internal Medicine : Official Journal of the Society for Research and Education in Primary Care Internal Medicine, 23*(4), 399-404.

[22] Weber, V., Bloom, F., Pierdon, S., & Wood, C. (2008). Employing the electronic health record to improve diabetes care: A multifaceted intervention in an integrated delivery system. *Journal of General Internal Medicine : Official Journal of the Society for Research and Education in Primary Care Internal Medicine, 23*(4), 379-82.

[23] Magrabi, F., Westbrook, J. I., Kidd, M. R., Day, R. O., & Coiera, E. (2008). Long-Term patterns of online evidence retrieval use in general practice: A 12-month study. *Journal of Medical Internet Research, 10*(1), e6.

[24] Varonen, H., Kortteisto, T., Kaila, M., & EBMeDS Study Group (2008). What may help or hinder the implementation of computerized decision support systems (cdsss): A focus group study with physicians. *Family Practice, 25*(3), 162-7.

[25] Young, A., & Beswick, K. (1995). Protocols used by UK general practitioners, what is expected of them and what solutions are provided. *Computer Methods and Programs in Biomedicine, 48*(1-2), 85-90.

[26] Liaw, S. T., & Schattner, P. (2003). Electronic decision support in general practice. What's the hold up?. *Australian Family Physician, 32*(11), 941-4.

[27] Liaw, S. T., Deveny, E., Morrison, I., & Lewis, B. (2006). Clinical, information and business process modeling to promote development of safe and flexible software. *Health Informatics Journal, 12*(3), 199-211.

[28] Simon, J. S., Rundall, T. G., & Shortell, S. M. (2007). Adoption of order entry with decision support for chronic care by physician organizations. *Journal of the American Medical Informatics Association : JAMIA, 14*(4), 432-9.

[29] Fung, C. H., Tsai, J. S., Lulejian, A., Glassman, P., Patterson, E., Doebbeling, B. N., et al. (2008). An evaluation of the veterans health administration's clinical reminders system: A national survey of generalists. *Journal of General Internal Medicine : Official Journal of the Society for Research and Education in Primary Care Internal Medicine, 23*(4), 392-8.

[30] Bott, O. J., Ammenwerth, E., Brigl, B., Knaup, P., Lang, E., Pilgram, R., et al. (2005). The challenge of ubiquitous computing in health care: Technology, concepts and solutions. Findings from the IMIA yearbook of medical informatics 2005. *Methods of Information in Medicine, 44*(3), 473-9.

[31] Reinhardt, ER. 2008. Technical paradigms for realizing ubiquitous care. *Stud Health Technol Inform* 134:129-134

[32] Plaza, V., Cobos, A., Ignacio-García, J. M., Molina, J., Bergoñón, S., García-Alonso, F., et al. (2005). [Cost-Effectiveness of an intervention based on the global initiative for asthma (GINA) recommendations using a computerized clinical decision support system: A physicians randomized trial]. *Medicina Clínica, 124*(6), 201-6.

[33] Lee, F., Teich, J. M., Spurr, C. D., & Bates, D. W. (1996). Implementation of physician order entry: User satisfaction and self-reported usage patterns. *Journal of the American Medical Informatics Association : JAMIA, 3*(1), 42-55.

[34] Kaushal, R., Jha, A. K., Franz, C., Glaser, J., Shetty, K. D., Jaggi, T., et al. (2006). Return on investment for a computerized physician order entry system. *Journal of the American Medical Informatics Association : JAMIA, 13*(3), 261-6.

[35] Tierney, W. M., Miller, M. E., Overhage, J. M., & McDonald, C. J. (1993). Physician inpatient order writing on microcomputer workstations. Effects on resource utilization. *JAMA : the Journal of the American Medical Association, 269*(3), 379-83.

[36] Ash, J. S., Gorman, P. N., Seshadri, V., & Hersh, W. R. (2004). Computerized physician order entry in U.S. Hospitals: Results of a 2002 survey. *Journal of the American Medical Informatics Association : JAMIA, 11*(2), 95-9.

[37] McInnes, D. K., Saltman, D. C., & Kidd, M. R. (2006). General practitioners' use of computers for prescribing and electronic health records: Results from a national survey. *The Medical Journal of Australia, 185*(2), 88-91.

[38] Ash, J. S., & Bates, D. W. (2005). Factors and forces affecting EHR system adoption: Report of a 2004 ACMI discussion. *Journal of the American Medical Informatics Association : JAMIA, 12*(1), 8-12.

[39] Bates, D. W., Kuperman, G. J., Wang, S., Gandhi, T., Kittler, A., Volk, L., et al. (2003). Ten commandments for effective clinical decision support: Making the practice of evidence-based medicine a reality. *Journal of the American Medical Informatics Association : JAMIA, 10*(6), 523-30.

[40] Ash, J. S., Berg, M., & Coiera, E. (2004). Some unintended consequences of information technology in health care: The nature of patient care information system-related errors. *Journal of the American Medical Informatics Association : JAMIA, 11*(2), 104-12.

[41] Weiner, M., Gress, T., Thiemann, D. R., Jenckes, M., Reel, S. L., Mandell, S. F., et al. (1999). Contrasting views of physicians and nurses about an inpatient computer-based provider order-entry system. *Journal of the American Medical Informatics Association : JAMIA, 6*(3), 234-44.

[42] Han, Y. Y., Carcillo, J. A., Venkataraman, S. T., Clark, R. S., Watson, R. S., Nguyen, T. C., et al. (2005). Unexpected increased mortality after implementation of a commercially sold computerized physician order entry system. *Pediatrics, 116*(6), 1506-12.

[43] Sittig, D. F., Ash, J. S., Zhang, J., Osheroff, J. A., & Shabot, M. M. (2006). Lessons from "unexpected increased mortality after implementation of a commercially sold computerized physician order entry system". *Pediatrics, 118*(2), 797-801.

[44] Cordero, L., Kuehn, L., Kumar, R. R., & Mekhjian, H. S. (2004). Impact of computerized physician order entry on clinical practice in a newborn intensive care unit. *Journal of Perinatology : Official Journal of the California Perinatal Association, 24*(2), 88-93.

[45] Keene, A., Ashton, L., Shure, D., Napoleone, D., Katyal, C., & Bellin, E. (2007). Mortality before and after initiation of a computerized physician order entry system in a critically ill pediatric population. *Pediatric Critical Care Medicine : a Journal of the Society of Critical Care Medicine and the World Federation of Pediatric Intensive and Critical Care Societies, 8*(3), 268-71.

[46] Upperman, J. S., Staley, P., Friend, K., Benes, J., Dailey, J., Neches, W., et al. (2005). The introduction of computerized physician order entry and change management in a tertiary pediatric hospital. *Pediatrics, 116*(5), e634-42.

[47] Campbell, E. M., Sittig, D. F., Ash, J. S., Guappone, K. P., & Dykstra, R. H. (2006). Types of unintended consequences related to computerized provider order entry. *Journal of the American Medical Informatics Association : JAMIA, 13*(5), 547-56.

[48] Classen, D. C., Avery, A. J., & Bates, D. W. (2007). Evaluation and certification of computerized provider order entry systems. *Journal of the American Medical Informatics Association : JAMIA, 14*(1), 48-55.

[49] Khajouei, R., & Jaspers, M. W. (2008). CPOE system design aspects and their qualitative effect on usability. *Studies in Health Technology and Informatics, 136*, 309-14.

[50] Eccles, M., Hawthorne, G., Whitty, P., Steen, N., Vanoli, A., Grimshaw, J., et al. (2002). A randomised controlled trial of a patient based diabetes recall and management system: The DREAM trial: A study protocol [ISRCTN32042030]. *BMC Health Services Research, 2*(1), 5.

[51] Liaw ST, Pleteshner C, Deveny E, Mulcahy D, Guillemin M, Arnold M. An Evaluation of the Clinicians Health Channel (2000-3*). Final Report to the Office of the Chief Clinical Advisor, Victorian Government Department of Human Services.* Health Informatics Research Group, Department of General Practice, University of Melbourne: 30 September 2003.

[52] Liaw ST, Tomlins R. Developments in information systems. Chap 12 in: *General Practice in Australia 2004*, page 569. Aust Gov Publishing Services, Commonwealth Department of Health & Family Services. May 2005

[53] Berner, E. S. (2003). Diagnostic decision support systems: How to determine the gold standard?. *Journal of the American Medical Informatics Association : JAMIA, 10*(6), 608-10.

[54] Ahearn, M. D., & Kerr, S. J. (2003). General practitioners' perceptions of the pharmaceutical decision-support tools in their prescribing software. *The Medical Journal of Australia, 179*(1), 34-7.

[55] Rochon, P. A., Field, T. S., Bates, D. W., Lee, M., Gavendo, L., Erramuspe-Mainard, J., et al. (2006). Clinical application of a computerized system for physician order entry with clinical decision support to prevent adverse drug events in long-term care. *CMAJ : Canadian Medical Association Journal = Journal De L'association Medicale Canadienne, 174*(1), 52-4.

[56] Avery, A. J., Savelyich, B. S., Sheikh, A., Morris, C. J., Bowler, I., & Teasdale, S. (2007). Improving general practice computer systems for patient safety: Qualitative study of key stakeholders. *Quality & Safety in Health Care*, *16*(1), 28-33.
[57] Kohn, L. T., Corrigan, J. M., & Donaldson, M. S. (2000). *To err is human: Building a safer health system.* Washington, D.C.: National Academy Press.
[58] Leape, L. L., & Berwick, D. M. (2005). Five years after to err is human: What have we learned?. *JAMA : the Journal of the American Medical Association*, *293*(19), 2384-90.
[59] Barraclough, B. H. (2001). Safety and quality in australian healthcare: Making progress. *The Medical Journal of Australia*, *174*(12), 616-7.
[60] Donaldson, L., & Philip, P. (2004). Patient safety: A global priority. In *Bull world health organ.* Switzerland.

Review Questions

1. What are the benefits of using clinical decision support systems?
2. What evidence and of what degree of accuracy is this available to convince decision makers to implement a CDSS?
3. How should a CDSS be evaluated for suitable local use?

Health Informatics
E.J.S. Hovenga et al. (Eds.)
IOS Press, 2010
© 2010 The authors and IOS Press. All rights reserved.
doi:10.3233/978-1-60750-476-4-312

24. Translational Bioinformatics

Fernando MARTIN-SANCHEZ PhD in Informatics, MSc, BSc (Biochemistry and Molecular Biology)[a] , Isabel HERMOSILLA-GIMENO DVM, MA, BA[a]
[a]Medical Bioinformatics Department, National Institute of Health "Carlos III", Ctra. Majadahonda a Pozuelo, Km. 2. 28220 Majadahonda, Madrid – SPAIN

Abstract. This chapter gives an educational overview of:

- The origins and evolution of bioinformatics from its beginning where it was a discipline mainly oriented towards the resolution of problems in biology to the present where it shows a clear interest on the field of translational research in medicine.
- The different aspects of bioinformatics, ranging from its application for the study of individual entities, such as a gene or a protein, through its role as support to the large sequencing projects, and the global approach to genomics to systems biology.
- Bioinformatics resources most used by researchers, distinguishing between the different information resources (databases) and the tools (programs) used to process them.
- The current relevance of bioinformatics in medicine, both in the field of biomedical research and in the fields of clinical practice and public health as well as its multiple connections with the field of medical informatics.
- The main lines for research and development in translational medicine, its main applications in the field of genomics medicine and future challenges raised by the new trends in medicine.

Keywords. Bioinformatics, genomics, medical informatics applications, genetics research, knowledge, database, public health informatics, data collection, computer systems, molecular medicine

Introduction

The convergence between biology and computer science started in the decade of the 1960's although it didn't received the name of Bioinformatics until the 1990s. This was the first of a number of fruitful synergies between apparently dissimilar disciplines that have had a great impact in Biomedicine. In its early years the application of computing to biology focused mainly on the use of algorithms to analyse the evolutionary relations between different organisms and the development of databases to store the growing number of DNA and protein sequences [1] [2]. Bioinformatics was essential to support the progress of the Human Genome Project (HGP) and became a consolidated discipline at this time [3]. The consensus agreement by the scientific community to make publicly available the sequences through Internet, itself experiencing a worldwide expansion at that time, was a key success factor.

The release of the sequence of the Human Genome in 2003 was only the beginning that opened new avenues for research. Post genomic research includes at least four different approaches, individual genomics, comparative genomics, functional genomics and proteomics. Individual and comparative genomics focus on the analysis of genome variation between different individuals or different species, respectively. Functional genomics and proteomics deal with the manner in which genetic information is expressed in the cell, either at the intermediate level (transcription) or at the final level (translation into proteins). The role of bioinformatics in these areas is to manage and analyse these massive volumes of data generated by systematic and global scale genomic studies with the aim of providing some insight into the relations between genome structure and function. Figure 1 shows some examples of databases storing genetic and genomic data.

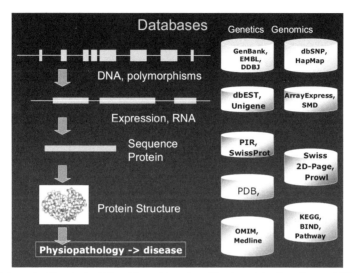

Figure 1. Information Flow in the Cell and Some Examples of Databases That Store Data at Different Levels

These relations are particularly interesting for medicine since the most prevalent diseases (cancer, neurodegenerative or cardiovascular diseases) result from a complex interaction between many genes and environmental factors.

Therefore, the latest trends point towards a central role of bioinformatics in biomedical research and clinical practice expanding its initial scope. The birth of what has been called molecular medicine or genomics based medicine is demanding the integration of genomic information with clinical information, a step that can only come through the collaboration and synergy of bioinformatics and medical informatics. The result of this synergy has given rise to a new discipline known as Biomedical Informatics [4].

The concept of translational biomedical research defines this attempt to achieve a fast application of experimental biological findings into routine clinical solutions; this is why the term "Translational Bioinformatics" has been adopted, mainly by the American Medical Informatics Association (AMIA), to refer to this new approach to bioinformatics, strongly based on a clinical perspective.

Translational bioinformatics is now considered one of the main branches of biomedical informatics (together with clinical informatics and public health informatics). Biomedical informatics has become an inclusive term that represents an established scientific discipline, being this fact shown by the large number of publications, congresses, scientific associations, projects, educational programs and research centres devoted to it. This chapter reviews the different contributions that bioinformatics is making to biomedical research and clinical practice following both a chronological pattern and a diverse focus analysis (genetics, genome, post genome, molecular medicine, translational medicine) that is briefly detailed in this introduction. Table 1 summarizes the types of data managed in each of these areas.

Molecular Genetics	Genome project	Post-Genomics	Molecular Medicine
- Sequences	- Genome fragments	- SNPs, haplotypes	- Physiology
- Alignments	- Annotations	- Complete genomes	- Pathology
- Patterns	- Genes and regulatory	- Microarray images and data	- Genetic Networks
- Structures	regions	- Proteomic data	- Metabolic Networks
			- Interactions

Table 1. Types of data that bioinformatics deals with in each of the areas

1.   Bioinformatics Before the Human Genome Project: Supporting Molecular Genetics Research

Watson and Crick described the double helical structure of DNA in 1953 setting the basis of modern biology. DNA research in those early years was known as molecular genetics and was restricted, due to existing available technologies, to the study of individual genes or proteins, a painstaking slow process at the time. Therefore, the development of informatics tools and methods was oriented towards extracting the maximum information from these experimental approaches.

1.1 Sequence Data Management and Analysis

The first informatics applications in molecular biology were databases that stored information about sequences. A sequence is the order in which the different bases are arranged in a DNA fragment, and this fragment will determine through the application of a genetic code, the constitution and order of the different amino acids that form a protein. Figure 2 shows an example of a DNA sequence.

The size of the most popular databases of DNA sequences such as GenBank, DDBJ and EMBL has grown exponentially since their creation. The management of these huge repositories represents one of the greatest achievements of bioinformatics. In addition to these three databases of DNA sequences that work in coordinated manner[1] there are hundreds of databases that store sequences of biological macromolecules. One example is SWISS-PROT[2] the most important database for protein sequences.

The letter chains corresponding to DNA and RNA sequences and the amino acids of the proteins are particularly suitable for informatics treatment. These are not only useful for storing sequences but also for comparing them, aligning them and to find common regions. The family of BLAST programs[3] shown in Figure 3 is the one most used for these purposes. When a research group obtains a sequence experimentally, they can, firstly, compare it with all the other sequences of the database and determine the degree of similarity they show. If the function of these similar sequences is known, this information can be essential for establishing the function of the problem sequence.

---

[1] http://www.ncbi.nlm.nih.gov/collab/

[2] http://us.expasy.org/sprot/

[3] http://www.ebi.ac.uk/Blast2/index.html

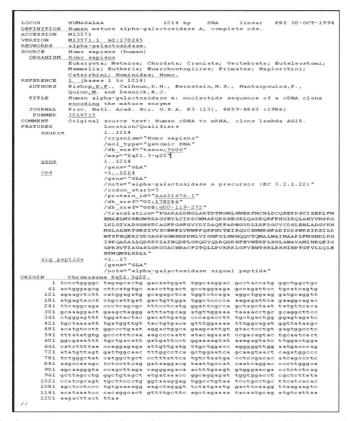

Figure 2. Example of DNA Sequence (Genbank record) Human Mature Alpha-galactosidase A, complete cds.

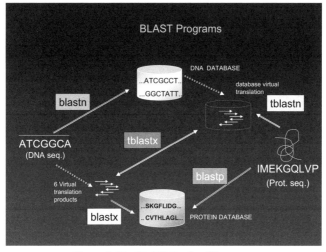

Figure 3. The BLAST Family of Programs

Alignment between groups of sequences can be also done, thus providing information about the degree of similarity among them. The complex algorithms used to align multiple sequences are very demanding computationally. They, through the comparison of different positions in the sequences together with the insertion of gaps, make it possible for the largest number of bases to coincide in the same positions. It is from multiple alignments that the common areas, most conserved, are deduced indicating the presence of functionally or structurally important regions in the sequences. Programs derived from CLUSTAL[4] are widely disseminated with this purpose.

Sequence alignments are essential for the study of evolution. It is believed that the more similar two sequences are, the greater the chances of them being homologues, this is, that they come from a common ancestor and that they have evolved through the accumulation of changes or mutations. Phylogeny is the study of the evolution of living organisms. Bioinformatics has been applied to the construction of phylogenetic trees that, taking into account all the genetic information, allow for the reconstruction of the evolution of a species or the diversification of the strains from a single organism. In these trees, the distance between the branches is proportional to the differences found between two forms. Phylogenetic studies represent an important tool in genetic and molecular epidemiology studies. Programs accessible through the Internet such as PHYLIP[5] are some of the most widely used in this environment. Another resource would be "Tree of Life" [6].

1.2 Bioinformatics Resources Related to Protein Structure and Function

Structural Bioinformatics has as its main goal to find out the manner in which the linear sequence of a protein (the chain of amino acids it is composed of) determines its three dimensional structure, and from this point, to understand how either the whole structure or part of it is associated to a specific function [5]. Characteristic patterns in the sequences can be studied, particularly important zones that have been conserved through evolution or regions with a regulatory function. PROSITE [7] is the most important database for patterns (regions of sequences of specific interest) and Protein Data Bank[8] is the reference resource for three dimensional protein structures as the one shown in Figure 4.

The relation between structure and function, although not yet deciphered in biology, poses a challenge for bioinformatics systems which have provided valuable clues to understand this process, and even solve it in very specific cases [6]. To further advance in this field, systems for the structural and functional classification of proteins have been developed; CATH is one of such systems[9]. Prediction systems are numerous and in many cases they work in intermediate steps, they first predict the secondary structure (characteristics due to the hydrogen bonds between amino acids) such as coil, alpha-helix or pleaded sheet from the sequence or primary structure. PREDICTPROTEIN is an Internet service that integrates several tools devoted to this purpose[10]. Then, they can try

---

[4] http://www.ebi.ac.uk/clustalw/index.html

[5] http://evolution.genetics.washington.edu/phylip.html

[6] http://tolweb.org/tree/phylogeny.html

[7] http://www.expasy.ch/prosite

[8] http://www.rcsb.org/pdb

[9] http://www.biochem.ucl.ac.uk/bsm/cath_new/index.html

[10] http://www.predictprotein.org/

to predict the folding of the complete molecule or tertiary structure. Special programs such as Rasmol or Cn3D have been developed to graphically visualise these three dimensional structures.

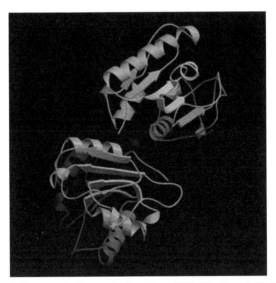

Figure 4. Structure of a Protein Retrieved From PDB. (Bacillus subtilis lipase)

Also in this area, sequences can be used to identify families of homologous proteins that might have the same three dimensional structure. If it is not possible to find related sequences, there are other methods such as "threading" in which the compatibility of each of the residues with a valid folding is examined, based on their biophysical properties (hidrophobicity, stability); an example of this type of systems is 3D-PSSM[11].

2. Bioinformatics in the Genomic Era

In recent years the development of automated methods of DNA sequencing have made it possible for scientists to carry out large scale sequencing projects, being the Human Genome Project the one that attracted most interest. This international program started in 1990 and ended in April 2003 although previously, in February 2001, the journals Nature and Science published a draft of the sequence with 97% total bases, 85 % in order) [7] [8]. The Human Genome Project had as its main goals the construction of detailed genetic and physical maps of the human genome as well as to determine its complete sequence. The remaining challenge is to locate and determine the function of all the genes and their role in the development of diseases.

Bioinformatics plays an important role in the storage and management of the genomic sequences, in the assembly of sequences and in the process of gene prediction and annotation.

---

[11] http://www.sbg.bio.ic.ac.uk/~3dpssm/

2.1 Sources of Genomic Sequence Data

Besides the genome sequences yielded by the different genome projects there are also other DNA sequences important for research such as STS (sequence tagged sites) and EST (expressed sequence tags). The first are short DNA sequences useful as markers because their exact location is known while the added value of ESTs is that they are sequences of genes or fragments of genes obtained through complementary DNA sequencing therefore known to be expressed in a cell. These sequences are available in National Center for Biotechnology Information (NCBI) databases [12]: Another useful resource is Unigene, a system that classifies dbEST into groupings of sequences, each related to a gene and offering information about the tissues in which these genes are expressed and their location in the genome.

Entrez Gene[13], provides a unified interface for queries to access curated information about a loci o a specific place in the genome. With the name of the gene we can get information about all related bibliography, diseases in which it plays a role, known mutations, its sequence, the protein it codes for, homology with other sequences and the reference sequence. Furthermore, there are several services that provide information about the current status of the different genome projects both finalised and in progress: GOLD – Genomes On Line Database[14] is one of them (the current version of the GOLD database contains 797 complete genomes, of which 658 are Bacteria, 86 Eukarya, and 53 Archaea).

2.2 Assembly of Partial Genome Sequences

Sequences generated in massive sequencing projects are automatically collected by the laboratory equipment known as DNA sequencers. These DNA sequences are then stored in databases in diverse formats for their later use. There are many programs specially designed to manage these sequences, controlling their quality and facilitating their posterior analysis. It is necessary to take into account that DNA sequencers can only read short DNA fragments (less than 800 bases), thus it is essential to keep track of the thousands of fragments in which the genome subject to study is divided, in order to be able to rebuild it, by assembling all the different partial sequences obtained, to finally render the complete sequence of the problem genome.

2.3 Gene Finding and Genome Annotation

Genome sequencing works provide the "raw" sequence of DNA bases that make up an organism's genome. It is now known that the Human Genome is made up of large areas with no known function, and the genes or functional units are located scattered along the whole sequence. Therefore, not only is it important to locate the beginning and ending of all genes, but also to find out which of the two DNA strands is the one that codes for a specific gene, where can the regions that regulate their function be found, and when possible, to establish the specific function associated to a given gene. In higher organisms the genes are not continuous entities but instead they are found fragmented throughout

---

[12] http://www.ncbi.nlm.nih.gov/genome/sts/ and http://www.ncbi.nlm.nih.gov/dbEST/index.html

[13] http://www.ncbi.nlm.nih.gov/sites/entrez?db=gene

[14] http://www.genomesonline.org/

the chromosomes, following a scheme of introns (areas that are discarded) and exons (that are transcribed). A level of additional complexity lays on the fact that one gene may include more than one pattern of fragmentation, a phenomenon called alternative splicing, thus generating several transcription and translation patterns.

Bioinformatics has found in this area and important niche of development, developing databases and tools that help predict all these characteristics, allowing for the annotation of raw DNA sequences. GENSCAN[15] and GeneID[16] are examples of programs that predict gene structures. ENSEMBL[17] is a good example of a system dedicated to the automatic annotation of genomes.

2.4 Genome Browsers

Genome viewers or browsers, are useful bioinformatics tools that allow navigating through all the available sequences in the different databases. Thus, it is possible to access the sequence of a gene beginning at the chromosome level by zooming in and changing the level of resolution by selecting one of the arms, down to the bands in which they are divided, and all the way to the gene level and their sequence. In the intermediate levels, the information is completed by other data of interest such as the position of the point mutations, the areas rich in gene number or the content of the bases G plus C. One of these systems (NBCI MapView) can be seen in figure 5. One such example of these navigators was developed by the University of California Santa Cruz[18].

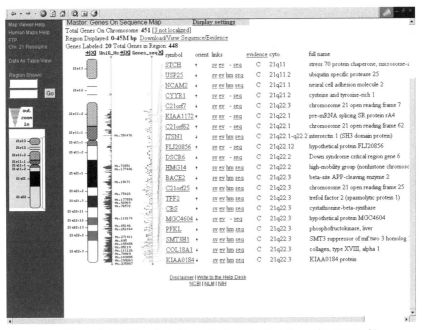

Figure 5. MapView. Main Screen for Browsing Data From Chromosome 21

---

[15] http://www.mit.edu/genscan.html
[16] http://genome.imim.es/geneid.html
[17] http://www.ensembl.org
[18] http://genome.ucsc.edu/cgi-bin/hgGateway

3. The Role of Bioinformatics in Post- Genomic Research

New challenges arose once the complete sequence of the Human Genome was obtained. The initial consensus sequence of the human genome led the way to the sequencing of individual genomes with the identification of genetic differences between them (SNPs and haplotypes). Research now is also focusing on the expression of complete sets of genes (cellular transcriptome) and the study of temporal proteomes present in a cell at a specific point in time and biological conditions. Proteins in a cell determine which metabolic pathways (metabolomics) are turned on or off and which physiological processes are taking place.

This way, the genomic era turned into a post genomic era, in which the most promising research lines pursue the use of the large number of structural information generated for its utilisation in functional analyses [9]. Genomes are analysed and compared to find out their existing relation and function. This new era is that of the "omics" studies, a suffix that relates to the work in genomics (study of the group of genes) proteomics (study of the group of proteins expressed by a genome) or metabolomics (global analysis of all or a large number of cellular metabolites) as it is graphically shown in Figure 6.

New laboratory technologies such as biochips allow researchers to study in more detail the fields of the individual genetics variations, the interactions between genes and the assessment of their dynamic behaviour in the cell, the ultimate responsible of the evolution of the different diseases. The great challenge of bioinformatics is to store, manage and analyse all these data to be able to effectively apply and translate this knowledge into measures, tools and methods for the improvement of healthcare.

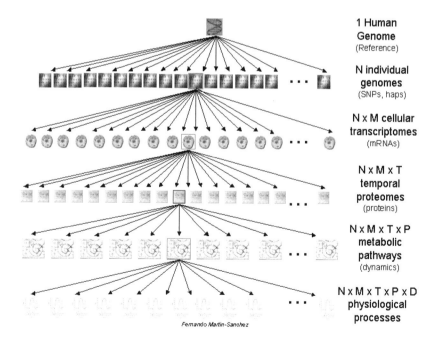

1 Human Genome (Reference)

N individual genomes (SNPs, haps)

N x M cellular transcriptomes (mRNAs)

N x M x T temporal proteomes (proteins)

N x M x T x P metabolic pathways (dynamics)

N x M x T x P x D physiological processes

Fernando Martin-Sanchez

Figure 6: Data Explosion in Post-Genomic Research

3.1 Individual Genomics

The sequence obtained through the Human Genome Project is just a consensus sequence of the human species because it corresponds only to a few persons whose genetic material has been sequenced. However, it is thought that there are lots of differences between the genetic material of different individuals due to mutations and polymorphisms that correspond to approximately 0.1% of the Human Genome (one in every thousand bases). These differences are precisely what determine the difference in susceptibility of different people to suffer diseases or to a specific therapeutic treatment. Sequences of the same gene may vary from some individuals to others by a mutation. SNPs (single nucleotide polymorphisms) are frequent changes in one DNA residue (present in more than 1% of the population studied), that when accumulated, might lead to the loss of the function of the gene or to a different susceptibility to a disease. Recently, other sources of human genetic variation have been described. They are known as structural variation o copy number variation and it has been postulated that they could increase the degree of interindividual variation to almost 3% [10].

Genetic variations and their relationship with the development of diseases had been subject of study for a long time but, the technology available before the genome project only allowed to tackle very infrequent changes (mutations) that produced a clear effect on the cells, such as the development of monogenic diseases due to a problem in a single gene. However, the diseases that are more prevalent (cancer, cardiovascular and neurologic diseases) are complex entities in which many genes are involved and therefore several polymorphisms are present [11]. The systems for rapid sequencing and new laboratory technologies (microarrays, mass spectrometry) allow to study all possible polymorphisms and to detect mutations in complex genes. The significance of human genetic variation is analysed by observing the mutations in sequences of normal genes and correlating them with specific diseases or with specific patterns of response to drugs[12].

Bioinformatics is indispensable for the work with SNPs at the stage of information storage and management. Among the databases that can be highlighted due to their importance is the one developed by the NCBI (dbSNP). All the information stored in other databases is used for annotating SNPs or to collaborate in associative studies in which SNPs are used as markers for complex diseases [13]. The latest tendency in works in human genomic variability is haplotype studies. It has been proven that SNPs are inherited in block between a generation and the next and, therefore the profile of SNPs in a specific gene only correspond to specific patterns or groupings. The prediction, storage of haplotypes and their integration with clinical data is a new challenge of bioinformatics in this particular area [14]. The Hapmap project specifically addresses this issue[19].

3.2 Comparative and Microbial Genomics

Many microbial genomes and some multicellular eukaryotes have been sequenced. The possibility of knowing these genomes and the experimentation with these model organisms provide numerous clues for deciphering the molecular bases of diseases in human beings. Studies based on the homology between sequences of genes or proteins permit to check hypotheses and to predict the response to drugs or toxic agents [15].

---

[19] www.hapmap.org/

Diagnosis based on the detection of microorganisms can be done by using genetic markers, and it is also possible to deepen into the mechanisms by which they cause disease. The goal is to help in the understanding of microbial biology, to study their mechanisms for developing resistance to antibiotics, the identification of strains, the identification of new genetic targets of therapeutic value and the development of preventive measures against infectious diseases [16] [17].

3.3 Functional Genomics and Microarrays

If structural genomics is the branch of genomics oriented towards the characterization and location of the sequences that make up the DNA, functional genomics is the systematic retrieval of information on gene function, through the application of global experimental approaches that assess the function of the genes. Molecular interactions in the cell are complex and are influenced in many diverse ways by both internal and external factors, triggering processes of differential genetic expression. This is, even though all the cells of an individual contain the same genetic information, there are differences in the intensity, the information expressed or the time at which the information is expressed.

Cellular differentiation is a result of these variations and they can also be the origin of certain pathologies. Several new technologies allow scientists to study thousands of genes at the same time in a single experiment. This not only permits the simultaneous quantification of the expression of a large number of genes, but also the qualitative approximation by checking the expression pattern. Gene function can be studied by identifying which genes are differentially activated when comparing healthy versus diseased tissue, cells in different stages of development or in different metabolic or environmental conditions.

One of the most important genomic technologies to collect gene expression data is the one known as Biochips or microarrays. They may be defined as small size devices (chips or slides) that contain biological material and that are used for obtaining genetic information. In general, the term microarray refers to the devices in the shape of an array in which minute quantities of biological materials (DNA, protein) are placed and chemically attached to a solid surface. It is also called biochip due to the analogy to high density electronic circuits present in a microelectronic chip.

The nomenclature used to refer to these technologies or "Biochips" uses more specific terms such as DNA chips, protein arrays, oligonucleotide arrays or tissue arrays that refer to the type of biological material placed on the device.

Due to the extreme miniaturisation of the system, the number of slots is very elevated, even reaching the number of hundreds of thousands. Thus, this technology of DNA biochips or microarrays allows for the detection of mutations [18] and the measurement of the expression of thousands of genes at the same time [19], having opened the field for the study of complex, multigenic diseases; this is why they have a big impact on research and why they have great clinical potential [20] [21].

The potential of these systems brings about the acquisition, in a short period of time, of large volumes of information (sequences, mutations, data about genetic expression, analyses of clinical interest, drugs screening) that need to be managed with bioinformatics techniques to extract knowledge of medical use [22]. The application of "Data mining" techniques [23] and of advanced visualization methods come together hand in hand with the need to manage the results obtained in microarray projects [24]. The application of these new technologies of genetic information in the biomedical research environment has given rise to the appearance of a new "term": in-silico biology: this is, the retrieval of knowledge through theory considerations, simulations and experiments carried out in a computer, a technology based in silica [25].

3.4 Proteomics

The proteome can be defined as the group of PROTeins expressed by a GenOME. PROTEOMICS, then, is the study of proteomes, just as GENOMICS is the study of genomes. It is an essential discipline in the post genomic era that aims to discover all the proteins that give the cell its structure and function [26]. Different technologies allow to obtain and compare "instant photographs" of the proteins that are being expressed in a cell at a specific moment (robotics, electrophoresis 2D, mass spectrometry, microchips) [27]. Bioinformatics provides tools for comparing and analysing images that result from two dimensional gels (as the program Melanie), as well as specialised databases in which experiments and sequences are stored, as it is shown in figure 7. These can be used to identify proteins that are of special interest when comparing different proteomes (for example, normal cells versus tumour cells).

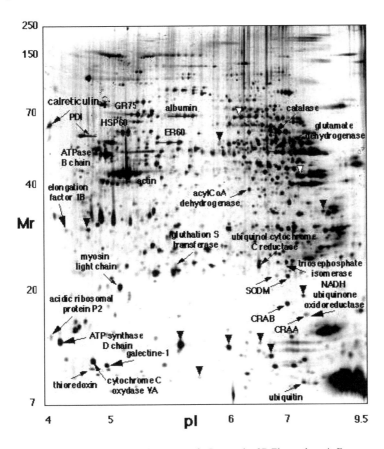

Figure 7. Resulting Image of a Proteomics 2D Electrophoresis Essay

3.5 Systems Biology

The development of genomic and proteomic technologies permits to carry out systematic global studies of multiple cellular entities. The next step in the study of physiopathological processes is the analysis of the interactions, and the regulatory networks that exist in cellular systems and control their behaviour. This is what systems biology does. Systems biology is the application of systems theory to genomics. It aims at developing a systems level understanding of biological processes. The final objective consists on explaining the complex phenomena of living organisms in terms of the theory of control and feedback network regulation. To advance in this systemic approach, complex mathematical models are applied to simulate and model chemico-physical events. Systems biology makes it possible to join the world of research, theory and computer simulation. In terms of medical research, systems biology represents a potential way to close the existing gap between microscopic measures proceeding from the biological research domain and macroscopic phenomena described at the individual (clinical) level.

4.   Toward Clinical Application: Translational Bioinformatics

4.1 Synergy Between Bioinformatics and Medical Informatics

Medical informatics, understood as the processing of clinical information [28] and bioinformatics, oriented towards handling (molecular and) genetic information [29] have come closer as information of the Human Genome Project was generated and linked with medical knowledge about diseases [30] [31] [32] [33]. It could be said that as genetics and medicine converge so do the disciplines that process the information that supports them. However, there are numerous difficulties when trying to integrate these two worlds that have developed almost independently from their respective origins. Apart from the technical and methodological difficulties inherent to the actual effective integration of genetic and clinical information there are others, such as cultural and formative barriers derived from the different focus that the two fields have. It was with this in mind that several international initiatives, such as the European Commission projects BIOINFOMED [4] and SYMBIOMATICS [34], tried to identify priority areas for research and support activities for overcoming these difficulties and to help make possible for information technologies to offer adequate answers to the challenges in the areas of data processing that molecular or genomic based medicine pose [35].

Figure 8 shows a scheme that proposes three approaches for the analysis of these aspects [36]. They would be: to expand bioinformatics solutions to manage clinical data, to adapt medical information systems to hold genomic data or the design of new systems through the collaboration of experts of both fields or even of new specialists in the interdisciplinary field of biomedical informatics. Following the BIOINFOMED White Paper, this discipline aims to create a common conceptual information space to further the discovery of novel diagnostic and therapeutic methods in the rapidly evolving arena of genomic medicine.

4.2 Molecular Medicine and Personalised Healthcare

The Human Genome Project was seen as an important source of knowledge about the relation between the structure of human genes and physiopathological processes. Research in genomics and proteomics will allow, on the one hand to increase knowledge of the molecular causes of diseases and, on the other hand to discover how genetic differences between people are the cause or contribute to the development of diseases. In this chapter we will distinguish between molecular medicine, defined as medicine that tries to explain life and disease in terms of the presence and regulation of molecular entities and personalised medicine that consists on the application of genomics to identify the individual predisposition to develop a specific disease and to design therapies adapted to the genetic profile of the patients making it possible to prescribe treatments with guaranty of security and efficiency. The first is more geared towards knowledge about the disease while the second tries to know and use in the clinic the genetic differences between people. They both pursue the improvement of healthcare, but applying different methods. In many cases it is not easy to distinguish these two approaches because there is evident overlap between them and the term genomics based medicine could be a good term to include them both. Figure 9 describes these two complementary approaches.

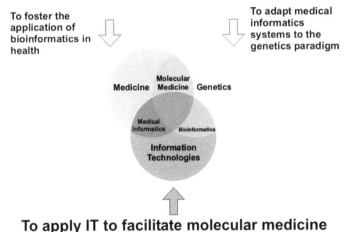

To apply IT to facilitate molecular medicine

Figure 8. Interdisciplinarity in Medicine, Genetics and Informatics

We describe below a few of the most important contributions of genomics to healthcare. The new tools used in genomic research are increasingly being applied to the clinical practice as diagnostic tools. The high performance of the new devices (biochips) permits the simultaneous monitoring of a large number of parameters that can be used as diagnostic markers. This will greatly affect the methods of genetic analysis [37]. The list of diseases with a genetic basis continues to grow [38]. However, the increasing attention that this area attracts is focused on predictive analyses that identify individuals with high risk of suffering a disease based on a SNPs or haplotype analysis before any symptoms appear. Proteomics will also offer new biomarkers of interest in the follow-up of patients.

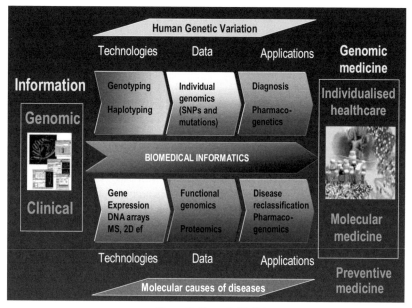

Figure 9: Genomic Medicine

Microarray studies are making it possible to compare differential expression patterns of genes between healthy cells and those from diseased tissue [39]. These studies make it possible to understand the mechanisms of diseases better and in some cases, they help identify different molecular forms and even suggest new classification for diseases that would help to improve in the diagnosis and prognosis [40].

New technologies that aim to understand the role of genes in diseases are revolutionizing the process of discovery and development of new drugs. Pharmacogenetics aims at the prescription of "personalised drugs" or drugs that are specific for different strata of patients that are classified depending on their genetic characteristics [41]. The use of biochips in the screening and toxicology of drugs make it possible to quickly analyse the changes in genomic expression that take place during the delivery of a drug as well as the location of new therapeutic targets and associated toxicological effects (pharmacogenomics) [42].

The use of new genetic information technologies will make it possible to perform cost-effective screening (genetic tests) at the population level. To transfer the genomic knowledge to the field of public health and epidemiology, it will be important to develop efforts in associative genetics, genotype-phenotype population studies, programs for disseminating genetic information and training health workers. Other examples of integration of information on the human genome in epidemiology include: -specific prevalence data on genetic variants, -epidemiological data on the relationship between genetic variability and diseases in different populations, and -evaluation of the validity and impact of genetic analyses [43].

For health professionals all these works mean an opportunity to carry out a more personalised medicine, that take into account the genetic makeup of the patients and that helps select the most effective treatment and also to apply preventive medicine strictly speaking, in which some diseases can be treated even before the first symptoms appear.

4.3 Bioinformatics Applications in Health

During these last years of genomic research, bioinformatics has reached its maturity and it has offered to the scientific community, models, methods and techniques for managing the avalanche of experimental data (sequences, biochips, proteomics, SNPs) and for extracting knowledge useful for biology. Lately, bioinformaticians have broaden their views by trying to show that the results obtained to date can also lead to the development of medical applications [44].

The work done in systems biology tries to characterize complex genetic and metabolic networks, their interactions and the role that they play in diseases [45]. The Pharmaceutical industry uses information from functional genomics to identify new targets useful for the development of drugs and it applies the knowledge obtained from studies of the genetic variation of individuals for the personalisation of drugs to the patients. The studies carried out with DNA microarrays and proteomics, Liotta, Kohn and Petricoin [46] show molecular patterns associated to different subtypes of diseases and can offer powerful diagnostic systems. Databases that integrate clinical and genetic information have been available for years (table 2 lists several of the most frequently used).

Table 2 – Main Clinico-Genetic Databases

Name	URL	Centre
OMIM	http://www.ncbi.nlm.nih.gov/sites/entrez?db=omim	NCBI - USA
Genes and Disease	http://www.ncbi.nlm.nih.gov/disease/index.html	NCBI - USA
Genecards	http://www.genecards.org/	Weizmann Institute - Israel
Geneclinics-Genetests	http://www.geneclinics.org	Univ. of Washington – Seattle - USA
dbSNP	http://www.ncbi.nlm.nih.gov/SNP/	NCBI - USA
Genetics Home Reference	http://ghr.nlm.nih.gov/	NLM-USA
HapMap	http://www.hapmap.org/	International HapMap Project

The work done in molecular evolution and microbial genomics make it possible to advance in the knowledge and understanding of pathogenic microorganisms and the course of the infections they cause. In a way, all these works are trying to provide support to what has been called "clinical genomics" or the study of genes in a large scale in the context of human diseases.

4.4 Molecular and Genetic Data Integration in Health Information Systems

It is now difficult to predict the medical alterations that a single gene or protein mutation can produce and, therefore, how to translate genetic discoveries into new clinical procedures. It has become clear that genes interact with many other genes and environmental factors. Thus, only combined studies of gene interactions in humans and other animals and large epidemiological studies from many different populations can discover the complex pathways of genetic diseases [47]. Biomedical informatics plays a central role in this aspect, as described in the graphic shown in figure 10.

Health records will include genetic data of the patients and their families [48]. The ongoing work by the HL7 Clinical Genomics Working Group[20] aims to define standards for representing and exchanging molecular information from patients and their families in clinical repositories. Protocols and guidelines for clinical practice will have to take into account the results obtained from genetic tests. Access to genomic information sources will be readily available for clinicians attending to medical criteria (symptoms, diseases) instead than to biological criteria for which they were initially designed for [49]. One such example is Disease card (figure 11), a system for information retrieval on diseases of genetic origin developed by University of Aveiro in collaboration with the Institute of Health Carlos III under the umbrella of the European projects INFOGENMED and the Network of Excellence INFOBIOMED. It includes more than 2000 diseases[21] [50].

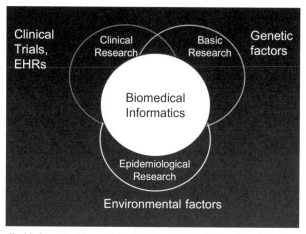

Figure 10: Biomedical Informatics Connects the Worlds of Clinical, Genetic and Environmental Data

Clinical trials will require a data infrastructure that allows to manage genetic profiles of patients. Coding systems for diseases and medical terminologies will have to include new concepts and entities coming from medical genomics and powerful decision making support systems will be required as well as virtual systems for continuing medical training on genetics [51].

---

[20] http://www.hl7.org/Special/committees/clingenomics/index.cfm

[21] http://www.diseasecard.com

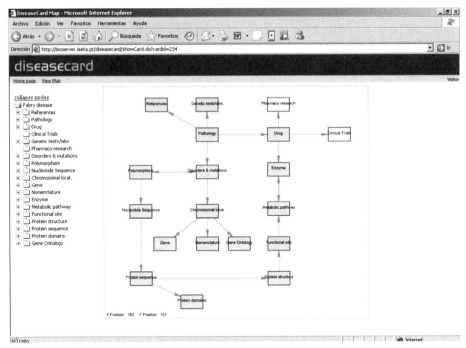

Figure 11: Screenshot from the Disease Card System

4.5 Current Research Topics

Some years ago, a few authors started to wonder about the implications that the convergence of clinical and genomic research might have for informatics [52]. The arrival of molecular medicine or genomics based medicine is demanding an integration of the genetic information (genotype) with clinical information (phenotype) that rises from the collaboration and the synergy between medical informatics and bioinformatics.

Just as described above, experts in medical informatics are trying to adapt their systems to the genomics revolution. At the same time, bioinformaticians lay a bridge to medicine. This is the reason why these two disciplines approach each other, collaborate and give rise to biomedical informatics, represented schematically in figure 12, allowing for a new approach to the processing of information about diseases and health.

In this new discipline all information levels are integrated (from the molecule to the population, through the cell, the tissue, the organ, and the patient) and the most appropriate methods and techniques for each case are applied, some from bioinformatics, some from medical informatics and others even from public health informatics or epidemiology as it is shown in figure 13.

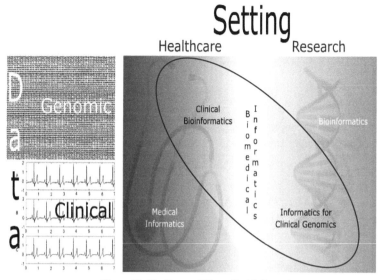

Figure 12. The Scope of Biomedical Informatics

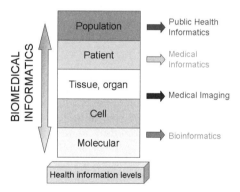

Figure 13: Integration of Information Levels in Biomedical Informatics

The objective is non other than to process, in the most efficient manner, all the information coming from biological, clinical, and environmental research and to advance in the development of molecular and personalised medicine. We could even add the concept of preventive medicine, this is, to practice healthcare interventions even before the symptoms of the diseases appear, since there is a possibility to predict genotype-environmental interactions that might lead to the phenotypes associated to diseases.

Some systems that integrate clinical and genomic data have already been developed in several areas: databases for pharmacogenetics, tumour banks, systems for molecular images or databases for genomic epidemiology and few others are on the works, such as clinico-genetic workstations, solutions for security and confidentiality of data, biobanks with populational data including clinical and genetic information [53] or systems for data and text mining and natural language processing for biomedical literature. In any case, it is evident that informatics will play a key role in the translation of all this knowledge that is generated in genomic and molecular research into diagnostic and therapeutic solutions allowing to improve healthcare and the wellbeing of people.

Currently among the major topics of research, as can be seen in the different work programmes of the main research funding agencies (NIH, UE) are:

- Development of models and digital simulations of human physiology and pathology: using computers, researchers aim to build integrated multi-scale models of the body, combining anatomic and functional details. These models link molecular (genes, proteins), and metabolic (pathways, cell assemblies) information to phenotype data. These models can be built by combining two approaches: (1) bottom-up, from molecules to clinical manifestations, or (2) top-down, from clinical manifestations to inner mechanisms. The first approach has been addressed by bioinformaticians and computational biologists whereas the second one has been an objective of medical informaticians.
- Design of new clinical decision support systems for the effective use of organ and disease models, integrated with actual patient data sources (from clinical settings)
- Integration of specific "omic" and clinical patient data to understand the mechanisms of disease and, discover and validate biomarkers of disease in the framework of personalized medicine
- Linking phenotype models and representations to the electronic health record
- Semantic organization, retrieval and interoperability of information (including images and text) from biomedical sources (both local and global) for clinical and health services research and practice.
- To enhance patient and professional biomedical education and continuous training using an "information-based" approach, including visualization and modelling tools, decision support and intelligent Web access to bibliographic and multimedia sources.

The importance that this field has acquired in recent years is shown by the fact that AMIA organised the first Summit on Translational Bioinformatics in San Francisco in March in 2008. Besides this, the NIH is funding a number of initiatives that specifically address relevant aspects of biomedical informatics. Some of them are the seven National Centers for Biomedical Computing, the Biomedical Informatics core of the Clinical and Translational Science Awards and the graduate educational programs in biomedical informatics in 19 universities all around the USA.

5.   Trends and New Challenges for Translational Bioinformatics Beyond Genomic Medicine

5.1 Disease and Health-omics

The definition of medical health is not only the absence of disease at a certain point in time of the person's life but it is also related to the risk of suffering future health problems. To obtain a global view point of the development of diseases the focus should be on both genetic and environmental factors and their interactions, e.g. the Genome, the Phenome and the Envirome [54]. The Genome relates to genetic personal information, the SNPs and mutations present and the interactions between all the genes. The Phenome characterises the phenotypes, including the concrete expression of disease in the individual and lastly the Envirome includes the knowledge about action mechanisms of environmental factors (toxic agents, drugs, food, etc) that might influence the other two. It is the combination of the three what compounds the health risk profile of the individual. Therefore, to advance in this scenario, integrated data environments for assessing the relative contribution of factors (genetic, environmental, phenotypic) that confer an individual a relative risk of developing a disease will be needed. Most probably all this information will be linked with the personal electronic health record as shown in figure 14.

In the next years, translational bioinformatics will have to focus also on the development of causal models that can aggregate and propagate what is known about the factors that confer an individual either relative protection or an increased relative risk of developing a disease, incorporating available evidence from literature and allowing the update of these systems as new data are published almost on a daily basis. These models will have to check for inconsistencies or even contradictions and will be connected with the personal health records and with the systems that collect actual values of these (risk) factors for each individual.

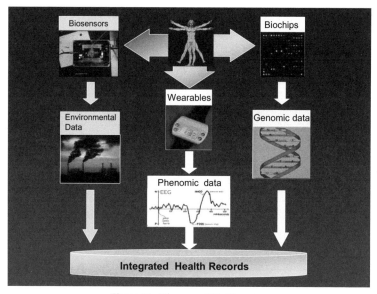

Figure 14: Disease and Health-omics

5.2 Nanomedicine and Regenerative Medicine

Among the most promising trends in medicine for the new future are nanomedicine and regenerative medicine. These two fields pose new challenges for informatics beyond those addressed under the realm of genomic medicine [55].

Nanomedicine is defined as the use of nanoscale tools and components for the diagnosis, prevention and treatment of diseases and for understanding their pathophysiology[22]. Several authors have postulated the need of a new discipline "to

---

[22] European Science Foundation 2005 http://www.esf.org/

organize, standardize, share, compare, analyze and visualize the vast amounts of data being gathered at the nanoscale" what is called Nanoinformatics [56].

Regenerative medicine seeks to develop functional cell, tissue, and organ substitutes to repair, replace or enhance biological function that has been lost due to congenital abnormalities, injury, disease, or aging. (NIH Definition, NIBIB, June 2004). Biomedical informatics can support regenerative medicine through the application of tools and information systems to characterize the molecules involved in selective mechanisms, including growth factors, hormones, cytokines or integrins.

Several requirements come also from the need of improved tools for designing, modelling, and visualizing the new nanomaterials and scaffolds for tissue engineering. Also new databases will have to be designed to store physical, chemical and biological properties of nanotechnology developments [57].

One such new project with a main focus on these new areas is ActionGrid. This project funded by the European Commission (2008-2009) has as its main objectives to analyse synergies between medical informatics, bioinformatics and nanoinformatics, to act as a multiplier of previous outcomes in Grid and biomedical informatics and to combine these results with data from an inventory of Grid/Nano/Bio/Medical methods and services developed by the consortium. This project includes partners form Europe, Latin America, Western Balkans and Northern Africa.

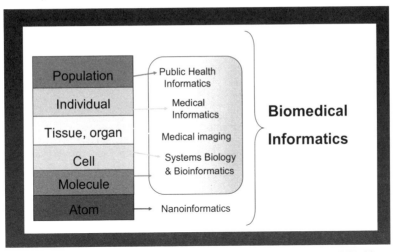

Figure 15: Expanding the Scope of Biomedical Informatics Toward the "nano" World

Figure 15 graphically shows an innovative framework for future biomedical informatics. Just as the genomic revolution brought about the connection of medical informatics with the molecular domain, is the discipline ripe now for exploring the nano world and expanding its scope to the atomic level?

References

[1]   Trifonov EN. "Earliest pages of Bioinformatics". Bioinformatics 2000, vol 16 no 1, pp. 5-9. FREE
       (http://bioinformatics.oxfordjournals.org/cgi/reprint/16/1/5)

[2]   Roberts RJ. "The Early Days of Bioinformatics Publishing". Bioinformatics 2000, vol 16, pp. 2-4. FREE (http://bioinformatics.oxfordjournals.org/cgi/reprint/16/1/2)
[3]   Bairoch A. "Serendipity in Bioinformatics, the Tribulations of a Swiss Bioinformatician through Exciting Times". Bioinformatics 2000, vol 16, pp. 48-64. FREE
[4]   Martín Sanchez F. et al. "Synergy between medical informatics and bioinformatics: facilitating genomic medicine for future health care". Journal of Biomedical Informatics. 2004; 37 (1) pp 30-42.
[5]   Levitt M. "The Birth of Computational Structural Biology". Nat. Structural Biology, 2001. vol 8, 5: 392-393.
[6]   Ponting C.P. Issues in predicting protein function from sequence. Briefings in Bioinformatics, March 2001, 2, 1:19-29 FREE
[7]   International Human Genome Sequencing Consortium. "Initial sequencing and analysis of the human genome". Nature. 15 February 2001, Vol. 409 (#6822) pp 860-921.
[8]   Venter C. et al. "The Sequence of the Human Genome". Science 16 February 2001 Vol. 291 (#5507) Pages 1304-1351
[9]   Gershon, D. "Bioinformatics in a post-genomics age". Nature, 1997. 389: p. 417-418.
[10] Estivill X, Armengol L. "Copy number variants and common disorders: filling the gaps and exploring complexity in genome-wide association studies". PLoS Genet. 2007 Oct; 3(10):1787-99.
[11] Mathew C. "Postgenomic technologies: hunting the genes for common disorders". BMJ 2001. 322. 1031-1034. FREE (http://www.bmj.com/cgi/content/full/322/7293/1031)
[12] Subramanian G, Adams M, Venter C, Broder S. "Implications of the Human Genome for Understanding Human Biology and Medicine". JAMA 2001;286:2996-2307
[13] Dutton G. "Computational genomics: The Medicine of the Future?". Annals of Internal Medicine. 1999, 131, 10 801-804.
[14] Lippert R.; Schwartz R.; Lancia G.; Istrail S. "Algorithmic strategies for the single nucleotide polymorphism haplotype assembly problem". Briefings in Bioinformatics, 2002, 3, 1:23-31. FREE (http://bib.oxfordjournals.org/cgi/reprint/3/1/23)
[15] Dubchak I.; Pachter L. "The computational challenges of applying comparative-based computational methods to whole genomes". Briefings in Bioinformatics, 2002, 3, 1:18-22. FREE (http://bib.oxfordjournals.org/cgi/reprint/3/1/18)
[16] Gingeras, T.R., et al. "Simultaneous genotyping and species identification using hybridization pattern recognition analysis of generic Mycobacterium DNA arrays". Genome Res, 1998. 8(5): p. 435-48. FREE (http://www.genome.org/cgi/content/full/8/5/435)
[17] Sintchenko V, Iredell JR, Gilbert GL. "Pathogen profiling for disease management and surveillance". Nat Rev Microbiol. 2007 Jun;5(6):464-70. Epub 2007 May 8.
[18] Hacia, J.G., et al. "Detection of heterozygous mutations in BRCA1 using high density oligonucleotide arrays and two-colour fluorescence analysis". Nat Genet, 1996. 14(4): p. 441-7.
[19] DeRisi, J., et al. "Use of a cDNA microarray to analyse gene expression patterns in human cancer". Nat Genet, 1996, 14(4): p. 457-60.
[20] Virtanen C, Woodgett J. "Clinical uses of microarrays in cancer research". Methods Mol Med. 2008;141:87-113.
[21] Martín-Sánchez, F., López-Campos, G., "Tecnologías basadas en Biochips. Aplicaciones en diagnóstico clínico e investigación biomédica". II Symposium Internacional sobre Diagnóstico Genético en Medicina. 1998. Madrid. (in Spanish).
[22] Wu T.D. "Large-scale analysis of gene expression profiles". Briefings in Bioinformatics, 2002, 3. 1:7-17 FREE (http://bib.oxfordjournals.org/cgi/reprint/3/1/7)
[23] Maojo V, Martín-Sánchez F, Crespo J, and Billhardt H. "Theory, Abstraction and Design in Medical Informatics. Application to Medical Data Mining". Methods of Information in Medicine 2002, 41:44-50
[24] Dugas M, Weninger F, Merk S, Kohlmann A, Haferlach T. "A generic concept for large-scale microarray analysis dedicated to medical diagnostics". Methods of Information in Medicine . 2006;45(2):146-52.
[25] Gardiner-Garden M.; Littlejohn T.G. "A comparison of microarray databases". Briefings in Bioinformatics, 2001, vol. 2, no. 2:143-158. FREE (http://bib.oxfordjournals.org/cgi/reprint/2/2/143)
[26] Lee K. "Proteomics: a technology-driven and technology-limited discovery science". Trends in Biotech. 2001, 19 6:217-222
[27] Persidis, A., "Proteomics". Nat Biotechnol, 1998. 16(4): p. 393
[28] Greenes, R.A. and Shortliffe, E.H "Medical Informatics: An Emerging Academic Discipline and Institutional Priority". JAMA, (1990): 263, 1114-1120. Boston, MA.
[29] Teufel A, Krupp M, Weinmann A, Galle PR. "Current bioinformatics tools in genomic biomedical research" (Review). Int J Mol Med. 2006 Jun;17(6):967-73.
[30] Altman, R.B. & Koza, J., "A programming course in bioinformatics for computer and information Science students". En L. and Klein Hunter T.E., Ed. Pacific Symposium of Biocomputing´96, Hawaii, 1996. p. 73-84. World Scientific, Singapore. FREE (http://helix-web.stanford.edu/psb96/altman.pdf)

[31] Altman, R. . "The Interactions Between Clinical Informatics and Bioinformatics". JAMIA 2000 Vol 7, 5: 439-443.   FREE
(http://www.pubmedcentral.nih.gov/articlerender.fcgi?tool=pubmed&pubmedid=10984462)
[32] Kohane I, . "Bioinformatics and Clinical Informatics: The Imperative to Collaborate". JAMIA 2000 7, 5: 439-443.   FREE
(http://www.pubmedcentral.nih.gov/articlerender.fcgi?tool=pubmed&pubmedid=10984470)
[33] Miller, P. . "Opportunities at the Intersection of Bioinformatics and Health Informatics". JAMIA 2000 7, 5:431-438.   FREE
(http://www.pubmedcentral.nih.gov/articlerender.fcgi?tool=pubmed&pubmedid=10984461)
[34] Rebholz-Schuhman D, Cameron G, Clark D, van Mulligen E, Coatrieux JL, Del Hoyo Barbolla E, Martin-Sanchez F, Milanesi L, Porro I, Beltrame F, Tollis I, Van der Lei J. "SYMBIOmatics: synergies in Medical Informatics and Bioinformatics--exploring current scientific literature for emerging topics". BMC Bioinformatics. 2007 Mar 8;8 Suppl 1:S18. FREE
[35] Altman, R.B., 1998. "Bioinformatics in support of molecular medicine". En C.G.Chute, Ed., AMIA Annual Symposium, Orlando. p. 53-61.
[36] Martín-Sánchez F., Maojo V., and López-Campos. G. "Integrating genomics into health information systems". Methods of Information in Medicine 2002, 41:25-30
[37] Collins F. S. "Medical and Societal Consequences of the Human Genome Project". 1999 New Eng. J. Med. 341:28-37.
[38] McKusick V. "The anatomy of the Human Genome. A Neo-Vesalian Basis for Medicine in the 21st century". JAMA 2001 286. 18:2289-2295
[39] Rhodes DR, Chinnaiyan AM. "Integrative analysis of the cancer transcriptome". Nat Gen. 2005 June, 37 Supp.: S31-7
[40] Sorlie T, Perou C M, Tibshirani R, Aas T, Geisler S, Johnsen H, et al. . "Gene expression patterns of breast carcinomas distinguish tumor subclasses with clinical implications". Proc. Natl. Acad. Sci. U. S. A. (2001) 98: 10869-10874.
[41] Phillips K, Veenstra D, Oren e, Lee J, Sadee W. "Potential role of Pharmacogenomics in reducing adverse drug reactions". JAMA 2001. 286-18:2270-2279
[42] Housman D. . "Why pharmacogenomics? Why now?" 1998. Nature Biotechnology 16:492
[43] Khoury M. J., HuGENet. "1st Annual Conference on Genetics and Public Health". 1998. http://www.cdc.gov/genetics/publications/abstracts.html
[44] Sander C, "Bioinformatics-Challenges in 2001". Bioinformatics 2001.17:1,p1-2
[45] Bayat A, Bioinformatics. British Medical Journal 2002; 324:p1018-22
[46] Liotta L, Kohn E, Petricoin E. "Clinical proteomics. Personalised molecular medicine". JAMA. 2001. 286:18 2211-2214
[47] Billhardt, H., J. Crespo, V. Maojo, F. Martín, and J.L. Maté. ."Unifying Heterogeneous Medical Databases". In "Medical Data Analysis". 2001. Lecture Notes in Computer Science 2199: 54-61, edited by J. Crespo, J., V. Maojo and F. Martín. Springer Verlag: Heidelberg
[48] Del Fiol G, Williams MS, Maram N, Rocha RA, Wood GM, Mitchell JA. "Integrating genetic information resources with an HER". AMIA Annu Symp Proc. 2006:904.
[49] Sikorski, R.& Peters, R., "Genomic Medicine, internet resources for medical genetics". JAMA 1997. 278(15): p.1212-1213
[50] Dias GS, Oliveira JL, Vicente J, Martin-Sanchez F. "Integrating medical and genomic data: a successful example for rare diseases". Stud Health Technol Inform. 2006;124:125-30.
[51] Collins F. S, 2001. "Genetics moves into the medical mainstream". JAMA 2001, 286.18:2322-2324
[52] Rindfleisch TC, Brutlag DL. 1998 "Directions for clinical research and genomic research into the next decade: implications for informatics". J. Am. Med. Inform. Assoc. 5(5):404-11
[53] Maojo V, Martin-Sanchez F. "Bioinformatics: towards new directions for public health". Methods Inf Med. 2004;43(3):208-14.
[54] Martín Sánchez F "Bioinformática" in Belmonte et at (Eds). Manual de Informática Médica. Editorial Menarini 2003 (in Spanish).
[55] Martín-Sanchez F, López-Alonso V, Hermosilla-Gimeno I and Lopez-Campos G. "A primer in knowledge management for Nanoinformatics in Medicine". (Accepted as oral communication in the 12th International Conference on Knowledge-Based and Intelligent Information & Engineering Systems. KES 2008. Zagreb, Croatia. September 2008.
[56] Ruping K.and Sherman B.W. "Nanoinformatics: Emerging Computational Tools in Nano-scale Research". In Nanotech 2004: Technical Proceedings of the 2004 NSTI Nanotechnology Conference and Trade Show, Volume 3.
[57] Schmidt KF. "Nanofrontiers: Visions for the future of Nanotechnology". 2007. Woodrow Wilson International Center for Scholars. Project on Emerging Nanotechnologies.

Review questions

1. Summarize, completing the following table the most important bioinformatics resources referred in the chapter:

	Databases	Programs
Molecular genetics		
Human Genome Project		
Post-genomic research		
Genomic Medicine		

2. Identify three possible applications of classical bioinformatics in medicine
3. List all the laboratory techniques that are generating molecular data and that could be used in medical practice
4. Describe three different health information systems that could be affected by the introduction of molecular information from patients
5. Discuss the main similarities and differences between systems biology and biomedical informatics

Further reading and information

Research centres

- NCBI – National Center for Biotechnology Information – http://www.ncbi.nlm.nih.gov
- EBI – European Bioinformatics Institute, http://www.ebi.ac.uk
- SIB - Swiss Institute of Bioinformatics, http://www.isb-sib.ch/
- Sanger Centre, http://www.sanger.ac.uk/
- Infobiogen, http://www.infobiogen.fr/

Books

1. Baldi P, Brunak S. Bioinformatics. 2nd ed. MIT Press, 2001. (Adaptive computation and machine learning series.)
2. Baxevanis AD, Ouellette BFF. Bioinformatics: a practical guide to the analysis of genes and proteins. 2nd ed. John Wiley and Sons, 2001.
3. Bishop, M. (Ed.). 1998. Guide to Human Genome Computing. 2th ed. San Diego : Academic Press.
4. Gibas C. and Jambeck P. Developing Bioinformatics Computer Skills. 2001. O'Reilly.
5. Higgins D, Taylor W. Bioinformatics. Oxford University Press, 2000. (Practical approach series.)
6. Lengauer T (Ed). Bioinformatics. Wiley-VCH Series, 2001. (Methods and principles in medicinal chemistry series.)
7. Mount DW. Bioinformatics: sequence and genome analysis. Cold Spring Harbor Laboratory Press, 2004.
8. Shortliffe, E.H. and Cimino J.J. (Eds). 2006. Biomedical Informatics: Computer Applications in Health Care and Biomedicine (Health Informatics) 3rd Edition. Springer Science
9. Coiera E., Guide to Health Informatics, Arnold Publication, London, (2003)
10. Campbell A.M and Heyer L.J. 2006. Discovering Genomics, Proteomics and Bioinformatics (2nd Edition) (The Genetics Place Series Published jointly by Cold Spring Harbor Laboratory Press and Benjamin Cummings. (ISBN 0-8053-8219-4)
11. Barnes M.R. (Ed). Bioinformatics for Geneticists: A Bioinformatics Primer for the Analysis of Genetic Data. Wiley & Sons Ltd. 2007 (reprinted with corrections April 2008)
12. Hoyt R. MD, Sutton M. PhD, and Yoshihashi A. MD Medical Informatics: Practical Guide for the Healthcare Professional 2007

13. Hu H. and Liebman M. <u>Biomedical Informatics in Translational Research</u> 2008. Artech House, Incorporated

Journals

- Bioinformatics - <u>http://bioinformatics.oupjournals.org/</u>
- Briefings in Bioinformatics - <u>http://www.henrystewart.co.uk/journals/bib/</u>
- Journal of Computational Biology - <u>http://www.liebertpub.com/CMB</u>
- In Silico Biology - <u>http://www.bioinfo.de/isb/</u>
- Bioinform - <u>http://www.bioinform.com/index.htm</u>
- Bioinformatics World - <u>http://www.bioinformaticsworld.info/</u>
- Methods of Information in Medicine - <u>http://www.schattauer.de/index.php?id=704&L=1</u>
- Journal of Biomedical Informatics - <u>http://www.elsevier.com/wps/find/journaldescription.cws_home/622857/description#description</u>
- Journal of the American Medical Informatics Association - http://www.jamia.org/
- BMC Bioinformatics - <u>http://www.biomedcentral.com/bmcbioinformatics/</u>

Conference Proceedings

- PSB – Pacific Symposium on Biocomputing , 2007 Edition January 3-7, Maui, Hawaii <u>http://psb.stanford.edu/psb07/</u>
- RECOMB – Research in Computational Biology , 2007 Edition, April 21-25; San Francisco, CA, USA <u>http://www.recomb2007.com/</u>
- Annual International Conference on Intelligent Systems for Molecular Biology (ISMB) & European Conference on Computational Biology (ECCB) , 2007 Edition, July 21-25, Viena, Austria <u>http://www.iscb.org/ismbeccb2007/</u>
- Summit on Translational Bioinformatics, 2008 Edition, March 10-12; San Francisco, CA, USA <u>http://www.amia.org/meetings/stb08/</u>
- MEDINFO, 2007 Edition, August 19 -24 ; Brisbane, Australia – IOS Press, Amsterdam
- American Medical Informatics Association, 2007 Edition, November 10-14; Chicago, IL, USA <u>http://www.amia.org/meetings/f07/</u>
- MIE 08 – Medical Informatics in Europe, 2008 Edition . May 25-29. Goteborg, Sweden <u>http://www.sfmi.org/home/index.asp?sid=63&mid=1</u>

Scientific societies

- ISCB – International Society for Computational Biology, <u>http://iscb.org/</u>
- IMIA – International Medical Informatics Association - http://www.imia.org
- AMIA - American Medical Informatics Association - http://www.amia.org
- EFMI – European Federation of Medical Informatics – http://www.efmi.org

Section 4

Supporting Health Care Service Delivery Management

Health Informatics
E.J.S. Hovenga et al. (Eds.)
IOS Press, 2010
© 2010 The authors and IOS Press. All rights reserved.
doi:10.3233/978-1-60750-476-4-341

25. Research, Forensics, Public Health, Injury Prevention and Policy Development

David RANSON[1] BmedSci, BZM, BS, LLB, MRCPath, FRCPA, DMJ(Path)
Deputy Director, Victorian Institute of Forensic Medicine, Clinical Associate Professor, Department of Forensic Medicine, Monash University, Director, National Coroners Information System, Melbourne, Australia

Abstract. This chapter gives an educational overview of:

- Management implications of information technology in research, public health and policy development
- Modern developments in death investigation, injury prevention and disaster management
- The dangers of applying global analysis to individual health care situations and vice versa
- Mechanisms that can be used to identify diffuse disaster in global and individual medical practice
- The impact of informatics in areas of medical services which rely upon observational studies rather than validated clinical trials to develop knowledge bases
- A paradigm shift in health care policy towards client driven services and the implications for medical informatics

Keywords. Medical Informatics, Risk Management, Health Policy, Health Care Systems, Safety, Health Care Quality, Database, Evidence Based Practice, Public Health Informatics, Epidemiology, Population, Telemedicine

Introduction

Today the health care sector is increasingly reliant on data to inform policy development, clinical audit, operational management and individual patient care provision. Global network services are increasingly available to the medical services sector and are critical to the success of modern health service provision. With current reliance on data and communications networks come issues surrounding the control and access to such data. In particular data on health care outcomes is increasingly being seen as something that should be available to patients and prospective patients as well as health care service providers and policymakers. This raises significant health care planning issues as well as legal issues touching as it does on matters relating to privacy and private versus public rights.

The management implications of information technology in research, public health and policy development are identified in this chapter with particular reference

---

[1] Corresponding Author: davidr@vifm.org

to modern developments in death investigation, injury prevention and disaster management. The dangers of applying global analysis to individual health care situations and vice versa are examined and the mechanisms that can be used to identify diffuse disaster in global and individual medical practice are explored. Modern trends in death and injury prevention are used as a model to demonstrate the impact of informatics in areas of medical services which rely upon observational studies rather than validated clinical trials to develop knowledge bases. The chapter concludes by noting that a paradigm shift in health care policy towards client driven services has occurred. The implications for medical informatics of this change are briefly discussed.

The avenues for research in medicine are almost unlimited as is the ability of medical data sets to grow in size. On an individual case basis the introduction of CT, MRI and other radiological scans as well as electrocardiographical data, clinical photographs and scans of tissue biopsies have vastly increased data storage requirements for an individual patient care record. While data storage technology has for the most part kept up with these developments when it comes to record keeping and clinical logs the expansion of the data set has had significant impact on the data communications infrastructure that is required for this data to be available for research. There is little doubt that information technology has made a major impact in the research carried out in many of the medical discipline areas.

The field of public health, injury prevention and related areas of health policy formation has benefited very greatly from the rapid developments that have been made in the area of health informatics. Indeed medical epidemiology as a specialist area probably could not have developed the way it has in recent years were it not for the rapid advancements made in the field of medical informatics at a technical and organizational level. It must be remembered, however, that advances in technology and information theory do not of themselves lead to changes to medical research or practice. It is the acceptance by medical professionals of such new technology and the integration of new information handling practices into medical research and practice that has resulted in the advances we have seen in the fields of public health, medical epidemiology and health policy development [1].

It could not be said that developments in information technology have been the underlying stimulus for the development of new directions in health policy. Whilst the field of public health and health policy formation is highly reliant upon information technology much of the drive to advance these areas has come from the changing economic structure of health care. The economic pressures now placed on health care resources allocation and national and international health care budgets have been considerable. The upward spiral of health care costs seems inevitable. This appears to have prompted an almost frantic drive towards rationalization of health resources which in turn has stimulated many of the advances in information systems related to health care [2].

The insatiable demand for health care information on the part of policy makers now faced with the economic reality of rising health care costs and effective reductions in health care budgets has artificially stimulated the field of health informatics. In layman's terms this scenario might be described as the field of health informatics having had a sudden rush of blood to the head. The explosion of ideas, network information systems, hardware and software platforms that resulted was both productive and destructive. Productive, in that new information systems were appearing almost every week but destructive, in that attempts to develop health informatics standards came too late. In many cases by the time the standards were published the health information field had moved ahead and developed in a way that made the new standard obsolete. This was particularly seen with regard to privacy and security of electronic data and was complicated by the integration of commercial systems for medical service billing into health care information streams. Finally we are beginning to achieve a level of integration between the emerging standards and the technology itself which is permitting appropriate security provisions to be imposed that protect patients, individuals providing health care and health care service organizations.

Today governments recognize that the provision of health care services to the community cannot be seen as an isolated health service function. Efficient total health care provision is reliant upon integration with other core government services. For example data on legal intervention orders in domestic violence from the courts could be integrated with health care information from emergency department data on intentional injury due to interpersonal violence. Such data integration between justice systems and health care service providers could provide health policy units with information on service need for health care planning and the courts with similar legal services data to assist with planning of court time and identification of the need for legislative reform. Some aspects of this information in turn may also be useful for social services agencies, volunteer support groups and emergency response agencies such as the police and ambulance services. However, as access to such highly personal data extends into these non medical areas and is integrated with other governmental, social and community data sets the need for sophisticated and secure systems for data interchange becomes a high priority. Indeed health informatics providers at a technical information service level are now required to provide varied levels of access for different classes of users across a large number of government and private agencies.

Medical health care providers have in the past been largely immune to the issues of cost efficiency at commercial level. Health care standards were set by professional medical bodies with little or no interest in the economic consequences of the health care policies. This attitude amongst health care professionals has almost completely died out. It is now clear to all that resources are limited and that governments will allow economic factors to have a significant role in shaping their health care policy. Like it or not, health care providers are having to accept the fact that health policy is being determined by individuals from the fields of business and economics whose attitudes to health care outcomes, resource allocation and medical effectiveness may be very different to that traditionally found in health care professionals [3].

The health power equilibrium has changed. If health care workers are to continue to play a part in health policy development they need to be empowered with the skills in data analysis in order for their voices to be heard amongst national and international policy makers. The development of health informatics as a specialty for health care professionals is at last providing them with a new role as stake holders in health care planning. In this chapter we will look at a few examples of areas in which health care priorities and goals are being influenced by the growing resource to be found in health informatics with particular reference to injury prevention and the information that can be gathered and used from death investigation.

1.   Communication and Data Processing

When considering some of the technologies involved in health informatics it is important to recognise the distinction between information networks (communication) and the technologies involved in data processing. Health informatics in its broadest sense involves a very wide range of information technology including data processing, communication, networking and telecommunication. Indeed today telemedicine is one of the new emerging fields of health informatics and one which has the capacity to significantly alter the delivery of health care, particularly in rural areas and communities that are geographically isolated. A recent study [4] predicted that in the United States of America 28 billion dollars could be saved in health care costs through the efficient use of telecommunications in the movement of patient management information. This study also identified that health care administrative costs could be reduced by 6.8 billion dollars through the use of modern electronic communications and data processing technologies.

Recognition of the importance of electronic communications and the value of networking has resulted in a number of initiatives around the world. In Australia the development of the Health Communications Network is a sign of the significance that is placed on networking by health care policy makers. Medical information networks today comprise systems with advanced developments of central hubs and main data trunk lines. Most of our major medical and health care institutions are already connected electronically and developments in the links between these central sites have lead to advances in the complexity and quality of the electronic data that can be communicated. Today complex medical procedures and clinical consultations can be supervised, and sometimes conducted over teleconference links.

Increasingly health care education services are being delivered via distance education and clinical skills are being gained through teleconference-based clinical consultations as well as 'face to face' consultations. These developments increase the opportunities for professional development of health-care workers and provide health service policy makers with an opportunity to improve the efficiency of their workforce for a far lower cost. Although telemedicine offers considerable advantages to health-care practice allowing patients to access a far wider range of specialists and allowing specialists to provide expert consultation services over a large geographical area, these initiatives still raise significant problems.

1.1 Telemedicine – Problems to be Resolved

Five major problems remain to be solved before telemedicine and the widespread use of such health care information networks becomes a universal reality.

The first of these is the need for education and training of health care professionals. A large commitment to training is required by health care institutions before these modern technologies become truly effective in the work place.   In addition health-care professionals themselves need to become clinically comfortable with engaging in medical practice by this non-traditional method. Medical practitioners providing such services need to be assured that the health care support staff, present with the patient at a remote location, are appropriately skilled and trained and aware of the limitations of telemedicine consultations.   Similarly the medical specialist themselves need to be made aware of the limitations and advantages of practicing in this manner. This change is more than an appreciation and understanding of the different requirements for a teleconference consultation. It involves a major cultural shift for health care workers that is probably best achieved in the long term by the introduction of these skill sets in undergraduate programs.

The second major problem to be overcome is that whilst the major institutions are well networked electronically and increasingly primary health care providers have access to local health care and government based information networks many of their patients are still relatively remote from health care information and communication systems. In the past this "last mile of wire" was a significant factor limiting the impact of medical informatics in primary health care and it is still a significant problem in remote communities and in underdeveloped countries. It is almost certainly the most important mile as far as electronic communication and networking in health care is concerned [5] but the paradigm has shifted in the developed world so that today it is the link with patients that is limited rather than the link between primary health care providers and the broader health-care sector.

The third major problem to be overcome relates to communication standards and electronic data interchange standards in health informatics. Today standards are increasingly being developed but are often implemented differently in particular countries. The absence of commonality in data dictionaries used in the healthcare sector is a significant impediment to global research. Whilst standards such as the ICD10 coding systems go much of the way to solving this issue there is always a lag between the development of a new standard and its global acceptance and implementation. As commented before, it is essential that technology and standards develop in concert and until such a balance is achieved the absence of implemented international standards will remain a significant impediment to the establishment of worldwide health care related communications.

The fourth problem in health communications that has the capacity to significantly impair the development of research and health care policy is the community and social attitudes to telemedicine and health care networking. In particular issues in relation to medical ethics with respect to privacy and confidentiality must be addressed and the clients of the healthcare sector need to become familiar and comfortable with using this technology. The irony is that it is the young in our community who are most familiar with modern communications and information technology and yet they are the sector in our community which makes relatively little use of health-care services. In contrast it is the rapidly expanding older population in our community who are perhaps less familiar with such technology who make the greatest demands on our health-care system and could arguably benefit the most from skill acquisition in the use of health care related communications and associated electronic resources.

Finally there are significant legal impediments to the expanding use of telemedicine that are associated with issues relating to medical registration and civil and criminal liability in medical practice. Telemedicine is not a new aspect of medical practice. Traditionally, communication between patients and doctors about diagnosis and provision of care has taken place through a number of media that in the past have included letters, telegrams, telephone and radio. In Australia perhaps the best-known example of telemedicine was, and still is, provided via radio telephony links with the Royal Flying Doctor Service. From a legal perspective telemedicine services confined to, and being provided solely within, a single state or local legal jurisdiction can be easily supported by the local administration making minor changes to their legislation.

However, where telemedicine services cross national, state and legal jurisdictional boundaries, problems can arise. "Out-of-hours" care provides a good example of the types of problems that can arise. In the practice of radiology, the move towards digital systems has facilitated radiologists being able to provide remote diagnostic services from their homes or from a nearby clinic, freeing them of the requirement to be colocated in the same hospital as the patient. However, the need for 24-hour diagnostic support raises issues regarding maintenance of high quality service delivery, in particular with regard to issues such as fatigue in medical staff. The opportunity for the reporting radiologist to work in a different world time zone has the potential to resolve some of these difficulties. For example, a radiology service in Australia may send a number of its specialist staff to Europe where they can review the digital images and so provide the Australian "out-of-hours" night-time reporting service during European daylight hours. Similar arrangements can be made with regard to other medical services although diagnostic reporting services such as pathology and radiology particularly lend themselves to this type of arrangement. The registration and regulation of medical practitioners in these arrangements can be problematic. Robertson, [6] in an article produced for the American Medical Association website, reviewed aspects of the legislative changes to medical licensing or registration in the United States implicit in these developments and commented:

"Until recently, a physician could provide an opinion or interpretation to a physician in another state who had primary patient care responsibility, and this practice was not regarded as practicing out of his/her state. Today, however, the out-of-state practice of medicine without a license is prohibited, whether the physician is treating the patient in person or from a distant location. In this day and age, a physician is considered to be practicing medicine in the state where the patient is located and is subject to that state's laws regarding medical practice, which typically means a license in that particular state is necessary. Thus, state boards have denied requests from out-of-state psychiatrists, for example, to conduct therapy with their patients located in another state via telephone or videoconferencing. Imprecise definitions regarding just what is "out-of-state" medicine (eg phone calls from patients who live in one state, but who seek care from an adjacent state, across a state line for care) also abound. Some states consider all out-of-state practice to be telemedicine, whether it utilizes phone calls, e-mail or online discussions. Even definitions from organizations such as the American Medical Informatics Association, the United States Department of Commerce, and various state and specialty medical societies vary considerably. Telemedicine in particular has crystallized the tension between the states' role in protecting patients from incompetent physicians and protecting in-state physicians from out-of-state competition, and the desirability of ensuring patients' access to the highest quality medical advice and treatment possible, wherever located."

Today cost factors associated with the provision of medical services have led to state and private health services often being outsourced to private providers based outside the jurisdiction. In Singapore, for example some radiology services are provided by medical practitioners based in India. The digital nature of radiology practice today facilitates such arrangements which are far less common in other diagnostic service areas such as pathology. Traditionally pathologists still send microscope slides for diagnostic opinions to colleagues via postal services. However, as the technology associated with the digitisation and communication of image data improves, we can expect to see a far wider use of diagnostic telemedicine in pathology. This issue has become significant for many of the craft groups within the medical profession who are increasingly coming to grips with these changes to their traditional medical practice for example The Royal College of Pathologists of the United Kingdom has issued specific guidance in the form of codes of practice for remote diagnostics [7].

The rapid development of telemedicine and, indeed, the requirement for medical services to be provided across State and national boundaries on economic and medical manpower grounds, mean that the traditional models for licensing and registration of medical practitioners may need to be substantially modified. At the same time, in the absence of agreed international standards in medical training that could be used to accredit the skills of a doctor for cross registration purposes seems to necessitate the continued existence of the somewhat muddled situation of variable registration rules being applied to medical practitioners who use telemedicine to provide health care services across State and national borders.

It must be said that medical ethicists and legal professionals have been slow to come to grips with modern information technology and the implication that it has for the regulation and education of medical practitioners. Again it is essential that these aspects of the implementation of new technology are integrated with the technical development of health communications networks for such systems to be accepted by the community at large

2.   For Whom the Bell Tolls

The ability of policy makers to formulate health policy is intricately bound to the health care information service which provides them with the data they need. It has to be remembered, however, that the source of such health data ultimately comes from the grass roots level of health care. As we have already noted this is the very area which is least developed and prepared with regard to information systems. Despite this, health care workers in the field recognise the importance of information for health care planning. Whilst the task of data collection is onerous, there is now an increased understanding of the need for information in order that health services might be improved.

Where health interacts with non-health related agencies recognition of the importance of interchange of core information is less well recognized. This network disconnection can be seen particularly in the area of mortality data and death investigation. In many cases the individuals with access to this information do not come primarily from the health care field but instead from the legal and administrative organs of government. For health care planning to be truly effective health policy makers must be informed and provided with data from both the health care community and the associated legal and administrative services that impact upon health. All death investigation takes place in a medical, scientific, administrative and legal environment that is specific to that type of community and legal jurisdiction within which the death occurred.

The differences among jurisdictions arise from a variety of interrelated factors including social, religious, political and legal influences, as well as the development of the medical profession and its specialties. At the most mechanical level, records are generated and retained about who has died. A cause of death is assigned within a registry office inside government bureaucracy, generally by recording on a death register the cause of death given in the report or certificate of the treating doctor. The maintenance of a death register and a birth register has important social implications. A community needs to know information regarding those who make up its population. From a practical perspective this is needed in order to ensure that community services are appropriate to the size and make up of the population. However, at a deeper level our concerns about threats to our safety generate a desire to find out more about deaths that occur in our community and to understand their causes so that we can feel less threatened. Community and personal grief involve important emotions that can have deep effects on the functioning of individuals, families and in some cases the whole community. In this environment a society's ability to independently investigate critical deaths from a perspective that is focused beyond that of any individual professional group such as scientists, the medical profession or the police is important.

The legal profession and the medical profession have at their roots a work practice that is related to the individual handling of cases so that work is carried out on a case by case basis dealing with each case as an isolated event. For many years, however, the medical profession in particular has reaped the benefits, in terms of research into the understanding of disease and health care planning, of the analysis of groups of cases that show similar features. Not only do such group analyses lead to increased understanding of disease processes, therapeutics and health care but they increase the efficiency in which medical professionals can undertake their work. The growth in medical informatics has facilitated the rapid development of such research. Such analysis of groups or collections of like cases is rare within legal systems including death investigation systems such as coroners or medical examiner systems. Yet if we are to learn from those defects in society that result in death and injury we need to be continually reminded of the risks and dangers in the community. Similarly those who have the responsibility and power to make our society safer including health care policy makers need to be reminded and continually charged with that duty and alerted to the information on community risks and hazards that is available from the organizational areas outside the health care sector.

The development of health care policy and health care plans for prevention of disease and injury remains at the forefront of public health. Many of the initiatives and directions taken to improve health and safety fall within the framework of community education. There are many clinicians, pathologists, epidemiologists and indeed lawyers who see this educational and preventative role as one of the most important goals of any health care information system. The reality, however, is that at the grass roots level those charged with the legal investigation of death and injury are not integrated with the health care information system. If each injury and death is to play a part in moulding and shaping public health policy leading to a healthier and safer community the information revealed by such tragedies has to be communicated and analysed by policy makers. The absence of such data communication makes us all vulnerable. As Donne[2] said "Ask not for whom the bell tolls, it tolls for thee".

---

[2] John Donne 17th Century author of a poem (Meditation 17) - http://www.online-literature.com/donne/409/

3.   Disaster and Diffuse Disaster

In examining the ways in which health informatics resources can contribute to public health and policy development it is useful to consider the notion of diffuse disaster. In a mass disaster the entire society including its medical, political and administrative officials is alerted. This in turn stimulates sympathy, concern and practical action in the form of response activities designed to deal with the injured, the loss of life and destruction of community and property. Inevitably in the case of mass disasters there is a post disaster investigation process that examines the cause and the response to the disaster. In addition detailed investigations are directed to determine processes and mechanisms to prevent the hazardous situation occurring again. Essentially it is the manner in which the extent of the disaster is communicated to the public and the response agencies that determines the nature of the eventual investigation and preventative processes.

The diffuse disaster is very different Deaths, injury and disease are with us every day. They form part of our unconscious acceptance of life in our community. Not all of us will experience deaths or severe injury, not all of us are informed of death or serious injury, not all of us are aware of the suffering deaths or injuries cause but nonetheless such morbidity and mortality is present throughout our community. It is the wide temporal and geographical distribution of these events that prevents them being perceived by the community as a disaster. Yet if one was to view the incidence and prevalence of such morbidity and mortality with the temporal and geographical factors removed they would indeed form a true mass disaster. For example if one-tenth of the murders in Australia were to occur at a single place at a single point in time from the actions of a single person there would be a national outcry yet murders and other forms of violence and non accidental injuries occur throughout our community all year round. As a result of this failure to identify the collective nature of such diffuse disasters, their investigation is impeded and their significance is lost on the community. As a result the drive from the community for action in relation to the prevention of such deaths or injuries never occurs.

The above issue is easy to comprehend when one examines death, non-accidental and accidental injury. However, the concept of the diffuse disaster can also be found in the area in natural disease. The concept of the diffuse epidemic is well recognized and much medical research today involves the identification of similar or like cases of disease. Such pattern based disease analysis forms one of the cornerstones of medical epidemiology. However, our ability to identify patterns and trends in disease in the community is strictly limited by the quality and quantity of the data that are obtained and analysed. A disease process may be so rare that only a single case occurs in the world each year. Yet if we have one hundred years' worth of data a pattern and trend might be identifiable. The information gained on the diseases aetiology and pathogenesis might have implications for a number of co-related disease processes whose origin continues to remain obscure.

4. Examples of Health Information Influencing Research, Public Health and Health Policy Development.

4.1 Infectious Diseases

Possibly the best example of the way in which health information has influenced research, public health and health policy development can be seen in relation to communicable diseases. Indeed the very foundations of medical epidemiology come from research that led to an understanding of the infectious nature and pathogenesis of communicable diseases. The outstanding success of organizations such as the Center for Diseases Control in Atlanta and the various Departments of Epidemiology, Community Medicine and Social and Preventative Medicine worldwide have established the place of medical epidemiology and statistics in medical science. Information gathering and data processing has certainly been one of the major tools employed in these disciplines. In recent years the rapid expansion in health informatics together with network and communications services has led to a transformation in communicable disease surveillance including the identification of infectious hazards. In 1984 an information system was established in France to provide for national surveillance of communicable diseases [8]. This information system allowed both data entry and information retrieval as well as interpersonal communications. The backbone of the system was a relational database and a telephone dial-up network to a Videotext server provided the access to the system. This network was established by the National Department of Health and the National Institute of Health and Medical Research in France and was based on the belief that

> "improving the quality, adequacy and rapidity of response of public health systems depends mainly on the ability to refine the processes implemented to collect, analyse and distribute needed information and reinforce interpersonal communication between different partners."

It should not be thought that the use of information and communication networks solves all problems with regard to the notification of infectious diseases. Studies from the Center for Diseases Control in Atlanta have demonstrated [9] that delays occur even when data is reported via the National Electronic Telecommunications Systems Surveillance in the United States. These delays were recognized to occur across a very wide geographical area and reinforce the difficulty for health care planning when there is little standardization between the organizations that provide the basic data. It is clear that the difficulties in timeliness of data on national electronic networks does not relate to the complexity of the technology employed nor to the network structure. Instead the major difficulties are experienced at the grass roots level with the data providers. Education of staff and standardization of human organizational procedures involved in the provision of primary data sources is an essential step to take in ensuring the success of these national networks.

4.2 Quality Assurance

Current economic models of health care delivery are looking more and more towards output measurement for identifying successful health programs and efficient health care services. Quality assurance and control are two essential elements in ensuring that health care provision is both effective as well as efficient. Whilst quality assurance systems can be found at all levels within the health care system they are most clearly identifiable within a hospital and laboratory environment.

Hospital information systems have in the past tended to concentrate upon the areas of financial management and patient administration. In recent years, however, there has been increased recognition that hospital based information systems have a role to play in health care quality assurance [10]. An important factor in these quality assurance systems is that if data are collected from the global health environment of a hospital it is possible to identify not only quality levels of individual items of health service but also information relating to total patient outcome. This whilst highly desirable in an economic and health policy sense carries with it a number of potential dangers if such global data taken alone is used to influence individual patient based health care practice. An example of this issue can be seen in the situation that arose in the Ford Pinto case.

Here a situation arose in relation to vehicle manufacture. The company identified that a minor increase in the cost of the vehicle would have led to increased safety for the occupants. Whilst this would add a very small amount to the cost of each car it amounted to a substantial overall sum for the manufacturer. An individual purchaser of a car may have been prepared to pay the small increased cost of the modification had they known of the risks of not having the modification to the vehicle. The manufacturer would not have seen this small purchase cost factor as they saw the cost in terms of the millions of dollars of additional manufacturing costs. In the final event, however, the manufacturer when looking at global costs decided not to proceed with the modification. Subsequently successful legal action was taken against the manufacturer by injured parties demonstrating the danger of taking this global cost saving approach.

Quality assurance issues in medical informatics also overlaps with the field of infectious diseases particularly in the area of infection control and antibiotic therapy [11]. Health informatics systems have much to offer in the area of monitoring of adverse drug reactions within hospital audit systems, patient outcome measures and planning of new or reviewed health care systems. Assessing the quality of health care is now a mandatory task in almost all major health systems. The financial limitations placed on the growth of the health care industry in modern times makes the need for information, that can be used for health care planning, all the more intense.

4.3 Death Investigation

Death Investigation takes place at many levels. Death investigation processes can be seen at their simplest level in the case where a medical practitioner assesses the death of their patient and signs a death certificate. In a hospital setting this same process can occur but with the added facet of a hospital autopsy and/or a clinicopathological audit process. Where formal external state based investigations are performed it is the coroner's or medical examiner's systems that bear the brunt of the detailed death investigation.

The legal process of such investigation processes, albeit carried out by medical practitioners, has in the past resulted in cases being investigated on a case by case basis with little concern given to the patterns of injury that might be identified by a systematic analytical approach to death investigation. The analysis of collections of like cases is rare within coroners' systems and yet if we are to learn from those defects in society that result in death we need to be continually reminded of the risks and dangers around us. On a random case by case basis this is extremely difficult for a coroner's system to identify potentially significant fatal hazards in our society and yet at the same time coroners and their supporting investigatory medical agencies are in a position of having access to a wide body of information relating to such groups of death. It is of particular interest that the coroners' and medical examiners' systems have within them the means to make public the issues and factors that have contributed to the death. While several countries today are attempting to collate and analyse national data from death investigation systems there is no coherent system available anywhere in the world.

Coronial systems were originally created to gain wealth for the crown. Despite this their potential use as agents for the identification of preventable hazards in society has been long recognized. In 1907 William Brend [12 p.140] wrote that:

"the value of the (Coroners) statistics is diminished by the absence of coordination ...... hence we have the anomaly that while a full enquiry is conducted into deaths from violent and unnatural causes, practically no subsequent use is made of the information for public health purposes"

In 1915 the same author [13] wrote

" .... the prevention of death is not now regarded as the main purpose to be served by inquest enquiry becomes of relatively little value."

In Australia today the role of the Coroner in the prevention of deaths is well recognized and medical informatics including data analysis, networking and communication systems is playing an increasing part in bringing together death and injury data for the benefit of the community. The National Injury Surveillance Unit is actively pursuing information system networking to allow investigatory agencies to analyse group death and injury data. National databases are becoming established with regard to particular health problems and Australia has the world's only national sudden infant death database which is available to researchers in the fields of medical epidemiology and basic medical science.

In 1991 the Australian Royal Commission into Aboriginal Deaths in Custody [14 para 4.7.4] stated that:

"moreover, in human terms, thoroughly conducted coronial enquiries hold the potential to identify systemic failures in custodial practices and procedures which may, if acted on, prevent future deaths in similar circumstances. In the final analysis adequate post-death investigations have the potential to save lives."

The construction of a national coroners database is now underway in Australia. Recent case studies in Victoria have demonstrated the success of such an approach.

In the three year period between 1987 and 1990, 20 fork lift related deaths occurred in Victoria. These deaths represented a significant increase over the 22 such deaths that had occurred in the previous ten years. Group analysis of these cases by the coronial systems led to identification of a number of risk factors resulting in these fatalities. Fork lift operation and design factors associated with fatal hazards were identified and a number of recommendations were made. The implementation of these recommendations have resulted in a significant reduction in such fatalities [15].

Analysis of deaths related to Methadone overdosage in 1989 in Victoria revealed a sudden and unexpected increase in fatalities amongst intravenous drug addicts who had just commenced a Methadone maintenance program. As a result of the identification of these, recommendations were made regarding the assessment of drug dependent persons admitted to the program. Medical education and training regarding drug addiction treatment programs was increased and deaths from Methadone toxicity were substantially reduced [16].

The difficulties of data collection and analysis in the area of death investigation are considerable. Countries with national death investigation systems are at a considerable advantage in having a uniform and consistent data source. The reality, however, is that legal death investigation systems are most commonly based on local jurisdictions which operate independently from each other. In the United States there are over 2,000 separate death investigation jurisdictions, each operating essentially independently of the other. Such a situation makes the task of integrating information systems almost insurmountable. The Center for Diseases Control in Atlanta has been working with the national association of medical examiners to resolve this problem. Today their stated goals [17[p.88]] are:

"(a) to obtain more timely, accurate and complete information on sudden unexpected deaths;

(b) to better understand the causes of those deaths; and

(c) to reduce the mortality from those causes that are amenable to public health intervention"

The development in Australia of the National Coroners Information System is perhaps the world's first comprehensive national database of coronial information. It contains data including all demographic information on each death reported to coroner throughout Australia and includes coronial findings and verdicts, specialist medical and toxicology reports, and other details regarding the results of specialist investigations. Operating through the medium of secure Internet database access the system has attracted international interest (from New Zealand, England and Canada).

Currently some 200,000 coroners' death investigations are contained within the National Coroners Information System. There are over 40 authorised organisations which have access to the system (equating to approximately 120 third party users), with around 250 death investigation users also registered to access the data (coroners, forensic scientists, pathologists, coroners police, researchers).

The most compelling justification for the existence of the coronial jurisdiction is its ability to contribute to the prevention of injury and death. This is achieved by identification of fatal hazards and risk factors combined with the making of recommendations to reduce the risk of injury and death. In this way, coroners' findings assist in developing public policy in areas such as product safety, health, transport, and workplace safety. They can also assist in the investigation of criminal offences. The National Coroners Information System enables the rapid identification of up to date information on deaths investigated by the coroners' jurisdictions. In broad terms the benefits of the National Coroners Information System in Australia not only include better information on deaths but also improvements in the operation of the coroners jurisdiction itself. The National Coroners Information System:

- makes inquests more efficient and effective by enabling coroners in each jurisdiction to quickly access up-to-date information about similar cases to those being investigated;
- assists in the early identification of systemic or wide ranging risk factors;
- informs policy makers both in government and non-government sectors about factors which contribute to preventable death and injury;
- enables researchers to access and analyse comprehensive national data.

In order to understand the significance of a death investigation database for research and public policy development it is perhaps interesting to explore the creation of the National Coroners Information System. The idea for a national database for coronial information had been considered in Australia for over 10 years. Australia's 8 separate coronial jurisdictions each have their own systems of data collection and storage. Prior to the establishment of the database in some Australian jurisdictions, coronial records had been based on a manual filing system without indexes which could have identified clusters of similar cases.

In 1994 the Australian Coroners' Society commissioned the National Injury Surveillance Unit of the Australian Institute of Health and Welfare to undertake a feasibility study on a national database for coronial information. This study was funded by the Australian Commonwealth Department of Health and Aged Care. The feasibility study recommended the establishment of a national database of coronial information. The recommendations of the study were taken up by the Australian Coroners' Society.

In September 1997 the Australian Coroners' Society endorsed a business plan for development and management of the National Coroners Information System put forward by a Monash University consortium called the Monash University National Centre for Coronial Information. The consortium was made up of the Victorian Institute of Forensic Medicine (a statutory agency of the Victorian Department of Justice and which is also the Department of Forensic Medicine at Monash University), Monash University's Department of Epidemiology and Preventive Medicine, and the Monash University Accident Research Centre.

In 2004 operation and management of the database was transferred from Monash University to the Department of Justice in Victoria with the database being operated by the Victorian Institute of Forensic Medicine. The governance structure now, comprises a three tiered structure. The three levels of governance are:

- the NCIS Committee (comprised of Victorian Institute of Forensic Medicine representatives, an injury prevention representative, and two State coroner representatives);
- the Victorian Institute of Forensic Medicine Council;
- the NCIS Board of Management (comprised of a representative of each of the funding agencies and chaired by a State Department of Justice chief executive officer).

The current line of responsibility can now be traced back directly to the Standing Committee of Attorney Generals of Australia which ensures that the information system has the backing of government at the political and operational level.

A number of injury/death prevention initiatives in Australia have either originated from, or been supported by, data sourced from the National Coroners Information System. These initiatives include:

5. Launch of a National Safety Campaign

A national safety campaign concerning working under vehicles was launched on February 18 2005 by the then Federal Minister for Ageing, Julie Bishop. This joint campaign by the Australian Department of Health and Ageing and the ACCC was prompted by new figures from the National Coroners Information System which showed that 19 home mechanics died in Australia in the previous four years as a result of incidents associated with the incorrect use of jacks. As part of this campaign, a safety alert brochure was produced and made available to be downloaded from the ACCC website.

5.1   TAFE Course for Farmers in All Terrain Vehicle Safety

In July 2004, an accredited TAFE training program was developed in Tasmania for farmers, to enrol in a 3 tiered program to increase awareness and safety concerning all-terrain vehicle use. Provided by "Stay Upright", the Tasmanian course received approval for development in part due to figures from the NCIS which showed 57 all-terrain vehicle related deaths had occurred in Australia since July 2000.

5.2 Increased Awareness of Dangers Associated with Blind/Curtain Cords

In July 2003, a request was made to the Research Centre for Injury Surveillance, Flinders University by the Commonwealth Health Department, to supply information regarding deaths of infants and young children due to strangulation by blind or curtain cords. They were able to use the National Coroners Information System to identify a number of these fatalities which occurred since the National Coroners Information System data collection began in July 2000. The number of the cases they found prompted them to lodge an "Issue of Concern" to the National Coroners Information System, which was subsequently passed along to all State and Chief Coroners around Australia. A brochure concerning Blind and Curtain Cord Safety was subsequently produced by the Commonwealth Consumer Safety Unit within Treasury and the Department of Health and Ageing.

In May 2004, the Blind Makers Association of Australia contacted the National Coroners Information System and requested de-identified case information concerning the nature of these fatalities, to present to their members at the Annual Conference. This material was used to demonstrate to manufacturers, the necessity of new regulations concerning the blind manufacture.

At the launch of the National Coroners Information System the Honourable Rob Hulls at that time be Attorney General of Victoria stated:

> "The NCIS represents a world first in providing an Internet accessible database of coronial information across Australia. Coronial data is a rich source of information about the causes of preventable deaths in this country. (The NCIS) will provide a means of accessing data in a timely way and will increase the potential for coronial information to contribute to a reduction in preventable death and injury in Australia and in doing so, it will reduce both the emotional and financial burden of lost life in our community. The NCIS will revolutionise the way we investigate and respond to preventable deaths in Australia".

Since the establishment of the database there has been very considerable interest in its operations from a number of jurisdictions around the world. There appears to be a recognised need for such data and given the international dimension of community and environmental hazards we may expect to see data linkage is being developed between a number of national coronial databases in the future.

6.   Informatics and Disaster Management

Incidents involving mass loss of life although rare present real challenges to the community. Events such as natural disasters, acts of terrorism, transportation accidents, building accidents and warfare are often associated with multiple deaths. These deaths pose particular problems for coroners. Coroners are responsible for the identification of deceased persons whose death is reported to them. In addition they are responsible for determining the cause of death and in some jurisdictions are required to delve more deeply into the circumstances surrounding the death and to identify the issues involved. With the increase in the movement of people around the world mass disasters often involve individuals from many different countries and death investigation jurisdictions. This can pose problems for international law and communication issues in relation to discovering personal information about those who may have died. In cases of mass death in warfare or as a result of acts of terrorism state security and intelligence issues may also complicate the picture and give rise to particular problems with regards to information management and data interchange.

Natural disasters have huge global implications for international cooperation, data exchange and disaster mitigation policy development. At 00:58:53 UTC on 26 December 2004 a natural disaster struck many of the countries around the Indian Ocean. An earthquake now thought to have measured 9.3 on the Richter Scale occurred along a 1200 kilometre fault line running approximately north to south in the Indian Ocean. It was an under-sea earthquake that involved vertical movement of the fault line that started just to the north of the western coast of North Sumatra. The shifting of the seabed resulted in a tsunami with waves measuring up to 30 metres in height. The waves caused coastal devastation that affected many countries in Southeast Asia. In places the damage extended inland for a distance of several kilomctrcs.

Although countries in South-East Asia were most affected, the tsunami also involved more distant regions with one death occurring in Port Elizabeth in South Africa some 8000 kilometres away. Because of the north-south orientation of the fault line, the predominant damage occurred in countries to the east and west of the earthquake epicentre. Some of the regions affected included areas of Indonesia, Thailand, Sri Lanka, India, the Maldives, Somalia, Myanmar and Malaysia. Occurring during the time of the northern hemisphere winter, European holidaymakers were present in large numbers at popular tourist destinations in Asia, particularly in Thailand. As might be expected, these tourists were based in holiday resorts on the coast, the very areas that were most badly affected by the tsunami.

Estimates of the direct human toll of this tsunami suggest that over 350,000 people died. However, the remoteness of some of the affected regions limited the availability of post- incident medical services. As a result, many others may have died later as a consequence of injuries or the ensuing health problems associated with the destruction of the infrastructure of their communities.

The worldwide response to the disaster was enormous. Citizens from a wide number of countries were among the victims and there was an immediate humanitarian response. This included both governments and charitable relief agencies that provided financial support, provision of specialist and expert services and volunteers. These procedures for disaster management and human identification are well established around the world - particularly in jurisdictions which have well-organised forensic and medico-legal services. International agreement on the use of standard documentation during the management of disaster victim identification had been established via the Interpol Standing Committee on Disaster Victim Identification. The use of such standard documentation facilitates international co-operation and information exchange for both disaster response planning and disaster response operations.

Standard documentation for disaster victim identification, such as that provided by Interpol, is inevitably complex and somewhat unwieldy. This is because the documents are designed to cover all potential scenarios in which the identification of human remains takes place. In addition a mass disaster incident could involve individuals from one race type or individuals from a variety of different ethnic backgrounds and nationalities. Indeed in different regions of the world one might often find that the victims are made up of a particular collection of racial groups defined by the region in which the incident occurred. In countries with less well-organised technical and communication services the capacity to respond to a mass fatality event requiring complex and sophisticated technological resources and expert scientific and medical personnel may be limited. This poses a number of significant problems for the international community when it comes to managing and responding to mass fatalities.

Modern disaster victim identification procedures often involve the entry of post-mortem and ante-mortem data into an electronic database to facilitate case matching. While specialist databases are available for individual disciplines, in particular forensic odontology, overall case data are usually collected within the structure and framework of the Interpol disaster victim identification forms. This is important because the level of international travel has resulted in an increased need to exchange data rapidly between countries whose nationals may be disaster victims. Electronic transfer of such data can considerably speed up the process of human identification although maintaining the standards of coding and data entry on an international basis is problematic. With the responsibility of the coroner for the identification of deceased persons and the current tensions in relation to disasters involving mass loss of life databases such as the National Coroners Information System may prove of considerable value in managing community problems such as missing persons and disaster victim identification.

Death investigation is of course only a part of the picture in identifying avoidable disease and injury in our community. However, it often represents the tip of the iceberg with respect to injuries and analysis of injury related fatalities provides valuable information with regards to injury prevention. Today injury analysis is receiving the increased attention from public health practitioners and medical epidemiologists. The National Injury Surveillance Systems are beginning to address these issues. The cost of injury to our society has been grossly undervalued in previous years and injury control and prevention is now becoming a core part of national health policy in many countries.

7.   Organisation Theory and Health Care

The organisation of health care systems have undergone a paradigm shift in recent years. Fiscal restraint, increasing commercialization of health care, community pressures and re-evaluation of health goals has led to a much changed environment. In many ways, changes in health care provision have followed the changes that have occurred in the world of business and commerce.

The shift towards client services and client satisfaction as a marker for the success of health care systems represents a fundamental change in the way health care is delivered. The classic centralized systems of state based health care where policy decisions percolate down to the periphery of the health care system, is being replaced by regionalized systems where much health policy is made at a local level in response to the stated needs of communities. This devolution of policy and control represents an enormous challenge for health informatics systems in the next decade. Indeed it could be argued that for such a diffusion of health policy and power to be successful, health information systems will have to play a major part in providing the glue that holds these regional health care systems together. Current analysis of modern information technology itself recognizes the way in which informatics systems are becoming a crucial component of modern organizational structures.

> "..... there are major strategic developments in IT itself which are now maturing to the point of practical commercial application. Of key importance are:
> - office systems and applications for the workplace.
> - communication technologies which provide open networks and value added network services.
> - information management techniques including imaging, hypertext and object orientated paradigms which enable the electronic capture and use of unstructured records and soft information, and also a richer interpretation of knowledge.
> - maturity in the management of IT with the recognition that this function should be managed in the same way as for other parts of the business. This includes the need to manage IT expenditures as investments with the assets generated being managed as are other assets, including the concept of return on investment and life cycle maintenance." [18]

Many of the old views of information technology including those originally applied in the area of health informatics are being eroded. Today we do not see health informatics simply in terms of databases to be used for research, hospital administration, patient record systems or appointment systems. The availability of new technologies for the electronic communication of images and the analysis of textural and relational information have radically changed the way in which health informatics can take part in the formulation of health policy and contribute to medical research and public health. In particular the use of health information systems is no longer considered to be the sole province of health care providers. Today it is the clients of the health care system, patients and their families who are demanding better information on health care service outcomes and are using that information with the public media to drive the debate on health care policy. On an individual basis patients are demanding to be informed as to the health care outcomes that have occurred in particular health care institutions and as a result of the work of particular medical practitioners. This demand is leading to a model of informed patient choice that far exceeds the traditional view of the involvement of patients in their own health care decisions.

References

[1] Paul-Shaheen P.A. "Overlooked Connections: Policy Development and Implementation in State Local Relations". *International Journal of Health Services,* Vol. 19, No. 3, 1989.

[2] Davis K. "Health Care Reform in the United States. The Contribution of Health Services Research to the Debate", *Annals of the New York Academy of Science,* 1993. December 31;703:287-90.

[3] Feinglass J. and J. Warren-Salmon "Corporatisation of Medicine: The Use of Medical Management Information Systems to Increase the Clinical Productivity of Physicians". *International Journal of Health Services,* Vol. 20, No 2. Pages 233-252, 1990.

[4] Schneider M.K., Mann N and Schiller A, "*Can telecommunications help solve America's health care problems?* (Boston: Arthur D. Little, July 1992)

[5] Blau, A"Bringing the Promise Home: policy options and Strategies to promote medical information networking" *Journal of Medical Systems,* Vol. 17, No. 6, 1993.

[6] Robertson J. *"Physician Licensure: An Update of Trends".* http://www.ama-assn.org/ama/pub/category/2378.html viewed 15 October 2007.

[7] Royal College of Pathologists of the United Kingdom. *"Code of practice for pathologists participating in remote reporting of histopathology or cytopathology."* August 2003

[8] Garnerin P, Valleron A The French Communicable Diseases Computer Network: A Technical View. *Comput. Biol. Med.* Vol. 22, No. 3, Pp 189-200, 1992.

[9] Birkhead G. et al, Timeliness of National Reporting of Communicable Diseases: the experience of a national electronic telecommunications system for surveillance. *American Journal of Public Health,* Vol. 81, No. 10, October 1991, pp 1313-1315.

[10] Selbmann H and Pietsch-Breitfeld P, Hospital Information Systems and Quality Assurance, *Quality Assurance in Health Care,* Vol. 2, No. 3-4, pp 335-344, 1990.

[11] Scott Evans R and S.L. Pestontnik S.L, *Applications of Medical Informatics in Antibiotic Therapy, Antimicrobial Susceptibility Testing,* Edited by J.A. Poupard et al, Plenum Press, New York, 1994.

[12] Brend, W.A. Bills of Mortality 5. *Trans. Med - Legal Society,* P 140 (1907).

[13] Brend, W.A. Enquiry into the statistics of deaths from violence and unnatural causes in the United Kingdom" *A thesis approved for the degree of Doctorate of Medicine in State Medicine at the University of London,* Charles Griffin and Co., 1915.

[14] *Royal Commission into Aboriginal Deaths in Custody - National Report.* Vol. 1, Para. 4.7.4, April 1991.

[15] *Coroners Case* No. 2272/89, Heard May 1990.

[16] Drummer O H et al, *American Journal of Forensic Medicine and Pathology*, 13(4):346-50, 1992.

[17] Medical Examiner/Coroner Information Sharing Program. *American Journal of Forensic Medicine and Pathology,* Vol. 10, No. 1, 1989, p 88.

[18] Lovell M and Olson M "IT Planning for the nineties: Designing new organizations" *Computer Control Quarterly,* No. 2 1991, pp 10-15.

Review Questions

1. What are the management implications of information technology in research, public health and policy development?

2. Describe modern developments in death investigation, injury prevention and disaster management.

3. What are the dangers of applying global analysis to individual health care situations and vice versa?

4. What Mechanisms can be used to identify diffuse disaster in global and individual medical practice?

5. Explain the impact of informatics in areas of medical services that rely upon observational studies rather than validated clinical trials to develop knowledge bases.

6. Have you observed a paradigm shift in health care policy towards client driven services?

7. What are the implications of this shift for medical informatics?

Health Informatics
E.J.S. Hovenga et al. (Eds.)
IOS Press, 2010
© 2010 The authors and IOS Press. All rights reserved.
doi:10.3233/978-1-60750-476-4-360

26. Resource, Quality and Safety Management

Evelyn J S HOVENGA, RN, PhD (UNSW), FACHI, FACS
Director, eHealth Education, Consultant, openEHR Foundation, and Honorary Senior Research Associate, Centre for Health Informatics & Multiprofessional Education, University College London, Honorary Academic Fellow, Austin Health, Melbourne, Adjunct Professor, Central Queensland University Rockhampton, Queensland, and Victoria University, Melbourne, Australia

Abstract. This chapter gives an educational overview of:
- Resource management relative to sustainability and the use casemix systems
- Types of resources and their information system needs to support their optimal management
- Quality, performance measurement options and associated information needs
- Casemix systems' characteristics, usage and need for enterprise systems

Keywords. Data Collection, Classification, Information Management, International Classification of Diseases, Statistics, Terminology, Outcome and Process Assessment (Healthcare), Health Care Systems, Health Facilities, Health Policy, Quality Control, Information Systems, Health, Decision Support Systems-Management, Nursing Informatics, Evidence Based Practice, Quality Indicators – Healthcare, Practice Guidelines

Introduction

Managing available resources, the quality of care and patient safety within any health care organisation constitute key functions enhanced by the good use of appropriate information systems. In chapter three we presented the requirements for sustainable health systems and in chapter four we demonstrated that electronic health records are central to all health information systems. Today's eHealth strategies need to include a strong focus on various health service delivery models and associated business processes including electronic home monitoring, electronic medication management, and the adoption of telehealth and web based technologies for multiple purposes. Every health care delivery organization needs to tailor these available technologies in a way that best meets their specific business needs within available resources and local technical possibilities. Health systems are complex highly connected social constructs that control funding, access to services, workforce supply and demand, availability and cost of drugs, supplies, equipment, physical facilities and technologies, research opportunities and adoption of research results, and that shape consumer expectations and ultimately clinical outcomes. All these processes and outputs are constrained by a nation's political, legal, workplace, cultural, financial and business systems. Individual health care enterprises need to function within such a system's environment. This chapter builds on those concepts focusing on the adoption of casemix and enterprise systems as these are central to supporting these many and varied management functions.

1. Resource Management

One fundamental principle underpinning resource management is the need to ensure entity sustainability. That is a health service delivery organization needs to manage its resources in a manner that ensures its ability to continue to provide the health services to meet the needs of the population serviced indefinitely. In real systems, a growing gap between resource supply and demand cannot be sustained for long, and corrections must be made to bring supply and demand into balance. Furthermore any healthcare enterprise consumes physical resources, and any analysis of the sustainability of healthcare must explore how effective and efficient such enterprises are in using what we take from the world and what we put back into it. Sustainable organizations have developed strategies that fine tune and maintain this balance in ways that avoid the need for periodic, reactionary, large and usually painful structural adjustments, or even collapse. To survive in the long run, organizations need to have sufficient resources to meet their objectives and

> "Sustainable organizations are able to adapt to their changing environment, and do so at a rate that is faster than the rate of change in their surrounding context. An inability to cope with rapid systemic change will mean that an organization ends up being overwhelmed by the demands made of it" [1p.12].

Health service managers are faced with cost control, technology and demographic demand as well as workforce capacity, funding, quality and safety challenges to maintaining sustainability [1p.12]. Almost two thirds of the growth in health costs comes from consumer demand for new technology and treatments. Consumers expect to receive newer, usually more expensive, diagnostic procedures and medications once they become available, yet one study has estimated that only 21% of health technologies in use are supported by controlled research evidence [2]. This suggests that health service managers need to carefully examine the likely cost benefits prior to introducing any new technologies. Characteristics of the population serviced directly impacts on costs incurred as for example it is well known that health expenditure rises sharply with advancing age, accounting for a third of health cost growth and the population aged 65+ years is projected to increase significantly in the next 20 years. On the other side of this equation is the knowledge that the resources needed to meet an increased demand for health services will decrease when they are needed most due to an ageing population while the demand grows for the delivery of high quality health services.

Thus from a health service managers' perspective there is a need to introduce strategies that reduce demand and increase resource availability and to be adaptive to accommodate unplanned changes fast. Resource management essentially requires the adoption of economic principles as it requires knowledge about how best to allocate/distribute scarce resource to unlimited possible uses, requiring many choices to be made. Such choices should be informed by the most up to date and relevant information regarding the best possible returns or benefits achieved (products, outcomes) relative to investments made (resources provided) so that allocative efficiency may be realised. These concepts and their relationships are now explored in greater detail.

1.1 Types of Resources (Input Measures)

From a big picture perspective, investments in the health industry consist of funds allocated by Governments, health insurance companies, private organizations, philanthropy, and individuals. Other resources are the capital infrastructure such as buildings and large equipment, a nation's communications infrastructure, the people employed to manage and deliver health care services, and all necessary supplies. The ways such resources are acquired and allocated vary between nations as this is dependent upon Government legislation, regulations, health policy initiatives, population characteristics, public health requirements, national health workforce education infrastructures and reporting requirements. Thus the external environment greatly influences how individual health care organisations best manage their available resources relative to possible health service delivery models. Enterprise information systems need to be able to accommodate these variations yet be interoperable within the health industry as whole.

1.2 Infrastructure, Supplies and Equipment

Any national e-health strategy requires the inclusion of access to a broadband communications network and the Internet and the provision of a national standards and knowledge management/representation and governance framework. Desired health service delivery models are to some extent dependent upon the available communications infrastructure and they influence capital works (buildings), medical and e-health technology needs. In addition national Governments need to ensure that there are no legislative or regulatory impediments to e-health technology adoption.

Organisational infrastructure includes, where relevant, the acquisition, management and supply of fuel, light and power, domestic services, food supplies/catering, care providers, drug, medical and surgical supplies to the point of care as well as administrative, financial, information and communication support services. In addition the overall infrastructure requires continuous property and equipment management, maintenance, repairs, regular reviews and updates, including building renovations or additions and an equipment replacement schedule, to ensure that it best meets current health service delivery model requirements. Overall the organisational infrastructure needs to provide a functional and safe environment for both staff and patients.

Another major infrastructure need is the management of patient records, paper based or electronic. Clinical records accumulate, and for chronically ill patients the size of the records being created become increasingly unwieldy, whether on paper or electronically stored. IT systems themselves can 'accumulate'. Most health services that extend over large communities and different sites accumulate different versions of clinical software, different mixes of departmental systems, and different interface solutions. Some legacy systems have been in existence for decades, and as time goes on, the expertise or resources to maintain them diminish – a classic sustainability trap. Further, the introduction of a new system will often demand that it interface with all relevant existing systems, and interfaces have the characteristic that their growth is a factorial in the number of systems being communicated - another sustainability trap. It quickly becomes clear why standards, and adherence to standards, is an essential strategy to get away from a growing burden of legacy systems, and an accumulation of interfacing and maintenance tasks that have the potential to overwhelm an IT support organization over time.

1.3 Workforce

The most significant resource is the health workforce consisting of a large number of separate professions, each with their own scope of practice and unique educational preparation. This workforce includes those who are employed to provide the many support services such as those identified in the previous infrastructure section. The biggest number of health professionals belong to the nursing profession although ratios between medical practitioners to nursing professionals vary significantly between nations as do the numbers of various other allied health professions such as physiotherapists, or dental practitioners. Most health professions need to be authorized to practice via various national registration requirements although there are many health workers who do undertake various activities directly associated with patient care who are not so credentialed. The available collective clinical knowledge, skills and capacity directly influence the quality of care provided, patient safety and outcomes. Consequently workforce planning, educational opportunities and outcomes as well as health professional staff allocation, scheduling and rostering practices are major contributing factors to achieving the desired quality and health service delivery outcomes. From an ehealth perspective it has become evident that we need an increased workforce capacity in this area although health informatics is yet to be formally recognized as an occupational discipline.

Workforce planning is about developing a strategy that aims to best match demand with supply. Demand is influenced not only by the burden of disease in any one population, access to health services by individuals and consumer expectations, but also by national health policy priorities as well as other policies such as those related to occupational health and safety, or road safety or the rate of violence or war. Supply is influenced by educational opportunities such as the number of students who can or seek to enrol in the various programs on an annual basis, the number who graduate and the number who continue to work in their profession.

In many instances the boundaries of practice between these professions need to be flexible to some extent to maintain efficiency, yet there is a need to ensure that anyone required to perform a specific role or task has the necessary knowledge and skills (competencies). Most health services require input from a number of different health professionals and health workers who essentially need to work as teams to optimize outcomes and efficiency. An imbalance in the health workforce, both an under and over supply, incurs additional costs.

1.4 Health Service Products and Outcomes (Output Measures)

Delivering health services results in discharged patients who have experienced an outcome. Outcome measures have a qualitative dimension, whereas output measures are used for quantitative purposes. They interrelate regarding the quality and cost of health care. Thus discharged patients may be described as health service 'products'. Such products then need to be defined to enable grouping so that such groups can be used as a means of capturing and managing the associated production processes and costs. Health service products and their classification or grouping are frequently referred to 'casemix'. Outcomes also need to be defined in some way as this is key towards enabling quality monitoring and management. We begin this section by first exploring the principles associated with performance and quality measurement followed by casemix and how this relates to resource and quality management.

2. Managing Quality and Safety – Linking Input With Output Measures

Resource allocation influences the ability to maximizing the benefits resulting from their use to deliver health services. Obtaining information about performance following the adoption of various delivery methods where each method uses its own unique set of resources assists resource allocation decision making. If the intended purpose was served in accordance with expectations then the performance could be regarded as highly effective. It needs to be recognized that in the health care industry the care of a particular patient type (production process) at minimal cost may be viewed as highly efficient but in fact may not be cost-effective as expectations may not have been met and/or the quality of care may not have been optimum with a poor outcome as the result. However, it is possible to achieve a better outcome at a lower than expected cost. Measuring such performances in a meaningful way requires standard definitions, valid and reliable data collection and an appropriate information system enabling data linkage and processing to produce meaningful reports.

2.1 Resource and Quality Management by Patient Type (Casemix)

Actual costs are influenced by the quality and quantity of all resources used to provide patient care towards achieving the desired outcome. As in industry, once costs are identifiable by product one can explore the most cost-efficient method to be employed to achieve the desired outcome. This requires us to identify and define outcome measures that are sensitive to subtle changes in a person's overall health status following discharge. The only way we can learn more about the relationships between staffing, care and treatment processes provided and outcomes is to have systems in place that can measure these concepts. Such measurement may take place continuously, periodically or at random.

3. Capturing Cost Data

Accounting costs are expenses classified by a standard chart of account. Costs are then allocated directly or distributed according to a uniform method of apportionment and transformed into unit costs by dividing the total costs by consistently defined and generally accepted units of service or work units. The sum of these units may be referred to as the departmental workload. The costs incurred in providing clinical services are directly related to the workload generated by patients, the staff provided to service these needs and materials used. For example nursing staff usage, is measured in terms of staff category (skill mix), the associated hourly cost and time. The cost per staff hour varies relative to staff category, shift and day of the week worked. The latter two variables may be dependent on penalty and shift allowances.

Thus both staff mix and rostering practices influence nursing costs. Such data should be captured as part of a nursing casemix system and is explained in greater detail later. Other clinical services have similar variables influencing costs.

The time taken by a health worker to carry out an activity or to provide a service is influenced by the nature of the work to be performed, the skill and knowledge of the staff member, the circumstances within which the work is performed, the methods employed, and the perceived time available. Actual costs will reflect all of these factors, including inefficiencies. These costs are then related to the output measure in use, eg. Australian Refined – Diagnosis Related Groups (AR-DRG). In this manner defined input costs relative to defined outputs are traced.

4. Quality

Quality is not a synonym for excellence; a quality service is the one best suited to the purpose intended and circumstances within which it is delivered rather than the best that money can buy. An appropriate level of quality may be determined by balancing factors such as performance, reliability, cost, consequences of failure, etc. A nation's quality health service may be evaluated based on the following key dimensions (adapted from [3]:

- Timely access to care
- Technical and allocative efficiency regarding resource availability
- Safety, technical proficiency and appropriateness
- Efficacy -capacity to provide the necessary services and their effectiveness
- Ability to meet provider and patient/client/consumer expectations
- Continuity of care via discharge planning coordination

Health service delivery quality may be defined as a service that suits the purpose, or conforms to requirements. These services are directly influenced by the quality of the national, organisational and environmental infrastructure within which these services are undertaken. The process of care in turn influences the outcomes and results obtained. Finally when this performance information is provided to health care consumers and individual care providers it influences the choices people make within the context of available treatment or care options. Consequently performance indicators need to be identified within the context of structure, process and outcomes.

At an institutional level quality may be measured in terms of the physical and organisational structures which contribute to or provide an appropriate environment for the delivery of quality health services. Consumers are concerned with getting the most appropriate service provided competently by a qualified person at an optimum time and place, within an acceptable timeframe, which achieves what it is intended to do and which meets consumer expectations at every encounter. Thus quality is the degree to which the above expectations are met.

Another perspective on the measurement of quality is through the examination of processes, procedures and outcomes. The adoption of what is known as 'best practice' or evidence based practice is seen as a sound strategy to enhance the quality of the services provided. However the rate of accumulation of new scientific information is a well-recognised bottleneck to evidence-based practice. In essence a health service needs to satisfy both the providers' and subjects' of care stated or implied needs, meet their expectations at the time of service delivery and base its practice on the best available evidence. Quality assurance requires evidence that the services provided will or have been provided consistently in accordance with best practice principles.

5. What is Evidence Based Practice?

The knowledge used as a basis for clinical, management and policy decision making to support healthcare varies in terms of quality, accuracy and soundness. Ideally such knowledge is based on reliable evidence however it is often clouded by values, opinions and other people's views, and consists of or comes from:

- tradition, 'we've always done it this way',
- authority, position power and perceived expertise
- borrowing from other disciplines
- what was learned during professional education and from textbooks
- reasoning, trial and error, 'let's try this and see'
- experience, 'this worked for me the last time'
- rules, regulations, procedures and protocols
- a role model or mentor, someone perceived as having expertise
- journal articles, popular press, the Internet, sales representatives
- processed data collected routinely, systematically such as trend data
- research results, both qualitative and quantitative and including randomised clinical trials usually conducted by others.

Evidence based practice (EBP) began with work by Cochrane [4]. Evidence based practice may be defined as a practitioners' ability to process critical evidence that supports their practice/activity to achieve an optimum outcome at least cost within the circumstances such care is provided. It requires every person working in the health industry to identify the best available evidence for every intervention and to use this as the basis for all decisions. Increasingly health care organizations make access to the Cochrane coloration and other sources of evidence available on-line to their health professional staff. Adoption of EBP is about less reliance on most of the above knowledge sources and a greater reliance on the best possible evidence available about what works and what does not. This requires an ability to look for, retrieve and assess what is good evidence and what is not. Health care professionals are required to have the ability to question plus possess the necessary skills to search out, retrieve, interpret and apply the evidence. Evidence is also needed to inform health policy development.

6. Practice Guidelines, Protocols and Standard Procedures

Guidelines are statements that define how desired results may best be achieved. Practice guidelines were originally defined by the US Institute of Medicine [5 p.27] as 'systematically developed statements to assist practitioner and patient decisions about appropriate health care for specific clinical circumstances'. They may also be used to educate individuals (providers, patients) or groups, as a component of continuing professional education, as a basis for resource allocation, to reduce the risk of legal liability for negligent care and to assess and ensure the quality of care. Clinical practice guidelines must be evidence based, valid, clinically applicable and flexible and need to have been developed by multi-disciplinary groups [6].

Guidelines, protocols and standard procedures are all process standards used to guide practice. They define expected performance and may be used as measures against which actual performance is evaluated. They are defined as a result of an analysis of practices used that are known to have resulted in the desired outcome. Clinical pathways or process standards define the most efficient and effective methods, service scheduling and organization needed to produce the desired results relative to clearly defined patient types within a defined length of stay or episode of care. Their use together with a continuous analysis of variation, provides an early indication about possible complications so that corrective action can be taken at the earliest indication of need.

7. Outcome Measures

The quality of a country's health service is generally speaking assessed by the mortality rates and incidents of morbidity. These types of statistics are reported worldwide as death rates, major causes of death, life expectancy, live births, maternal and infant mortality rates and others. Such measures are indicators of ill health and provide the big picture. This information may lead to the identification of areas warranting closer scrutiny. Two types of outcome measures are required, disease-specific to permit comparisons to be made between treatment options and generic outcome measures such as the degree of functional improvement, pain relief or improved general well-being. All outcomes need to be expressed relative to a time dimension ranging from immediate to long-term as the time taken to realise the results of care is in itself a quality measure. The most significant unresolved issues associated with quality measurement in health are issues of definition. The concept of health is subject to many different interpretations. Perspective or the position from which we view health influences the definitions used. There are healthy but disabled people for example.

Another way of looking at outcome from a quality perspective is to examine what constitutes health. After all, health services aim to promote, maintain and restore health. The Australian Institute for Health and Welfare defines health as social, economic, environmental, spiritual or existential well being. It also includes life satisfaction and other characteristics valued by humans. The World Health Organisation (WHO) defines health as 'a state of complete physical, mental and social well-being and not merely the absence of disease or infirmity'.

7.1 Health Status

Health status may be defined in many different ways. The concept of health varies between people. A patient's health status should be assessed on both admission and discharge as part of the admission, patient assessment and diagnosis processes adopted. Ideally an individual's health status has improved following the receipt of health and nursing services. This represents a good outcome measure although there is a need to define this in a measurable manner. For example the Apgar score is a health status indicator of newborns, the adoption of this score has supported the introduction of many new care processes and services resulting in significant improvements.

Individuals will place different values on health. Concert pianists are likely to value their ability to hear and their dexterity more than others where a hearing impairment does not significantly impact on their chosen career or lifestyle. Loss of function creates greater problems for some than for others. The value individuals place on health stems from whether our state of health allows us to lead a fulfilling and satisfying life. For some this leads to more risk taking behaviour than for others. Thus individuals contribute to their own state of health. The value of any health status is also age related. What is effective functioning for some individuals is not for other; it depends on one's perception and values. So another significant issue regarding quality measurement is the fact that there are many variables which influence health as it is perceived by individuals. There is no obvious direct cause and effect relationship in many instances, however measures of health may be used as indicators of quality. If we assume that customers of the health service industry expect to achieve or optimise their general health, then evidence of health status needs to be provided as a measure of quality.

7.2 Performance Indicators

Indicators are signs, flags or signals, some of which may indicate desirable events where others indicate negative events. There are two types of quality performance indicators. The first is a rate based indicator which designates a level of occurrence; the second is a sentinel event. Rate based indicators are measured against predetermined acceptable thresholds, whereas sentinel events are so serious that no rate of occurrence is considered acceptable. Thresholds must be achievable.

Performance indicators are used to identify areas which would benefit from further investigation so as to improve performance and quality. Indicators are chosen as much for their data availability and collection feasibility, as for their relevance or established link with the concept desired to be measured. Where the quality of a service cannot be measured directly, it may be measured indirectly through the use of any number of indicators. Such indicators are pointers from which one may infer that the desired quality and outcomes were achieved. Alternatively they are used to indicate areas for further investigation. Workload (demand for service) and service utilisation (services actually provided) statistics together with cost and outcome data may be used as indicators of quality.

There are a number of possible cost efficiency performance indicators for acute hospitals. Examples are: average inpatient unit cost, average length of stay, relative length of stay indicator, occupancy rate percentage of registered beds, total admissions, etc. None of these are very precise measures, but when compared over time or with other hospitals should indicate trends and relative cost efficiency. Such indicators do not assist in explaining cost variations, rather they indicate where further investigation is warranted. These data need to be associated with outcome data, including patient satisfaction or discharge health status data, to get a sense of the quality and effectiveness of services provided.

Other possibilities as outcome performance indicators are the adoption of the quality of life measure known as QALYs that indicate quality adjusted life years defined by Culyer [7] as a multi-dimensional concept that encompasses the physical, emotional and social effects of an illness or treatment. Another possible performance indicator is the saved young life equivalent (SAVE) [8]. Another is the Activities of Daily Living Scale (ADLS). Of course care needs to taken not to confuse such outcomes from a performance measurement perspective with those associated with untreatable natural disease progression where health services focus on achieving symptom relief and optimum life quality within normal disease progression constraints.

8. Measuring Performance

Many nations have systems in place to track critical incidents such as the emergence of side-effects associated with new drugs. The importance of reducing error in health delivery has also seen the introduction of critical incident monitoring systems in many countries. Underpinning all these systems is a basic requirement that we develop some electronic means for collecting, storing, linking and retrieving standard patient data elements. The electronic health record thus becomes a basic plank in our sustainability infrastructure, because many of the crucial data feeds needed to monitor health system behaviour and performance come from such records, wherever they are held, or however they might be structured. However a failure to adopt a national standard record structure impedes linking data and the ease of data retrieval possibly compromising the size of data samples for reliable analysis. In such instances middleware may be used to overcome this problem but this adds to the data collection and processing costs.

Operational effectiveness requires the ability to evaluate performance not only in terms of quality and safety of clinical care but also in terms of overall service quality, cost, dependability, flexibility and speed. Thus, sustainable practice also requires significant amounts of data about clinical and administrative processes, describing for example the flows of patients through a system, the status of clinical staff numbers, the availability and utilization of resources such as drugs and beds. With increasing monitoring of process data, we are better able to see the actual dynamic behaviour and performance of organizations, and use that data to first build meaningful models of the ways different processes interact, and then track any changes we make to the system.

Sustainability requires us to see clinical work in different ways, and measure variables not traditionally associated with health informatics. For example, only recently have we realised that it is just as important to measure the communication loads on clinical staff, the number of interruptions they have, and the level of multitasking load they are under, because of the significant impact human to human communication traffic has on the quality and safety of clinical care [9]. Sustainability requires us to look widely at organisational processes, and identify bottlenecks and inefficiencies wherever they might arise, not just at the moment of clinical care.

Better-informed decisions usually result in better clinical outcomes and reduced costs. With the merging of electronic health records and decision support systems, clinicians are increasingly in a position to make decisions based both upon the best scientific evidence, as well as patient-specific data. For this to happen, experience repeatedly shows that health information systems need to be designed and used in a manner that integrates them with daily workflows within any organization to achieve operational effectiveness at all levels. Many now argue that optimum efficiencies can only be achieved with the widespread adoption of *semantically* interoperable information systems i.e. systems capable of transferring, sharing, exchanging and meaningfully using information for decision support, regulatory reporting, population surveillance, clinical practice evaluation, outcome analysis and more. In other words, interoperability should enable the reuse (and avoid the 'waste') of data for multiple, often very different purposes.

One study of information sharing and integration in the public sector [10] supports this view, identifying that the primary integration problems are semantic issues, relationships between information and decision rules, data quality, interorganisational interactions, collaboration and trust. Semantic interoperability is required for the reliable transfer of clinical data as this is where the meaning of the data must be retained to validly enable the transferred data to be processed by the computer and used for decision support systems. All healthcare applications need to establish the functions they need to be able to perform so that the required degree and level of interoperability can be established enabling the identification of which standard they need to be compliant with.

Finally, it is important to recognise that information technology is not a universal panacea, and poor design and use of IT can itself lead to unsustainable practices and system behaviours. IT is only one component of any clinical service, and not the end goal itself, a maxim forgotten enough to be restated *ad nauseam*. Sustainable services require significant emphasis on change management and organisational process [1$^{p.17}$). Now that we have explored various principles associated with performance and quality measurement we'll examine the relationships between resources used, costs, quality, treatment and care processes, outputs and outcomes or put another way, health service 'products', as defined using Australian 'casemix' principles.

8.1 Linking Cost, Quality, Process and Outcome Measures

The adoption of casemix systems has the benefit of providing more detailed information than has traditionally been available. By linking cost, quality and process data relative to output measures new information is obtained that begin to explain some of the variations which may previously have been identified by performance indicators alone. Casemix refers to output measures that lend themselves to scrutinising all planned and systematic treatment and care processes as well as the management of the production process itself that was associated with each case or case type.

9. What is Casemix?

Casemix refers to a mix of patients classified in some way. It describes a system which groups patients by predetermined factors and an agreed 'grouping logic' using clinical, demographic and resource usage data into clinically meaningful and resource homogenous groups to describe any hospital or health service's output. In other words, a discharged patient is classified into a casemix category reflecting the types of patients treated and cared for by any health facility. Admitted and discharged patients can be classified based on a variety of criteria. These criteria are selected to suit the purpose for which this is done.

In Chile an admitted patient may be classified as fitting with an AUGE plan condition following initial assessment so that a standard care plan may be used as the basis upon which ongoing care is managed. However we know that such a provisional assessment may need to change once more tests have been undertaken and treatment/care options are implemented. Such changes especially occur following a patient's adverse reaction to the care or treatment given or when complications occur. For example the nursing process requires that a re-evaluation of all patients' nursing care needs is regularly undertaken based on patient responses to their illness/injury and treatments received and the nursing care plan is adjusted accordingly. Consequently once patients are discharged the treatment/care processes actually undertaken throughout a patient's journey (episode of care or hospital stay) can be used as criteria to determine the most appropriate casemix category as this will more accurately reflect resource usage and be more clinically meaningful.

We will now examine the most common criteria used for this classification, how such data are collected, the value of adopting a casemix system, the relationship between a casemix system and information systems that need to be in place to support casemix adoption within any healthcare facility. The Casemix Development Program funded by the Australian Government[11] commenced in 1989; a number of other countries have adopted and modified this system to meet their specific requirements. The Australian casemix system will be used to serve as a robust example of how casemix can be used to benefit a nation's health system.

9.1 Types of Casemix Systems

The casemix system now in use by Australian acute care hospitals to define their 'products' is the Australian Refined Diagnosis Related Groups (AR-DRGS). Many countries now use similar systems and there are a number of other casemix systems developed specifically for different types of patients such as aged residential care or intensive care or for neonates. In fact a casemix system can be developed and applied to any patient receiving any health service. For example the National Health Service in the United Kingdom uses Healthcare Resource Groups (HRGs) [12]. Canada has adopted their own Case Mix Groups (CMGs), as well as Day Procedure Groups (DPGs), and the Comprehensive Ambulatory Care Classification System (CACS) used to classify different patient populations. Descriptions of these are available at the Canadian Institute for Health Information's (CIHI) website [13].

Similarly patients may be grouped to represent homogeneity in terms of nursing resource usage. Such classification systems are therefore 'nursing casemix systems' also known as patient acuity or dependency systems. Other departments may also use a system to classify their patient services on the basis of resource usage in order to identify other AR-DRG component costs. Such departmental patient or activity classification systems can then also be used as components of the national or organizational casemix categories. This will be explained in some detail in another section.

9.1.1 Australian Refined Diagnosis Related Groups (AR-DRGs)

AR-DRGs apply to acute in-patients only. AR-DRGs are modelled on the Diagnosis Related Groups (DRG) system which has been used as a basis for allocating resources via the United States Medicare prospective payment system since 1983. This DRG patient classification system was developed during the 1970s by Fetter et al [14[p.107]] at the Yale School of Organisation and Management and the Yale School of Public Health "to attempt to discern and identify discrete kinds of illness for which one could expect, in a statistical sense, a relatively consistent response from any one physician or any one set of physicians with respect to the diagnostic and therapeutic services ordered to deal with that". On the basis that physicians are primarily responsible for determining the process and hence the cost of patient care, this grouping was used in an attempt "to establish the statistical similarity and significances of differences in resource consumptions and patterns from one kind of patient to another" [14[p.107]). Physicians were considered to be accountable for approximately 80% of total hospital expenditure [15]. The United States of America (USA) now has several different DRG systems in use.

The first version of DRGs contained 327 groups, these have expanded over the years as a result of many revisions to over 600 groups. Advantages of grouping are that there are considerably fewer case types (products) than ICD-10-AM codes, making the use of AR-DRG codes for reporting and statistical analysis purposes so much more feasible and useful. Grouping occurs by means of a simple classification algorithm using a few data items available on a patient's discharge abstract. Over the years all casemix systems in use have evolved based on continuous refinements. Australia releases a new version of the AR-DRGs every two years. As the use of casemix systems has expanded, new classification systems have also emerged.

9.2 Purpose of Adopting Casemix Systems

Once there is a defined 'product' it can be used for a variety of statistical analyses about health services delivered to gain a better understanding about the impact of health policy, available resources, a population's disease burden, best practices and changes over time. Outputs need to be defined not only in terms of the product as expressed by casemix but also in terms of outcomes. The latter is an essential prerequisite to the evaluation of service cost effectiveness. An understanding of the production relationships is necessary when using cost data as a basis for management decision making aimed at improving both efficiency and effectiveness of services provided.

Most commonly casemix information is used for costing and resource management purposes. The use of casemix for decision making, frequently centers around the financing aspects of the health system. Details of the financing of health services tend to change over time and differ between Countries as well as between Australian States and Territories and between the private and public sectors. One needs a good understanding of the issues, principles and details associated with both casemix data requirements and financing relative to different organisations in order to use casemix data optimally for decision making purposes. From a systems perspective such details determine system specifications. Formulae using casemix as a basis for funding public hospitals are heavily influenced by existing relationships between the funders and the providers of hospital services and by government policy objectives or other funding agencies. Tracking departmental costs by output measure(s) serves a number of different purposes. Systems need to support a wide range of clinical and financial analysis of data selected from an integrated database such as:

- analysis of operating costs, contribution margins, marginal costs;
- cost benefit/cost effectiveness analysis;
- trend analysis;
- resource utilization analysis; and
- productivity (efficiency) analysis.

A Casemix system provides management information to assist with improving cost efficiencies and health care effectiveness. It is used to compare identical health services provided by different facilities to identify 'best practice'. There are a number of reasons why the total costs for individual cases in any AR-DRG will vary between hospitals. These include demand and supply conditions in each local area, staff skill mix, differences in models of care delivery or practice patterns, staff scheduling, variations in the quality of care, and the availability of specialised facilities.

In Australia the primary purpose continues to be the determination of cost per AR-DRG category as it is used as the foundation for funding hospitals. Governments have recognised the need for consistent tools to assess quality, compare costs and understand the relationships between inputs and outputs for some time. These initiatives have had major implications for health information systems used for data collection and to provide management decision support at multiple levels of decision making. Examples of national casemix data reporting are provided at the Australian Government's casemix website.

The use of casemix data lends itself to be retrospectively aligned with the use of clinical pathways as well as the adoption of the nursing process which is a component of any clinical pathway. Such pathways may also be referred to as a 'patient journey' through the health system or any health service. Clinical pathways need to be constantly updated to accommodate the needs of new service delivery models such as "Hospital in the Home" and Shared Care/Integrated Service delivery models or health service delivery programs that operate across a number of hospitals, such as for oncology care. There is an expectation that community health care will play a bigger role in years to come as individuals become their own case managers. As a consequence there needs to be a different emphasis on information system requirements for the measurement of outcomes relative to resource usage. Casemix data is then used to evaluate the cost effectiveness of such new health service delivery models. Clinical studies using casemix data need to be able to access the patient level data whereas management studies use the cost centre level data, that is, data representing a total ward or department such as changes in the mix of patient types over time [16[p.63]].

For example ward nursing casemix systems enable nurses to compare patient types, ie categorized into any way relative to AR-DRG, cared for across organisations or across wards within an organization, by examining the relationships between nursing process activities and patient outcomes. Such analysis enables nurses to identify best nursing practice and to use that information for developing a standard nursing care plan for patients provisionally identified as being in that AR-DRG category. A good example may be the care of patients with diabetes but who are admitted for other reasons as demonstrated by Bozzo, Carlson and Diers [17].

Nurses may also use these data to demonstrate that where there is a great variety of AR-DRG type patients in one ward their care is not optimum as nurses cannot be experts in all areas of practice. Consequently it is beneficial to allocate similar patient types to the same ward or department to be cared for by nurses who have a lot of experience in caring for such patients. Casemix data then enables an evaluation of the impact of such a change.

10. Clinical Pathways, Patient Journeys and Casemix

In project planning terms a critical path is the shortest possible length of time within which a project may be achieved. One could view every patient's hospital admission as a project and aim to discharge each case within the shortest possible time. Many hospitals have begun to develop clinical paths for high volume or high cost AR-DRGs to assist management to achieve this. Managing each case relative to the clinical path is referred to as case management. Case management includes the adoption of the nursing process from which a nursing care plan is developed as well as discharge planning. It uses a multidisciplinary approach to account for all types of health services provided during the length of stay.

Historical casemix data may be used to first develop each clinical path and secondly to modify these as required based on best practice. It is the nursing care plan which determines the nursing resources required, both in quantity and quality. The Trend Care™ system includes the use of multidisciplinary clinical pathways. Its clinical outcome options enable clinical staff to define the standard of care required for patients, and the expected patient outcomes. The clinical pathway system facilitates variance tracking and analysis, and contains automated patient history, risk management assessments and outcome assessments. TrendCare™ provides comprehensive clinical pathway reports and graphs which can identify potential areas for improvements in care planning, pre surgical patient preparation and clinical processes. This enables corrective action to be taken as soon as possible. This is one way by which to manage individual length of stay and patient throughput as a whole. It is an important tool for using casemix data for decision making. The use of clinical paths is expected to increase productivity, improve quality and control costs. Obsolete or unnecessary practices may be identified during the development and evaluation processes. Such pathways are also useful tools for discharge planning. It is a mechanism for achieving financial objectives without compromising the standards of care.

Clinical path care plans are developed so as to achieve high quality care, effective communication between all disciplines, collaboration and optimum resource utilisation. The use of standardised care plans and terminologies facilitates automation of clinical data and as a result improved capacity for clinical research at less cost than is the case with a paper based system. If casemix data is intended to be used to allocate a standard critical path then the necessary data elements need to be collected on admission based on the initial patient assessment, planned care processes and an estimated length of stay so that a provisional casemix category can be allocated. If the use of casemix data is confined to retrospective data analysis then it is appropriate to collect the necessary data following discharge. The intended use of casemix data determines what data need to be collected when and how. Remember that a person's health status on admission becomes the benchmark against which outcomes may be measured.

11. Discharge Planning

Discharge planning is about assessing patient needs and obtaining or coordinating appropriate resources for patients and clients in a timely manner as they move through the health care system (patient journey). The aim is to provide care continuity and to ensure that patients move through the system in the shortest possible time without adverse effects or the need for re admission. For many hospital cases this requires follow up care by community based services. Such care needs to be anticipated and organised in advance. Casemix-based funding provides an incentive for effective discharge planning. This may require a specifically appointed person to be responsible for discharge planning on a case by case basis.

Problems following discharge can occur where a patient or the family are unable to support daily living needs or do not understand directions for follow-up care or are unlikely to comply with advice given. Also the home environment may not be suitable for satisfactory self care. The home location relative to the treating centre may prevent care on an outpatient basis. Discharge planning must occur in consultation with the patient, the home based care givers if present, community based services and the health professionals providing inpatient care. An interdisciplinary approach is highly desirable. Discharge planning needs to commence on admission and in some cases prior to admission. Length of stay can be reduced only in conjunction with effective discharge planning. A discharge planning program may identify specific groups of patients who have specific needs which could be met more cost effectively as an outpatient or in the home compared with inpatient care. However in some instances this may require the establishment of new community services or joint ventures to enable the adoption of new health service delivery models.

12. Casemix Data Following Discharge

Data needed to enable the categorization of discharged patients must be extracted from medical and nursing records. It consists of all data needed to be entered into the grouper software so that each patient can be classified into a case type such as an AR-DRG. This includes demographic data such as age, gender, date and time of admission and discharge, discharge primary and secondary diagnosis, all clinical interventions, operations, tests and diagnostic services undertaken as well as discharge status. These parameters all need to be coded. Health information managers who have the necessary coding skills, code the conditions treated and the procedures performed using for example the International Classification of Diseases - 10th Revision Australian Modification (ICD-10-AM) system. Other ICD versions may still be in use in other countries. These codes, denoting the principal diagnosis, significant secondary diagnosis and procedures, are then used by grouper software to classify the in-patient episode. There needs to be consistency between organisations so that casemix data can be aggregated and compared.

12.1 Coding and Classification Systems Used

Two types of data are used to group patients, clinical (diagnosis, procedures) and demographic (age, gender etc). The current grouping logic has been arrived at based on clinical edits and resources used (activity based costs) as identified via clinical costing systems. Clinical data need to be coded into a major diagnostic category, then into a diagnosis as defined using the International Classification of Diseases (ICD) system. For some patients there may be more than one diagnosis. In addition clinical data are needed to identify medical procedures and other factors that differentiate care processes such as severity of illness and resources used. In 2008 Australia used the sixth edition of the ICD version ten with Australian modifications (ICD-10-AM) to code clinical data. These codes are then used to classify discharged patients into AR-DRG groups based on hierarchies of diagnoses and procedures within major diagnostic categories and distributed between surgical, medical and other partitions using 'grouper' software. Each group contains several different diagnoses that are clinically meaningful as a group and that usually require the use of a similar amount of resources, that is all variations are statistically insignificant. As there is a strong correlation between resource usage and length of stay or episode of care, this is often used as a proxy cost indicator.

The ICD-10-AM classification system uses an alphanumeric coding scheme for diseases. It is structured by body system and aetiology, and comprises three, four and five character categories [18] to reflect a code for a diagnosis. Also used is the Australian Classification of Health Interventions (ACHI) developed by the NCCH. This system's codes have seven digits. The first five digits are the Medical Benefits Schedule (MBS) item number. The two-digit extension represents specific procedures included in that item. The classification is structured by body system, site and procedure type. Procedures not currently listed in MBS have also been included (for example allied health interventions, cosmetic surgery). Some of these health interventions may well be performed by nurses. Coding manuals may be purchased from the NCCH. Other national data standards, some of which are also used by the casemix system, are defined in the Metadata Online Registry (METeOR) maintained by the Australian Institute of Health and Welfare [19]. Associated issues were presented in previous chapters on important health information concepts and clinical terminology.

Once casemix based funding is introduced there may be an associated desire to maximise income and minimise costs by manipulating casemix data. This possibility raises ethical issues which one will need to be aware of. It suggests that regular auditing of coding is required. Accurate coding of clinical data is extremely important as reliable casemix information depends on it. This task is still undertaken manually by 'coders', that is staff [in some countries medical staff] who have been trained to extract the right clinical information from the medical record and to convert this into codes for entry into the grouper system. Once we have well designed electronic health record systems in use this activity can be automated.

Defining hospital products in casemix terms makes it essential to adopt a cost centre accounting process in a manner that enables these cost centres to track and allocate their costs by these products. It should be noted that some hospitals also undertake teaching and research in addition to providing health care, the products of these activities require their own definition. In addition some services are provided which do not directly contribute to the organisation's main product. For example a hospital kiosk or the local meals on wheels service provided for other organisations or individuals. Such activities can provide additional income and also incur costs.

12.2 Obtaining Cost Data by AR-DRG

A National Costing Study was first conducted in Australia during 1992, this work is now regularly updated. Such studies identify the following casemix component costs from a number of nationally representative hospitals: Ward Nursing, Medical, Pathology, Imaging, Operating Theatre, Drugs, Critical care, Allied health, Medical and Surgical supplies, Overhead allocation, Patient catering and Other [20]. Individual organisations may decide to break this down further into individual responsibility centres or departments. Such breakdowns or unbundling of total costs is also dependent upon the funding or resource allocation formula in use. For example if the organisation is funded separately for intensive care or medical services or for non acute patients or outliers etc., then there is a need to identify costs associated with the components of every such output measure in use. This will vary depending on the health service delivery methods adopted. All of these factors have implications for casemix information system development.

There are essentially two different approaches which may be used to cost the products of health services. The first is referred to as clinical or product costing. It uses a bottom up approach by capturing data about all cases and the many services provided or activities undertaken during an episode of care. This is known as activity based costing. Clinical costing relies on the use of departmental feeder systems such as nursing workload monitoring systems in order to provide detailed information which is useful for all levels of decision making. These feeder systems use Relative Value Units (RVUs), as a basis of distributing total departmental costs on a per patient basis. These units are explained in the section on service weights.

It is relatively expensive to implement and maintain a clinical costing system in large organisations. However each country needs to have a selection of facilities that do have this capacity as it is needed to form the basis of any national funding allocation formula. It takes some time from system implementation before meaningful information becomes available. Initially decisions tend to be made solely on length of stay (LOS) as there is a strong correlation between cost per case type and LOS so this is used as a proxy performance indicator. Consequently every effort is made to simply discharge patients sooner to reduce the LOS and hence reduce costs. This in turn has an impact on quality as there are likely to be some patients who need to be re-admitted having been discharged too early.

The second option is to use what is referred to as cost modelling. In Australia the Yale Cost Model was originally used for this purpose, again this model has been refined over the years. It is a top down approach where all costs associated with the organisation's service provision are distributed to the products, however defined. The relationships between costs, activities and casemix products are modelled. These distinctions are not clear cut as some cost modelling does occur in the first approach as well to overcome the difficulties associated with activity based cost accounting in hospital departments including nursing.

12.3 Costing Departmental Services

To cost departmental services, accounting systems need to be merged and related to information pertaining to:
- all paid staff hours used by that department
- actual services provided per patient type (intermediary products or work units).

The quantification of any departmental workload monitoring system requires the measurement or estimation of staff hour usage from which a model is developed. The model then continues to be used as a proxy for that workload. A departmental workload monitoring system thus quantifies available paid staff usage and is a prerequisite to cost accounting. This is particularly useful in costing nursing services as this is the single biggest department contributing to the total product cost in hospitals. However not every health care agency has such sophisticated information systems.

Other departments also need to identify how best to relate their services and associated costs to individual patients. For example pathology departments undertake individual tests. Each test requires a certain amount of resources to produce the results. Such test can then be grouped on the basis of resource usage based on actual measurement or expert opinion, to produce relative value units (RVU). These data then need to be collectable by patient so that the cost can be related to the AR-DRG. In other words departmental casemix systems are feeder systems to the organisational casemix system.

12.3.1 Nursing Cost Centre Level Data for Casemix

Once a casemix system is in place there are many ways to make good use of the available data within an organization. However the benefits improve exponentially once several hospitals use casemix systems with the same data structures. As nursing is usually the biggest and most complex hospital cost centre we'll use this to illustrate the value of such cost centre data. Ward nursing costs may be derived once a nursing casemix system, described below, is in place. According to Picone et al [21$^{p.26}$] valid and reliable measures of nursing service must be established before the cost of nursing services can be determined. These comments apply equally to other departments. The importance of the validity of the source data used for the costing of such departmental services is directly related to the proportion contributed to the total product cost. This will vary for each category. Because nursing costs comprise a large proportion of the total costs for most AR-DRGs, the tracking and accuracy of nursing costs are very important. Valid nursing casemix systems such as Trend Care™ do this very well.

Nursing Casemix Systems

Nursing casemix systems are better known as patient acuity, dependency or nursing intensity systems. Such systems have been around since the 1950s and were primarily used to assist nurse managers with staff allocation to meet a ward's patient care needs. Once casemix systems were introduced, these nursing casemix systems formed the basis for identifying nursing costs per length of stay or episode of care for each case type however these were defined.

The Patient Assessment and Information System (PAIS) was developed during the early 1980's to facilitate efficient management of nursing resources relative to defined patient populations. The research underpinning this system measured how nurses distribute their time between activities and patients [22]. Patient characteristics and care requirements are used as a means of classifying patients into groups on the basis of average nursing resource usage. Thus each patient group represents a level of patient/nurse dependency. PAIS provides a good estimate of nursing resource requirements for each patient's category which may be compared with the caring staff resources actually provided. However this estimate is provided in total staff hours required and does not differentiate between different categories of caring staff based on skill mix. PAIS is used as a nursing resource allocation decision support system for management. The time values indicating nursing resource usage by patient dependency category were reviewed, validated and updated for all Queensland public hospitals during 1995 [23]. Such systems are also used to capture nursing costs by case type. PAIS was used for this purpose for the first Australian casemix costing study. Subsequent national costing studies have used a combination of systems then in use.

More recently data from the Trend Care™ system[1] has been used as this system is now used by many Australian and Asian health care facilities. This is a clinical decision support and workload management system specialising in; patient acuity / patient nurse dependency measurement, similar to but more advanced and automated than PAIS, clinical pathways and care plan management, patient assessments, and outcome measures. Recent versions of the TrendCare™ system have included many other functions providing reliable and up to date information to support the management of high quality care. This system has advanced HL7 messaging and interfacing capabilities enabling data to be imported and exported from and to other information systems so that there is only one entry point for patient and staff data. In this way data reliability is maximised. The TrendCare™ acuity, clinical pathway and care planning system caters for a wide range of patient types. Many TrendCare™ user sites have achieved significant improvements in quality care, staff satisfaction and efficiencies by using the system. Reports generated by the system enable nurse managers to measure the impact of identified trends and changes in patient activity and acuity over time and enables nurse leaders to work collaboratively with finance managers to appropriately resource nursing services for the future.

Measuring Nursing Resource Requirements

The development of Nursing casemix systems requires a researcher to measure nursing work relative to patient characteristics and nursing care needs. A similar process needs to be undertaken when an existing nursing casemix system such as when TrendCare™ is introduced to ensure that this system reflects actual nursing resource needs appropriately. When selecting a nursing casemix system it is important to evaluate the degree of accuracy and the appropriateness of the time values to the local situation. There are a variety of ways to do this, some methods are more reliable and accurate than others. First of all it is critical to arrive at an appropriate taxonomy describing the world of nursing practice before any measurement can take place. Existing systems such as TrendCare™ have done this and they have a system in place that enables such studies to be undertaken as part of the system implementation process.

Actual measurement studies are complex; industrial engineering or workstudy principles need to be applied. Nursing casemix systems provide valuable information enabling better nurse staff and quality management. Such systems also enable nurse managers to explain why more or less nurses are needed as it enables the monitoring of trends regarding patient mix and impacts following the adoption of various nurse practices. From an AR-DRG type of casemix perspective, the nursing casemix system needs to be able to classify patients on the basis of average daily nursing time requirements for that patient type, that is such systems must be able to determine individual patients' degree of nursing dependency.

Diers [16 [p.59]] was able to produce six DRG 'clusters' that shared similar nursing resource requirements, with estimated average times per patient day. These clusters were clinically credible. This work was repeated in Australia based on PAIS data. It was then demonstrated that where no time measurements were available, expert nurses were able to arrive at a nursing service weight per patient type based on their

---

[1] Trend Care Systems Pty Ltd http://www.trendcare.com.au/index.html

expert knowledge by consensus using a Delphi method [16 p.59]. This method is therefore an acceptable alternative to actual work measurement.

Nursing Service Cost Weights

There is a high correlation between length of stay and total nursing hours required to care for patients so that the average length of stay is a good indicator of the total nursing cost relative to other patients. The total cost of providing care for any patient type, such as any AR-DRG, during any one length of stay as an in-patient consists of many cost components, one of which is a nursing cost. One needs to be able to differentiate between the products or output measures of the organisation as a whole (that is by AR-DRGs) and departmental products such as nursing services delivered. Such departmental or intermediary products including nursing, imaging, critical care and others, contribute to and need to be incorporated in the final product. Departmental service weights based on relative value units (RVUs) are used for this purpose.

A nursing service cost weight is the measure of the mean cost of providing a nursing service for any patient type relative to the cost of nursing other patient types. To capture that total cost there is a need to know the average number of nursing hours provided each day. This information comes from the nursing casemix system, such as PAIS or TrendCare™, in use. For example if the average length of stay for an AR-DRG is 6 days, and typically such patients are grouped into a nurse dependency level 3 (4hrs) for 2 days, level 2 (3hrs) for 2 days and level 1 (2hrs) for 2 days then the total nursing hours for that length of stay equals 18 nursing hours. For another AR-DRG the total nursing hours for the mean length of stay may be 27 hours. The average of all patients in the study co-hort, that is using a sufficiently large sample to represent all patients in the country, area of interest or organization, is then allocated a cost weight that equals 1. All other patient type cost weights are then calculated relative to that. In other words each AR-DRG is allocated an average nursing relative value unit (RVU) from which the nursing service weight is calculated. Each AR-DRG needs to have data from a reasonable sample size, say a minimum of 20 patients, from which such averages are calculated, refer Table 1.

Table 1 Nursing Service Weight Description – an example

Patient types	Relative Value Unit (RVU) (Nursing Time/Length of Stay)	Nursing Service Weight
Average of all patients	20 hours	1.00
AR-DRG xx1	18 hours (18/20)	0.90
AR-DRG xx2	27 hours (27/20)	1.35

This information enables either the time to be multiplied by an hourly rate, as is done for clinical costing, where these data are used as a feeder system to capture the nursing cost component of an AR-DRG, or it is used to distribute the total allocated nursing costs proportionally using the nursing service weights (cost modeling) to arrive at the total nursing cost per AR-DRG for the study co-hort. Picone et al [21 p.59] also developed a model of relative nursing intensity by regressing nursing time on length of stay to produce a beta weight. Note the difference between the two, the former is used as a basis for cost modeling used by clinical costing systems, a bottom up approach, and the latter is ultimately used for cost modeling using a top down approach. Australia regularly undertakes a national casemix cost study and updates the nursing cost weights as part of that process as these data are used in the costing models that form the basis of hospital funding as part of the Australian Government policy initiatives. The latest such study used data obtained from Trendcare ™ systems as these are widely used around the country.

12.4 Casemix Information Systems

Information systems associated with casemix may be described as grouper software, costing systems, morbidity systems, hospital information systems, electronic health records, departmental (feeder) systems including nursing casemix, pathology, organ imaging systems and executive information systems. Given that all of these systems need to able to share data these may collectively be referred to as Enterprise systems[24]. Three determining factors for casemix system implementation are 1) economic considerations, 2) technical advances in medicine, computing and communications and 3) changes in philosophies regarding health service delivery. The latter is directly influenced by Government health policies. For example there may be a strong focus on primary health care requiring a reduction in acute hospital care services.

12.4.1 Casemix Implementation Requirements

Adopting 'casemix' is not a simple process as there are many factors that need to be considered by a number of different stakeholders who all need to work together. First it requires a decision about which classification system should be adopted nationally? It is recommended that an existing valid system such as the AR-DRGs, be adopted and later modified to meet local needs. The next decision is about which version of the ICD classification system should be used and how to ensure that there is the necessary workforce capacity to undertake clinical data coding, unless of course it is decided to implement appropriate electronic health record systems so that the necessary data extraction can be automated. Then there is a need to consider the financial information structures such as the charts of accounts in use, do these need to be modified? Before any nation considers implementing a casemix system it is necessary to fully consider all the cost and potential benefits of doing so. This chapter has explored these issues to enable you to make a start towards successfully implementing a casemix system within an overall enterprise system so that resources, quality and patient safety can be routinely measured and appropriately managed.

However it needs to be realised that there are other methods that may be adopted either in conjunction with casemix systems or as an alternative to manage resources, quality and patient safety. For example Chapter 31 describes a clinical practice improvement strategy. The ISO 9000 standards reflect principles of good management practices on which to base one's own quality management system design consolidating improved practices and procedures resulting from an ongoing policy of continuous improvement of all areas of work practice. In any event it is highly desirable if not essential to link quality with financial, personnel, process, output and outcomes information producing enterprise wide system as this produces meaningful new information on which to reliably base many important management decisions.

13. What Are Enterprise Systems?

Any enterprise can be viewed as a system where the many patterns of staff activity, the variety of work processes and information flows collectively represent that organisation's business processes. An enterprise information system is one that integrates all the information flows associated with these organizational business processes. An analysis of such business processes enables the many parts to be identified and documented within the context of the whole system. This forms the basis for system design. Ideally such analysis is undertaken from an ontological perspective such that all key organizational entities, ideas and events, are viewed together with their properties and relations so that they can be structured according to a system of categories. In other words the knowledge about the enterprise is represented by a structured identification of key entities, concepts, attributes and relationships.

Enterprise systems integrate information associated with all operational business activities across multiple sites as appropriate. From a health system perspective we argue that the basic underlying concept to underpin any enterprise system is the electronic health record of any individual for whom a health service is provided. All other business activities, particularly service delivery models in use or desired to be adopted, need to relate in some way to this fundamental concept to form the basis for an effective enterprise system design. Only well designed fully interoperable enterprise systems are able to adequately support resource, quality and safety management at minimal cost. The purposes for which casemix data is expected to be used determines the data processing and reporting requirements. Consequently it is essential that business processes, data flow and connectivity requirements are analysed to determine information needs and to document casemix system functional requirements. This in turn determines desired system architectures and other specifications.

13.1 Business, Data and Information Architectures

Casemix systems need to be within enterprise wide systems , controlled centrally in accordance with an enterprise wide IT strategy, be standards compliant and have adopted an open systems approach to enable network connectivity and the ability of various database management systems to span multiple networks and multiple data bases. An open system is one in which multiple software applications from multiple vendors work seamlessly across multiple computing platforms, driven by common interfaces. It is important for healthcare organisations to adopt system architectures that can handle all its business complexities yet have sufficient flexibility and expandability to accommodate future changes and associated information needs.

Ad hoc system acquisition and deployment within organizations for the purpose of meeting specific, usually departmental, requirements have resulted in variations in hardware and software adoptions for multiple software applications within one resulting in silos of information due to system incompatibility. In such instances the integration of such applications requires the development and maintenance of middleware to enable data transfer (messaging) between systems. This is costly and not as effective as the adoption of fully integrated enterprise systems. Within the health industry it is also highly desirable to have compatible enterprise systems so that information flow can cross organisational boundaries with ease. This is certainly a requirement for effective supply chain management and for the successful adoption of individual e-health records within a nation.

However health care service providers are not easy to define or be uniquely identified. In today's world there are multiple enterprise variations to be considered. For example a single organization can provide any mix of services from multiple locations; several organizations can provide services from a single location; a single service can be provided by multiple facilities (e.g. telemedicine); and a service or capability can go to a person (e.g. ambulance, home care). In addition each organization has its own funding structure based on ownership and legal responsibilities.

Healthcare enterprises are 'open' systems in that healthcare services are not delivered in isolation; they are part of a bigger national health system that provides it with funding, a capital infrastructure, an educated workforce, equipment, supplies, information and knowledge resources. Enterprise system development requires successful coordination, integration and sharing of information in a context of changing work processes, significant organizational change and forever changing external political and institutional environments. One associated aim is to reduce the carbon footprint by electronically supporting all business processes such as by moving from paper to electronic records and cutting down on travel costs through telehealth and maximizing efficiency by creating the right tools, redesigning service delivery models and/or restructuring service processing. Information and communication technologies are crucial tools to enable any large and complex modern enterprise to model, measure and then manage business processes, and target sustainable practices.

14. Conclusion

Resource management within any health service needs to undertaken in a sustainable manner. This requires a careful analysis and monitoring of all operations so that strategies may be adopted to continuously ensure that changing demands for health services along with changes in delivery models and treatments can continue to be accommodated in a safe, effective and efficient manner. This requires the implementation of suitable enterprise wide information services, including the adoption of a national casemix schema and workforce planning. It is highly desirable for nations to establish a suitable health policy and governance infrastructure that supports a reduction is health service demands ,via the adoption of health promotion, illness and injury prevention strategies[2], and the provision of safe quality health services via the national adoption of foundational health informatics standards and associated legislatures.

References:

[1] Coiera E and Hovenga E.J.S Building a sustainable health system. IMIA Yearbook of Medical Informatics 07, Methods of Information in Medicine 2007 Vol.46 Suppl 1 pp.11-18

---

[2] Australian Council for Safety and Quality in Health Care, http://safetyandquality.org

[2] Buchan H. Gaps between best evidence and practice: causes for concern. *MJA* 2004;180:S48-9. http://mja.com.au/public/issues/180_06_150304/buc10752_fm.html cited August 2008
[3] Boyce N, McNeil J, Graves D, Dunt D, 1997 Quality and outcome indicators for acute healthcare services: a research project for the national hospital outcomes program, Australian Government Department of Health and Family Services, Canberra
[4] Cochrane A.L 1972 Effectiveness and efficiency. Random reflections on health services. London: Nuffield Provincial Hospitals Trust (reprinted in 1989 in association with the British Medical Journal).
[5] Fields M.J and Lohr K.N (eds) 1992 Guidelines for clinical practice – from development to use. National Academy Press, Institute of Medicine, Washington D.C.
[6] McCormick K.A and Fleming B 1992 Clinical practice guidelines, Health progress, December pp.30-34
[7] Culyer A.J (ed) 1990 Standards for socioeconomic evaluation of health care products and services, Springer-Verlag, Berlin
[8] Nord E 1992 An alternative to QALYs: the saved young life equivalent (SAVE), British Medical Journal, Vol.305, 10 October pp.875-877
[9] Coiera E When conversation is better than computerization. Journal of the American Medical Informatics Association 2000; Vol.7 No.3 pp.277-86
[10] Australian Government, Department of Health and Ageing – Casemix http://www.health.gov.au/internet/main/publishing.nsf/Content/Casemix-1 cited July 2008
[11] Dawes S, Cresswell A, Pardo T, Tompson F. Modeling the social and technical processes of interorganisational information integration. ACM International Conference Proceedings Series Vol.89 – Proceedings of the 2005 national conference on Digital government research 2005 pp.289-90
[12] National Health Service in the United Kingdom - Healthcare Resource Groups (HRGs), http://www.ic.nhs.uk/casemix cited July 2008
[13] Canadian Institute for Health Information's (CIHI) – casemix http://www.cihi.ca/cihiweb/dispPage.jsp?cw_page=casemix_e cited July 2008
[14] Fetter R.B. 1985, DRGs - fact and fiction, *Australian Health Review Vol.8 No.2 pp.105-115*
[15] Young D.W and Saltman R.B, Hospital Cost Containment and the Quest for Institutional Growth: A Behavioral Analysis", *Journal of Public Health Policy,* September 1983, pp.313-334.
[16] Diers D 1999 Casemix and Nursing, *Australian Health Review Vol.22 No.2 pp56-68*
[17] Bozzo J, Carlson B, Diers D 1998 Using hospital data systems to find target populations: New tools for clinical nurse specialists, *Clinical Nurse Specialist, vol.12, No, 2 pp 86-91*
[18] National Centre for Classification in Health (NCCH) – ICD-10-AM http://nis-web.fhs.usyd.edu.au/ncch_new/2.6.aspx accessed July 2008
[19] Australian Institute of Health and Welfare (AIHW) - METeOR http://www.aihw.gov.au/dataonline.cfm cited July 2008
[20] KPMG 1993 National Costing Study 1993, Report to the Commonwealth Department of Health, Housing, Local Government and Community Services. KPMG Peat Marwick, Adelaide
[21] Picone D., Ferguson L., Hathaway V. et al 1993, *NSW Nursing Costing Study*, Sydney Metropolitan Teaching Hospitals Nursing Consortium. September.
[22] Hovenga E J S 1995 Casemix, Hospital Nursing Resource Usage and Costs. PhD thesis, University of New South Wales, Sydney
[23] Hovenga E.J.S and Hindmarsh C 1996 Queensland PAIS Validation Study, CQU and Qld Health, Brisbane.
[24] Hovenga E J S and Whymark G 1997 Health Information Systems in a Casemix Environment in: Courtney M (Ed) *Financial Management in Health Services*, Maclennan Petty, Sydney

Review Questions

1. What are the critical characteristics of quality management?
2. How is organisational performance best measured?
3. Why should a country/organisation consider introducing a casemix system?
4. Can you explain the significance of coding accuracy?

Health Informatics
E.J.S. Hovenga et al. (Eds.)
IOS Press, 2010
doi:10.3233/978-1-60750-476-4-385

27. Health Supply Chain Management

Rolf ZIMMERMAN[1a] , Pat GALLAGHER[b]

aConsultant, SMS Management & Technology Limited, Melbourne, Australia
bDirector, Casprel Pty Ltd, Northbridge, NSW, Australia

Abstract. This chapter gives an educational overview of:
- The actual application of supply chain practice and disciplines required for service delivery improvement within the current health environment.
- A rationale for the application of Supply Chain Management (SCM) approaches to the Health sector.
- The tools and methods available for supply chain analysis and benchmarking.
- Key supply chain success factors

Keywords. Computer Communication Networks, Information Management, Medical Informatics Applications, Medical Order Entry Systems, Safety, Health Care Systems, Health Services Administration, Materials Management-Hospital, Quality Control,Decision Support Systems-Management, Database, Systems Analysis

1.   What is Supply Chain Management?

This chapter serves primarily as an introduction to supply chain practice and disciplines. It is by no means exhaustive, but hopefully provides some stimulation for health practitioners to seek further understanding and reap the clinical and efficiency benefits from opportunities offered in the "Walmart" disciplines [1]. Every health service is dependent upon the availability of a wide variety of equipment, products and supplies (physical items) at the point of care. Such physical items need to be purchased from and delivered to the organization by a large number of suppliers. Making these supplies available at the point of care in the right quantities in a timely fashion to meet specific needs requires good management, especially given the many factors such as shelf life and unknown variations in demand that also need to be considered during this process. It's about integrating key business processes between many suppliers and many end users. Supply chain management is about:
- planning based on demand and supply needs,
- sourcing stocked, made to order or engineered to order products,
- making use of products such as preparing substances in a pharmacy in accordance with a prescription,
- delivery of products needed at the point of care, and
- returning unused or faulty supplies.

The consideration of health informatics is usually focused upon the application of

---

[1] Corresponding Author: RZimmerman@smsmt.com

Information Systems to clinical process improvement, knowledge management and patient administration. What is often not understood is that all these activities are united by the requirement to identify or transfer information about physical items between them. This in itself is far from revolutionary, since patient details, diagnoses and procedural information also need to be transferred between procedures. There is presently considerable cutting-edge work being conducted on the development of common standards for the transfer of information between clinical and Patient Administration Systems (PAS), and advanced knowledge management and diagnostic support systems. This is not occurring in the supply-chain discipline for one fundamental reason....'It's all been done before by the worlds' top 900 companies' via the Supply Chain Council (SCC)[2], a global non-profit consortium established in 1996 to make dramatic and rapid improvements in supply chain processes. One only has to visit a hotel chain or retail grocery outlet, to witness automated reprovisioning and the application of simple stock item data to the customer management processes. The high order "clinical" outcomes for these two businesses include:

- The ability to track a variety of services in a hotel and tally a bill of everything from the mini-bar use to meals in the restaurant to your room bill. The hotel can also see your room preference for your next booking.
- The matching of your shopping profile against a loyalty scheme, and the provision for rewards for customer behaviours.

Once we start to apply these common outcomes to health care, some outstanding opportunities begin to present themselves. The key issue is that there are no secrets to the achievement of improved supply chain driven outcomes. We just need to apply the lessons of those many pioneers in the retail and manufacturing sectors and implement suitable e-commerce systems supporting supply chain management in the health industry.

1.1 How Does Supply Chain Management Apply to the Health Industry?

Here we argue that every clinical decision is a procurement decision. Gallagher [2] noted that to date little progress has been made so far in fundamentally improving general hospital clinical and process outcomes yet patient safety can be significantly enhanced by linking supply chain process improvements to patient care in all health sectors. Whilst there are many seemingly insurmountable issues in health care management, supply-chain disciplines offer substantial opportunity for realistic process improvement in core support processes and potentially clinical processes. A hospital supply chain goes well beyond medical products; that is we are not just dealing with pharmaceuticals and devices. Aside from over the counter (OTC) products and toiletries we should also include: cleaning, beds, food, tools and equipment procurement in the mix. The same rules apply to all types of merchandise and equipment: create a unique numbering system and hold that core data in a central database from which all participants download information when they need it, and when they need it to exchange that information internally and externally to or from a hospital.

To help the reader better understand the basic differences between say, a retail supply chain community commitment to supply excellence and the vastly different

---

[2] Supply Chain Council (SCC) http://www.supply-chain.org

view in the ehealth sector one needs to understand the 'people' factors. Which is that clinicians and 'business people see the same thing in a different light. A retail community is reasonably harmonised and well informed about the importance of customer facing performance and their role in having the right product at the right place and at the right time. Whereas that is not so in the health industry. In health the attitudes are generally more inward looking to the needs of 'my patient' in 'my department' and not the bigger picture. While health people understand the 'five rights' of product availability for a patient; *right product, right delivery, right patient, right place and right time,* few concern themselves with how the first element, right product is actually achieved.

Hospitals are not hotels and are not shops. Management of these enterprises strive to manage the cost of inventory as a mission critical responsibility. In a hospital the nurse's focus (quite rightly) is on patient care. Furthermore, we are often told that "health is complex' in the context of change in adopting and adapting to technology based business processes, such as e-commerce. This is not really true. What is complex, in this case, is the interaction of people towards their professional skill delivery and patient care responsibilities compared to the non-clinical process of supply issues. This is a real problem. The core goal is to establish the mindset that the supply chain is a legitimate link to the clinical chain, and not a separate system, operated and run by 'different' people in parallel to care givers and other clinical professionals. This requires us to examine the existing systems, standards and technologies in use together with experience sharing to turn a manual, largely paper based legacy process into an automated service. Systems include e-commerce platforms, an example of standards is the purchase order templates and catalogue structure. A technology could be a barcode. Experience comes from a wide range of sources including publications such as this book The aim is to deliver a service that allows full visibility of product movement and location, from the source of supply to the point of patient care or consumption.

Who is the core user/client of a hospital supply chain system? A nurse. It is a nurse who is the pivotal point of data reticulation and it is the nurse who is the primary conduit for most products directly or indirectly consumed for patient care. Traditionally people play a major role in the outcomes of a good or bad supply chain. If there is no trust from the nursing community, that the supply people will support them adequately, then all sorts of complicated trouble looms. For example nurses will hoard supplies if they fear there is likely to be a period of non availability.

However the major factor and the major goal of a supply chain is to deliver, over and above the expected criteria, this may be expressed in one word – and that word is *convenience.* There should be total convenience in the work load asked of a nurse to undertake supply related tasks that help their care giving role rather than add a burden to their care giving role and time.

Australia has undertaken a major six year Pharmaceutical electronic Commerce and Communications (PeCC) project researching and implementing information technology systems into the health sector supply chains emulating the retail industry's methodologies adapted slightly to suit the healthcare community [3]. Seventy-four companies contributed about one third of the project's costs as stakeholders for this exploratory and communications effort moving forward only when change management issues had been addressed. There were many beneficial achievements, key findings were that when fully implemented the major advantages arising from PeCC will be reduced waste through improvements to supply chain management, timely, accurate and useful availability of actual costs of health consumables and better cost management. One large teaching hospital case study undertaken during the PeCC project examined the impact on clinical services and patient care. Over a two-year period this effort was a fantastic success and delivered incredibly good statistics. Built on trust and communication the supply people instituted and maintained a total promise of full stock availability in every ward and theatre without any nurse needing to lift a finger or phone/fax to make it happen. Using EAN/GS1 barcodes the new supply chain methodology delivered 99% service levels and at the same time decreased the overall stock holdings and errors, waste and obsolescence by incredible amounts. The memorable comment from a senior NUM (Nurse Unit Manager) was this telling line:

"My staff are whistling at work – I haven't heard a happy nurse whistling for years"

This hospital also adhered to the 'static' catalogue functionality. And over time the instances of medical errors relating to product selection and supply fell way dramatically because the supply person and the nurse were involved in reading the same product barcodes and then the nurse reading the patient wrist bands, as a routine. Key points of this case study are presented in Box1 (based on [3^{p. 43}]).

Box 1 Large Teaching Hospital e-Commerce Implementation Case Study

<table>
<tr><td colspan="3">Large teaching hospital had spent four years searching for cost effective measures and new processes, including the IT component, for using e-commerce to manage medical consumable products.</td></tr>
<tr><th>Problem Statement</th><th>New Process</th><th>Results</th></tr>
<tr>
<td>
<ul>
<li>Large ageing and depreciating stockpile,</li>
<li>Multiple storage areas for stock along the patient care chain</li>
<li>Large infrastructure within the Stores department</li>
<li>Labour intensive, paper based system highly prone to error</li>
<li>Most telling was that research found that the average Australian nurse spent up to 20% of their time on other tasks.</li>
</ul>
</td>
<td>
<ul>
<li>Barcoding all items</li>
<li>Allocating 1.4% of annual budget on IT expenditure</li>
<li>Adopted e-commerce practices</li>
<li>Re-engineering existing system</li>
</ul>
</td>
<td>
<ul>
<li>Reduced time to replenish stock from 3hrs to 20 min</li>
<li>Hospital deficit of $6M turned into $1M surplus</li>
<li>Nurses were freed from previous tasks related to purchasing, supply, logistics matters and related paperwork</li>
<li>Culture change, effective union negotiations</li>
<li>Reduced wastage and inventory from $600,000 to less than $57,000</li>
<li>Moved from a 'just in case' mindset to a 'just in time' approach</li>
</ul>
</td>
</tr>
</table>

1.2 Rationale for Supply Chain Improvement

So where does the supply-chain fit in any nation's health industry? The Australian government noted that the United States, Europe and Japan were in the process of redesigning hospital supply chains and developing supporting foundations for e-commerce whilst the United Kingdom and Canada were also committed to an e-commerce agenda for health in 2002 [4^{p.6}]. Australia represents a small market so needs to position itself to be responsive to global trends. More recently the Australian National eHealth Transition Authority (NeHTA) has published the business architecture for e-Health procurement [5^{p.6}] in which a number of direct and indirect benefits to be gained were published. These are summarised as cost reductions, quicker order fulfillment, automated order tracking, lower disputed invoice rate, logistics integration, better demand and supply matching.

Whilst NEHTA and the Health jurisdictions are struggling with the macro –

issues, supply-chain reform is already benchmarked (globally across all industry sectors), achievable (many case studies) and can be used as a tool to influence related activities. Some of the touch points where supply chain activities touching specialist Health Care issues, these are:

- Patient Safety
- Process improvement, and
- Provision of metrics, benchmarks and measures for harvesting the "value" from process improvement

These "value propositions" for health will be explained shortly. Firstly, let us consider the broad reasons why supply chain reform is so compelling for the health sector. In simple terms it is because the world's supply chain problems have largely been solved by retail and distribution businesses. Whilst the population has been ageing, national medical costs have been growing and clinicians have been developing better cures and procedures, the product / service delivery mechanisms have become increasingly ripe for major reform. The value proposition is simply to free-up increasingly scarce resources for a focus on better health outcomes. To make the proposition even more compelling, the top 900 global supply chain managers have documented all the best practices required to make this happen via the SCC by developing the supply chain world's most widely accepted framework for evaluating and comparing supply chain activities and their performance (SCCRv9.0:2008)[3] A combination of information technology advances and a development of process maturity, (standards) allowing increased sharing of information between organisations, has revolutionised the distribution and supply of material.

In the book by Thomas L Friedman, "The World is Flat", the supply chain revolution is highlighted with examples from Walmart and UPS, the world's largest package delivery company and a leading global provider of specialized transportation and logistics services. Friedman [1] explains how IT advances and some innovative thinking has allowed these two companies to relentlessly improve competitive positioning and, in the case of UPS provide completely new services. Walmart has used the principles of supply chain management to drive out costs and unnecessary process steps from its business. One percent here, a couple there, and before long they have a major cost advantage. This is effectively what Woolworths (grocery stores) has achieved in Australia with its' project Refresh. Incremental process improvements have built up to deliver a $220 million dollar per year advantage over their similar sized rival – Coles. UPS initially followed the process improvement path, and then found it was in a new business space - insourcing. Once they had developed a business that could provide scale logistics services to small and medium businesses alike, they also found that they had developed competencies for re-engineering and management of whole specialist logistics operations. UPS now manages warranty repairs for Toshiba laptops, distribution of Ford motor cars and many other specialist logistics activities, on behalf of their parent companies. They are so good at it, that none of us have noticed it happening. So what about the management of health supply chains? No problem. It is just like any other, with considerable opportunity for those organisations that become first movers, and apply the basics.

---

[3] Supply Chain Operations Reference (SCOR) Model contains process maps and benchmarked best practices, from member organisations, at: www.supply-chain.org.

2. Measurable Benefits of Supply Chain Improvement

What are the benefits for the Health industry and population at large? The projected outcomes based on our experiences are significantly compelling and ironically perhaps reasonably 'easy' to accomplish.

Money: world wide the Health sector opinion makers believe that about 15% of all products purchased for a hospital are never used on, or by a patient. In broad terms, in Australia, that is around $2 billion of wastage that could be re-directed to other uses. The money that disappears is distributed between:

- Waste - thrown out at end-of-batch life, or part used dosage/packs. This is quite common in environments where medication is highly subsidised. It is also a symptom of a lack of systems support to account for partial product delivery and enable redistribution of the residual (ie: over prescribed).
- Theft – may be more significant then at first believed. Australia loses $7mil in PBS drug sent off-shore. The benchmarked "good" hospital used in this chapter found that after gaining stock visibility, that their transportation contractors we stealing 10% of all stock dispatched by their wholesaler.
- Miscounting and mistakes – Common where manual processes exist. API lost sight of 16% (and had to publicly write it off) of their wholesale stock recently.

Accounts payable: essentially the accounts payable department is a quality measure of a supply chain. If an invoice can be paid without error, query or delay, then the system is effective. If not, then paying suppliers becomes problematical. Here in Australia this leads to suppliers refusing to deliver product until their account is paid. Why is this relevant? If that is a crucial catheter, that is not available, it will affect patient care with total certainty. So the link between – *supply, payment, patient care and record keeping* is demonstrably important (but undervalued and under managed) not just by administrators but by clinicians as well

Shrinkage: similarly, the general consensus is that theft is the core reason for wastage; this is not so. There are many reasons why money goes 'missing' and only some are due to illegal activity. The remainder are caused by carelessness, overbuying, hoarding, dated stock, transcription errors and notably the inability to have electronic visibility of a products location and value at anytime. The old saying being –*'if you do not know the problem, you cannot fix the problem'*

The fact that a hospital accountant cannot reliably locate and value the entire inventory available for use is a hidden problem in most hospitals. This can be as low as 5%, an average of 10% or in very large and poorly run sites as much as 15% to 20%. Using the retail comparison again their 'shrinkage' is usually under 3% and often less than 2%.

Errors: across the board and in every facet of a hospital mistakes reduce dramatically when data is aligned and not re-worked; dropping from double digit rates to one or two percentage points.

Productivity: nurses become ever so much more effective when other people undertake supporting tasks that deliver trust and certainty for nurses, in a convenient manner, rather than under constant aggravation that requires constant re-working.

Patient care: a result of better supply visibility, less errors, more nurse time and product availability, is the beneficial focus on a patient, all at a lower cost than any manual supply system

3.   Patient Safety

By far the most prominent health supply chain issue is associated with patient safety. The main risk being: medication mis-management. Many think that medical incidents are all the result of an interrelationship of complex clinical processes. In reality the administration of incorrect medication or dosage is invariability a supply-chain issue. Fixed by more accurate facility level data management and streamlined record/dispensary processes. Hopefully, NeHTA will deliver a National Medical Product Catalogue, but in the mean time it behoves us to maintain an accurate list of products by facility and organisation. Many organisations have up to five times the number of items listed, as actually exist (in hospitals up to 300,000 listed items to 60,000 valid ones). One organisation conducted two years of progressive data cleansing, to find that they had to delete another 8,000 items (of 24,000) after they conducted a data match with their suppliers. This impacts on the delivery process, because it greatly increases the risk of ordering the wrong product or dosage and mis-identifying at dispense, by up to the ratio of data inaccuracy. This is before one accounts for any process 'mistakes'. The potential for improvement is profound. Due to the voluntary incident reporting regime in Australia, it is hard to get confirmed figures on medication incidents. Based on US data Bates, Cohen et al [6] reported that drug complications represent the most commonly occurring adverse events. In addition they noted that costs of inefficiencies related to error that do not result in injury are also great. One example given that has relevance to supply chain management is about when a medication dose is not available for a nurse to administer, this tends to produce a delay of at least two hours or the dose is missed. Nurses spend a lot of time tracking down such medications.

The US Department of Health and Human Services Food and Drug Administration (FDA)[4] began monitoring medication error reports in 1992[8]. As a result they recognised the significance of the high incidence of medication error and noted contributing factors. In 2004 the FDA finalized a rule requiring bar codes on the labels of thousands of human drugs and biological products. This measure's aim is to protect patients from preventable medication errors by helping ensure that health professionals give patients the right drugs at the appropriate dosages. The rule also requires machine-readable information on container labels of blood and blood components intended for transfusion. The FDA estimates that these rules will help prevent nearly 500,000 adverse events and transfusion errors while saving $93 billion in health costs over 20 years. This makes the effort involved in improved management seem like a small price to pay to protect the public against this issue.

3.1 Improved Processes

One of the universally accepted figures for measured errors is 16% for each manual transaction in a value chain. It gets more interesting when you also consider that each error made takes an average of three times the effort of the original transaction to rectify. This is a Supply-Chain benchmark that has been the basis for the introduction of barcode technology and automated data entry. How does this apply to health care?

---

[4] http://www.fda.gov/

Too often processes are not automated and there are key bits of information passed on paper, by voice or not at all. The result is compound errors at the rate of 16% compounded by the number of instances a manual transaction occurs. Rework and lost efficiency can be significant. For example one hospital ward was found to have 25 manual processes to interface with a patient. This Hospital, in Melbourne, underwent a Supply-Chain improvement project, which provided products direct to ward without manual stock-takes by nurses. This released 20% more nursing time for the same staff. The automation of rationing, medication and services tracking also provides opportunity for accurate cost apportionment and automated reordering. The same disciplines are equally valid for automating report generation (for the many different agencies requiring them). Hotels have done this for years, and as a result they rarely furnish the wrong mini-bar bills to their clients. They also maintain outstanding visibility over their operating margins.

3.2 Metrics for Cost Savings

"Show me the money", is always the core question for process improvement. Supply Chain advocates have been benchmarking the opportunities for years. The commonly provided international benchmark figure for each transaction costs greater than $50 in process costs to raise a manual (paper) transaction document (PO, Invoice etc) [7]. This shrinks to less than $5 for the generation of an automated electronic document. At $45 difference this amounts to $45,000pa savings if you produce 1,000 purchase order to your suppliers. One organisation known to the author spent $275,000 on a new system for ordering and dispensary. It automated 20,000 purchase orders p.a. with a Net saving of about $900,000p.a. Add to this saving our previous issue of errors reduction. Not only is wastage reduced following automation but the total cost savings may also be estimated. The cost to fix each transaction error is US $70 each. It doesn't take many to create a business case for process simplification and automation. Now add a greater risk of possible death, on your watch.

4.   Other Opportunities

Like the United Parcel Service (UPS) there are opportunities to be harvested from this new "Flat Earth" of global connectivity and standards. Consider the future. One day there will be a common electronic medical (health) record, combined with e-scripts and e-ordering. No longer will the patient be considered only in terms of the treatment they are presently receiving, or their current demographic. It will now be possible for governments and health funds to manage cradle-to-grave healthcare. This will create a whole new model for combined funding or health, retirement, nursing homes and death benefits. For now we will focus on the basics.

4.1 How Do We Achieve It? (Tools for the Practitioner)

1. *Data alignment*. We need to catalogue the patient and the product. That is we need lists of patients and products, each with unique identifiers and structured in a manner that enable electronic access and accurate identification of the right patient and product. The procedure will look after itself. One of the key issues

compromising patient safety is the assignment of the wrong product, dose or timing.

2. *Standards* come into play here, as the mechanism for ensuring data alignment between process partners.

3. *Process improvement* is not a black art for supply chains. Supply chain operations reference (SCOR) process maps can serve as a template to compare and update existing processes. An overview booklet and quick reference guide to version 9 (released March 2008) of this model is available to the public via the SCC website (http://www.supply-chain.org). Compare your own processes against these. If you have a process that is genuinely unique due to clinical reasons, use the equivalent SCOR process as a benchmark. If it is not unique, use a template. You will be in good company – the top 900 supply managers globally. Alternatively, if a process does not appear in this reference model – review it to determine if it is needed at all.

One of the most practical and compelling aspects of a detailed supply chain process model, is the opportunity to use it in the measurement of performance. Each of the processes in the SCOR process matrix is linked by the data transferred between them and the standardisation of performance metrics. This enables an organisation to map the links between internal processes and to other organisations in their supply chain. It is the latter that is truly empowering. This is because it has enabled the measurement of performance across supply chains. Large retailers have needed standards metrics to work with trading partners and to allow them to share the benefits of efficiencies. Box2 lists the 13 core high level metrics defined by the SCOR model. These provide a basis for agreement on measures between trading partners, and they provide some very interesting data when applied to existing supply chains.

Box 2 Benchmarking - map the gaps - 13 SCOR measures

- Delivery performance
- Fill rate
- Perfect order fulfilment
- Order fulfilment lead time
- Supply chain response time
- Production flexibility
- Supply chain management costs
- Cost of goods sold
- Value added productivity
- Warranty cost or returns processing costs
- Cash to cash cycle time
- Inventory days of supply
- Asset turns

4.2 Practical Comparisons

When we apply the metrics to a "real" supply chain, we often find that it is the first time anyone has actually attempted to measure performance. Without going into the organisational or cultural issues behind this, it suffices to say that the magnitude of outcomes can provide an initial impetus to further consider supply chain improvement. Table 1 provides an example comparing processes between similar sized hospitals. The differences are substantial.

Table 1 Process Comparison Between Two Similar Sized Hospitals

Process	Hospital 1	Hospital 2
Deliveries per week	800	50
Invoices per month	20,000	3000
Pay reconcile and settle	30% 1st time	95% 1st time
Hard & soft shrinkage estimate/measured	18%	8%
Internal fill service level	90%	99%
Delivery errors	+5%	Less than 1%
Stock turnover	4 yrs	Average 10 times per Annum
Clinical time spent on supply management	Up o 20%	Almost nil

Be aware that rarely are all the SCOR measures quantifiable. In many organisations three measures, out of thirteen, are the only possible ones to be confirmed. The result is that we measure what we can, as a basis to further improve. In the example above we can see that hospital 1 generates many more invoices for the same amount of net activity. They have less bulk deliveries, have trouble settling payments 70% of the time. Shrinkage or wastage, internal service levels and delivery errors are all considerably higher. Finally it takes four years to turnover their stock and the clinical staff (nurses) spend 20% of their time on managing local (ward) supply issues. By adding the incremental costs of each process issue will show an enormous efficiency gap between hospital 1 and 2. The most compelling figure is the final one. Hospital 2 nursing staff spent 20% more time on the core business of looking after patients.

4.3 Industry Level Benchmarking

Opportunity analysis can be undertaken when we look at the industry as a whole. This approach can be less confronting for organisations, allowing senior management time to see supply improvements as an opportunity. The advantage of seeing that the whole health sector does not perform to the level of the retail sector is two fold.

Firstly, the opportunity to improve is easily confirmed by benchmarking against the best practitioners, and the magnitude of the potential to improve can be assessed. Secondly, the opportunity is able to be seen less as "showing our dirty laundry" to publishing improvements against industry best practice. In pure competitive terms, senior management can be enthused about the opportunity to quickly lead the industry in efficiency gains, with low risk, by applying proven methods. If we apply the SCOR metrics to both retail and health industries as shown in Table 2, the opportunities in health are clear. The retail industries have long contributed to global benchmarked best practice in supply-chain management. To compare their industry sector performance to health (using the standard benchmarks) we can easily assess the magnitude of possible gains. This can be partly by direct comparison between known performance figures (ie: fill rates at 9% difference) or by inference in those areas where no performance measures are available (SCM costs are generally not accounted for in health, hence figures like 20% more time nursing are the closest quantifiable figure of SCM effort). The first step to realising these opportunities is to understand what is not measured, indicating where to look, and what measures to apply to these target areas.

Table 2 Comparing SCOR Metrics Applied to Retail and Health Industries

Metric	Retail Industry	Health Industry
Delivery	80% correct	Less so
Fill Rate	Known/98%	Unknown/89%
Fulfillment	Few back orders/larger	More/random
Lead time	Slot times	Any/many times
Response	Customer driven	Supply – 'too good'
Flexibility	End to end	Dysfunctional
SCM Cost	Benchmarked	Vaguely aware
COGS	Margin focus	Accounting focus
Value add	Higher productivity	More tribal
Credit/returns	1.5%	+/- 10%
Cash Cycle	11, 28, 40 days	30, 64, 92 days
Days of stock	Counted in weeks	Counted in months
Asset Turns (annual)	12 to 30 times	3 to 12 times

5. Australian Experiences in Applying Health Supply Chain Practice.

Australian experiences over the last ten years in developing the necessary health specific practitioner tools and applying the concepts contained in this chapter are presented here as a demonstration of the various difficulties encountered during such a process. There are a number of lessons to be learned from these experiences in Australia and Turkey.

   The PeCC project mentioned previously became the catalyst for at least five follow up projects on:

1. Development of Health e-commerce technical standards (Standards Australia IT-14-10 sub-committee)[5]
2. Building a central Australian catalogue for medical products (Medical Coding Council of Australia (MCCA)
3. A nationally focused hospital based project undertaken by the Hacateppe University Research Project based in Ankara Turkey, to introduce a single patient numbering system, introduce a single costing system and to create a single (TGA-like) product catalogue.
4. The Pharmaceutical Extranet Gateway (PEG) to create an integrated e-commerce network across all points of supply to the point of sale
5. The Pharmaceutical Integrated Logistics (PIL) system, a sister project to PEG operating to meet the needs of the Surgeon General in the Australian Defence Force's medical and dental supply and records requirements for the Army, Navy and Airforce.

5.1 Case Study 1: PeCC project

The PeCC project (1996-2000) was an Australian Government initiative under the auspices of the Department of Industry, Science and Technology and a DIST branch known as NOIE (National Office for the Information Economy) (More, McGrath 2000). The primary task was (and still is) to get the entire re-supply and consumer community to accept the use of a unique product identifier and to use this number without exception throughout the supply process.

---

[5] http://www.e-health.standards.org.au/cat.asp?catid=14

Of course we refer to the GS1 (barcode) numbering system then known as EAN. Supply chain systems cannot deliver any benefit at all unless a GS1 number is the sole identifier of product information exchange and reticulation. And as you will read further on, this simple concept requires an investment in cataloguing and other tools to make and deliver end-to-end electronic visibility of product as it moves from the supply environment into the clinical sector and to a patient and a patient's record

The simple plan was to firstly implement demonstration outcomes in retail pharmacy, transfer that knowledge and skill into hospital pharmacy and then move into medical surgical and other supply requirements in a hospital. Broadly speaking the pharmacy model worked perfectly and the other sectors are only now becoming partly compliant.

Was PeCC successful? The answer is a qualified 'yes', primarily because PeCC became the catalyst for other projects. On the other hand there was a level of failure to recruit the entire community to accept and think 'e-commerce' as a daily benefit to their function within a hospital.

5.2 Case study 2: Standards Australia IT-4-10 Health e-commerce Sub-committee

In 2000 the PeCC 'team' with its knowledge was recruited to form a new working party at Standards Australia's Health Informatics IT-014 Committee that became the IT-014-10 (Health e-commerce) sub-committee. The Australian Government's department of health and ageing asked this group to develop and publish e-commerce document standards to underpin the gradual move from manual and proprietary systems to global standards and e-enablement of the entire chain. The entire chain? Yes, this means the clinical chain as well in recognition that supply chains are in fact an integrated part of the clinical chain. This understanding can be best expressed in two example questions: –

1. *'if a nurse reaches for a critical item and it is not there, who do we blame, and is this a supply or is this a clinical problem?'*

The answer is we blame the supply people and yes it is a clinical problem at this point. The other question was –

2. *'if a medical misadventure occurs due to wrong product use and consumption, who is at fault?'*

The answer to this question is provided in an Institute of Medicine (IOM) report [9] that urged the adoption of unique product identifiers for both supply and clinical use. In the former context it was to save an estimated 15% waste of money and stock in USA supply chains and to help minimise medical misadventure, then quoted as 90,000 deaths a year. Of these 90,000 deaths over 53% were related back to a product supply problem and/or mistake.

Was IT-014-10 successful? Absolutely, in two short years the 30-person group published a (worlds first) complete set of e.commerce EDI and XML trading documents, notably the:

PO	*Purchase order*
POA	*Purchase order acknowledgement*
ASN	*Advanced shipping notice Invoice*
RA	*Remittance advice, and above all the*
PRICAT	*The standard format of population a central controlling catalogue*

The secret to achieving effective supply systems and safe clinical supply systems is to use a single catalogue, with aligned and harmonized data based on a unique identifier (like a car number plate). The basis of this catalogue was the acceptance that the supplier, the manufacturer 'owned' the core identification data and only the supplier should ever populate or amend this single source of shared information. As we will see below some of this message was heard and others chose and still choose, sometimes, to ignore it.

5.3 Case study 3: Medical Coding Council of Australia (MCCA)

A natural occurrence from the PeCC and IT-014-10 activities was for government and stakeholders to see the need to build Australia's central catalogue for medical products. Hence the *Medical Coding Council of Australia* was formed. Chaired by a industry CEO the committee had over thirty members from every facet and part of the health sector as well as the IT and telecommunications industries and logistics and transport representatives. It took three long years and some serious argument and debate to finally publish a report as a consensus recommendation to the then Federal Health Minister to create implement and operate a single national database. This MCCA database was to be populated only by suppliers, and then quality assured by medical professionals and operated under a joint industry and government controlling Council. The MCCA was (still) born.

A fundamental thesis of the report's recommendations was to refer heavily to the existence in Australia of the Therapeutic Goods Authority (TGA)[6]. The TGA (similar to the USA FDA) is the custodian and protection agency charged with registering details (the static information on the label) of every product consumed in the Australian health system. It is illegal to supply non-TGA authorised products in Australia.

Briefly the report said that over time the sensible outcome would be to convince the TGA to accept the merger of a MCCA catalogue into the TGA database system. This would require the TGA to accept a supply chain, overseeing database role, as well as a medical focus at some future date. As you will read in the next section, this is a highly desirable solution to any national cataloguing model.

The basic conflicts and central issues that (still) bedevil this concept is the failure of people to accept simple, but ruthless disciplines. Primarily that the *GS1* number is the *LINKING* identification number between supply and medical uses. The other, as we will also see below) is the inability of some people to understand the difference between *static and dynamic* catalogue data and how best to utilize a central catalogue of *static* data to be then valued added with differing *dynamic* data streams to sub-catalogues

Was the MCCA successful? In theory it was a grand success, but in practice not so much so. Why? Firstly the departmental officers ignored the recommendation calling for a joint industry and government council to be formed. Rather they went forward on their own. Soon afterwards the original decision to use the IT-014-10 PRICAT structure was abandoned entirely to use an academically influenced, medically inclined version. This was known for some years as the *ACOM, the Australian Catalogue of Medicines.*

This diluted the concept of the GS1 high level hierarchy in favour of a mixed and mapped version to medical terminology codes. This immediately broke the 'supplier

---

[6] http://www.tga.gov.au/

only' populating rule. Not surprisingly the interest and enthusiasm for change in the supplier community faded fast when, after years of PeCC, IT-014-10 and MCCA led logical debates and reasoned decision making, the ACOM model ignored this consensus and went their merry way. Was ACOM successful? No. it was and is not working today as a standalone entity, but is now incorporated into its replacement system known as the National Product catalogue (NPC); more on the NPC later in this chapter.

5.4 Case study 4: The Hacateppe University Research Project (HUAP)

The *Hacateppe University Research Project (HUAP)* is based in Ankara Turkey. The author was recruited by Medicare Australia to be the project manager for the development of a single product catalogue. HUAP has a committee and working group structure with over fifty (mostly medical professional) members. These committees work for and report through to three government ministries: Minister for Health, for Labour and for Treasury/Insurance. An eminent professor and CEO of Turkey's largest (1200 beds) hospital chairs HUAP.

Was Component C of HUAP successful? Yes, very much so. From a standing start in March 2005 the central database was fully functional and fully staffed in March 2007. Today the HUAP *National Product Database* is undoubtedly the best example of its kind and purpose anywhere in the world. Other countries have FDA and TGA databases for civilian medical purposes but none, to the authors knowledge, combine both supply and clinical use as well as third element of insurance claims processing (similar to Australia's Medicare Australia)

Why was this outcome so relatively spectacular? Solely because of three key facts:

- HUAP Component C members were convinced by, and then totally embraced the concepts, theories and lessons from the many overlapping years experience from PeCC, IT-014-10, MCCA and other aligned programs in Australia
- Notably a 100% acceptance of the PRICAT structure of static (and not dynamic) data being solely initiated by suppliers, and
- A government 'decree' mandating the use of the NPD by all suppliers wishing it sell product into the Turkish Health System via the master NPD downloading data to sub-catalogues

So there was a plan, there was a method and there was above all else a central authority demand that the NPD be the sole source of all electronic product data used in Turkey today. While this is a demonstrably effective outcome there is still work to do in Turkey towards a fully linked supply, clinical and claims based network. The Turkish leadership has a three phase priority use of the NPD in hospitals: a) the tool for Component B (the costing project), then b) as the central controller and linking mechanism for patient insurance claims and payments to suppliers from these claims, and c) the supply chain. While the supply chain task is the third priority for hospitals it is now being used 100% by Turkey's retail pharmacies. All drug wholesalers and in turn their chemist clients use the NPD to align, via the use of the GS1 number and barcode, information across the closed loop of the supply cycle.

Starting with the pharmacist dispensing and/or over the counter (OTC) point of sale using the scanned barcode to record the sale. This unique number is then used by every point of the replenishment process right back to the supplier/manufacturer. This transaction system is now the base for Turkey's eventual *Electronic Health Record* system in contributing the *Patient Medical Record* component of the more complex 'Health' repository.

It is time to return to the previous mention of '*static*' and '*dynamic*' data structures used in national or central database. The fundamental premise is a lesson learnt from the retail sector and it has to do with the sharing of common data and the separation of specialist data. Think of it this way. A buyer needs different information on the same product than does a nurse or a pharmacist, as well as a person doing insurance processing or to an accounts payable person. None of these people need to download, see, use or store every byte of data across the entire personality and attribute of each and every product. It is a waste of time, waste of computer memory space and is confusing.

The *HUAP PRICAT* master database management staff therefore asks the supplier and the supplier only to populate just the *static* data on their product. The GS1 number, description, size, strength and so forth as well as category codes for pharmaceuticals (ATC code) or GMDN for medical devices. This commonly used data set is mandatory to meet all the needs of supply, patient safety and accurate recording applications. The PRICAT has thirty-five fields of data. Therefore separate users will all download just these 35-fields. Then they are responsible to add the dynamic data fields they require; like price, pallets, clinical terminology or other specialist information to sub-catalogues. Not only is this simple and sensible it is also sensitive to the supplier's point of view in asking them to only commonly share static data that is not a) commercially sensitive (price) or b) not their responsibility (terminology) as well as c) increasing their workload.

The Turkish experience validates these core issues:

- Electronic supply and electronic health applications CANNOT function without a common database
- Only suppliers must be responsible for the core, shared static data, and
- The less the suppliers are required to contribute the more certain they will perform cooperatively and effectively

And as a result the NPD currently (mid 2008) contains *170,000 GS1 identified products.* For further details you need to visit their website at www.huap.com.tr

5.5 Case study 5: Pharmaceutical Extranet Gateway (PEG)

The *Pharmaceutical Extranet Gateway* takes us back to the late PeCC and early MCCA days. This project had steering committee of suppliers, wholesalers and pharmacists whose goal was to create an integrated e-commerce network across all points of supply to the point of sale. This would have and will one day electronically exchange $6 billion worth of product, seamlessly and without re-keying or re-working. It is this mention of re-keying that is pivotal to the most basic lesson of the PeCC to HUAP journeys; if GS1 is not the only number used universally then someone, at sometime has to re-key data from one computer to another. The certain result will be medical misadventures as well as less control over timely, accurate and useful management information on product use and investment. PEG has never been a total success because Australia is still without a NPD.

5.6 Case study 6: Pharmaceutical Integrated Logistics Syste (PILS)

The best case study to last. Can anything be better than the HUAP story? Well, yes as long as we are mindful of the differences in scale and that the PILS example is the total answer to health supply performance needs and criteria. Like HUAP's NPD, the PILS system adopted by the Australian Defence Force (ADF) uses an IT-014 compliant catalogue version database. It contains around 40,000 GS1 identified medical, OTC and medical device products. It is worth noting the difference between HUAP's 170,000 and PILS 40,000 products on file. An average Australian hospital will typically hold or need, at some time, a product from a choice of 50,000 to 70,000 products depending on type and size of a hospital. So while 40,000 reflect this smaller need of a military unit the 170,000 in Turkey covers a unique multiple tender and supply platform.

Why is PILS so good? On the supply side of the system it delivers central control total over instant and accurate visibility on all products in all military establishments. Any purchasing person can drill down by any logical criteria to see and obtain information of movement, location, use, costs and totals over the entire inventory. All without the re-keying or re-working of core and uniquely held data. More significantly PILS also has integrated doctor prescribe and pharmacy dispensing inputs, thereby truly linking the supply chain to the clinical chain as was expressed as highly desirable at the 2000 Australian Government's *Health Online Summit* held in Sydney.

Better still the PILS system then ties this together into a *personal medication record*. As a result whenever a soldier moves from a location to report to new location his or her medical record is instantly available. Pre-PILS this could take 'months' and was highly inaccurate. So PILS delivers on all fronts:

- A central database of unique aligned and harmonised product data.
- Complete e-commerce compliant supply chain
- Linked to some clinical functions, and
- Delivering a *personal medication record* for each service person and for some family members as well

The Australian case studies have shown that we have the technologies to be successful but that the failure of some people, organisations or politicians not to grasp the significance of key success factors is the primary impediment to success and our inability to attain very significant benefits to be realised from the Health e-procurement and supply chain management. Australia's achilles heel is the lack of a national comprehensive catalogue.

6. Supply-Chain – Why Bother?

We have argued that every clinical decision is essentially a procurement decision as clinical decisions tend to be influenced by available resources (products, supplies and services). Consequently improvements in procurement can only lead to improvements in health service delivery, but that's not the only reason to bother implementing improvements in supply chain management. I would have to say do it.....because you can. The supply chain management disciplines are well documented. The standards are mature and the process improvements can be benchmarked. Better still the cultural impact of seeking 'best-practice' in this arena will carry over into other more complex and less mature areas. This is an approach that has been practiced and can be consistently applied. Box 3 presents some basic maxims for improved supply chain performance. These are based on the hard won lessons from supply chain professionals. Use them to validate the improvement targets chosen. The key lesson is that there is no secret to supply-chain practice. It is one of the few practice areas that has well documented processes and standards. They are available to all to apply for improved health outcomes.

Box 3 Supply-Chain Maxims

- **Lesson 1 - forecasting**
  The very beginning is for the supplier to get manufacturing forecasts in a timely, accurate and useful manner
- **Lesson 2 - don't re-key**
  At the complete other end, for the supplier to understand, is that the number of credit notes is a direct measure of performance. IT standards for data sharing are one of the core enablers for coordinating the flow of supply chain information between trading partners.
- **Lesson 3 - cash flow**
  Mistakes make credits notes that delay accounts receivable and incur three bad cost events
- **Lesson 4 - Data owner**
  As the supplier, don't reinvent cataloguing. Religiously align data with its' source. Catalogue management is another of the key data enablers for consistent supply information between trading partners.
- **Lesson 5 - Knowledge owner**
  As the buyer, empower them, and provide mechanisms for feedback.
- **Lesson 6 - Share the data, share the knowledge, share the benefits** Walmart supply chain mantra. Their success is based on marginal improvements for all parties in the supply-chain.

---

7. Conclusion

We will close this subject with a focus on the 'user' audience for a medical products supply chain and some further comment on catalogues and standards. The first thing to acknowledge is the significance of adopting **Standards, databases and catalogues.** We have seen that without standards electronic methods cannot work. Computers can't 'think' and cannot cope with a different identification and document regimes for one product. Having a single, reliable, aligned and harmonized source of common data is also mandatory to ensure that every point of data capture and point of data usage is a seamless exchange of information without re-working or re-keying.

So what is the problem? We have seen that the Turkish authorities and the ADF have implemented a working cataloguing platform. Around the world all health jurisdictions are working towards a central resource database solution; the problem is what should the central resource look like and how should it function and for whom?

An example of a good idea being undertaken the wrong way is the situation currently in Australia. While this is clearly the opinion of the authors and not anyone else, the case is demonstrable that 'big' databases working as a catalogue don't work. The National Product Catalogue (NPC) in Australia has a PeCC, MCCA and ACOM hereditary. In one way or another all were dedicated to linking supply to clinical functionality with the twin goals of financial performance and patient care. Broadly speaking this was to design master databases with approximately thirty character fields as the core repository and then let separate parts of the system add their different data as required independent of a central source but receiving downloaded static data from this source, to a sub-catalogue.

For reasons to do with a focus on tendering and high level procurement, the Australian NPC is now designed to represent over one hundred character fields of data. The difference between the practical relevance of thirty fields to all people and a hundred fields to all people is pretty clear:

- It is too much to expect the suppliers to populate and indeed threatens their perception of confidentiality (sensitive price dissemination)
- For all but the catalogue controllers over one hundred fields of data is just not necessary for any one sub-function; therefore people will download and store unnecessarily large files

What are the benefits? The outcomes are significantly compelling and ironically perhaps reasonably 'easy' to accomplish, as the HUAP and PILS platforms suggest. These benefits may be summarised as saving money, improved effectiveness of accounts payable systems, reduction is waste (shrinkage), reduction in errors, improved clinical productivity, improved patient safety. In closing it can be said that to ignore the e-enablement of supply is to fundamentally threaten the capacity to create and operate other e-health applications; including prescriptions and patient records for example. A medication record is vital to many of these other systems and a medical record system cannot work without a seamless supply chain link. Therefore the ability to exchange product information in a timely, accurate, useful and safe manner is mandatory for any other health informatics application that contains the use of a product. A visibly functioning e-commerce based supply chain platform will deliver countless invisible benefits as well as being a foundational platform for other e-health systems.

References

[1]   Friedman T 2005 The World is Flat, Penguin
[2]   Gallagher P 2007 Health Care Supply Chain: every clinical decision is a procurement decision. Presentation at the Information Technology in Aged Care Conference (ITAC 2007), Melbourne refer http://www.agedcareassociation.com.au/organisation/page.cfm?id=79 cited 24 June 2008
[3]   More E, McGrath M. 2000 The PeCC story, Commonwealth of Australia, Canberra
[4]   Commonwealth of Australia 2002 National Action Plan to facilitate the take-up of e-commerce in Australian hospital supply chains: A report by the National Supply Chain Reform Task Force, Canberra
[5]   NEHTA 2007 e-Procurement Business Architecture: supply chain version 1 12-7-2007 from http://www.nehta.gov.au/index.php?option=com_docman&task=doc_download&gid=290&Itemid=139. cited 25 June 2008.
[6]   Bates D W, Cohen M, Leape L L, Overhage J M, Shabot M M, Sheridan T 2001 Reducing the frequency of errors in medicine using information technology Journal of the American Medical Informatics Association Vol.8 No.4 pp.299-308
[7]   Kearney A T 2006 International Consultants http://www.atkearneypas.com/
[8]   Food and Drug Administration (FDA) Center for Drug Evaluation and Research, Medication Errors http://www.fda.gov/oc/initiatives/barcode-sadr/default.htm cited 7 October 2008
[9]   Kohn L T, Corrigan J M, and Donaldson M S, Editors; Committee on Quality of Health Care in America, Institute of Medicine 2000 'To Err is Human: building a safer health system, National Academies Press, Washington DC

Review questions

1. What is your understanding of supply chain management and how does this relate to the organization you work for?
2. What are the potential benefits of automating the supply chain in your country?
3. What are the critical aspects of supply chain management that must be complied with?
4. Can you write up a case study relating to an organisation of your choice and identify the major areas requiring change?

Health Informatics
E.J.S. Hovenga et al. (Eds.)
IOS Press, 2010
doi:10.3233/978-1-60750-476-4-404

28. Change Management – An overview

Sebastian GARDE[1] Dr. sc. hum., Dipl.-Inform. Med., FACHI
Senior Developer, Ocean Informatics, Düsseldorf, Germany

Abstract. This chapter gives an educational overview of:
- The need for systematic and comprehensive change management in health that involves everybody
- Various change management types, models, best practices, and techniques, and how to plan and execute change management
- Some of the common mistakes with change management in healthcare

Keywords. Medical Informatics, Health Facilities, Health Services Administration, Socioeconomic Factors, Information Systems, Health, Risk Management, Communication

Introduction

This chapter explores the necessity for change management and aims to serve as an introduction to some of the most common mistakes as well as best practices.

Change management is one of the tasks absolutely necessary when for example an existing (information) system is adapted or new software is to be introduced anywhere in the health care sector. In fact, this is true for many changes (no matter of which nature) because systematic change management can significantly increase the success of a desired change.

Until recently, change management has often been overlooked with sometimes disastrous consequences for a project. For example, the costs for failed Information Technology projects have been estimated at 75.000.000.000 US-$ in the US [1]. Certainly not with all, but certainly with some of these projects, it would have been possible to prevent the failure and turn the project into a success.

Nowadays, the necessity of systematic and continuous change management is no longer overlooked as frequently. Unfortunately however, too often change management is only being paid lip-service to, its importance is emphasized, but in the end not taken advantage of. A typical reason is that the project is late anyway and that it is thought that no more time can be spent (read: wasted) on systematic change management. However, the opposite is true: Not taking advantage of what change management has to offer, will almost certainly delay the project further, whereas systematic change management throughout the project can significantly speed up the project.

---

[1] Corresponding Author: sebasti@ngar.de

1. Types of Change Management

There are at least three different types of change management with different purposes used in different areas [2].

1. The first type is change management in systems engineering. This is mainly a formal process to request, plan, implement and evaluate changes to a system in order to support the processing and traceability of these changes.

2. The second type of change management can best be described as an Information Technology (IT) Service Management Discipline. It ensures that standardized methods and processes are in place for efficient and prompt handling of all changes to a controlled IT infrastructure. Changes may arise in response to any problems with the infrastructure or externally imposed requirements such as, to name just one, legislative changes.

3. The third type of change management is a structured approach to the change in individuals, teams, organizations and societies that enables the transition from a current state to a desired future state. "Change Management is the process, the tools and methods to manage the people-side of business change in order to achieve the required business outcome, and to realize that business change effectively in the social infrastructure of the workplace." [3].

While certainly all types of change management are important, the one that seems to be most relevant to Health Informatics is often the third type. Or as Lorenzi and Riley put it:

"Certainly, technical challenges still exist; they always will. However, as our new systems affect larger, more heterogeneous groups of people and more organizational areas, the major challenges to systems success often become more behavioral than technical" [4[p. 116]].

Hence, this chapter deals primarily with this third type of (people-focussed) change management and when from now on change management is mentioned, the third type of change management is being referred to.

2. Levels of Change Management

Change management can refer to a number of different levels, for example:

- One individual: the change may be a new behavior of this individual.
- A team: the change may be a change in the communication within the team
- An organisation: The change may be a new business process or the introduction of a new IT system.
- A society: The change may be new legislation.

No matter on what level, all the previous levels need to be considered for a change to be successful, in essence it requires the engagement and participation of the people involved. Change management provides a framework for managing the people side of these changes, which includes both an organizational perspective as well as models for individual change. This chapter can only serve as a short introduction to change management.

3.   The Map is Not the Territory

Whenever talking about the importance of change management, it is important to realise that "the map is not the territory". The meaning of this map/territory relation is that individual people do not have access to absolute knowledge of reality, but in fact only have access to a set of beliefs they have built up over time, about reality. This idea has been introduced by Chris Argyris as the Ladder of Inference [5] and elaborated by Senge and colleagues [6] [7]. Figure 1 presents an example of a simple Ladder of Inference.

As a consequence of the map/territory relation and the Ladder of Inference, any communication in change processes needs to make sure that information about the change and its consequences is presented in such a way that people with different belief systems can access and understand the information. According to Senge and colleagues [7], change managers need to make sure that a conscious effort is made to move back down this ladder in order to:

- become more aware of their own thinking and reasoning (reflection),
- make their thinking and reasoning more visible to others (advocacy), and
- inquire into others' thinking and reasoning (inquiry).

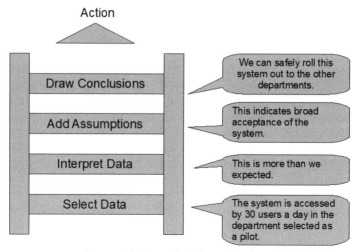

Figure 1: An Example of the Ladder of Inference

4.   Change Management – Does it Concern Me?

Depending on the size of a project, it can be very beneficial to employ dedicated change managers. It is important however to recognize that change management cannot be separated from the rest of the project – but needs to be an integral part of the project. Hence, in essence, everybody is a change manager – consciously or not. Hence the question only is whether you are a good change manager – or not. This chapter aims to provide you with some of the basic ideas of change management as a first step towards improving your personal change management skills.

5. A Selection of Best Practices

Whenever there is a change that you are responsible to conduct, there are several best practices that are summarised as follows:

- **Communicate, communicate, communicate**
- **Aim for continous improvements**
- **Aim for a couple of 'Quick Wins'** – and celebrate them! There is evidence that simple and cost-efficient additions or adaptations can be decisive for efficiency and user friendliness. Aim to implement these! (see e.g. [8]
- **Experiment**, and try until it works
- **Involve users and create ownership**
- 'Walk the talk' (Do exactly what you say you are doing)
- **Be clear about who is responsible for what**
- **Systematically use experiences from existing systems** (which includes people as well as software!)
- **Build up a Critical Mass**: A critical mass is the number of people that is sufficient to collectively bring about the desired change. It must be big enough to overcome the inertia and resistance. It is important to invest in the development of a critical mass as this makes changes less painful and faster.
- **Be clear about the rationale for improving a system and who benefits or loses** (and what can be done to minimize or compensate these losses if required). For example, the introduction of new software can considerably move workloads from one profession to another. Don't hide this – you will be found out – but rather show how this fits together with your overall plan. If there is more (or different) effort involved in using a new system (e.g. DRG documentation), ensure that the persons given this effort, get something back in turn, for example more and better possibilities to analyse their own data.
- **Within your circle of influence, any change introduced should aim to decrease the amount of time required by health professionals – not increase it** [9]. Health care workers are under permanent time-pressure due to increasing patient numbers, increasing documentation requirements, and increasing complexity of today's healthcare [10].
- **Continuously ,manage' the expectations of users about the change** – or they will be disappointed in the end and resist.

5.1 Most Important Success Factors

In 2003, the Research company Prosci asked 288 organisation from 51 countries about the most important success factor. The following are the top 5 [11]:

1. Efficient support from top management
2. Support from future users through early involvement
3. Exceptional team
4. Continuous, targeted communication
5. Good planning and organisation

This is also consistent with a more recent report [12] where participants stated that the most important thing they would change in their next project is to engage senior leaders earlier and more proactively in order to obtain buy-in, sponsorship at the right level in the organization and enable senior leaders to participate actively.

5.2 Most Important Barriers

According to the same report, the most important barriers that prevent a change in an organisation are:

- Resistance of staff
- Resistance of mid-management
- Insufficient support by top management
- Time frame, budget and/or resources insufficient
- Inertia of the organisation

The factors include top management that is not directly involved with the project, does not keep up to date with the project's progress and thus usually does not intervene soon enough when problems occur. Apart from not providing adequate resources, underestimating the effort required by everybody (including the effort required by top management), insufficient or inconsistent communication or dictating change without communicating the benefits, ignoring the impact of change on employees by focussing on the business issues of the change and neglecting the employee side of things and thus causing employees' fear and confusion; shifting project priorities midway in the project, or changing their own attention too soon are all common barriers to successful completion of a project.

6. Change Management Models and Techniques

There is an abundance of change management models and techniques (see Further Reading) and this chapter can only pick up a small exemplary selection of these models and techniques.

6.1 Lewin's Basic Stages of changes

Kurt Lewin, one of the most famous psychologists of his time, identified three stages of change that are still the basis of many change management approaches today [13]:

Unfreeze: Many people like to live with the conception of safety and control. This is a stable (or frozen) basis, however, even changes that offer considerable benefit will be discomforting. Often "push methods" can be required initially to 'unfreeze' people's mind and start them to move away from their current position. After this, usually "pull methods" can then be used to keep them going, which is often the better approach. Although pulling is more difficult than pushing, it is often more effective. While push-methods are based on leaving no choice (e.g. but to leave the current position), pull methods are based on creating a desire for a change (and seek to optimize it with everybody's input.

Transition: Once people are unfrozen or 'change ready' (which can take a considerable amount of time), it is time to move from one state to another. It is important to note, that a transition should not be considered as one step – but as a whole trip or journey. This is true for the leaders of a particular change, who may have spent months on the details of the change as well as for the mass which is usually involved later and cannot be expected to have the same understanding of for example the necessity for a change just like that. Thus transition consumes some time as well. However, importantly, the transition journey needs to end, otherwise people get too comfortable (for example of not really being accountable) or too frustrated (e.g. being afraid of losing a job) and no real action is being taken.

Refreeze: In the end, it is important to "refreeze" the new state and establish stability and harmony. In modern organizations of the "flat world" [14] this step is often only very tentative as the next big change may well be already into planning, which can be dangerous and impact on the efficiency of staff.

6.2 The ADKAR Model

The ADKAR model for individual change management [15] describes five required building blocks for change to be realized successfully on an individual level. The building blocks of the ADKAR Model include:

- Awareness – of why the change is needed
- Desire – to support and participate in the change
- Knowledge – of how to change
- Ability – to implement new skills and behaviors
- Reinforcement – to sustain the change

Without Awareness, Desire, Knowledge, Ability and Reinforcement at the individual's level, it is unlikely that a permanent change will be realized - even if the problem is big and the offered solution is good.

6.3 Force Field Analysis

Force field analysis [16] provides a framework for looking at the factors (forces) that influence a situation, originally social situations. Force field analysis takes into account forces for and against a specified changed. After having described the desired change in some detail, it is helpful to list all the negative and positive forces in separate columns and indicate the strength of each change on a scale of 1 (not so strong) to 5 (very strong). Usually this involves brainstorming by a selection of stakeholders. The strength can also be indicated by the length of arrows used to indicate the strength of the force (see Figure 2 for an example). Once these forces are identified, it may be time to decide if the project is viable at all. If negative forces are too strong, the effort may be in vain. However, if one decides to continue, the force field can be used to identify

- Negative forces that can be weakened
- Positive forces that can be strengthened

While both weakening negative forces and strengthening negative forces is important, often it is more effective to reduce negative forces: Just pushing a project through with positive force may simply not be enough.

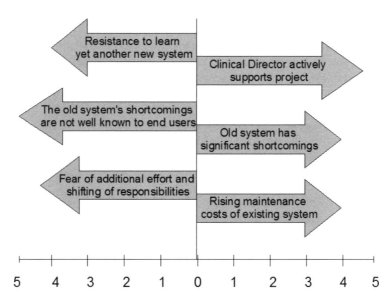

Figure 2: A Simple Example Force Field for the Introduction of a New Clinical Software System. Forces against change are towards the left, whereas forces for the change are towards the right. The longer the arrow, the stronger the force (on a scale from 1-5).

6.4 The Speed of Trust

Stephen M.R. Covey in his book „The Speed of Trust: The one thing that changes everything!" Covey [17] argues that in the end the most important thing to make any change happen is trust. According to Covey, trust comes in 5 waves:

1. self trust
2. relationship trust
3. organisational trust
4. market trust
5. societal trust

Covey argues that self trust can be gained by increasing one's credibility consisting of a person's integrity, intent, capabilities, and results. In order to build relationship trust it is essential to talk straight, demonstrate respect, create transparency, right wrongs, show loyalty, deliver results, get better, confront reality, clarify expectations, practice accountability, listen first and understand then seek to be understood, keep commitments, and extend 'smart' trust. Organisational, market and societal trust can be gained by proper alignment, a good reputation, which is hard to build up but very easy to lose, and contributions to the society.

7.   A Word of Caution: Change Saturation

There seems to be a limit to how much change people can cope with in a given period of time. This is referred to as change saturation and the limit depends on many factors including cultural ones. There are ways of recognizing change saturation and strategies to deal with them. Generally speaking, change saturation may have been reached when the amount of change that is happening is high and disruptive and the inherent organisational change capacity (determined by e.g. culture, history, structure and the change management competency within the organisation) is low [18]. Short term strategies for dealing with change saturation usually reduce the number of changes required by priorisation and decrease the disruptive nature of the change through effective change management. Long term solutions can address the organizational capacity issue by building change management competency throughout the organization [18]. This emphasises again the need for increasing everybody's change management skills.

8.   Conclusion

This chapter can only serve as a very brief introduction to what is involved in change management. It is important to remember that:

- Change management occurs on many levels from individual to societal.
- No matter what, you are a change manager (within your circle of influence) – the only question is, are you a good or not so good one.
- A formal and integrated change management approach can decide whether a project is successful or not.
- That at least a basic knowledge in Change Management techniques will help you considerably to understand and anticipate people's reactions to change and be proactive in leading the way right (however, if it is the right way, is not a question of change management).
- Trust you have built up with the stakeholders involved in any change, is important for a fast and successful implementation of that change.
- Due to the complex nature of health care, health care systems, and health care organizations, a comprehensive and integrated approach to change management is even more important.

References

[1]   Keil, M, Tiwana, A & Bush, A. Reconciling user and project manager perceptions of IT project risk: a Delphi study. Info Systems J. 2002, vol. 12, pp. 103-19.
[2]   Wikipedia 2008, Change Management, http://en.wikipedia.org/w/index.php?title=Change_management&oldid=186871110.
[3]   Jeff Hiatt Tim Creasy cited by Johnson, BL & Davis, VR. Change Management: A Critical Factor in EMR Implementation. For the Record Magazine. 2004, vol. 16, no. 5, p. 32.
[4]   Lorenzi, NM & Riley, RT. Managing change: an overview. J Am Med Inform Assoc. 2000, vol. 7, no. 2, pp. 116-24.
[5]   Argyris, C. The Executive Mind and Double-Loop Learning. Organizational Dynamics. 1982, vol. Autumn 1982.
[6]   Senge, P. The Fifth Discipline: The Art and Practice of the Learning Organization. New York, NY, Doubleday/Currency. 1990.
[7]   Senge, P, Kleiner, A, Roberts, C, Ross, R & Smith, B. The Fifth Discipline Fieldbook - Strategies and Tools for Building A Learning Organization. New York, NY, Doubleday/Currency. 1990.
[8]   Marinakis, HA & Zwemer, FL, Jr. An inexpensive modification of the laboratory computer display changes emergency physicians' work habits and perceptions. Ann Emerg Med. 2003, vol. 41, no. 2, pp. 186-90.
[9]   Giere, W. Electronic Patient Information -- Pioneers and MuchMore. A vision, lessons learned, and challenges. Methods Inf Med. 2004, vol. 43, no. 5, pp. 543-52.

[10] Hasman, A, Safran, C & Takeda, H. Quality of health care: informatics foundations. Yearbook of Medical Informatics. 2003, vol. 2003, pp. 143-52.

[11] Prosci (Research Company) 2003, 'Best practices in Change Management Benchmarking Study 2003'.

[12] Change Management Learning Center - Prosci 2007, Change saturation, http://www.change-management.com/tutorial-bp-2007-saturation.htm.

[13]   ChangingMinds.org   2008,   Lewin's   freeze   phases http://changingminds.org/disciplines/change_management/lewin_change/lewin_change.htm.

[14] Friedman, TL. The World is Flat - The Globalised World in the Twenty-First Century, 2nd Edition. London, Penguin Books. 2006.

[15] Hiatt, J & Hiatt, JM. ADKAR: A Model for Change in Business, Government and Our Community. Loveland, Colorado, Prosci Learning Center Publications. 2006.

[16] Lewin, K. Defining the "Field at a Given Time". Psychological Review. 1943, vol. 50, pp. 292-310 (Republished in Resolving Social Conflicts & Field Theory in Social Science, Washington, D.C.: American Psychological Association, 1997).

[17] Covey, SMR. The SPEED of Trust: The One Thing that Changes Everything. New York, NY, FreePress. 2006.

[18] Change Management Learning Center - Prosci 2007 Best Practices in Change Management Report, http://www.change-management.com/best-practices-report.htm.

Further reading

- A good and comprehensive overview of various change management techniques is presented at http://changingminds.org/.
- Also the Prosci's Change Management Learning Center at http://www.change-management.com is a good starting point for further reading.

Review Questions

1. Why is systematic and comprehensive change management important?
2. Does change management concern you?
3. What types and levels of change management do you know?
4. What does "The Map is not the Territory" mean?
5. What are some principles and best practices for change management and some of the most common mistakes with change management in healthcare?
6. Name and describe the 5 stages of the ADKAR model using an example from your own personal or professional experience.

Health Informatics
E.J.S. Hovenga et al. (Eds.)
IOS Press, 2010
413
doi:10.3233/978-1-60750-476-4-413

29 Project Management in Health Informatics

Jessica HO[1] DipPM, BN, RN, GradDipIT(software), MHlthSc, MACS, PhD
candidate
*Director of Interagency Information Policy Development (DIIPD), Australian
Government Department of Defense, Canberra, Australia*

Abstract. This chapter gives an educational overview of:
- the concept of project management and its role in modern management
- the generic project lifecycle process
- processes used in developing a plan for the management of resources –
  time, cost, physical resources and people
- the concept of managing risk in projects
- communication processes and practices that are important to the
  management of projects

Keywords. Medical Informatics, Health Services Management, Risk Management,
Socioeconomic Factors, Communication, Information Systems, Health, Critical
Pathways,

Introduction

Most people have far more involvement in the management of projects than they
realise. Buying a car or renovating a house is a project, and must be managed as such
where the purchase is done at the right time, at the right price and to the quality, the
buyer has specified. Similarly, this can be applied to erecting a new building
structure, building a new computer program or even carrying out a surgical procedure.
Identifying what needs to be done, by when and at what cost and risk are just as
important to an architect designing a major construction as it is to a teacher planning
next year' study guide.

Therefore, projects may come in many sizes from small activities that might take
only a few hours to complete to major items of work that are carried out over several
months and involve thousand of staff and contractors. In some instances, you may not
even be aware that you are participating in the process of completing a major project.

The most common definition for project is given in the Project Management
Body of Knowledge - PMBOK [1[p.4]] which states:

> *"A project is] a temporary endeavour undertaken to create a unique
> product or service and organised in such a way as to achieve a set of
> objectives."*

Every project has a start and finish point. No project is a continuous process,
which explains the term 'a temporary endeavour' from the definition above.

---

[1] Corresponding author: jessicaho@grapevine.com.au

Therefore, an easy way to identify if whether something is a project or process is to look for its finishing point. If there is none then what you have is a process and not a project.

In addition, the term "to create a unique product' indicates that no two projects are the same, as the management of projects often is very different and requires varying technical skills and philosophy, hence requiring the development of different approach to tackle them.

## 1.	Project Management Role in Health Care Industry

Project management is the discipline of planning, organising, monitoring and controlling all aspects of the project in a continuous process in order to achieve its internal and external objectives. The project manager is responsible for taking the organisation's strategic direction and turning it into tangible, achievable project outcomes. However, the project manager is quite often just a client representative and has to determine and implement the exact needs of the client, based on knowledge of the healthcare organisation he/she is representing. More than often this particular individual does not participate in the activities that produce the unique product or service, but rather strives to maintain the progress and productive mutual interaction of various parties/organisations in such a way that the overall risk of project failure is reduced.

Therefore the ability of the project manager must include the adaptation to various internal procedures of the contracting party, and to form close links with the nominated stakeholders, which are all essential in ensuring that the key issues of cost, time, quality and above all client satisfaction can be realised.

In whatever field, a successful project manager must be able to envision the entire project from start to finish and to have the ability to ensure that this vision is realized.

The uniqueness of project management in health care industry lies within the realm of mastering one's understanding of the health care sector information needs and the procurement of the fit for purpose IT product or services as identified by the contracting organisation. Many IT products and/or services within the health care sector are purchased from a third party software vendor nowadays. The nominated project manager has to be able to represent and translate the client/organisation's vision and objectives across to ensure a successful project outcome.

## 2.	Project Life Cycle and Approaches

There are many different approaches to managing a project, and different organisation/industry may utilise different approaches to deliver their IT product. Nevertheless, the common concept of initiation, development or planning, production or execution, and closing/maintenance exists among all the identified approaches below:

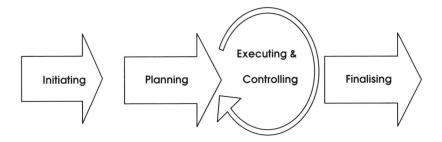

Figure 1 Project Life Cycle and Approaches

2.1 The Traditional Waterfall Development

A traditional phased approach identifies a sequence of steps to be completed. IT projects typically progress through these stages in a linear fashion:

1. project initiation stage – Requirements Analysis of project
2. project planning or design stage – Design widget
3. project execution or production stage – Code and Unit test Widget
4. project monitoring and controlling systems – Integrate and System test widget
5. project completion stage – Widget completed

Waterfall is conceptually straightforward because it produces a single deliverable. It assumes that events affecting the project are predictable and that tools and activities are well understood. Once a phase is complete, it is assumed that it will not be revisited. The strength of this approach is that it lays out the steps for development and stresses the importance of requirements [2]. The fundamental problem of this approach is that it pushes risk forward in time, when it is costly to undo mistakes from earlier phases [3]. Therefore, the real risk of the project is masked until the end of the project lifecycle. This late discovery of design/code/requirement defects most often will result in costly overruns and/or project cancellation.

2.2 PRINCE and PRINCE2

PRINCE (PRojects IN Controlled Environments) was first developed by Central Computers and Telecommunications Agency, now part of Office of Government Commerce, in 1989 as a UK Government standard for IT project management. Initially developed only for the need of IT projects, the latest version, PRINCE2, is designed for all types of management projects.

PRINCE2 is a process-driven project management method [4] which contrasts with reactive/adaptice methods such as Scrum described below. PRINCE2 defines 45 separate sub processes and organises these into eight processes as follows:

- Starting up a project (SU)
- Planning (PL)
- Initiating a Project (IP)
- Directing a Project (DP)
- Controlling a Stage (CS)

- Managing Product Delivery (MP)
- Managing Stage Boundaries (SB)
- Closing a Project (CP)

Each process is defined with its key inputs and outputs together with the specific objectives to be achieved and activities to be carried out. The following PRINCE2 Process Model Diagram (Fig2) illustrates the PRINCE2 processes attached to this methodology.

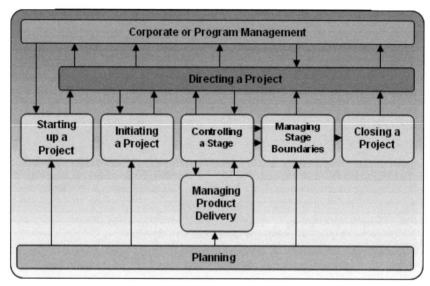

Figure 2 PRINCE2 Process Model Diagram [4]

2.3 Agile Project Management (Scrum)

Traditional project management can be ineffective since the requirements are elusive, volatile and subject to change. However an emerging concept – Agile Project Management may be applied to IT projects which require a highly iterative and incremental process to allow developers and project stakeholders to actively work together to understand the domain, identify what needs to be built and prioritize functionality.

Agile methods are used when these conditions are present: project value is clear; the customer actively participates throughout the project; the customer, designers, and developers are co-located; an incremental feature-driven development is possible; and visual documentation (cards on the wall vs. formal documentation) is acceptable [2].

"Scrum" is an iterative incremental process of software development intended to be for management of software development projects [5]. Scrum process skeleton includes a set of practices and predefined roles, including the main roles of:

1. ScrumMaster – who maintains the processes and works similar to a project manager
2. ProductOwner – who represents the stakeholders and writes user stories (system requirements), prioritises them and places them on the product backlog and

3. Team - which include the developers, designers, testers, in a small cluster multi-skill team of 5 – 9 persons.

The team creates an increment of potential usable portion of the software, in each 'sprint' (15 – 30 day period as decided by the team). The set of features that go into each sprint come from the product backlog, which prioritised the set of high level requirements of work to be done. During the sprint, no one is able to change the backlog, which means that the requirements are frozen for sprint.

Many processes within the above mentioned sprint phase are unidentified and uncontrolled [6]. There is however the first and last phase consisting of defined processes. The knowledge of how to do these processes is explicit and the workflow is linear. The following (Fig 3) is a methodological diagram of a Scrum process [6]:

SCRUM Methodology

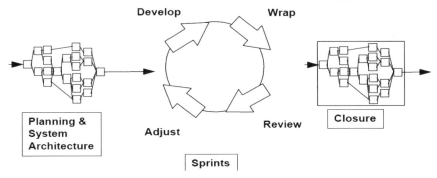

Figure 3 a Methodological Diagram of a Scrum Process [6]

There are several good implementations of systems for managing the Scrum process and the "sprints". One of Scrum's biggest advantages is that it is very easy to learn and requires little effort in general terms to start using.

2.4 The Rational Unified Process (RUP)

RUP iterative processes were developed in response to waterfall characteristics. With an iterative process, the waterfall steps are applied iteratively. Instead of developing a whole system in one-go, an increment (eg: subset of system functionality) is selected and developed, then another increment and so on [7]. In a sense, this process can be classified as agile project management.

In brief, there are four distinct stages to RUP:

1. Inception - The goal of the Inception phase is to achieve concurrence among all stakeholders on the lifecycle objectives for the project. The Inception phase establishes that the project is worth doing and that one or more feasible candidate solutions exist.
2. Elaboration - The goal of the Elaboration phase is to achieve sufficient stability of the requirements and architecture; to select and acquire COTS packages; and to mitigate risks so that a single, high-fidelity solution can be identified with a predictable cost and schedule.
3. Construction - The goal of the Construction phase is to achieve a production-quality release ready for its user community on a regular, incremental basis.

4. Transition - The goal of the Transition phase is to field the selected solution to the user community and provide necessary support.

An iteration is one pass through all stages above. The deliverables of a stage vary, depending on its position within the overall lifecycle, and the nature of the project. An iteration can be seen as a mini project with a plan, deliverables and assessment, in which periodic assessments and corrections are applied to the remainder of the project.

From this you should be able to develop a methodology for the management of your project in line with the wider needs of your organisation. The success of any individual project relies heavily on the project manager constantly reviewing and monitoring the project as it moves through the lifecycle.

3.   Managing Project Resources

There are many activities and resources that a project manager has to manage in order to achieve the project objectives. The functional approach to project management prescribes a mode of action or activity through which the project objectives are achieved. The Project Management Body of Knowledge, commonly known as PMBOK identifies nine main functional elements as knowledge areas that are important to the successful achievement of a project's objectives. These resources and activities are similar to the processes that would be found in other areas of your organisation and as such can be easily aligned with them. These elements are as follows:

3.1 Scope of the Project

This is one of the most important elements of all in a project. The scope of the project is one part of the element most often referred to throughout the project lifecycle. It will be able to make or break the project. Most likely it will be constantly revolving and updated as more information and requirements are uncovered. A project manager has to be able to develop strategy to deal with the demand of changes involving the project scope.

Like all project plans, there are no specific rules about what must go into the scope definition, or how it should be presented and laid out. But as a minimum, PMBOK [8] suggested the following should always be included – not necessarily in this order but certainly in this detail:
- Background or overview of the project
- Objective/s to be achieved
- Scope Statement covering the broad areas of work to be carried out
- Broad strategy for the achievement of the project
- Constraints around which the project is to work
- Exclusions showing what work is not being done as part of the project
- Assumptions and questions yet to be answered
- Related projects that may have an effect on, or be affected by, this project.

It is crucial however that engagement with the end-user should begin at this point if not earlier. Usually this is performed by interviewing them. Other important considerations during the end user's interrogation is the gathering of information regarding what connection this new system has with other health information systems in the organisation, how their wishes can be accommodated into the arrangements of their organisation and most importantly how this new system is expected to improve their work processes. An early buy-in from end users would definitely improve the implementation process of the new health information systems at a later stage.

3.2 Time Management

Time is vital to all projects as it dictates how successful the project is through using the metrics of whether the widget/product was delivered on time. Unfortunately, it is also extremely variable because although the project manager may have control over their project, he/she may not have any means of controlling other project deliverables that he/she depends on. In fact, we can safely describe time as being a constraint to projects rather than a resource. Project managers need to be aware that time unlike funds and people, is the one resource or commodity that can never be replaced if it is used wrongly.

Therefore, how do we manage time? Time management can be conducted using a variety of techniques and activities such as:

- Early planning – deciding what has to be done, how it will be done and what will be used to do it
- Estimating – determining the duration of an activity
- Scheduling- analysing the effect an activity has on other activities and resource restraints and from this determining the best time to carry it out
- Controlling – ensuring that planned or expected time-related outcomes are maintained

3.3. Cost Management

Cost is another important element in the achievement of project objectives. The management of costs includes an analysis of those resources needed to successfully achieve the project's objectives and the costs of acquiring and using them [8]. Costs are usually measured in monetary units eg: $ dollars $. The following common required processes are described by PMBOK as ensuring that the project is completed within an approved budget [8]:

1. Resource Planning: determining what resources and quantities of them should be used
2. Cost Estimating: developing an estimate of the costs and resources needed to complete a project
3. Cost Budgeting: allocating the overall cost estimate to individual work items to establish a baseline for measuring performance
4. Cost control: controlling changes to the project budget

This results in the need to develop a budget, where the Project Manager has to apply a dollar value to each task based on the cost of the resources as a unit value, and the number of units used for each task. The sum total of this becomes the project budget.

3.4 Project Quality Management

"Quality is a matter of opinion" Managing project quality is like flying a plane. You are the pilot and our objective is to get your passengers to their location safely and

most comfortably. The passengers are the people who would sign off on whether or not you have achieved this objective. Your aim is to take the plane to the exact destination as specified on the route, and in accordance with any rules, guidelines and legislation in force at the time. And the aim of your passengers is to go to the same point in the most comfortable and cost effective way. Hopefully they would not tell you how to fly the plane and hopefully you won't tell them to "Shut up, sit down and enjoy the flight".

Therefore, managing quality within a project means looking after all those activities needed to ensure that the requirements of the client (regardless of who this is) are delivered within the constraint of cost and time. Along with scope, time and cost, quality is one of the four important key elements of project management.

The management of project quality includes an identification of all elements of the project that demand a quality process or outcome. Quality Management is all about applying project management procedures, application of industry standards, ensuring there are checklists and signoffs, following OH&S standards, how documentation is controlled, how meetings are conducted and how variations are managed.

This involves the management of [8]:

- Product – the quality of the outcomes desired by the customer/s and defined (and agreed) in the project team
- Processes – the planning and management of all these processes aimed at producing the product to the desired quality and
- People – those who will be responsible for ensuring that the processes are well-defined and managed to achieve the desired product.

3.5 Project Risk Management

Risk is defined in Merriam Webster Online Dictionary [8] as "a possibility of loss or injury". Risk is a concept that denotes a potential negative impact to some characteristic of value that may arise from a future event. Exposure to the consequences of uncertainty constitutes a risk.

Risk Management in a project involves identifying, analysing and responding to risk factors and events throughout the life of a project. There are 6 processes included in Project Risk Management [1]:

1. Risk Management Planning – the main output to this is a risk management plan
2. Risk Identification – understanding what potential unsatisfactory outcomes are associated with a particular project. Several risk identification tools and techniques include brainstorming, the dephi technique, interviewing and SWOT analysis. The key output being the Risk Register
3. Qualitative Risk Analysis – Cost effective process to prioritise the identified risk. The key output being the updates made to the Risk Register
4. Quantitative Risk Analysis - This process assigns a numerical rating to risks. PMBOK has an example of a cost/risk simulation diagram (page 259). Project managers could use this cost/risk diagram to demonstrate risk impact of various project funding levels.
5. Risk Response planning- This process develops options, determines actions, and assigns responsibilities to enhance opportunities and reduce threats. The key output being the updates made to the Risk Register.

6. Risk Monitoring and control - This process monitors newly arising risks, and tracks existing risks and trigger conditions during the project. The key output being the updates made to the Risk Register.
7. Risk Management Planning – is a continuous process throughout the lifecycle of your project and your assessment of whether or not it worked should be taken into account

The output of this exercise ensures risk management is commensurate with the project risk and importance. It provides sufficient resources and time for risk management activities and establishes an agreed basis to evaluate risks. Therefore, it is important for the project team and stakeholders to review project documents and understand the organisation's and the sponsor's approach to risk.

Some of the risks common to all projects are:

- Parts of the project steps left out - Eg: Project Manager being presented with a project brief that says little to address the problem
- Late completion – Projects or part of it could be completed late (if at all) to the wrong quality, or over price
- Changes to procedures – either post contract signatory or the customers changes his/her mind making a mess of the schedule, objectives and/or budget
- Lack of clarity in scope of plan – there may be a lack of or even missing a real objective other than some fuzzy picture of what the client wants as a result of the project or it may be totally incorrect
- Project tasks incomplete at end date – there are quite often many finalisation activities that still need to be done after the actual objective has been achieved at the end date that may not have been considered during the planning phase
- Quality objectives not met – end product may not be to the required standard
- High rectification or follow-up costs – including ensuring sufficient funds are allocated to recruiting the best team to the project

While in themselves these risks may not bring the project to a complete halt, they will require close management to ensure that the project doesn't stray too far from what is originally set out to achieve.

3.6 Project Procurement Management

All projects need goods and services of varying quantity and quality to achieve the desired outcome. These consist of [9[p236]]:

- Procurement Planning: determining what to procure and when
- Solicitation planning: documenting product requirements and identifying potential sources
- Solicitation: obtaining quotations, bids, offers or proposals as appropriate
- Source selection: choosing from among potential sellers
- Contract administration: managing the relationship with the seller
- Contract close-out: completion and settlement of the contract, including resolution of any open items.

Such goods and services can range from stationery and copying services to major contractor and specialist services. Regardless of their type or the use to which they will be put, the procurement of these must be planned and managed throughout the project's lifecycle.

3.7 Project Human Resource Management

Without skilled and knowledgeable staff no plan can ever be successfully implemented and carried out. This highlights the need to identify, select and lead those who play a role, large or small in the achievement of the project's objectives.

But in a project environment people are more than a resource to be used to achieve a project's objectives. They are a pool of competencies that, if applied correctly, can see the project take on its own momentum and achieve outcomes that create far greater value to the planning and implementation of current and future projects.

3.8 Project Communication Management

Effective communication is the vital link between people, ideas and information throughout a project's lifecycle. Communications management provides the identification and implementation of the processes needed to ensure that this link is developed and maintained for the duration of the project. It consists of [9 p235]:

1. Communications planning – determining the information and communication needs of the stakeholders, who needs what information, when will they need it, and how will it be given to them
2. Information distribution – making needed information available to project stakeholders in a timely manner
3. Performance reporting – collecting and disseminating performance information. This includes status reporting, progress measurement and forecasting.
4. Administration closure: generating, gathering and disseminating information to formalise phase or project completion.

3.9 Project Integration

This is the management of the overall project scope to ensure that the desired objective is achieved in a way that meets or exceeds everybody's expectations. A project that comes in under time, within budget and above the desired quality can be guaranteed to please the client, provided it is not at the cost of alienating your team and the organisation for whom you work.

Project Success and Failure

Studies have shown that project success and failure is a question of perception [10]. A project may be perceived to have failed in one environment but not another. Customers may produce different evaluations when asked about the outcome of the project. Hence, project failure is not solely based on whether the project objectives were met, or whether the project was on time and on budget, but also related to the expectations of the customers.

Unfortunately, IT projects have certain characteristics that make them different from other more conventional projects (eg: civil works, engineering) and therefore increase the chances of their failure. Most of the specifics are related to the fact that IT projects involved software which generate the following constraints [11]:

- Abstract constraint – IT projects are often poorly defined, codes of practice are frequently ignored, and in some cases not many lessons are learned from past experience
- Difficulty of visualisation
- Excessive perception of flexibility
- Hidden complexity
- Uncertainty – rapid pace of technological change
- Market pressures demand delivery in the shortest timeframe which compromises software quality
- Tendency to software failure – tendency to re-write codes to perform well established functions
- Goal to change business processes

The ambiguity can be avoided if a single goal is set and if it is set by the customer and not the project team. This means that ultimately the success or failure of a project is determined by the satisfaction of the party that requested its development.

4. Conclusion

One of the crucial factors for ensuring the success of any project is the degree to which its project resources are effectively managed. It is clear that the development of a computerised health information system of a considerable size requires much time, money and the most appropriate project management approach. All approaches described in this chapter (Waterfall, RUP, Scrum, PRINCE2) allow the Project Manager to reach the same conclusion – stakeholder/ client/ customer's satisfaction with the end product produced.

Success requires good planning, appropriate allocation of resources, and effective monitoring and control. PMBOK concentrates on that which is common: practices which are applicable to most projects most of the time using nine areas that contain a relevant body of knowledge. They are:

- Project Integration Management
- Project Scope Management
- Project Time Management
- Project Cost Management
- Project Quality Management
- Project Human Resource Management
- Project Communication Management
- Project Risk Management
- Project Procurement Management

Managing health information systems development in health care organisations is not a small feat. If the health information system is to be of substantial use, changes in the way health care organisations operate may be necessary. This has not usually been the case, partly because of the many inherent factors in a complex organisation where project managers may neglect to see that the users come from diverse professional backgrounds. Underestimating the enormity of the task is perhaps the single contributing factor to the failure of any project before it even begins [12].

Experience in Australia and overseas shows that IT projects in general, have had significant failures which are very costly. It is useful to learn from these failures, by refining project management approaches that could potential be used to address demanding organisations such as those found in the health care sector.

References

[1]   Project Management Institute (PMI), 2004 *A Guide to the Project Management Body of Knowledge: (PMBOK® Guide)*, 3rd Ed., Project Management Institute, Pennsylvania.
[2]   Hass, K., 2007 " The blending of Traditional and Agile Project Management" *PM World Today*, Vol.IX, Issue V, http://www.pmforum.org/library/tips/2007/PDFs/Hass-5-07.pdf cited on 15 April 2008.
[3]   IBM, 2005 "Rational Unified Process" *Training Course Workbook*, IBM/Medicare Australia, Canberra.
[4]   ILX Group, 2008 "PRINCE2 Processes", http://www.prince2.com/prince2-process-model.asp cited on 15 April 2008.
[5]   Rising, L & Janoff, N, 2000 "The Scrum Software Development Process for Small Team" *IEEE Software*, July/August, http://members.cox.net/risingl1/Articles/IEEEScrum.pdf cited on 15 April 2008.
[6]   Schwaber, K., *SCRUM Development Process*, http://jeffsutherland.com/oopsla/schwapub.pdf cited on 15 April 2008
[7]   Peraire, C. & Pannone, R., 2005 "The IBM Rational Unified Process for COTS-based projects: An introduction",   http://www.ibm.com/developerworks/rational/library/aug05/peraire-pannone/index.html, cited on 14 Jan 2008.
[8]   Merriam-Webster Online, 2008 *Merriam Webster Online Dictionary*, http://www.merriam-webster.com/dictionary/risk accessed on 15 April 2008.
[9]   Bennatan, E.M., 2000 *On Time Within Budget*, John Wiley & Sons, Inc., Canada.
[10] Pinto, J.K. & Mantel, S.J., 1990 "The Causes of Project Failure" *IEEE Transactions on Engineering Management*, vol.37, no.4, November.
[11] Rodriguez-Repiso, L, Setchi, R. & Salmeron, J.L., 2007 "Modelling IT projects success: Emerging methodologies reviewed" *Technovation*, vol.27, pp582-594.
[12] Heeks, R, *2006* 'Health information systems: failure, success and improvisation', International Journal of Medical Informatics, vol.75, no.2, pp125-137.

Review Questions:

- Review the PM Body of Knowledge Guide (it is available on the Internet)
- List other common project failures
- Identify the common Project lifecycle approaches

Section 5

Supporting Health Informatics and Clinical Research

Health Informatics
E.J.S. Hovenga et al. (Eds.)
IOS Press, 2010

doi:10.3233/978-1-60750-476-4-427

30. Evidence Based Health Informatics

Elske AMMENWERTH PhD[1]

Professor for Health Information Systems, Head of the Department of Health Information Systems, University for Health Sciences, Medical Informatics and Technology (UMIT), Austria

Abstract: This chapter gives an educational overview of:
- The need for a systematic evaluation of health information systems
- How to plan and execute an evaluation study
- How to select adequate quantitative and qualitative evaluation methods
- How to judge the quality of an evaluation study
- The idea of evidence-based health informatics

Keywords. Evidence Based Practice, Information Systems, Health, Medical Informatics Applications, Evaluation, Research Methods, Data Collection, Risk Management, Safety, Technology Assessment, Biomedical, Internet

1. Introduction

Health Information Systems are intended to support health professionals and organisations in delivering healthcare. Their introduction can radically affect health care organisation and health care delivery and outcome. It is evident that the use of modern information and communication technology (ICT) offers tremendous opportunities to support health care professionals and to increase the efficiency, effectiveness and appropriateness of care. For example, valuation studies on CPOE systems (computerized physician order entry) showed that such system can strongly reduce medication errors [1].

However, there can also be hazards associated with information technology in health care. ICT can be inappropriately specified, have functional errors, be unreliable, user-unfriendly, ill-functioning or the environment may not be properly prepared to accommodate the ICT in the working processes [2]. For example, there are several case studies on negative effects of CPOE systems on medical care, often relative to sub-optimal practice of information management (see, for example, [3]. Given the significance of health information systems and both the intended beneficial effect as well as the unintended negative effects on patients and professionals, it is morally imperative to ensure that the optimum results are achieved, and any unanticipated outcomes identified [4].

The objectives of evaluation studies can be according to Friedman, Wyatt [5]:
- To learn from experiences, to improve local systems
- To support decisions with regard to further introduction or improvement of systems

---

[1] Corresponding author: elske.ammenwerth@umit.at

- To justify expenses related to system introduction
- To prove that systems are safe for patients and users
- To support further development of health informatics as a science

According to [2], evaluation can be defined as "the act of measuring or exploring properties of a health information system (in planning, development, implementation, or operation), the result of which informs a decision to be made concerning that system in a specific context." This definition highlights the fact the evaluation can comprise both quantitative ("measuring") as well as qualitative ("exploring") aspects. Friedman and Wyatt [5] call this "objectivist" and "subjectivist" approaches to evaluation. Objectivist studies make use of experimental designs and statistical analysis, focusing on quantitative data derived from quantitative methods such as time measurements (see below). They are trying to answer questions such as "how large is the effect" or "is the effect due to the introduced system". Subjectivist studies rely primarily on qualitative data derived from qualitative methods such as qualitative observations (see below). They focus on description and explanation of situations, trying to answer questions such as "what did happen" and "why did it happen".

A recent literature review [6] of publications between 1982 and 2002 found 1,035 evaluation studies. This means that around 1% of all scientific publications in health informatics are evaluation studies. Most studies evaluated decision support systems and expert systems (24% of all studies), tele-consultation systems (20%) and general clinical information systems (15%) (see Figure 1). More than 80% of all studies could be clearly classified as objectivist studies.

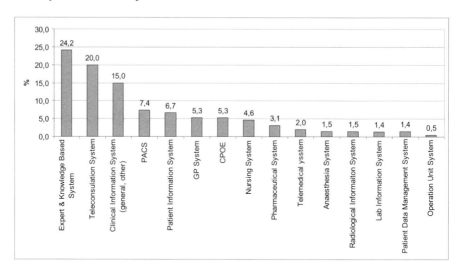

Figure 1: Evaluated Types of Information Systems 1982- 2002 (n = 1,035)

2. Planning and Executing of An Evaluation Study

When planning an evaluation study, it is necessary – as in any empirical investigation - to follow a systematic, step-wise approach. The following steps are recommended (slightly adapted from [7]:

    1.   Study Exploration
    2.   First Study Design

3. Operationalisation of Methods and detailed Study Plan
4. Execution of Study
5. Report and Publication of Study

2.1 Study Exploration

The Study Exploration Phase forms the basis for an evaluation study and results in a preliminary outline of the study. Identify the major sponsors for the evaluation, i.e. who wants the information from the evaluation study? What is the strategic objective of the study? What is the intended audience? What is the organizational and political context for the evaluation studies to take place? What are the major stakeholder groups that should be involved in the preparation of the study? What is the available budget? Is there sufficient political acceptance to go on? This phase should end with a written approval by the relevant decision-makers before going on.

2.2 First Study Design

The First Study Design Phase has the purpose of sketching the foundation for study. Establish the evaluation team; formulate in detail the study questions you want to answer; identify any constraints the study may have (e.g. budget, location, time, political aspects); select the (quantitative or qualitative) methods you want to apply to answer your study questions; describe the organizational context and technical setting your study will take place in; outline the time plan for the evaluation study and inform the involved user groups; pay attention to any legal or ethical aspects that may occur; decide on a strategy for reporting the evaluation results. At the end of this phase, you should have a written agreement on the study outline.

Please note that different groups may have different evaluation questions in mind. As it is impossible to evaluate all possible questions, you typically will have to select the most important ones. There are several evaluation frameworks that may help you to decide on important evaluation questions. For an overview on those frameworks, see [8]; for a list of possible evaluation criteria see [6].

2.3 Operationalisation of Methods and Detailed Study Plan

This phase is dealing with the selection of an appropriate design and methods to answer the leading questions (the information need), in accordance with the setting, the resources (available competences, staff, time, money, readiness of the participants to take part, etc.) and the objectives of the study. You will have to decide on study design, outcome measures, on details of the quantitative and qualitative methods (see also next section for more details on evaluation methods), on participants, whether it is a laboratory study or a field study, on study flow, and on project management and risk management aspects. The result of this phase is a detailed study plan that will be followed in the next phase.

Please note that several experimental, quasi-experimental and non-experimental study designs can be applied to IT evaluation studies. The study design has to be carefully selected depending on the study questions you may have. For quantitative studies that want to prove a hypothesis (e.g. on the effect of an information systems), experimental designs (such as randomized controlled trials) are typically seen as having a higher internal validity than quasi-experimental designs (such as before-after trials or time series analysis). For an overview on quasi-experimental designs, consult [9]. For qualitative studies, non-experimental designs such as case studies are normally chosen, but there also exist approaches of qualitative experiments.

2.4 Execution of Study

During this phase, the study plan is followed, i.e. qualitative and/or data is gathered and analysed as planned. Depending on the study design, data will have to be gathered at several locations and/or at several points in time. Special attention should be given to quality of data and to any unintended factors that may influence the findings of the study. Observations will be analysed and interpreted to answer the original study questions.

2.5 Report and Publication of Study

The results of the study should be published in a report for the decision-makers and stakeholders of the study. In some cases, international scientific publication may also be done. In any case, publication should follow established reporting guidelines such as the STARE-HI guidelines [10]. Figure 2 summarizes the described steps of an evaluation study.

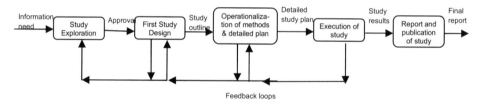

Figure 2: The Major Steps of An Evaluation Study (Adapted from [7]). Boxes comprise activities; arrows into a box from left are input; arrows out from a box are output. Feedback loops indicate that earlier steps may have to be redone or refined.

3. Quantitative Evaluation Methods

Quantitative methods deal with quantitative data, that is with numbers. Numbers have the advantage that they seem to be exact; they can easily be processed, aggregated, compared and presented - even in large numbers. The basic idea of quantitative methods is that objects have attributes (such as duration or amount) that can exactly be measured. To get data representative for a predefined population, a sampling is selected and then analysed.

Typical quantitative evaluation methods comprise:
- Time measurements (e.g. time-motion and work-sampling)
- Event counting
- Quantitative questionnaires

3.1 Time Measurements

The time-motion analysis is based on trained observers that measure the duration of observed events (e.g. tasks) while using a pre-defined list of event categories. Typically, for time-motion analysis, one observer for one observed actor (e.g. one user) is needed. This disadvantage is resolved by the work sampling analysis. Here, trained observer document which task is just being executed only at pre-defined (e.g. every 5 minutes) or randomly selected time intervals. By this, they can observe several actors in parallel. By counting the number of observed task in each category, the overall distribution and thus the duration of each task can be calculated. However, to get precise numbers, a relative large number of observations have to be done here. For details on work-sampling see e.g. [11]. Please note that both approaches (time-motion and work sampling) are typically conducted by external trained observers, but can principally also be conducted by the actors (e.g. users) themselves – this, however, may endanger the quality of the data.

3.2 Event Counting

This comprises observations of clinical situations or processes or analysis of available data (e.g. log files), counting the number of events that occur in a given time period. This can, for example be counting of medication errors (based on an analysis of patient records), counting the number of clicks when using certain software, counting the number of physician-patient interactions or counting the number of patients entering a department. As for any measurement, special attention should be given to train the observers and to use standardized observation protocols to achieve inter-observer reliability.

3.3 Quantitative Questionnaires

Questionnaires that use standardized, closed questions lead to quantitative results. For questionnaires addressing subjective opinions and feelings, the 5-point Likert scale is typically used ("strongly agree" – "agree" – "neither/nor" – "disagree" – "strongly disagree"). The quality of data achieved by questionnaires depends on a thorough formulation of questions and answers and an intensive pre-test of the questionnaire. The available literature (see e.g. [12] should thus be consulted before planning a questionnaire to ensure objectivity, reliability and validity of results. If possible, available and validated questionnaires should be reused.

Please note for all methods: The quality of quantitative data depends on whether data acquisition was objective, reliable and valid. Objectivity refers to whether the results are independent from the observer (e.g. different observers would have come to the same measurements results). Reliability means whether there was no measurement error. This can be tested for example by re-doing the measurement. Finally, validity means whether the measurement did really measure what the observer intended to measure (that is, the time measurement really reflects the time needed for a certain activity and nothing else).

4. Qualitative Evaluation Methods

Qualitative methods deal with qualitative data, that is with text and any other non-number data. Qualitative data has the advantage that it is rich in information, it can describe individual situations and contexts, and it can be analysed even when available only in a small number. Typical qualitative evaluation methods comprise:

- Qualitative interviews
- Qualitative observations
- Qualitative content analysis

4.1 Qualitative Interviews

This comprises all forms of semi- or unstructured interviews that use open questions, thus generating free-text as results. This allows the respondent to answer freely, and it allows interaction between interviewer and respondent. The interview can be conducted with one or more respondent at the same time. Group interviews support interaction between respondents, but should only be done in groups without hierarchical dependencies. In any case, a pre-tested interview instruction is needed that describes how the interviewer should conduct the interview and document the results. Answers are typically recorded by tape and later transcribed in verbal or aggregated protocols. The analysis of the data can be done by for example qualitative content analysis (see below).

4.2 Qualitative Observations

This comprises open, less-standardized, non-quantitative observations of processes or events. In contrary to quantitative observations, the aim is not to count and measure, but to get insight into a situation. The observations are typically documented in a field diary and/or on predefined observation protocols. Qualitative observations generate text (such as observer notes) that can be analysed by qualitative content analysis. Please note that for qualitative observation, there should be a certain familiarity of the observer with the observed field (for example with the situation in the clinical department).

4.3 Qualitative Content Analysis

Text obtained from qualitative interviews or observations can be analysed by a methodological, planned approach based on categories. Here, the material is stepwise analysed and coded into several available categories. The categories can either be defined beforehand (deductive approach), they can be developed only while reading and analysing the text (inductive approach), or they can be defined beforehand and refined while analysing the text (mixed approach). The coding of text into categories should be reproducible; it must therefore be clearly documented and explained by so-called anchor examples. Typically, the text material is read and coded more than once to make sure that nothing is overlooked, and that the categories are homogeneous and all filled with text examples. Based on the categories and the text passages that are related to them, the text can then be further analysed to identify larger patterns and to answer the study questions.

Please note for all qualitative methods: The quality of qualitative data depends on the following aspects: Is it clearly documented how data were gathered and analysed? Is any interpretation reproducible for the reader? Is any aggregation of data based on pre-defined rules? Is there – after some time – no new information from further analysed data (so-called data saturation)? Has the validity of interpretations been checked with the interviewed and/or observed persons (so-called member checking)? Does data from several sources point to the same results (triangulation)? For further reading on qualitative methods, please consult e.g. [13].

5. Conclusion: The Emergence of Evidence-Based Health Informatics

This chapter presented some basic information on how to conduct evaluation studies (both quantitative and qualitative ones) in health informatics. Evaluation studies contribute to the further development of health informatics as a scientific discipline. In other words, they contribute to Evidence-Based Health Informatics. Evidence-based health informatics (EBHI) can be defined as the conscientious, explicit, and judicious use of current best evidence to support decision with regard to IT use in health care (based on EBM-definition by [14]).

EBHI means that decisions with regard to IT introduction or IT development in health care should be based on available evidence. This evidence comes from IT evaluation studies that have to be published and made available to the IT decision-makers to support EBHI. The Evaluation Database [15] is one attempt to make evaluation publications easily available.

However, for the individual decision-maker, it may be difficult to keep track of all published evidence. Therefore, in medicine and nursing, which have a longer tradition in evidence-based practice, systematic reviews and meta-analysis are used to aggregate knowledge from individual trials and to come to evidence-based recommendations. While narrative reviews are quite frequent in health informatics, quantitative reviews in the form of a meta-analysis are currently seldom undertaken. Reasons may comprise the heterogeneity of studies and clinical contexts and the often quasi-experimental study designs leading to low study quality. In addition, there are frequent objections against conducting evaluation at all by decision-makers and stakeholders (for details, see [16]). Another problem may be that of publication bias in health informatics. There are estimations that around half of the evaluation studies that have been done never get published [17].

Overall, there seem to be several challenges with regard to the emergence of Evidence-Based Health Informatics. These challenges should be addressed by the health informatics community, to make Health Informatics a mature and scientific discipline that is willing and able to understand and optimize the effects of their systems on health care practice. Evaluation, if done in a systematic and professional way, provides evidence both for local improvement of health information systems as well as for the emergence of evidence-based health informatics.

References

[1] Feldstein AC, Smith DH, Perrin N, Yang X, Simon SR, Krall M, et al. Reducing warfarin medication interactions: an interrupted time series evaluation. *Arch Intern Med 2006;*166(9):1009-15. http://archinte.ama-assn.org/cgi/content/full/166/9/1009

[2]   Ammenwerth E, Brender J, Nykänen P, Prokosch H-U, Rigby M, Talmon J. Visions and strategies to improve evaluation of health information systems - reflections and lessons based on the HIS-EVAL workshop in Innsbruck. *Int J Med Inf 2004*;73(6):479-91.
[3]   Han YY, Carcillo JA, Venkataraman ST, Clark RS, Watson RS, Nguyen TC, et al. Unexpected increased mortality after implementation of a commercially sold computerized physician order entry system. *Pediatrics 2005*;116(6):1506-12. http://pediatrics.aappublications.org/cgi/content/full/116/6/1506
[4]   HIS-EVAL. Declaration of Innsbruck, *Results from the ESF Exploratory Workshop on Systematic Evaluation of Health Information Systems*, April 2003, Innsbruck. Available at http://bisg.umit.at/e/projekte/project9.htm; 2004.
[5]   Friedman C, Wyatt JC. *Evaluation Methods in Medical Informatics*. New York: Springer; 2nd edition. 2006.
[6]   Ammenwerth E, de Keizer N. An inventory of evaluation studies of information technology in health care: Trends in evaluation research 1982 - 2002. *Methods Inf Med 2005*;44:44-56.
[7]   Nykänen P, Brender J, et al. *GEP-HI - Guidelines for Best Evaluation Practices in Health Informatics*: EFMI-WG on Evaluation of Health Information Systems; 2009 - version 0.16 - Available at http://iig.umit.at/efmi/.
[8]   Yusof M, Papazafeiropoulou A, Paul R, Stergioulas L. Investigating evaluation frameworks for health information systems. *Int J Med Inform 2008*;doi:10.1016/j.ijmedinf.2007.08.004.
[9]   Harris A, McGregor J, Perencevich E, Furuno J, Zhu J, Peterson D, et al. The use and interpretation of quasi-experimental studies in medical informatics. *J Am Med Inform Assoc 2006*;13(1):16-23.
[10] Talmon J, Ammenwerth A, Brender J, de Keizer N, Nykänen P, Rigby M. STARE-HI - Statement on Reporting of Evaluation Studies in Health Informatics. *Int J Med Inform 2009*; 78(1): 1-9. http://iig.umit.at/efmi/starehi.htm
[11] Sittig DF. Work Sampling: A Statistical Approach to Evaluation of the Effect of Computers on Work Patterns in The Healthcare Industry. *Methods of Information in Medicine 1993*;32(2):167-174.
[12] Friedman C, Wyatt J. Publication bias in Medical Informatics. *J Am Med Inform Assoc 2001*;8(2):189-191. http://www.pubmedcentral.nih.gov/articlerender.fcgi?artid=134558
[13] Denzin N, Lincoln Y. *The SAGE handbook of qualitative research*. 3. ed. ed. Thousand Oaks: Sage; 2005.
[14] Sackett D, Rosenberg W, Gray J, Haynes R, Richardson S. Evidence based medicine: what it is and what it isn't. *BMJ 1996*;312(7023):71-72. http://www.bmj.com/cgi/content/full/312/7023/71
[15] EvalDB. *A web-based inventory of evaluation studies in medical informatics 1982 - 2002*. 2004; Available from: http://evaldb.umit.at
[16] Rigby M. Evaluation: 16 Powerful Reasons Why Not to Do It - And 6 Over-Riding Imperatives. In: Patel V, Rogers R, Haux R, editors. *Proceedings of the 10th World Congress on Medical Informatics (Medinfo 2001)*. Amsterdam: IOS Press; 2001. p. 1198-202.
[17] Ammenwerth E, de Keizer N. A viewpoint on evidence-based health informatics, based on a pilot survey on evaluation studies in health care informatics. *J Am Med Inform Assoc 2007*;14(3):368-71.

Review questions

1.   What is the definition of an IT evaluation study?
2.   Why are IT evaluation studies performed in health care, what are typical objectives?
3.   What are the major steps of an evaluation study, and what is the result of each steps?
4.   What are typical quantitative evaluation methods?
5.   Which major types of time measurement methods exist?
6.   What are typical qualitative evaluation methods?
7.   What do we mean when talking of evidence-based health informatics?

Health Informatics
E.J.S. Hovenga et al. (Eds.)
IOS Press, 2010
doi:10.3233/978-1-60750-476-4-435

31. Assessing and Improving Evidence Based Health Informatics Research

Jeremy WYATT   DM (Oxon), FRCP (London), FACMI[1]
Professor & Director, Health Informatics Centre, University of Dundee, Scotland

Abstract: This chapter gives an educational overview of:
- health informatics research, its aims and scope and how is distinguished from other activities
- quality criteria for health informatics research
- past research in health informatics and how it could be improved
- critically appraised published research to motivate readers to carry out research themselves
- online resources to support and improve their research

Keywords. Evaluation, Medical Informatics Applications, Research Methods, Information Systems, Quality Control, Documentation, Software, Information Management

Introduction

Research is a key element of commercial and public sector innovation and helps policy makers and practitioners make decisions about whether to purchase and adopt new technologies. However, as Sullivan said, *"Uncritical adoption of new systems based on the pressures of technological push continue to discredit policy makers... There are great opportunities for researchers interested in evaluation to fill the vacuum left by informatics practitioners who are too busy writing their next line of code."* [1]. This chapter considers the nature and kinds of research in health informatics, some quality criteria for research and how we currently match these criteria, before discussing methods to improve the quality of research in our discipline.

1. Definition and Aims of Research in Health Informatics

One definition of research is:
"The process of finding facts. These facts will lead to knowledge. Research is done by using what is already known. Additional knowledge can be obtained by proving (or falsifying) existing theories or systems, and by trying to better explain observations." [2].

Another is: *"The attempt to derive generalisable new knowledge by addressing clearly defined questions with systematic, rigorous methods."* [3]

In health informatics we study health information, communication and decisions and technologies to improve these [4]. So, to be generalisable, health informatics

---

[1] Corresponding author: j.wyatt@chs.dundee.ac.uk

research should contribute knowledge that applies to information, communication, decisions or technologies to improve these in contexts distinct from that in which the research was carried out. This could include a different information system, different users of the system or its application to different patients from those studied.

The main aims of carrying out research in health informatics include:

- To question existing theories and assumptions about the principles of health informatics and to build a set of tested theories about what works, when and for whom
- To make progress towards evidence based informatics, ie. contribute rigorous, generalisable evidence to inform decisions by system developers, users and purchasers to help them all provide safe and effective systems for health services
- To help train the next generation of health informatics professionals and researchers
- To contribute to the health informatics research process, for example by developing and validating new measurement instruments (eg. [5] [6]

2. Quality Criteria for Health Informatics Research

The definitions of research set out above require activity that is more systematic than the search for knowledge - which may be as simple as consulting a colleague. There are three main kinds of systematic health informatics research:

1. Theory formulation: Attempts to discover and formulate new hypotheses, theories or laws of health informatics
2. Theory testing: Attempts to disprove existing theories
3. Evaluation studies: Attempts to learn lessons about information, communication or decision making or systems to improve these that may be of value to others.

If the researcher is aiming to discover and formulate a new theory or hypothesis, the following quality criteria apply:

- The theory or hypothesis is clearly stated, in a format that can be tested and disproven, since this is the only way that science progresses [7]. Vague wording or concepts that are not clearly defined have no place in a theory or hypothesis
- There must be a plausible reason or argument why the theory or hypothesis is true
- The theory or hypothesis must be of general interest with clear implications for at least some workers in some areas of health informatics - the more workers or areas, the better
- The theory must be non trivial. For example, the theory "*more information means better decisions*" is both banal and tautological, since information is defined as the commodity that supports decision making [8]

As an example of applying these criteria, the hypothesis "*Some data entry forms are better than others*" might be useful and could be tested, at least by an opinion survey. However, it is too vague to be useful to system developers or users. A more useful theory would be "*Forms in which each data entry field appears in a consistent place lead to more accurate, faster clinical data entry*". This theory about data entry was in fact tested by 15 users in a series of elegant experiments [9]. These studies showed that the fastest data entry tool was one with a paging rather than scrolling form, which made all findings from the controlled vocabulary available at once rather than displaying only a subset of findings tailored by the patient's problem list, and which used a fixed palette of modifiers rather than a dynamic "pop-up" list.

If the researcher is seeking to test an established theory as Poon [9] did, the following criteria apply:

- The theory is correctly stated and has not already been disproven
- The theory is important, in the sense that disproving it would make a difference to the decisions made by a significant number of workers in the field
- The methods used to test the theory do genuinely test it and, if successful, will disprove it

The last point about the methods used is key, and can be restated as requiring that the research methods must have both high internal validity and external validity. Internal validity means that the results obtained on the users, processes, information system, clinical setting etc. are true and not the result of some mistake by the researcher or accidental bias. To meet this criterion, the researcher needs to define the question carefully and to choose study methods that minimise bias. Textbooks on evaluation methods cover these issues in some depth [10] [11], while Box 1 provides an example of a study with poor internal validity, and shows how a better research question and more rigorous study design could improve this.

Box 1: A Research Study With Poor Internal Validity, and How to Improve It: [12]

Research question: Do the patients of doctors who use medical libraries spend less time in hospital ?
Study design: Case-control study, comparing the length of stay (LOS) in patients whose doctors use the library often versus patients whose doctors do not.
Result: Mean LOS was significantly less in library-using doctors
Alternative explanations of the study results:
a. Library use by doctors is the *cause* of reduced LOS (the authors' interpretation)
b. Use of library is a *marker* of a certain kind of hard working doctor, who also tend to keep their patients in hospital for a shorter period
c. Library use by doctors happens because some doctors keep their patients in hospital for less time, so that they have more time to spend in the library
A better research question: What is the impact on patient LOS of providing a typical sample of doctors with easy access to a library ?
A better study design: Randomise a sample of at least 30 typical doctors to easy access to a library (eg. a free access to a full text web library) versus normal access; measure the LOS of their patients in the following months, correcting for cluster randomisation.

The second, often neglected, criterion for study methods is external validity. Even if the results of a study are correct ie. internally valid, it is also necessary for the results to be important, ie. generalisable to other systems, users, clients, clinical settings or processes. To meet this criterion, the researcher again needs to define their question carefully so that it is likely to interest others, even if the answer is negative. Ideally, a researcher sets out to disprove a popular, accepted theory fundamental to the discipline [13]. However, since health informatics is largely an engineering discipline, we tend to lack theories [14]. This means that researchers usually settle on more modest aspirations, choosing typical users, processes, clinical settings, measurement methods, etc. so that whatever their results they can be safely applied elsewhere. Box 2 illustrates a randomised trial that, despite being a rigorous design with high internal validity, failed to answer a question of broad interest to others. It also suggests how the original research question and study design could be improved to increase external validity.

Box 2: A research Study With Poor External Validity, and How to Improve It: the ACORN field trial [15]

Research question: Does the ACORN decision support system (DSS) lead to faster, more accurate cardiac care unit (CCU) admissions for chest pain patients in the Westminster hospital accident & emergency (A&E) department ? *Study design:* Randomised controlled trial comparing the time to admission and false negative admission rates in 153 patients randomised to use of ACORN versus control patients *Results:* ACORN's advice was only available in 51% of cases before the doctor saw the patient; there was no difference in the accuracy of patient management nor the delays experienced by high risk cardiac patients. *Limitations on the generalisability of the study results:* a)   The results only apply to the ACORN DSS, a Bayesian DSS developed in that institution and tailored to those patients using a database of 500 past patients b)   The results only apply to the specific group of chest pain patients studied and the small group of ACORN users, with the training and skills they brought to the study c)   The results only apply to that specific hospital with its catchment area, case mix, admission procedures, CCU bed allocation, etc. *A better research question:* What is the impact on chest pain patient management in a typical hospital of providing a typical sample of users with a more generic chest pain DSS ? *A better study design:* Recruit a sample of at least 30 typical doctors spread across several hospitals which are typical in their catchment areas, patient mix, staffing and CCU bed allocations; randomise the doctors to access to a generic, widely available DSS which requires no specific tailoring versus no DSS access; measure the management of their patients, correcting for cluster randomisation

These issues of internal and external validity have been discussed at length because they are key to research and also apply to the third type of more applied research that aims to carry out an evaluation study to produce robust, useful results. The two essential criteria are again internal and external validity, as described above and explored in the previous Chapter.

3. What Health Informatics Activities Are Not Research ?

Table 1: Health Informatics Activities That Are Not Considered Research, and Reasons Why

Activity	Reason why this is not health informatics research
Developing information systems to support clinical research, eg. for a clinical trials office, or to link clinical datasets	Use of informatics to support clinical research, not research in health informatics
Developing information systems to support biological research, eg. to match gene sequences or visualise proteins	Use of informatics to support biosciences, not research in health informatics
Focus groups or an audit carried out in one site to characterise a clinical problem for which an information system may be the solution	Not enduring or generalisable beyond that site; if multi site, would be health services research, not health informatics research
Systems analysis and modelling for a specific piece of software	Not generalisable beyond the specific uses, users and software scope studies, of limited and fleeting interest to others
Formative evaluation of a system, such as usability testing of a software prototype carried out as part of the design and development process	Rarely enduring or of interest to others
Qualitative or quantitative study of reasons for a system's success or failure	Results apply to the system, setting and users studied, unless the study is specifically designed to capture generic lessons likely to apply to similar systems, users and settings

If research in health informatics is systematic investigation of the process or products of health informatics activity to generate knowledge that can be applied by those carrying out the activities or using the products elsewhere, then we need to understand which other health informatics activities would not be considered research. Perhaps the most frequent confusion is with audit, which has been defined as *"A structured process to ensure we are carrying out best practice by reviewing what we are doing and comparing it with what we should be doing".* [16]. So, for example, assessing the usage of a system or the skills of its users to allow improvements to be targeted would not be considered research, as it is of very limited interest outside the time and place where the study was carried out. Research in health informatics should also be distinguished from a number of other activities listed in Table 1.

4. Matching Research Questions and Methods to System Development

The scope of research in health informatics is wide, ranging from conceptual and qualitative studies to the use of quantitative methods in psychological experiments, cohort studies, randomised trials, and synthesis of primary studies using the methods of systematic review, economic modelling and policy analysis. The reason why we include so many disciplines and types of study in our research is because many of interventions we investigate are complex, ie. *"built up from a number of components, which may act both independently and interdependently."* [17].

Carrying out research on complex interventions is challenging and requires substantial thought and resources. Although it is tempting to rush in to a "definitive" trial before the intervention is sufficiently developed, this is usually unhelpful. If the trial result is negative, we are left unsure about whether the intervention is truly ineffective, whether it was implemented badly or in an inappropriate setting, or whether the study simply used an inappropriate design or outcome measures. Even if the trial has a positive result, it can be hard to know how to apply it in a different setting [18].

Table 2: Health Informatics Research Aims, Methods and Outputs by System Development Phase

System development phase	Aim of research	Typical research methods	Output
1. Problem formulation	To describe a problem	Introspection, ethnographic methods	A rich description of the problem
2. Theory generation	To formulate and test a predictive theory	Modelling, simulation, testing using case studies	A tested theory of how to address problem
3. Develop, formative test	To develop and improve a prototype solution	Lab studies of usability, accuracy, etc.	A tested prototype based on theory
4. Summative test	To test if / when system solves the problem	Prospective field trials using controlled before after, interrupted time series or RCT designs	Evidence about the system
5. Policy analysis	To choose between interventions	Systematic review, economic modelling	Advice on cost effectiveness

There is therefore a strong argument for basing the design of all clinical interventions on relevant theory and using studies to test the applicability of the theory in that clinical setting. Table 2 suggests five distinct stages of health informatics research that set out to: describe a clinical problem, develop a theory of how to solve it and a prototype system to address it, test the prototype in a formative setting, use the results to develop a more robust system which is then tested in a summative setting, and finally use the totality of evidence about the system to inform policy. At each stage the kinds of questions and research methods used differ, as do the disciplines involved. In some ways these stages resemble the levels of Friedman's *"Tower of achievement" in health informatics*" [19].

5. How Well Have We Pursued Health Informatics Research in the Past ?

"Huge sums of money are spent annually on research seriously flawed through inappropriate designs, unrepresentative small samples, incorrect analysis and faulty interpretation. Errors are so varied that a whole book on the topic is not comprehensive… We need less research, better research & research done for the right reasons." [20] (Altman 1994)

This indictment of research and researchers addressed clinical research, but it is reasonable to ask if health informatics also has these problems. The figure shows how all 165 *"research"* papers from the 1997 AMIA Fall symposium were classified [21]. Soon after Altman's comments [20], less than a quarter of the research studies presented at this prestigious conference were considered to have generalisable results.

Figure: Breakdown of 1997 AMIA Fall Symposium "Research" Articles Reported by [21]

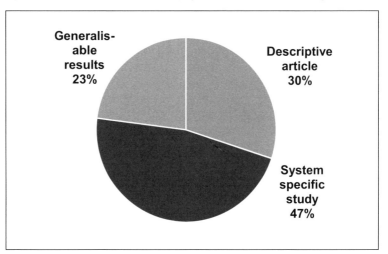

In a more exhaustive study of 1035 evaluation papers published in journals between 1982 and 2002, the authors found that over the period the number of laboratory studies and technical evaluations declined while the number of studies focusing on the impact of information technology on the quality or outcomes of care increased. The authors interpreted this as a sign that evaluation research in medical informatics was gradually maturing [22]. However, in a follow-up study on a random subset of 120 articles [23], scientific quality was assessed independently by two observers using a checklist, with excellent agreement. Unfortunately this showed that research quality improved only slightly over time, and only 19% of the variance in quality was accounted for by the year of publication. Worse, the apparent improvement may be because more of the research studies recently were randomised trials, and the quality of RCTs was rated significantly higher than that of other studies.

In conclusion, there are doubts about the quality of research in many areas, and health informatics is no exception. How can we improve the quality of health informatics research ?

6. Changes in Health Informatics Culture and Practice

We believe that some broad changes in the culture of health informatics need to take place, based on greater awareness and clarity about the three fundamental kinds of research: theory formulation, theory testing and evaluation to generate practical lessons. This will require a shift in emphasis from constructing artefacts to science [14] In addition, action is needed to improve the quality of health informatics research by three stakeholder groups: leaders in the field, researchers and research funders.

6.1 Actions by Leaders in the Field, Such as Journal Editors and Referees

We need more leadership on the part of senior members of field to enhance research quality, for example by a shift in conference and journal editorial policies. This might include editors and referees ranking a paper describing a well expressed and important hypothesis as highly as one describing the evaluation of a completed system with generic lessons. Studies that use a specific evaluation method should conform to the specific reporting standards for the method, such as CONSORT for RCTs – see Table 3 - as well as to the broader STARE-HI (Statement on Reporting of Evaluation Studies in Health Informatics) guideline[2].

PhD examiners should consider carefully whether a student who has simply implemented a clinical system using established principles has really made the original and substantial contribution to knowledge that a PhD requires.

Journals should consider how they can help improve the quality of the research they publish as well as the ability of peer reviewers to recognise it. Use of the above reporting guidelines may help. Methods of Information in Medicine has set up a Student Editorial Board to which international graduate and post-doctoral training programs can propose members [24]. This should help new researchers to learn how to review manuscripts early during their career, under the supervision of experienced journal editors.

Editors have complained that too many manuscripts submitted to their journals describe engineered artefacts without a scientific purpose [25]. They argue that the quality of results reporting should be increased and that impact studies should be more frequently performed to strengthen the methodological underpinnings of our field. The reporting standards in Table 3 and the STARE-HI initiative may help this.

---

[2] http://iig.umit.at/efmi/

Table 3: Reporting Guidelines for Different Kinds of Studies

Study design	Name of reporting guideline	URL
Survey or cross sectional study	STROBE	http://www.strobe-statement.org/Checklist.html
Prospective cohort study	STROBE	http://www.strobe-statement.org/Checklist.html
Case control study	STROBE	http://www.strobe-statement.org/Checklist.html
Assessment of accuracy	STARD	http://www.equator-network.org/index.aspx?o=1050
Randomised trial	CONSORT	http://www.consort-statement.org/index.aspx?o=1011
Randomised trial of non-pharmacologic treatment	CONSORT Extension for Non pharmacologic Treatment	http://www.consort-statement.org/index.aspx?o=1417
Cluster randomised trial	CONSORT extension for cluster trials	http://www.consort-statement.org/index.aspx?o=1047
Qualitative study	BMJ qualitative research checklist	http://resources.bmj.com/bmj/authors/checklists-forms/qualitative-research
Health economic study	BMJ health economic study checklist	http://resources.bmj.com/bmj/authors/checklists-forms/health-economics
Systematic review of trials	QUOROM (Quality Of Reporting Of Meta-analyses	http://www.consort-statement.org/mod_product/uploads/QUOROM%20Statement%201999.pdf
Systematic review of observational studies	MOOSE	http://www.equator-network.org/index.aspx?o=1052

6.2 Actions by Researchers

Researchers need to address important, enduring questions, which in health informatics tend to be about communication, decision making, people, teams and organisations. They need to de-emphasise fleeting questions about specific technologies or, worse, a specific information system whose answers will be of limited interest even in one year's time. With the wide range of questions that occur in health informatics, researchers also need to avoid a Procrustean approach in which the research question is adjusted to fit their favourite research method. This means being eclectic and either training in a wide variety of methods, or working with a wide group of collaborators. Otherwise there is a risk that, to the methodologist with a sample size calculator, every question becomes the null hypothesis for a trial or to a qualitative researcher, every question becomes an invitation to participant observation !

Researchers also need better skills in searching the literature for past studies of similar systems or theories, validated measurement instruments, methods to overcome biases and evidence to support or deny important theories. Reading about the errors and failures of the past eg. [26] should help to expose researchers to the need for careful choice of system development options and study methods to maximise internal and external validity. Reference to the reporting guidelines listed in Table 3 and the supporting material that accompanies each may also help improve researcher understanding of internal and external validity.

Where time allows, as in PhD research projects, students should be encouraged to identify and focus on fundamental health informatics principles and construct systems and experiments to test these, rather than building and testing ad hoc software applications, even though this can be a demanding activity in itself.

Researchers should avoid trying to market a research project to an audience who is not competent to judge its quality. Thus, they should not approach a medical funder for a project they believe addresses important technical questions, nor a technical funder to support a project with no technical innovation, but that may have clinical benefits.

Finally, to ensure that those trying to summarise the literature by carrying out systematic reviews can include both negative as well as positive studies, it is important for all researchers to publish negative as well as positive studies [14] [27] and to register their studies prospectively. Since July 2005 at least one health informatics journal, the Journal of Medical Internet Research, will only consider trials for publication that have been registered in a trial registry before it started, to reduce publication bias and selective reporting of positive outcomes. The journal has created the free International eHealth Study Registry to support this activity [28].

6.3 Actions by Funding Bodies

We believe that bodies who fund research in the area need to become clearer about whether they are aiming to fund science (the formulation and testing of important theories) or evaluation studies. They therefore need to debate and understand the nature of health informatics and of scientific progress in the field, which means recruiting experienced health informatics researchers to support their policy and funding decisions. Such researchers need to be unbiased in their approach, able to identify which questions and requests for funding represent truly original and important work and which are replicating well known studies or systems with little added value.

There is another issue that besets our field, lying as it does on the interface between medical and technical disciplines. Unfortunately, some researchers approach medical funders with proposals that embody no new technical insights but claim technical novelty; medical funders find it hard to detect this untruth, and may fund it even though there is no obvious clinical application. Other researchers approach technical funding bodies with proposals for an apparently useful application that a medical referee would rapidly detect as implausible. Again, the funding body will find it hard to detect this and funds the application even there is no technical innovation, as the health benefit appears plausible. Usually the researchers in both cases are simply naive about where the value of their proposal lies, but in others cases they unfortunately exploit the lack of awareness of technical issues by medical funders and clinical issues by technical funders. Better relationships between funding bodies and joint funding programmes are ways to address this issue.

7. Some Online Tools to Support Researchers

All parties can benefit from a range of online tools and information to support research and improve its quality. The reporting guidelines listed in Table 3 include a wealth of methodological advice, in the shape of supporting articles. There are also a wide range of other online resources to support researchers, some of which are listed in Box 3.

Box 3: Some Other Sources of Methodological Advice on the Web

- Home page of the EFMI Working Group for Assessment of Health Information Systems
- http://iig.umit.at/efmi/ This includes a searchable inventory of published evaluation studies in medical informatics 1982 – 2005 http://evaldb.umit.at/index.htm
- The AHRQ Evaluation Toolkit. Casack CM and Poon E (Eds) *Evaluation Toolkit (version 3)*. Agency for Healthcare Research and Quality, National Resource Centre for Health Information Technology, Washington DC, US. http://www.ahrq.gov/
- The IS World searchable database of validated measurement methods in computing and informatics
- http://www.isworld.org/surveyinstruments/surveyinstruments.htm
- The Missing data web site http://www.lshtm.ac.uk/msu/missingdata/index.html
- Other ESRC research methodology support sites linked from http://www.ccsr.ac.uk/methods/

8.   Summary and Conclusions

Successful and productive health informatics research often appears to be a combination of luck, creative art, and science [14]. However, the most important element is clarity about what the research is for and how it meets the criteria for high quality research discussed earlier. Then researchers can ask questions that are likely to be of broad and enduring interest and choose methods that ensure the maximum possible internal and external validity.

We must not forget that the point of research is to improve health informatics knowledge, practice, health information systems and ultimately patient outcomes. We need to identify and target weak points in this knowledge chain, exploring potential methods to help translate informatics theory and research results into practice. Specialist journals may have a contribution here [29].

Finally, we must avoid excessive focus on merely developing and improving research methods, as opposed to identifying and answering important health informatics research questions. In conclusion, if our discipline is to thrive and take root in firm ground, research activity needs to be taken seriously by all, otherwise we could end up building edifices on sand.

References & further reading

[1] Sullivan F. What is health informatics? J Health Serv Res Policy. 2001 Oct;6(4):251-4.
[2] www.simple.wikipedia.org/wiki/Research
[3]   UK   Department   of   Health   Research   Governance   Framework http://www.dh.gov.uk/en/Researchanddevelopment/A-Z/Researchgovernance/index.htm
[4] Wyatt JC, Sullivan F. ABC of Health Informatics 1: What is health information ? BMJ 2005; 331:566-8
[5] Staggers N. The Staggers Nursing Computer Experience Questionnaire. Appl Nurs Res. 1994 May;7(2):97-106
[6] Demiris G, Speedie S, Finkelstein S. A questionnaire for the assessment of patients' impressions of the risks and benefits of home telecare. J Telemed Telecare. 2000;6(5):278-84
[7] Popper K R . Conjectures and Refutations: the growth of scientific knowledge. Oxford: OUP 1965
[8] Shortliffe E, Perrault L, Wiederhold G, Fagan L (eds): Medical Informatics, 2nd Edition. New York: Springer Verlag 1998
[9] Poon AD, Fagan LM, Shortliffe EH. The PEN-Ivory project: exploring user-interface design for the selection of items from large controlled vocabularies of medicine. J Am Med Inform Assoc. 1996 Mar-Apr;3(2):168-83
[10] Friedman CP, Wyatt JC. Evaluation methods in biomedical informatics (2nd edition). New York: Springer-Publishing, October 2005. 386 pages, ISBN 0-387-25889-2

[11] Brender J. Handbook of Evaluation Methods for Health Informatics. Academic Press 2005.

[12] Marshall JG. The impact of the hospital library on clinical decision making: the Rochester study. Bull Med Libr Assoc 1992; 80(2):169-178

[13] Kuhn T S. The Structure of Scientific Revolutions. Chicago Univ Press 1970.

[14] Wyatt J. Medical informatics, artefacts or science? Methods Inf Med. 1996 Sep;35(3):197-200

[15] Wyatt J. Lessons learned from the field trial of ACORN, an expert system to advise on chest pain. In Proceedings of Sixth World Conference on Medical Informatics, Singapore. Barber B, Cao D, Qin D, Wagner G (eds); Amsterdam: North Holland, 1989: 111-115

[16] Leicester Primary Care Audit Group 1996 – now The Clinical Audit Support Centre http://www.clinicalauditsupport.com/aboutus.html

[17] Campbell M, Fitzpatrick R, Haines A, Kinmonth AL, Sandercock P, Spiegelhalter D, et al. Framework for design and evaluation of complex interventions to improve health. *BMJ* 2000;321:694-6

[18] Campbell NC, Murray E, Darbyshire J, Emery J, Farmer A, Griffiths F, Guthrie B, Lester H, Wilson P, Kinmonth AL. Designing and evaluating complex interventions to improve health care. BMJ. 2007 Mar 3;334(7591):455-9

[19] Friedman CP. Where's the science in medical informatics? J Am Med Inform Assoc. 1995 Jan-Feb;2(1):65-7

[20] Altman D G . The scandal of poor medical research. BMJ 1994; 308: 283-4

[21] Krishna S, Andrews J E, Craven C.K, Patrick T.B An Analysis of MEDLINE Indexing of Medical Informatics Literature Proceedings AMIA Symposium 1998 p.1030 https://www2.amia.org/pubs/symposia/D004947.PDF

[22] Ammenwerth E, de Keizer N. An inventory of evaluation studies of information technology in health care trends in evaluation research 1982-2002. Methods Inf Med. 2005;44(1):44-56

[23] de Keizer NF, Ammenwerth E. The quality of evidence in health informatics: how did the quality of healthcare IT evaluation publications develop from 1982 to 2005? Int J Med Inform. 2008 Jan;77(1):41-9. Epub 2007 Jan 5

[24] Aronsky D, Haux R, Leong TY, McCray A. The Student Editorial Board of Methods of Information in Medicine--an opportunity to educate tomorrow's peer reviewers. Methods Inf Med. 2007;46(6):623-4

[25] Talmon JL, Hasman A. Medical informatics as a discipline at the beginning of the 21st century. Methods Inf Med. 2002;41(1):4-7

[26] Koppel R, Metlay JP, Cohen A, Abaluck B, Localio AR, Kimmel SE, Strom BL. Role of computerized physician order entry systems in facilitating medication errors. JAMA. 2005 Mar 9;293(10):1197-203

[27] Tierney WM, McDonald CJ. Testing informatics innovations: the value of negative trials. J Am Med Inform Assoc. 1996 Sep-Oct;3(5):358-9

[28] Eysenbach G. Tackling publication bias and selective reporting in health informatics research: register your eHealth trials in the International eHealth Studies Registry. J Med Internet Res. 2004 Sep 30;6(3):e35

[29] Lehmann CU, Altuwaijri MM, Li YC, Ball MJ, Haux R. Translational research in medical informatics or from theory to practice. A call for an applied informatics journal. Methods Inf Med. 2008;47(1):1-3

Review questions

1. What is research ? Why do we undertake it ?
2. What are the three main kinds of research ? How do they differ from one another ?
3. What are the main quality criteria for research in health informatics ?
4. Explain the term "internal validity" and how to maximise it
5. Explain the term "external validity" and how to maximise it
6. How can those working in health informatics improve the quality and quantity of research activity ?

Health Informatics
E.J.S. Hovenga et al. (Eds.)
IOS Press, 2010
© 2010 The authors and IOS Press. All rights reserved.
doi:10.3233/978-1-60750-476-4-446

32. Practice-Based Evidence for Clinical Practice Improvement: An Alternative Study Design for Evidence-Based Medicine

Susan D HORN PhD[a,1,2], Julie GASSAWAY MS RN[2,b], Leah PENTZ B.Sc[2,c], Roberta JAMES M.Stat[2,d]

[2] *International Severity Information Systems, Inc, Institute for Clinical Outcomes Research, Salt Lake City, UT 84102 United States of America*
[a] *Senior Scientist*
[b] *Director of Project Development,*
[c] *Formerly Research Associate*
[d] *Formerly Data Systems Specialist*

Abstract: This chapter gives an educational overview of
- The limitations of evidence-based practice.
- Strengths and weaknesses of RCT and observational studies.
- The general PBE-CPI study design.
- Benefits of PBE-CPI studies and how they can enhance our ability to discover and establish standards for best practice.
- The relationship between CIS and PBE-CPI studies.

Keywords. Evidence Based Practice, Research Methods, Information Science, Information Management, Knowledge, Quality Indicators-Healthcare, Statistics, Medical Informatics Applications, Information Systems, Data Collection, Data Management Systems, Clinical Trials, Practice Guidelines

Introduction

As clinical settings move from paper to electronic records, well designed clinical information systems (CIS) are becoming more important to both clinicians and researchers. Health care professionals are starting to look past the value of data storage and ease of access and are beginning to explore how the data can be leveraged to guide better clinical decision making starting with more research [1]. This chapter reviews limitations of current clinical research study designs, describes a new study design called practice-based evidence (PBE), compares it to other study approaches, and then discusses the relationship of CIS and PBE to improve clinical care.

---

[1] Corresponding Author: shorn@isisicor.com

1. Evidence-Based Practice

A recurring criticism in medical care is the lack of adequate high-level research evidence with which to establish evidence-based practice. Tunis, Stryer, and Clancy [2] write:

"The current clinical research enterprise...is not consistently producing an adequate supply of information to meet the needs of clinical and health policy decision makers... [due to] a systematic problem in the production of clinical research. ...A consistent finding of [systematic literature] reviews is that the quality of evidence available to answer the critical questions identified by experts is suboptimal. ...These gaps in evidence undermine efforts to improve the scientific basis of health care decisions...[such that] clinical practice guidelines may not be able to develop clear, specific recommendations."

These authors call for new research methods to address practical questions about risks, benefits, and costs of interventions as they occur in routine clinical practice. New methods would address questions such as 'Does the treatment work in the real world of everyday practice?' and 'For whom does the intervention work best?' This approach is in contrast to explanatory clinical trials or efficacy studies (for example: Randomized Controlled Trials (RCTs)) that are concerned with questions such as 'Does the investigational treatment cause an effect?' and 'How and why does the intervention work?' Explanatory trials are designed to maximize the chance that some effect of a new or existing treatment will be revealed by the study. They are a form of confirmatory analysis of suspected relationships discovered in previous research.

Berguer [3] discusses problems with the evidence in evidence-based medicine (EBM). The main tools of EBM are randomized trials and meta-analysis, but he states that these methods are unlikely to lead to discovery of new and best treatments for specific types of patients. "*[Rigorous] observational and inductive clinical intelligence should be stimulated and published because a therapy needs to be invented before it is proven effective.*" To paraphrase Berguer, RCTs are important to the *confirmation* of new and/or current interventions and practices, not to the discovery of more effective and efficient interventions or practices.

There are additional calls for new approaches to evidence-based medicine and performance in quality and costs of healthcare systems. Porter and Teisberg [4] observe that medical services are restricted or rationed, many patients receive poor care, and high rates of preventable medical errors persist. There are wide and inexplicable differences in costs and quality among providers and across geographic areas. Competition in healthcare is operating at the wrong level. "*System participants divide value instead of creating it.*" This form of zero-sum competition must be replaced by competition at the level of preventing, diagnosing, and treating individual conditions and diseases and determining the best treatments for specific types of patients [4]. Westfall and colleagues [5] remark "*What is efficacious in randomized clinical trials is not always effective in real world, day-to-day practice. Practice-based research provides the laboratory that will help generate new knowledge and bridge the chasm between recommended care and improved care.*"

Practice-based evidence for clinical practice improvement (PBE-CPI) research methods are a variant of the new designs called for by others [6]. Methods such as PBE-CPI can liberate us from the straightjacket that has constrained our ability to discover and establish standards for best practice and as will be discussed later, the ability to improve the development and refinement of CIS.

2. Randomized Controlled Trials: Features and Challenges

The intellectual origins of RCTs come from agriculture. In agricultural hothouses, the environment can be reasonably controlled and various interventions tested. RCTs were developed in simpler times when we did not have powerful multivariate statistical tools and, even when we had them, we lacked the computational power that readily accessible computer-based statistical packages have brought us over the last 30 years. As a research model, the RCT allowed one to make relatively simple computations using fairly small sample sizes; it was well suited to computational constraints of an earlier era. Today, RCTs do not harness the full power of multivariate statistics in which many variables can be considered simultaneously and covariates can be identified and neutralized to evaluate intervention effects.

A hallmark of an RCT is the random assignment of study participants into a treatment arm and a control arm to control for participant differences that might otherwise affect the outcome. By neutralizing participant differences through randomization, RCTs help to isolate the effect of the treatment under review. Nonrandomized comparison groups present the risk that some non-treatment effects remain unaccounted for and thus compromise one's ability to have full confidence that the outcome is truly a consequence of the treatment or intervention under study.

When designed and conducted properly, RCTs are considered the gold standard to establish causality in scientific research. Clinical and health services research communities have come to accept hierarchies of evidence where randomized controlled trials (RCTs) are considered the highest level of evidence and anything less than RCT-level evidence is considered somewhat suspect. However, a true clinical setting is much less controllable than an agricultural hothouse and this difference leads us to question the applicability of this pre-established hierarchy in the medical field.

From the clinical perspective, using RCTs presents several major challenges that are not easily overcome. We mention a few here and later discuss how a PBE-CPI approach is not bound by many of the same constraints.

2.1 Standardization and Artificiality.

RCTs require use of standardized treatment protocols and hold all other variables constant in order to isolate the effects of the intervention and to reduce "noise" in the data. One result is that the intervention setting can become artificial and may not reflect what would otherwise transpire under less-controlled, real-world clinical environments. Standardized treatment protocols require extensive quality control to decrease error rates about the treatment. Treatment purity is difficult to maintain over time, across centers, and across clinicians; if compromised, an "intent-to-treat" analyses, which keeps everyone in the study and in their assigned groups even if the treatment protocol or control is not followed as prescribed, may be the best remaining analysis option. Unfortunately, "intent-to-treat" analyses no longer reflect efficacy.

2.2 Selection Criteria, Patient Recruitment, and Generalizability.

Selection criteria for RCTs are often quite restrictive in order to reduce variation stemming from differences among study participants. Restrictive selection criteria limit the generalizability of the study's findings ("external validity") to the types of individuals represented in the study. The study's findings may not apply to the types of individuals excluded from the study such as individuals with comorbidities. Clinicians often dismiss RCT findings, since they deem their patients to be quite different from those seen in a clinical trial. Restrictive selection criteria can result in studies with very small numbers—drawn from a much larger pool of otherwise eligible participants. Typically, only a small percentage of patients—usually 10 to 15 percent—are eligible for a trial. Enormous resources must then be expended to recruit large pools of potential participants in order to locate individuals who meet the selection criteria and thus achieve the sample size needed to power the analyses.

2.3 Blinding.

RCTs assume some degree of "blinding." Ideally, all three actors—the study participant, the clinician, and the researcher/observer—are unaware as to whether the participant is in the treatment or control arm. Double blinding means that two of the three are blinded—both the participant and one of the other two actors. However, some interventions are not easily disguised and others are impossible to disguise.

RCTs present other challenges including ethical challenges to randomization and lengthy planning and approval processes that can sabotage even the best-designed studies. Most formidable is cost: An RCT can be very expensive, since it may require an elaborate protocol to screen patients, coordinate care, and collect data, in addition to providing the intervention or treatment to participants.

All of this leaves clinical research with a dilemma. On one hand, clinical practice needs the validation that sound scientific evidence can provide. On the other hand, its highly customized, multi-factorial approach does not lend itself well to RCTs that require a limited set of interventions and selection criteria that can make participant recruitment difficult and expensive, while making study findings less generalizable. Over the years, many variants of the RCT have evolved to address one or more of the challenges identified but none have overcome the limitations inherent to an RCT.

2.4 Observational Data and Causal Inferences

Confidence in a treatment depends on belief that supporting evidence implies a causal connection, not accidental association. Randomization underlying the RCT provides a relatively high degree of confidence in this regard, but remains tied to the limitations of cost, relevance, and design. An attempt to make the design more clinically applicable is to use naturalistic data representing the population and circumstances of interest. But in such data, subjects are not randomized into various treatment groups; consequently, analyses often cannot discern whether differences in outcomes are due to different treatments or to other differences between subject groups.

The limitations of RCTs have generated considerable effort to create methods that identify treatment effects using observational data. In the last 30 years, a large literature base has developed on causal inferences and observational data [7] [8] [9] [10] [11] [12] [13] [14] [15] [16]. Methods have been created that allow for unbiased estimates of treatment effects by controlling for unmeasured confounders 10] [11] [12] [13]. Unfortunately, these methods cannot identify all treatment effects of interest and are often sensitive to assumptions that are not testable. Also, they require considerable knowledge in statistics to understand and adjust sufficiently for nuisances, making them less useful to researchers and less comprehensible to decision makers.

In contrast, methods that bypass unobserved confounding have been developed. Specifically, instrumental variables allow for estimation of treatment effects in the presence of otherwise unobserved confounding [14]. However, the treatment effect is instrument-specific and may not be one of interest. In addition, it can be difficult to identify and measure the required variables, and similar to the preceding methods the necessary assumptions are not testable. As another alternative, the observed data can be analyzed as if there are no unmeasured confounders and then subject to a sensitivity analysis of potential confounding [9]. To be useful, however, this approach requires assumptions regarding the unknown confounding, and little is gained if results are determined to be sensitive to assumptions. Treatment effects can be identified from observational data without the need for sophisticated statistical models and untestable assumptions only if all factors influencing the distribution of both interventions and outcomes of interest are measured and controlled for in analysis and enough data are available. Unfortunately, when confounding factors are not statistically controlled, treatment effects may be indistinguishable from patient characteristics.

In real world settings it is not likely that all confounders can be identified and measured, ultimately leaving a researcher with three options: (1) pursue a costly RCT that may not address the clinical context of interest, (2) embark on statistically sophisticated methods that trade one set of untestable assumptions (i.e., the identification of all confounders) for another set of untestable assumptions (the necessary distributional or correlational assumptions underlying selection and instrumental variable models), or (3) report an analysis that does not account for confounding, mention the deficit as a limitation, and let the user beware.

3.   Practice Based Evidence

If the goal, however, is to produce useful information and reduce uncertainty for decision makers, the situation may not be so constrained. We suggest a paradigm shift toward the pragmatic: structure research to minimize the potential for accidental associations to improve its usefulness.

Rather than focus on meeting conditions for statistically unbiased causal effect estimates, we propose designing observational studies that focus on minimizing the plausibility of alternative explanations while estimating the complex associations between treatments and outcomes within a specific context of care. The identified associations are not equated with causal parameters but nonetheless inform such judgments to the extent that the design minimizes alternative explanations. The goal is to structure carefully the design to capture the salient information bearing on the research question. The proposed design trades uncertainty regarding generalizability in the case of the RCT, or uncertainty in necessary assumptions underlying the statistical methods mentioned above, for uncertainty regarding the potential for alternative explanations while explicitly minimizing the plausibility of such explanations. This proposed PBE-CPI method is available for use by most researchers with access to the standard computational power of today's PCs and a knowledge of basic multiple regression techniques.

3.1 Clinical Practice Improvement: Features and Challenges

PBE-CPI harnesses the complexity presented by patient and treatment differences, offering a naturalistic view of treatment by examining what actually happens in the care process [6]. It does not alter the treatment regime to evaluate efficacy of one particular intervention as is done in an RCT. The PBE-CPI approach offers the advantage of large numbers of patients—numbers that often cannot be attained in an RCT due to stringent selection criteria.

PBE-CPI is an observational study design whose measurements encompass a comprehensive view of clinical care by assessing: (1) key patient characteristics, (2) all treatment and care processes, and (3) outcomes. All three classes of data are considered simultaneously. See Figure 1. This comprehensive measurement framework provides a basis for meaningful analyses of significant associations between process and outcome, controlling for patient differences.

PBE-CPI designs include detailed measures of patient factors (physiologic severity of illness and psychosocial abnormalities presented at each visit or admission), care process factors (e.g., medications, treatments, therapies, interventions), and outcome factors (e.g., functional gain, severity of illness at discharge, discharge disposition, etc.). The results allow clinicians to objectively evaluate associations of care processes and outcomes based on treatment of similar patients. Without all three types of data (e.g., if one has only process and outcome data, but not detailed patient data), clinicians cannot tell if the outcomes achieved are due to process steps or differences in patient factors.

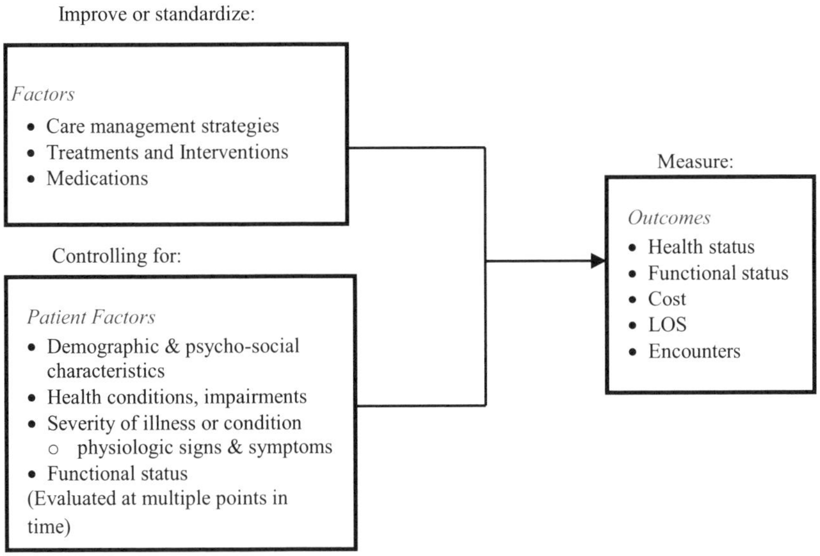

Improve or standardize:

Figure 1. Three Essential Components for a PBE-CPI Study

Patient Factors. Patient factors are the key characteristics of the study population: demographic characteristics, specific indications for treatment, severity of illness, initial functional status, psychosocial factors, etc. In PBE-CPI studies these patient characteristics address a central feature in RCT design, namely the need for randomization to neutralize the effect of patient differences. Randomization is used when patient differences cannot adequately be taken into account. In contrast, PBE-CPI studies incorporate detailed information about patients and account for these differences through statistical analyses. Detailed patient profile data include condition-specific physiologic data, such as those contained in the Comprehensive Severity Index (CSI®), a unique severity of illness measure used in PBE-CPI studies [6] [17] [18] [19] [20] [21] [22].

Care Process Factors/Treatments. A process of care is a sequence of linked, usually sequential, steps designed to cause a set of desired outcomes to occur. The goal is to find a measurable factor that describes each major process step. Examples include which drugs are dispensed, at what dose and frequency, what therapies are performed and for how long, etc. A data collection instrument records the process steps in detail, including dates and time. Thus, PBE-CPI studies require that clinicians and researchers work together to ensure actual interventions are characterized fully and accurately in the study. The high level of detail collected on processes and interventions during PBE-CPI studies is unique to its study design.

Outcome Factors. Medical treatments are designed to achieve specific outcomes. Among outcomes commonly assessed are condition-specific complications, condition-specific long-term medical outcomes (based on clinician assessment or patient self-report), patient functional status, patient participation in society, patient satisfaction, and cost. Outcome factors may be thought of as analogs to assessment endpoints in an RCT, but RCTs are usually powered for one primary outcome. In comparison, PBE-CPI studies usually encompass many outcomes.

To capture the required level of detail, PBE-CPI studies entail the creation of a large study database that includes all patient, process, and outcome variables of interest. Many details may already exist in medical records, but many require additional data collection tools that are implemented prospectively. The content of the tools is developed using a bottom-up approach, meaning front-line clinicians work together to develop the tools so their interventions can be documented standardly between clinicians and across facilities. It is important to note that standard interventions are not implemented but that interventions are documented in a standardized format. For example, if gait therapy is performed by multiple physical therapists, the study does not implement one specific type of gait therapy but requires the therapists to document details about the gait therapy such as the length of the therapy, the equipment used, and the level of assistance required, etc., in order to measure and describe the differences used in practice.

Multivariate statistical methods are then used to compare alternative treatments while controlling for other variables that may be driving observed differences between treatments and outcomes. These statistical methods allow the researcher to examine relationships far more complex than those using a single explanatory or treatment variable at a time. The coefficients of the significant independent variables in regression equations identify key process steps that, when controlling for patient factors, are associated with better outcomes.

PBE-CPI focuses on actionable findings that can be implemented in real-life clinical settings to improve outcomes. This focus on implementation governs who is involved in designing the study, what data are collected, what questions are answered during analyses, and who designs protocols for improvements in routine practice. Thus, PBE-CPI studies place a premium on the participation of front-line clinicians in the study design, variable selection and definition, study execution, analyses of data, and implementation of study findings. Those actually providing care are involved in all phases of a PBE-CPI project and that involvement helps facilitate buy in needed to overcome the RCT hierarchy and turn PBE-CPI findings into actual care improvement processes.

4. RCT and PBE-CPI Studies Compared

Table 1: RCT & PBE-CPI Studies Compared

Variables	RCT	PBE-CPI
Patient Variables	1. Patient eligibility and stratification factors 2. Eliminate patients who could bias results: comorbidities, severe disease, etc. 3. About 10-15% of patients qualify	1. Minimal patient eligibility and stratification factors 2. Use severity of illness to measure comorbidities and disease severity 3. All patients qualify by measuring patient differences; none excluded
Process variables	1. Treatment protocol 2. Specify explicitly every important element of the process of care for both treatment and control arms 3. Informed consent	1. Measure or record all treatments and interventions 2. Abstract information from charts based on existing practice 3. Informed consent often not needed[*]
Outcome variables	1. Powered for primary outcome 2. Change based on evidence	1. Many outcomes assessed-relevant to patients and providers 2. Improvement based on evidence
Measurements/ documentation	1. Limited number of patient variables, treatments, outcomes measured 2. Variables specified precisely for all patient, treatment, and outcome measures	1. Comprehensive holistic framework 2. Variables specified precisely for all patient, treatment, and outcome measures
Sample Size	• Typically small	• As large as desired
Database	• Limited to the variables needed	• Comprehensive and detailed
Result	1. Efficacy 2. Assigned causality	1. Effectiveness 2. Association and assumed causality
Hypotheses	• Typically one hypothesis • Clearly defined at the start • Narrow and focused	• Typically many hypotheses • Many and broad at the start • Refined and new hypotheses generated by analytic findings
Local knowledge	• Local knowledge excluded	• Local knowledge contributes and valued; entails participation by practicing clinicians
Confounders	• Assumed not relevant to study or outcome, excluded	• Affect outcomes and are relevant to include
Cost	• Very costly	• Moderate cost – depends on study design

[*] *Informed consent may not be required if there is no experimental intervention and if there are no data collected beyond what is ascertained from medical records and from reports prepared by clinician in the course of usual care.*

Table 1 compares RCT and PBE-CPI studies across several dimensions. PBE-CPI-like observational studies can help overcome many of the limitations that are inherent in RCTs. Despite conventional wisdom that RCT studies provide superior evidence relative to observational studies, there is growing empirical evidence that supports the use of well-designed observational studies akin to PBE-CPI studies to discover what works best in medicine. Three studies found that treatment effects from observational studies and RCTs were remarkably similar [23] [24] [25]. These studies concluded that well-designed observational studies do not systematically over-estimate the magnitude of the effects of treatment as compared with those in RCTs on the same topic. In addition, " the popular belief that only RCTs produce trustworthy results and that all observational studies are misleading does a disservice to patient care, clinical investigation, and the education of health care professionals" [25].

PBE-CPI has demonstrated the ability to identify important associations in many diagnostic groups. Table 2 gives examples of PBE-CPI studies and selected treatments that were found to be associated with better patient outcomes, their positive impact on patients, and their positive impacts on health care systems (e.g., reduced LOS and/or cost) [26] [27] [28] [29] [30] [31] [32] [33] [34] [35] [36] [37].

A key advantage of a PBE-CPI study is the naturalistic view of medical treatment that is provided by data recorded routinely by medical providers. This view is critical to determine implications of treatment alternatives. In everyday practice, patients are assigned to different treatments based on the provider's medical judgment, patient compliance is not artificially influenced, and monitoring of results is based on the provider's need for information about how a patient is doing. All these factors can impact the effectiveness of medical treatments. PBE-CPI analyses evaluate current practices and use the results to develop evidence-based improvements. Changes to the process of care rest on clinical data rather than on clinical opinion.

This approach is in direct contrast to the approach of traditional RCTs. Because RCT participants are screened, selected, and subjected to scrutiny and intervention control beyond that occurring in everyday treatment, RCTs report results that may not be broadly applicable in everyday medical treatment. For example, a recent study described a little-used 40-year-old drug, spironolactone, which was shown in a landmark clinical trial in 1999 to significantly reduce death and hospitalization for patients with [Congestive Heart Failure] [38]. There was a four-fold jump over 18 months in prescriptions for the generic drug. That surge in use was accompanied by a tripling of hospital admissions and of deaths resulting from dangerous elevations of potassium. Many patients given the medicine likely would have been excluded from participating in the original clinical trial. The authors note, "The new findings offer a provocative look at the difference between clinical trials and real-world medicine – and the potential dangers of applying trial results too widely. Patients in clinical studies typically are selected carefully to maximize the chance of showing a benefit and minimize side effects. Thus, trial patients represent only a subset of the types of patients doctors treat in their offices. Patients given the medicine in the aftermath of the 1999 study were on average 13 years older than participants in the original trial and more likely to have diabetes. Also the average dose in actual practice was 30 mg while 25 mg was used in the study." Alternatively, PBE-CPI studies can provide evidence to determine those medications and interventions that work best for the different patient types found in real-world practice.

Another key advantage of PBE-CPI study methods is cost. Using data from medical records and computerized databases is generally less costly than implementing a prospective RCT, while allowing for a much larger number of observations available for analysis and further hypothesis generation and refinement.

Table 2: Examples of PBE-CPI Studies, Selected Findings, and Their Effects

PBE-CPI Project	Selected Significant Findings	Associations	Implications
Abdominal Surgery [32]	Early feeding (start within 48 hrs after surgery) Sufficient feeding (>60% of protein and calorie needs)	Shorter LOS Lower Hospital Cost	Even though they had higher average severity of illness, patients fed early and sufficiently had between 1.4 and 2.9 days shorter average LOS and between $1,940 and $5,281 lower average cost per case than patients fed either not early and/or not sufficiently
Abdominal Surgery [29]	Use of PCA pump	Higher rate of post-operative surgical wound infection	10.7% infections for PCA users vs. 4.0% for non- PCA users
National Pressure Ulcer Long-term Care Study [31]	Disposable briefs Supplement use Combination medications	Fewer pressure ulcers	Less suffering and lower cost to treat in nursing homes
Formulary Limitations in the Elderly [35]	Greater formulary limitations	Higher health care resource utilization – more doctor office visits, more ED visits, and more hospitalizations per year	Common cost-containment strategies are associated with higher health care resource utilization
Asthma Drugs [36]	Use of newer asthma drugs	Lower overall drug costs and fewer PCP visits per year	Common cost-containment strategies are associated with higher health care resource utilization
Diabetes Study [37]	Self-monitoring of blood glucose along with consistent provider discussion	Better serum glucose control and fewer hospitalizations	Monitoring alone is not sufficient; discussion of results with providers is essential
Infants hospitalized with RSV [30]	33-35 weeks GA infants hospitalized with RSV	Higher intubation and longer ICU and hospital LOS	Consider prophylaxis for 33-35 week GA infants
Severely disabled stroke patients [34]	Earlier gait and tube feeding	Faster and more improvement in functioning and more home discharges	Even for low-functioning stroke patients, start gait and tube feeding in 1st 3 hours of rehabilitation
RN staffing in nursing homes [27,28]	RN direct care time 30-40 min/resident/day	Fewer hospitalizations, pressure ulcers, UTIs, and $3,200 cost savings/resident/year to society	Higher levels of RN direct care time/resident/day can lower overall costs and suffering for frail elderly nursing home residents

Observational studies do not scientifically prove causality of any underlying relationships, but can point to hypotheses that can be evaluated clinically. There are three ways to ascertain *causality* from PBE-CPI studies:

1. No added confounders cause the significant association to disappear,
2. A change in outcome follows a change in treatment as predicted by the PBE-CPI model [6],
3. Repeated studies on the same topic yield the same findings.

In summary, PBE-CPI studies have demonstrated predictive validity by observing that outcomes improve as predicted when practices change to align with those associated with better outcomes in PBE-CPI analyses. Thus, RCTs and PBE-CPI should be considered complementary. Practice effects of RCTs can be tested in PBE-CPI studies and PBE-CPI can be a progenitor of new RCTs.

4.1 PBE-CPI and CIS

PBE-CPI study data normally are abstracted manually from existing paper and electronic medical records or documented prospectively on standardized tools. This process is costly due to the labor-intensive nature of data entry and can include many errors. As we move forward in the information technology world, our goal is to use existing CIS data that can be exported for analysis. Unfortunately, to date we have had little success with exporting existing data (e.g., assessments for severity of illness signs and symptoms, nutrition treatments, medications that have been administered, development of complications, etc.) or programming standard prospective tools into a system and then exporting those data at the time of analysis. The problems stem from how CIS is developed and the main purposes for implementation, which are clinical data storage, ease of access to data, and monitoring of processes to reduce errors. Typically CIS software products have been created by vendors who developed the software with a top-down approach, i.e., programmers and clinical experts develop general user-requirements with the intent that the software will be used 'off-the-shelf' by multiple consumers. However, most consumers need to have the software customized because the product content is too general to capture their processes and work flow. The result is that many consumers may use the same software package but as a result of all the site specific customization, vendors end up supporting very different versions and there is no standardization across facilities. Our experience with these types of systems have motivated us to, yet again, call for a paradigm shift where CIS is:

1) developed with a bottom-up approach,
2) provides clinicians with reports and summaries of assessment and treatment data to assist with clinical decision making, and
3) allows easy access to data for research purposes.

The bottom-up approach concept should be used when creating requirements during development of CIS software because of its ability to create comprehensive data collection modules. The process benefits from having multiple clinicians from multiple centers describe what assessments and interventions they perform on specific types of patients. The back-and-forth dialogue between the clinicians assures that assessments and interventions called one thing at a facility and another thing at a different facility are defined together so the modules are standardized. For example, a byproduct of our efforts to create prospective data collection tools in an acute care post-stroke rehabilitation PBE-CPI study across seven facilities was the development of therapy taxonomies. The clinicians realized that the tools' list of activities and interventions was so comprehensive that it could be used on all patients and not just study patients. Creating minimum requirements using this approach around what each type of clinician should collect across software applications will encourage more standardization. This does not mean practice has to be standardized but how data are documented is standardized.

Once the content of data to be collected is determined, the bottom-up approach can be taken one step further to create feedback reports to help with clinical decision making. Many CIS packages contain some reporting features but they tend to focus on billing needs, submission of data to national databases (e.g., FIM in acute care rehabilitation, MDS in long-term care, etc.), and system or patient alerts (e.g., after a weight is entered a message may be displayed if the patient lost 10 pounds in one week, after a high systolic blood pressure is entered a message is displayed indicating a physician should be contacted, etc). Few have reports to summarize key assessment and treatment data over time for single patients or groups of patients who meet certain criteria. Combining these types of reports with research findings to inform clinicians when patients should or have received an intervention associated with better outcomes allows for improved implementation of protocols. Impact of using feedback reports can be monitored to assess implementation and success of protocols on improving overall outcomes for patients.

For this process to be successful, research needs to be a primary user of clinical data. A characteristic that allows for continued research is flexibility. The CIS software must have a database schema so that as new variables are identified as important to collect, they can be added to existing data collection modules or incorporated into new ones. In addition the database must be able to interface with statistical software or must be exportable. Research is an iterative process. As treatments are identified as being associated with best outcomes, they should be monitored over time and continually re-evaluated against new and existing treatments. The powerful relationship between CIS and PBE-CPI studies has the potential to change clinical care enormously over the next few decades making the practice of medicine a science.

An example of how this process has been affective is through multiple projects funded by the US Agency for Healthcare Research and Quality (AHRQ). The first project started with the implementation of protocols based on significant findings from the National Pressure Ulcer Long-Term Care Study (NPULS), a PBE-CPI study. Eleven long-term care facilities worked together to standardize their daily CNA documentation, which contained a subset of required variables to monitor pressure ulcer prevention protocol compliance. Weekly feedback reports based on the CNA documentation showed residents at risk of developing a pressure ulcer by displaying trended assessment and treatment data that assisted with care planning activities. This was the first time that many of the participating nurses used trended data to monitor patients' health status and then recommend interventions based on those data. The project was successful enough to warrant additional funding to take this approach and implement CIS that was programmed to contain the required variables and feedback reports. The CIS ranged in level of technology from digital-pens and forms to full electronic medical record systems. Additional funding has been granted to monitor not only the compliance and success of the pressure ulcer prevention protocols but to expand the research to start a new PBE-CPI study in pressure ulcer healing treatments. There is hope that this continuous process of improvement and research will be perpetuated in the long-term care facilities even after the AHRQ projects are completed.

We envision the future of PBE-CPI studies where patient, process, and outcome data will exist electronically in clinical CISs eliminating our current dependence on manual data abstraction. In addition, variables identified by clinicians as important to the study, but not already collected, could easily be added to the CIS without requiring additional, separate data collection tools. The efficiency and logistics of this new data acquisition modality will ease the conduct of iterative PBE-CPI studies to determine best practices, making them less costly and decreasing the clinician-turned researcher burden. Another benefit of this new electronic era is more consistent implementation of clinical practice guidelines and their protocols.

5.   Summary

PBE-CPI studies constitute a rigorous form of quasi-experimental research. Although they are weaker than RCTs on internal validity, they are stronger on external validity. Overall, PBE-CPI studies better represent actual conditions of practice, cost less, and increase research efficiency. They do not require homogeneous patient populations, so allow for inclusion of patients with comorbidities or complications. To avoid confounding the link between interventions and outcomes, PBE-CPI studies measure relevant patient characteristics using severity assessment tools and statistically adjust for patient differences. Further, they accommodate departures from rigid treatment protocols by carefully monitoring and measuring actual treatments; then use these data in statistical analyses. As this approach does not disqualify large numbers of patients, it facilitates the generation of the number of cases needed for statistical comparisons, while simulating the real world. Using multiple regression and other statistical techniques, researchers test treatments associated with clinical and cost outcomes sought for different kinds of patients.

Although PBE-CPI studies tend to focus on short-term outcomes, these outcomes include effects that are noticeable and holistically important to patients rather than only those that are physiologically measurable through laboratory or other tests. By design, PBE-CPI studies are replicated easily so they can be implemented at multiple sites.

The most appropriate design for a specific study depends on the nature of the research question and the type of knowledge needed. Methodology alternatives such as PBE-CPI do not replace the RCT, but rather provide additional sources of systematic outcomes information that improve on the anecdotal and informal knowledge base that underlies much of clinical practice. PBE-CPI studies have enormous power to enable health care providers, managed care organizations, payers, and individuals to evaluate current practice and improve clinical decision making. These studies answer questions in the real world where multiple variables and factors can, and do, affect patient outcomes. Appropriately designed clinical information systems will facilitate these efforts by improving the data collection process, assisting in more consistent implementation of study findings and their protocols, and allowing continued evaluation of the protocols over time.

References

[1] Powell J, Buchan I. Electronic Health Records Should Support Clinical Research. J Med Internet Res 2005;7(1):e4
[2] Tunis SR, Stryer DB, Clancy CM. Practical Clinical Trials: Increasing the Value of Clinical Research for Decision Making in Clinical and Health Policy. JAMA September 24, 2003;290:1624-1632.
[3] Berguer R. The Evidence Thing. Ann Vasc Surg April 21, 2004;18:265-270.
[4] Porter ME, Teisberg EO. Redefining Competition in Health Care. Harvard Bus Review June 2004;1-13.
[5] Westfall J M, Mold J, Fagnan L. "Practice-based Research—'Blue Highways' on the NIH Roadmap." *JAMA* (January 24/31) Vol 297, No. 4, 2007: 403-410.
[6] Horn SD. Editor. Clinical Practice Improvement Methodology: Implementation and Evaluation. Faulkner & Gray, New York, New York, September 1997
[7] Pearl, J. (2002). "Causal inference in the health sciences: A conceptual introduction." Health Services and Outcomes Research Methodology 2: 189-220.
[8] Pearl, J. (2003). "Statistics and causal inference: A review." Test 12(2): 281-345

[9]   Rosenbaum, P. R. (2002). Observational studies. New York, Springer.

[10] Heckman, J. J. (2001). "Micro data, heterogeneity, and the evaluation of public policy: Nobel lecture." Journal of Political Economy 109(4): 673-748

[11] Little, R. J. and D. B. Rubin (2000). "Causal effects in clinical and epidemiological studies via potential outcomes: Concepts and analytical approaches." Annual Review of Public Health 21: 121-145

[12] Winship, C. and S. L. Morgan (1999). "The estimation of causal effects from observational data." Annual Review of Sociology 25: 659-706.

[13] Winship, C. and R. D. Mare (1992). "Models for sample selection bias." Annual Review of Sociology 18: 327-350.

[14] Newhouse, J. P. and M. McClellan (1998). "Econometrics in outcomes research: The use of instrumental variables." Annual Review of Public Health 19: 17-34

[15] Heckman, J and Navarro-Lozano S (2004). "Using matching, instrumental variables, and control functions to estimate economic choice models." The Review of Economics and Statistics 86(1):30-57.

[16] Rosenbaum PR, Rubin DB (1985). The bias due to incomplete matching. Biometrics 41(1): 103-116.

[17] Averill, R.F., McGuire, T.E., Manning, B.E., Fowler, D.A., Horn, S.D., Dickson, P.S., et al. (1992). A study of the relationship between severity of illness and hospital cost in New Jersey hospitals. Health Services Research, 27(5), 587-617

[18] Horn, S.D., Torres, A. Jr, Willson, D., Dean, J.M., Gassaway, J., Smout, R.. (2002b) Development of a pediatric age- and disease-specific severity measure. Journal of Pediatrics, 141(4), 496-503

[19] Willson, D.F., Horn, S.D., Smout, R.J., Gassaway, J., Torres, A. (2000). Severity assessment in children hospitalized with bronchiolitis using the pediatric component of the Comprehensive Severity Index (CSI®), Pediatric Critical Care Medicine, 1(2), 127-132

[20] Ryser DK, Egger MJ, Horn SD, Handrahan D, Gandhi P, Bigler ED. Measuring Medical Complexity during   Inpatient Rehabilitation following Traumatic Brain Injury Arch Phys Med Rehabil (to appear - 2008)

[21] Horn, S.D., Sharkey, P.D., Buckle, J.M., Backofen, J.E., Averill, R.F., Horn, R.A. (1991). The relationship between severity of illness and hospital length of stay and mortality. Medical Care, 29, 305-317.

[22] Gassaway JV, Horn SD, DeJong G, Smout RJ, Clark C. Applying the CPI Approach to Stroke Rehabilitation: Methods Used And Baseline Results. Arch of Phys Med Rehabil. December 2005 supplement.

[23] Benson K, Hartz AJ. A comparison of observational studies and randomized, controlled trials. NEJM 2000;342:1878-86 (June 22, 2000).

[24] Concato J, Shah N, Horwitz RI. Randomized, controlled trials, observational studies, and the hierarchy of research designs. NEJM 2000;342:1887-92 (June 22, 2000).

[25] Ioannidis JPA, Haidich AB, Pappa M, Pantazis N, Kokori SI, Tektonidou MG, et al. Comparison of evidence of treatment effects in randomized and nonrandomized studies. JAMA August 2001;286(7):821-830.

[26] Bartels, S.J., Horn, S.D., Sharkey, P.D., Levine, K. (1997). Treatment of depression in older primary care patients in Health Maintenance Organizations. International Journal of Psychiatry in Medicine, 27(3), 215-231

[27] Dorr DA, Horn SD, Smout RJ. Cost analysis of nursing home registered nurse staffing times. J American Geriatrics Society 2005;53:840-845

[28] Horn SD, Buerhaus P, Bergstrom N, Smout RJ. Association between registered nurse staffing time and outcomes of long-stay nursing home residents. Amer J Nursing November 2005;105(11):58-71.

[29] Horn, S.D., Wright, H.L., Couperus, J.J., Rhodes, R.S., Smout, R.J., Roberts, K.A., et al. (2002a). Association between patient-controlled analgesia pump use and post-operative surgical site infection in intestinal surgery patients. Surgical Infections, 3(2), 109-118. Abstracted in Year Book of Surgery, 2003.

[30] Horn, S.D., Smout, R.J. (2003). Effect of prematurity on respiratory syncytial virus hospital resource use and outcomes. Journal of Pediatrics, 143 (5 Suppl), S133-141.

[31] Horn, S.D., Bender, S.A., Ferguson, M.L., Smout, R.J., Bergstrom, N., Taler, G., et al. (2004). The National Pressure Ulcer Long-term Care Study (NPULS): Pressure ulcer development in long-term care residents. Journal of the American Geriatrics Society, ; March 2004;52(3):359-367.

[32] Neumayer, L.A., Smout, R.J., Horn, H.G.S., Horn, S.D. (2001). Early and sufficient feeding reduces length of stay and charges in surgical patients. Journal of Surgical Research, 95(1), 73-77

[33] Willson, D.F., Horn, S.D., Hendley, J.O., Smout, R., Gassaway, J. (2001). The effect of practice variation on resource utilization in infants hospitalized for viral lower respiratory illness (VLRI). Pediatrics,108(4), 851-855

[34] Horn SD, DeJong G, Smout R, Gassaway J, James R, Conroy B. Stroke Rehabilitation Patients, Practice, and Outcomes: Is Earlier and More Aggressive Therapy Better? Arch Phys Med Rehabil 2005;86(12 Supplement 2):S101-S114.
[35] Horn SD, Sharkey PD, Phillips-Harris C. Formulary Limitations in the Elderly: Results from the Managed Care Outcomes Project. The American Journal of Managed Care (August 1998): 1105-1113.
[36] Horn SD, Sharkey PD, Kelly HW, Uden DL. Newness of Drugs and Use of HMO Services by Asthma Patients, Annals of Pharmacotherapy 35 (September 2001) 990-996.
[37] Blonde L, Ginsberg BH, Horn SD, Hirsch IB, James B, Mulcahy K, et al. Frequency of Blood Glucose Monitoring in Relation to Glycemic Control in Patients with Type 2 Diabetes, Diabetes Care 25:1 (January 2002) 245-246.
[38] McMurray JJV, O'Meara E. Treatment of Heart Failure with Spironolactone-Trial and Tribulations. New England J of Medicine 2004;351:526-528

Review Questions

1. What are the limitations of evidence-based practice?
2. Describe the strengths and weaknesses of RCT and observational studies
3. Explain the general PBE-CPI study design.
4. What are the benefits of PBE-CPI studies and how they can enhance our ability to discover and establish standards for best practice?
5. What is the relationship between CIS and PBE-CPI studies?

Health Informatics
E.J.S. Hovenga et al. (Eds.)
IOS Press, 2010
doi:10.3233/978-1-60750-476-4-461

33. Integration of Data for Research

Marienne HIBBERT M.App.Sci, PhD[1a], Jason LOHREY BSc (Physics & Computing)[b], Steve MELNIKOFF PhD[c]

[a] *Director, BioGrid, Melbourne Health, University of Melbourne and VPAC, Australia*
[b] *Chief Technical Officer, Arcitecta Pty. Ltd., Honorary Research Associate, Howard Florey Neuroscience Institutes, University of Melbourne , Australia*
[c] *Deputy Director, The Victorian eResearch Strategic Initiative (VeRSI),The University of Melbourne, Australia*

Abstract. This chapter gives an educational overview of:

- The clinical research lifecycle
- Sources of research data
- The need for contextual data standardization to retain meaning
- Information management principles for sustainable data
- Data linkage technologies used to support collaborative research aimed at improving health outcomes
- Making use of identifiers in health

Keywords. Computer Communication Networks, Software, Information Science, Data Collection, Documentation, Information Management, Information Services, Knowledge, Statistics, Terminology, Safety, Health Facilities, Research Methods, Ethical Issues, Code of Ethics, Personal Information, Information Systems, Outcomes Assessment (Healthcare), Semantics, Quality Indicators –Healthcare, Ontology, Systematised Nomenclature of Medicine (SNOMED), Logical Observation Identifiers Names and Codes (LOINC), Privacy, Personal Information, Informed Consent.

Introduction

The convergence of healthcare, life sciences, and information technology is revolutionising research in health. Researchers have the capability to analyse human biology at the finest levels through genomics, and link to health information sourced from clinical outcome data. The search for new treatments and the optimal use of available therapies is driving research today, and accelerating this convergence.

Previously data was stored 'in silos' so that extracting data from each data source was a nightmare of ethics approvals, comparability and logistics. Being able to collate data from multiple sources about an individual gives researchers the potential to both understand the fundamental causation of human disease and predict outcomes. This will enable the development of new drugs, new diagnostics, and lead us to the optimal use of therapies.

The key to studying and making the associations between all data types is access to detailed clinical data in sufficient numbers of patients. Studies need to review their sample size to ensure there is enough statistical power for the research questions being studied. Institutions may not have sufficient numbers to perform meaningful analyses

---

[1] Corresponding author: Marienne.hibbert@biogrid.org.au

by themselves, particularly where stratification is required to look at specific disease attributes. Clinical researchers are now looking beyond their own specialty into data from other disease groups, analysing the impact of co-morbidity as well as other factors. Figure 1 below shows a linkage of two lifecycles, on the left, a lifecycle diagram of the clinical research process and on the right, an analogous lifecycle for clinical/healthcare informatics research. In part, the linkage of the two is between the data produced by clinical research and its utilization in informatics.

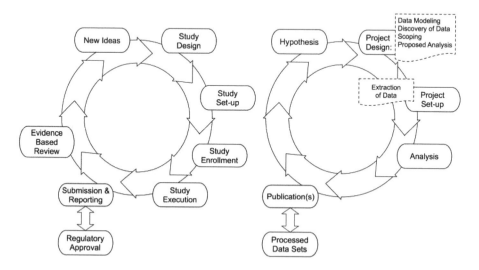

Figure 1 – Linkage of Two Life Cycles. *The left, lifecycle diagram of the clinical research process, is used with permission, Michael G Kahn MD, PhD, University of Colorado and Carol Broverman PhD, Partners Healthcare System.*

Types of research that can be addressed by linking to available data sets include:
- Screening activity - Genetic predisposition
- Environmental exposures
- Genetic influences
- Co morbidities
- Treatment strategies
- Drug discovery
- Quality and health outcomes research
- Longitudinal analysis
- Geographic and environmental influences
- Social and educational influence.

Understanding the steps in the life cycle of clinical research shown in Figure 1 will help in the successful design and execution of research. New and emerging data sets can broaden the scope of research questions and the use of technology and standards as outlined in this chapter can facilitate research in numerous fields. The technologies discussed in this chapter will help collaborative research across the health and non-health sectors will ultimately improving health outcomes in the future.

1.   Sources of Research Data

Clinical research requires access to as much data as possible and that data can be harvested from a variety of sources including relational databases, spreadsheets, Picture Archiving and Communications Systems (PACS) and paper-based records. Data may take two forms: a) exist in its own right, or b) exist in conjunction with some other data, such as a set of Magnetic Resonance Images, to provide context and description.

Data that exists to describe some other data is referred to as "metadata". Metadata may be embedded in the data itself or may be kept separately. For example, photos from a digital camera in JPEG format have embedded metadata describing the data, time, and camera settings at the time the digital photo was taken. DICOM[2] files include information describing the name of the patient, their age, sex, the acquisition parameters et cetera and the binary data itself.

Metadata is often stored separately to the data itself, in some form of database to help with indexing and searching, since the data files themselves are often too large to search efficiently and/or the processes that generated additional metadata may be costly to repeat. Depending on the type of research, the associated data files, may be retrieved for analysis after discovery through metadata searching.

Typically, information about the patient is of interest for clinical research, rather than information about the data set itself. Measurements and data acquisitions are done to assess the state of the patient and so information describing the data set itself may be required to assess the quality of assertions about the patient.

There may be significant differences in the quality of data that is available. Data quality may be affected by a number of factors including incomplete information, data entry errors, measurement errors, the quality of the devices used to acquire data and environmental conditions at the time of acquisition.

A diagnosis can vary depending on the person making the diagnosis and the criteria used. For example, a General Practitioner (GP) doctor may use a less precise or different set of qualitative and quantitative measures than a neurologist for assessing a person as having had a stroke. Consequently, general practitioners may report a different number of cases of stroke than specialists. Such differences must be taken into consideration when using different systems as sources of research data.

It is valid to use data of varying quality, provided the quality is understood. Every data repository should have an accurate assessment of the quality of data to enable the researcher to determine the quality and error in the derivative research. However, interesting associations in low quality data can be a trigger to improve data quality in the future, or can be useful for hypothesis generation.

Clinical data is stored in a variety of information models and databases. Established clinical systems used for patient care are expected to have well defined information models and databases. However, these information models are often established for a particular area of health care and may inconsistently overlap with other areas of health care. Research projects often develop numerous customised information models and databases, which may evolve over time. Databases may range from enterprise managed relational databases through to tabular information maintained in spreadsheets. Significant data is often only available in paper-based records that can go back for decades. These need to be transcribed into electronic form.

---

[2]Digital Imaging and Communications in Medicine, http://medical.nema.org/

Yet the structure and even legibility of such information can vary significantly, often a function of the clinician that designed the data collection for their area of research.

Ideally, clinical researchers should not have to deal with the underlying method of data storage. This presents a number of challenges for information management systems to a) make data from a large number of heterogeneous sources accessible and b) meaningfully combine data from different sources. There will be differences in terminology, differences in the structure and in the amount of information available. This problem is compounded when combining data across different disciplines of health care, and further amplified when using data from non-clinical systems such as demographic databases.

2.   Standardisation

As described in the preceding section, data of interest can come from a variety of sources. In order to meaningfully combine and analyse data, every research datum must be mapped to consistent information models with agreed semantics (its meaning).

A simple example, such as patient sex, needs clear definition. Some systems may use "male" and "female" while others use "m" and "f" and some systems may have a different number of variants for patient sex. For instance, some systems define "male", "female", "hermaphrodite", "male pseudohermaphrodite" or "female pseudohermaphrodite" [1]. Hermaphrodites, male pseudohermaphrodites, and female pseudohermaphrodites may be grouped as "intersex".

There are two key processes related to standardisation: a) agreement on common terminology and semantics and b) transforming data in arbitrary form to the canonical form (the simplest form without loss of generality). Common terminology requires the establishment of a reference ontology - this may take the form of a simple glossary and make use of established terminologies such as SNOMED[3]. Preferably, the ontology should provide complete usage and semantic context such as that provided by MeTEOR[4]. There are also formal languages for expressing concepts such as Archetypes with its associated Archetype Definition Language (ADL)[5]. Archetypes enable the representation of a concept relationship between different concepts, and rules for application of those concepts are expressed using ADL. Each such term in a concept can have a number of language translations allowing the same concept to be expressed in any number of languages. Formal expression languages, such as ADL, enable machine validation and subsequent machine interpretation of concepts allow precise, rigorous and language independent definitions of concepts to be shared across databases.

Data is likely to be retrieved from sources that utilise one or more of these standards. There is currently no single standard for data representation, especially across international boundaries. Consequently, linkage systems need to account for data in many different forms.

Data structures in the source system must be mapped to a common terminology and this may require case-by-case mapping. Hopefully, the same disciplines of health care will have the same, or at least similar, data structures requiring a once-off

---

[3] Systemized Nomenclature of Medicine-Clinical Terms, http://www.ihtsdo.org
[4] Australian Institute of Health and Welfare metadata registry, http://meteor.aihw.gov.au
[5] http://www.openehr.org/clinicalmodels/archetypes.html

mapping. Transformations of data can be done on the fly by extracting data and converting it as part of the query or may be done in batch and stored in an intermediate database.

In addition to SNOMED [2], MeTEOR [3] and OpenEHR [4], several other standards organizations are working towards the implementation of a common shared Electronic Health Record (EHR) environment: HL7, CEN, ISO/IEC, ASTM, DICOM, OMG, IHE, IEEE, OASIS, Regenstrief (LOINC), WHO, UN/CEFACT, W3C[6], CDISC [5] [6] [7] [8] [9] [10] [11].

There are continuing efforts to standardise, particularly within the same disciplines of health care but the development of standards often lags behind new clinical practice and innovative research. In addition, there are multiple overlapping standards, as well as standards yet to be developed. Unless there is a single standard that to describes everything now and can accommodate new data, there will always be a need to translate data to forms that allow cross-discipline discovery, analysis and interpretation. Paper was once the primary method of recording and storing clinical data and even this has the issue of possible changing context over time. Who can envisage how information will be captured, represented and stored in the next hundred years?

3. Information Management Principles for Sustainability of Data

Information management in clinical research aims to efficiently turn data collected from researchers into a form that is without error available for analysis, presentation, review, and subsequent long-term storage. This is especially important in an era of large volumes of *ephemeral* research data that cannot be reproduced, or reconstructed [12].

In accordance with good research practice, providing a robust mechanisms for the sustainability and archiving of data, over an appropriate period of time, will support the scientific objectives of the research, and the legal and ethical responsibilities of the investigators. The goal is research data that: is accurate, complete, timely, verifiable, secure and available.

Archiving is the long-term storage of data and documentation in a safe, secure location. An *archival program* is a well-defined process, and set of protocols, whereby data records progress from creation through to storage and preservation [13].

Sustainability of data can have various meanings [14]. From the World Council on Environment and Development it is information that: "meets the needs of the present without compromising the ability of future generations to meet their own needs". This definition challenges any research management system to be adaptable to future technologies, and anticipate and cope with the constant changes in health care and clinical research, while fulfilling the current, goals of the research.

Sustainable information management systems are needed for the timely translation of clinical research into useful health care practice. The lifetime of clinical research and associated data can be measured in decades, and can incur costs of hundreds of millions of dollars. It is the role of information management systems to provide the technological basis for successful completion of the research from the point of creation to final archive.

---

[6] W3C XSL Transformations (XSLT), http://www.w3.org/TR/xslt

Sustainability encompasses a number of key activities and issues [15] in the care of data for future use. These activities engender a degree of trust that the data will be viable for a long time.

A first step is to *select the data* for retention. What criteria should be used to keep a set of records, or discard another? What is the scope and purpose of the archival program, is it clearly defined and well documented? Questions of cost, risk, technical feasibility, and provenance all need to be balanced in deciding whether to archive all the data, or just a portion. Some answers lie in the legal and ethical obligations, in addition to the technical and scientific requirements.

The core activities of a sustainable clinical research information system centers around three areas:

1. *Archiving* ensures that the data has been properly selected and stored. Ensuring the security and validity of the information are specific objectives of archiving activities.
2. *Preservation* or *technological maintenance* makes sure that the data can be accessed and understood over time as the technology changes.
3. *Curation* is the management and promotion of data utilisation.

Curation considers data from its creation, with the promise that it will fulfil its stated purpose, as well as availability for: discovery, analysis, reuse, annotation, and publication. As the scope of clinical research continues to grow, new avenues of investigation are appearing where informatics, how information and information technology support research and research data, are a central part. The data management systems underpinning informatics will help in the sustainability of the data which is a continuous, on-going process.

4.   Linkage of Clinical Data Records

Record linkage is the general task of integrating information belonging to the same *entity* but derived from one or more independent sources. In the case of a single source, it might involve chronologically based data for correlation analysis. Or, for the case of multiple sources, relating disparate clinical records that belong to the same individual patient. Figure 2 – Illustrates linkage of data from four 'Mary Smith' records with a common 'linkage key' into a single data record which aggregates all the data fields from the individual source records.

Medical records serve a number of purposes in any health care system, and are a mirror of the health care process. They function as the main vehicle of communication between clinicians and services about patients, and as the primary body of evidence of a patients' clinical presentation, assessment, care and referral.

Clinical data record linkage can enhance the over-all quality of health care delivery by improving accessibility to information, and the lines of communication, but is also playing an increasingly pivotal role in medical research.

At the level of an individual patient the possibility of integrating large clinical datasets with records from other systems, such as community, welfare and education programs opens up new research opportunities addressing the holistic nature of health previously impossible or impractical to explore.

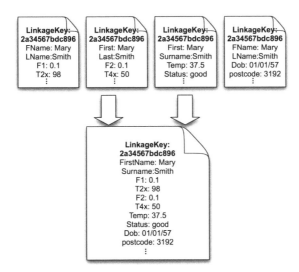

Figure 2 – Illustration of Linkage From Four 'Mary Smith' Records Into a Single Data Record

4.1 Issues of Identifiers in Health

All techniques for record linking patient records require using a set of common patient identifiers. This set may include: names, birth date, death date, sex, residence, hospital admission date and, or various unique identifiers, such as a health insurance number.

If a unique identification variable is accessible and shared by all the data sources, for instance a health insurance number, then the process of linkage is *deterministic* and an *exact matching approach* can be automated in a straightforward manner. Some countries, such as Chile, Denmark, Greece and others, have unique national identifiers for each citizen that can be used as an input to generation of a deterministic linkage key. To protect the privacy and ensure the individual cannot be identified, national identifiers should never accompany research data. Rather, they should be used to generate a one-way encrypted linkage key.

The crucial issue for clinical data record linkage is that such *mutual*, unique identifiers rarely exist, necessitating use of one or more identifying variables, such as surname, given name, date of birth, and the like, that may or may not correctly, and uniquely, identify an individual.

From the patient's point of view the quality of a health care system and their confidence in it depends on whether their personal health information is safe, secure, accurate, and confidential. Building a clinical record linkage capability directly tests these requirements, as the consequences of a breach of confidentiality could have grave personal impact and legal ramifications for researchers..

Consideration must also be given to the array of existing and emerging standards around health informatics and electronic health records (EHRs). These are typically applicable to the local context, but take into account policy developments, internationally and leverage the expertise of health agencies, researchers and other health related organizations world-wide. These standards are important guides for the development of reliable record linkage schemes, and the underpinning record identifiers.

4.2 Requirements for Clinical Data Record Identifiers

A number of identifying variables are usually needed for clinical data record linkage. Unfortunately these identifiers may not be unique to a particular individual, may be inaccurate, missing, and, or change over time. This forces record linkage to shift from a deterministic process to one of likelihood estimation. It becomes a *probabilistic measurement* of whether the identifying 'code' obtained from a set of identifying variables is a 'true' one. Even in the case of unique identifiers, there may be a situation of multiple exact matches needing resolution for a 'best' link via a likelihood estimator.

The need to engage statistical methods in the record linkage process establishes a set of ideal requirements on the types of identifying information [16]:

1. The identifying information should be *permanent*; that is, it should exist at the birth of a person to whom it relates or be allocated to him/her at birth, and it should remain unchanged throughout life.

2. The identifying information should be *universal*; that is, similar information should exist for every member of the population.

3. The identifying information should be *reasonable*; that is, the person to whom it relates and others, should have no objection to its disclosure for medical purposes.

4. The identifying information should be *economical*; that is, it should not consist of more alphabetic, digits and other characters than necessary.

5. The identifying information should be *simple*; that is, it should be capable of being handled easily by a clerk and computers.

6. The identifying information should be available.

7. The identifying information should be *known*; that is, either the person to whom it relates or an informant acting on his/her behalf should be able to provide it on demand.

8. The identifying information should be *accurate*; that is, it should not contain errors that could result in its discrepancy on two records relating to the same person.

9. The identifying information should be *unique*; that is, each member of the population should be identified differently.

4.3 Deterministic Record Linkage

Given a sufficient number of identifiers, linking clinical records can become a deterministic problem of formulating the level of 'agreement' between them before a 'match' or 'no-match' determination is made. The most restrictive, and simplest rule would be to require all the identifiers to perfectly agree. Less restrictive, would be a match between a subset of identifiers, for example, only requiring a match on surname and date of birth out of an identity set that includes first name, sex, and address. In either case deterministic record linkage strategies are easily adapted for computerized processing.

In a more realistic situation the data may contain missing or incorrect values, pointing to an inherent limitation of deterministic linkage schemes, that is there is no way to rank the identifiers in terms of their 'quality'. Each provides the same level of information, no more reliably than another, and a single miscoded item can drastically affect the overall result. For the same reason, it is also impossible to resolve multiple links between record matches.

4.4 Probabilistic Record Linkage

To take into account the differences in record identifiers, probabilistic record linkage provides a likelihood estimate of a correct match using a weighting for each identifier. The weight or *strength* of an identifier might be dependent of the amount of information conveyed, and how well it separates the space of all possible values for that identifier. For instance a variable like sex, having only two values (mostly), might be assigned a lesser weight as compared with a birth date, with a few hundred values. Consequently a record pair match on the single value, sex, would be assigned a smaller probability of a true match, relative to one on a single value of birth date. Weights can also be assigned measuring both agreement and disagreement between identifiers. In general, identifying information with the largest range of values, hence spectrum of agreement, carry the largest weights.

Record linkage identifiers together with a weighting system enable probabilistic record linkage to quantify an *outcome* probability of a match, mis-match, or near-match between record pairs. Once established, thresholds can then be set that set tolerance limits on the accuracy of a true or false record linkage.

4.5 Uses of Record Linkage

Either deterministic or probabilistic record linkage methods have their specific strengths and weaknesses, both enabling the linkage of large datasets at the level of individual records. From which researchers can begin to answer questions not possible from any of those databases separately, spanning multiple fields of inquiry and areas of health care.

5.   Technology Approaches

There are four key technology issues to be addressed:
   a)   how can information systems adapt to changes in the available information,
   b)   how should data be stored to ensure it is available at any time in the future,
   c)   how and at what point should data be transformed from the original format to the canonical forms, and
   d)   how can the identity of the patient be protected and never available to any researcher whilst allowing aggregation of data from multiple sources?
These issues are addressed using the following approaches.

Adaptive systems can accommodate changes in the methods of data storage, the systems and the structure of information. Adaptive systems can be achieved by using a Service Oriented Architecture (SOA) and flexible data representations such as the Extensible Markup Language (XML)[7].

Service-oriented architectures are primarily concerned with the definition of a service, not the way the service is fulfilled. That is, the consumer of a service does not know whether data was computed, transformed, or simply retrieved. This provides significant flexibility to change the way services are fulfilled without changing any other part of the system. It also means that federated systems are not concerned with

---

[7] http://www.w3.org/XML/

the underlying representation and structure of the data since that responsibility lies with the service provider.

XML, with associated schema definitions, provides one method for sustainable representation of data. XML uses simple, non-proprietary text that is both human and machine readable. Even without an associated schema, sensibly named elements and attributes and hierarchical representation provide useful context to the meaning of the data. Primary source of data can be converted into XML (provided the source system provides a method of access), and once converted, the data can be retained beyond the lifetime of the original systems.

The typical service components for a federation for clinical research is shown in Figure 3. Services for Clinical Data Research Federations form a cooperating set of functionality delivered to researchers. Starting with de-identified records from Data Providers, Linkage Services supply a key for data linkage to enable data from different providers to be combined for the same patient. The Ontology Services are critical for mapping diverse data dictionaries to a uniform reference set enabling data searching across the entire domain of data providers.

The Data Provider Services represent the institutions and repositories containing data of clinical interest. Data Provider Services can provide de-identified patient or codified data, or a subset of data, based on a query or direct retrieval using a given linkage key. For example, "what was the *age* at *diagnosis* of *Lupus*"? The terms "age", "diagnosis" and "Lupus" will all appear in the reference ontology, which is maintained by Ontology Services. The conversion of patient identity to a key is performed by the Linkage Services.

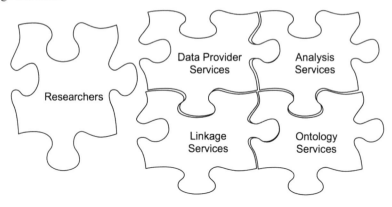

Figure 3 - Typical Service Components for a Federation for Clinical Research

Linkage Services are used to create a patient identifier (linkage key) that is hopefully unique for all sources of data. Currently there are three types of linkage approaches: a) manual linkage of data, b) automatic linkage based on linkage keys maintained in a central database, or c) automatic linkage based on distributed linkage keys. The manual approach requires an authorized agency to construct data sets upon request by researchers. A linkage chain key is allocated to all data sets and the master key curated and managed securely by the agency with temporary linkage keys assigned for each 'project'. Data is then extracted across the data sources, that is data extraction is authorized using the assigned 'project' keys [17]. Automated linkage using a centralized identity database is a variation on the manual service which creates a key from probabilistic matching of the identifiers. The generated identity information along with the generated key is stored in a secure master database and at the source in encrypted form. This establishes the platform for dynamic queries for authorized users[18].

The third approach works for probabilistic matching to removes the need for any identity information to leave the data source. A proxy for the identity of the patient is established by creating a one-way hash key at the data source and requesting a centralized service generate a linkage key for that hash identifier[8] [19]. The hash should be the same for the same identity information at different institutions. The data source maintains the mapping of patient identity to hash key and linkage key. It is possible that the patient identity changes, in which case the source will generate a new hash key. The central service can then be notified that a new hash (identity) exists for a given linkage key and the centralized service can notify other data sources of the alternate identity for that patient.

An Ontology service should maintain the definition of every datum within the federation. The definition with the name of the datum, its description and context for use as well as any agreed set of values should be included. Two approaches can be taken to managing the definition of terms: a) the Ontology Services which maintains the definition of datum and values at each Data Provider or b) each datum and values are mapped into an agreed definition and set of values before leaving the Data Provider. Method (b) is preferable, because it removes the need for the researcher to perform the potentially tedious and error prone step of mapping terminology from different sources into a unified data set for analysis.

The Analysis Services includes data access and query and allow researchers to distribute requests for data to all of the participating Data Providers and combine them using linkage keys. In order to know what to search for, and the meaning of resultant data, the researcher will refer to the Ontology Services. The Analysis Service can dynamically retrieve data from each Data Provider to present a view of the data which the researcher has permission to access and reflects the data available at the time. Since the result set for a given query is a function of time, any data sets supporting research must be temporally qualified or extracted and saved for future reference.

As well as user driven research, the Analysis Service can be configured with automatic analyses for purposes such as surveillance. For example, pattern matching might be used to send alerts of emergent diseases that might require a cross-institution response.

With such diverse source data, any data representation must be adaptive. One significant step to dealing with this complexity is to leverage XML which allows arbitrary and complex data to be hierarchically organised. The extensible nature of XML allows the inclusion of additional information without impacting on the calling applications, and the structure of XML need not be the same for all data providers. In addition, there are standard tools for processing XML data that allow it to be automatically transformed into other formats, such as web pages (HTML), spreadsheets, PDF documents, other XML schemas, et cetera. The basic tool for transformation is XSLT[9]. Extending the example of patient sex above, an XSLT transformation could be used to convert sex from different repositories into a canonical

---

[8] Ghranite™ uses this approach. See http://www.conduit.unimelb.edu.au/GRHANITE/index.html

[9] http://www.w3.org/TR/xslt

form. Transformation to a structure and semantics which can be understood by the researcher should be undertaken by the Data Providers.

Protecting the identity of the patient is of paramount importance. No data for research should ever be visible, nor leave the originating institution that identifies the patient. That is, the identity of the patient must be kept separate from the associated data. There are distinct pieces of information to consider: a) the patient identity, b) linkage keys generated from the patient identity and c) the clinical data for the patient. The Data Provider institution that manages the data is the only place where all three pieces of information can ever be associated.

These distributed systems often involve public communications networks. It is prudent that those transmissions be encrypted using either a Virtual Private Network (VPN) or Transport Layer Security (TLS).However, this only establishes the authenticity of the communicating systems. The authenticity of the researcher and other users accessing the system must also be established using means such as user name and passwords, digital certificates or other means A Data Provider may provide different information to different people. For example, a clinician operating at an institution may be able to see additional information that is not available to other researchers. This also illustrates the power of Service Oriented Architectures and flexible data interchange using XML because a) the Data Provider service decides what information is to be accessible based on the identity and associated authority of the requesting researcher and the service may return different information based on the context. Privileged data sent to other systems should never be cached, and if it is, guaranteed inaccessible to anyone other than the authorised users.

6.   Collaboration

In addition to technical requirements, there are also social requirements for collaboration that must be considered as sources of data transcend project, domain and institutional boundaries. While there are many ingredients required to foster collaborative research it is not just resources that are required. Often the greatest factor is the motivation and social skills to work with their colleagues, and a respect that together there is more to gain than individually. The process of collaboration can take many paths, but in health informatics it is helpful that the collaborating group:

- forms a working group which appoints a 'leader'
- meets regularly for communication and issue resolution
- specifies data items, definitions and methods of collection (what already exists and what needs to be collected)
- ensures each collaborator specifies levels of access to 'their' data
- defines research questions - those to be answered in 12 months as well as those possibly in 5 years time
- defines what resources are available for data entry and cleaning, analysis and report writing

The collaboration can only work when the researchers are committed to the project. In addition to the fundamental drive to answer the research questions, the following foundation areas will need consideration:

- Intellectual Property
- Ethics

- Security of data and information, and sustainability
- Governance and agreement of the collaborating parties.

Intellectual Property in this context can be regarded as '... the property of your mind or intellect [20].' and most researchers wish to have appropriate recognition and reward for their discoveries and endeavours. Many organisations have IP principles to guide a collaboration[10], but agreement up-front to authorship of publications and presentations and any patents and commercialisation can prevent disputes at a later stage.

Approval of the research by a constituted Ethics Committee is required when dealing with patient information. Issues that must be addressed are privacy of the individuals, validity of the research, risk to patients, consent and legislative requirements. There are many considerations involved and individual countries may have statements, regulations and charters on the Ethical conduct of Research in Humans [21] [22] [23] [24]. In the area of data and databanks there needs to be consideration of how the data is collected, stored and disclosed, in particular whether the data allows a patient to be readily identified (e.g. a name or image), re-identifiable (e.g. a code can be used to ascertain the identity), or non-identifiable – where all identifiers have been permanently removed.

Security, archival and sustainability of the data is required to protect the privacy of the data, the embodied value of the data and preserve the information so the validity of the research can be tested for a number of years after the studies completion (at least 10 years).

Many research bodies have templates for collaborative research projects which detail the intellectual property rights, the management structure, communication and reporting obligations as well as risks, indemnities and insurances. Such agreements protect researchers and their organisations as well as explicitly setting 'the rules of engagement' so that there should be no surprises and minimise disagreements. Many organisations have lawyers that assist with the development of these agreements and they should pass through all the collaborating parties' lawyers before sign off.

7.   Conclusions; Tomorrow, Today

It might be fitting to conclude a chapter on the integration of data for research with a perspective of how we should be engaging, and how we might work together in an ideal world that successfully joins together healthcare research, life sciences, and information technology to improve healthcare research and health outcomes.

This ideal calls for research information management systems to implement archives of *usable, addressable, linkable,* and *persistent* data. Such repositories will be adaptive systems acting to merge data services, metadata, and data, as part of what is being called the *semantic web* [25].

The ability to readily access and extract data from disparate and heterogeneous sources for integration, filtering, and analysis via metadata increases the value of the data to the researcher enormously. Planning repositories around international standards, ontologies, and the use of 'best practice' information management principles helps to ensure its sustainability and adaptation to future technologies.

---

[10] http://www.nhmrc.gov.au/funding/policy/ipmanage.htm

A challenge to building *collaborative* research systems is with the process of record linkage across systems. Addressing the issues raised when trying to associate records from different sources lead to a future where viable solutions have been found to sharing electronic health records and patient identification keys without compromising privacy concerns, or ethics requirements.

Communication and communication technologies are some of the keys to fostering collaborative research. They underpin a collegial environment that respects the individual scientist while fostering a team approach across geographic, and many times, ethnic, and political divides. Social networking tools, like *Skype*[11] for voice over internet (VoIP) telephone calls, or *SecondLife*[12] are connecting individual researchers as well as research teams worldwide.

There are many challenges to building the ideal world for healthcare research:

- Understanding the effects from the convergence of healthcare practice, with life sciences research, and information technology.
- Accessing, extracting and analysing data from distributed, heterogeneous sources through standards-based record linkage schemes.
- Building sustainable data repositories for long-term archiving.
- Developing practical data models for collaborative research.
- Solving, or at least making good progress on, the problem of ontologies.
- Managing research standards on a global scale.
- Planning for new, emerging technologies.
- Fostering collaborative teams that bridge geographic and geopolitical boundaries.

As these challenges are met, and future investigators achieve building a workspace environment that integrates data and tools from around the world, then the greater efficiency and efficacy of clinical research will translate into improved clinical practice and health outcomes.

References

[1] Fausto-Sterling A, The Sciences March/April 1993, p. 20-24.
[2] International Health Standards Development Organisation, SNOMED CT Systemized Nomenclature of Medicine-Clinical Terms, http://www.ihtsdo.org
[3] Australian Institute of Health and Welfare (AIHW) metadata registry, http://meteor.aihw.gov.au
[4] OpenEHR Foundation, http://www.openehr.org/clinicalmodels/archetypes.html
[5] DICOM Digital Imaging and Communications in Medicine, a division of the Association of Electrical and Medical Imaging Equipment Manufactures (NEMA) http://medical.nema.org/
[6] Dixon Hughes R (DH4) 2006, Review of Shared Electronic Health Record Standards; Final, National E-Health Transition Authority NEHTA www.nehta.gov.au/ cited 8 October 2008
[7] Ocean Informatics, Standards and the shared EHR - Applicability and impact, Prepared for NEHTA and DH4 review, September 2005.
[8] HL7 2.5 2000. HL7, Application Protocol for Electronic Data Exchange in Healthcare Environments, Version 2.5, ANSI Standard. Ann Arbor MI, USA.
[9] Beale T, Heard S, Kalra D, Lloyd D et al, 2002 The openEHR EHR reference model, Release 1 draft, www.openEHR.org
[10] ASTM E1714, ASTM International, Standard Guide for Properties of a Universal Healthcare Identifier (UHID), http://www.astm.org/
[11] Clinical Data Interchange Standards consortium, www.cdisc.org
[12] Gray J, Szalay A S, Thakar A R, Stoughton C, and van den Berg J, Online Scientific Data Curation, Publication, and Archiving, Microsoft Research Technical Report MSR-TR-2002-74, July 2002.

---

[11] Skype http://www.skype.com
[12] Second Life http://www.secondlife.com

[13] McCartney G. 2007 The Heritage Documentation Management System (HDMS), private communication IMCC-2007-02-12

[14] Garde S, Hullin C, Chen R, Schuler T, Granz J, Knaup P, Hovenga E 2007 Towards Sustainability of Health Information Systems: How Can We Define, Measure and Achieve It? In: Kuhn K, Warren J, Leong T (Eds) MEDINFO, 2007 Proceedings of the 12th World Congress on Health (Medical) Informatics, IOS Press, Amsterdam.

[15] Lord P, MacDonald A, Lyon L, Giaretta D, 2005 From Data Deluge to Data Curation; The Digital Archiving Consultancy Ltd. & the Digital Curation Centre, 2005 http://www.ukoln.ac.uk/ukoln/staff/e.j.lyon/150.pdf. cited 8 October 2008

[16] Fair, M. (1995). An Overview of Record Linkage in Canada, presented at the American Statistical Association Annual Meetings in Orlando, FL, August 1995

[17] Holman CDJ, Bass AJ, Rouse IL, Hobbs MST. 1999 Population-based linkage of health records in Western Australia: development of a health services research linked database. Australian and New Zealand Journal of Public Health 23 (5): 453-459

[18] Hibbert M, Gibbs P, O'brien T, Colman P, Merriel R, Rafael N, Georgeff M 2007 The Molecular Medicine Informatics Model (MMIM). Studies in Health Technology Informatics. 2007; 126:77-86

[19] GeneRic HeAlth Network Information Technology for the Enterprise (GRHANITE™) http://www.conduit.unimelb.edu.au/GRHANITE/index.html

[20] IP Australia (2000). http://www.ipaustralia.gov.au/ip/index.shtml

[21] Intellectual Property Management, National Health and Medical Research Council (NHMRC) Australia http://www.nhmrc.gov.au/funding/policy/ipmanage.htm

[22] US Federal Department of Health and Human Services, PART 46 Protection of Human Subjects http://www.hhs.gov/ohrp/humansubjects/guidance/45cfr46.htm

[23] European Commission http://ec.europa.eu/research/index.cfm

[24] The National Statement on Ethical Conduct in Human Research 2007 (Australia) . http://www.nhmrc.gov.au/publications/synopses/e35syn.htm

[24] Antoniou G, Van Harmelen F, 'A Semantic Web Primer, 2nd Edition', MIT Press 2008

Review Questions

1. Describe the clinical research lifecycle.
2. Identify possible sources of research data in your local health care organization.
3. Why is there a need for the adoption of contextual data standardization to retain meaning?
4. What are the information management principles for sustainable data
5. Explain available data linkage technologies in use to support collaborative research aimed at improving health outcomes.
6. Explain how identifiers in health are used.

Section 6

Health Informatics Education

Health Informatics
E.J.S. Hovenga et al. (Eds.)
IOS Press, 2010
© 2010 The authors and IOS Press. All rights reserved.
doi:10.3233/978-1-60750-476-4-479

34. Clinical Health Informatics Education for a 21st Century World

Siaw Teng LIAW[1], MBBS, PhD DipObst, GrDipPHC, FRACGP, FACHI[a], Kathleen
GRAY PhD, MEnvSc, MLibSc, BA[b]

[a]*Director, SSWAHS General Practice Unit, Professor of General Practice Faculty of
Medicine, The University of New South Wales, Australia*
[b]*Senior Research Fellow in Health Informatics, Faculty of Medicine, Dentistry and
Health Sciences & Department of Information Systems*

Abstract. This chapter gives an educational overview of:
- health informatics competencies in medical, nursing and allied clinical health professions
- health informatics learning cultures and just-in-time health informatics training in clinical work settings
- major considerations in selecting or developing health informatics education and training programs for local implementation
- using elearning effectively to meet the objectives of health informatics education

Keywords. Computer literacy, medical informatics, curriculum, credentialing

Introduction

This chapter focuses on medicine and nursing, but also makes reference to other clinical professions where there is significant interest in health informatics education. It is relevant to health informatics education at and for various educational levels including preclinical education, clinical training pre- and post-initial qualification, specialist training and continuing professional development. It offers various perspectives on health informatics educational provision, in consideration of the diverse needs of tertiary education institutions, in-house training units in healthcare organisations, professional accrediting bodies, and ICT services vendors and systems implementers.

One major theme running through this chapter is that health informatics education to build clinical competence is required for sustainability in healthcare, for three main reasons. Firstly, health informatics capability throughout the clinical workforce is required to sustain regional and national healthcare systems. Clinicians need to be able to achieve improvements in the safety and quality of care as new technology-based management tools are implemented within and between healthcare organisations. Secondly, health informatics capability is required to sustain the standing and influence of the clinical professions. Clinicians need to be able to work with integrity and uphold standards in applying technologically sophisticated advances in patient care, such as

---

[1] Corresponding Author: siaw@unsw.edu.au

advanced telehealth service delivery or medical robotics. Thirdly, health informatics capability is required to sustain a skilled clinical workforce that needs to update its professional practices continuously. Clinicians need to be able to use ICT-based collaboration and training methods to share knowledge and teach efficiently – for example, through the use of virtual environments and mobile communication systems.

Another major theme in this chapter is that historical and geographical divisions are becoming increasingly irrelevant to education for clinical health informatics competence. Worldwide online open-access information about advances in healthcare means that clinicians need to be prepared to address consumer expectations about ICT-enhanced quality of care. In an era where large multinational organisations are major players in ICT in healthcare, clinicians must be enabled in the course of their careers to integrate their professional activities across a changing array of ICT systems and standards. Moreover, an internationally mobile clinical workforce needs to be competent with uses of ICT in ways that are responsive to a range of local protocols and cultural values. Finally, clinical professionals need to be empowered to work with technology tools and resources in response to major global health issues such as epidemic outbreak or natural disaster.

1. Health Informatics Competencies for Clinicians

The foundation for many currently favoured sets of health informatics competencies was laid by the work of the International Medical Informatics Association Working Group 1: Health and Medical Informatics Education [1]. Although most effort internationally has gone into determining competencies for professional health informaticians, nevertheless detailed health informatics competency sets have been put forward also for practitioners in many clinical professions - notably nursing, radiography, dentistry and pharmacy - and in many medical specialties, such as emergency medicine and family practice.

This section begins with an overview of two base-level health informatics competency frameworks that are applicable for multiple clinical health professions. Each of these generic frameworks is endorsed by a national health informatics peak body, has been developed through wide cross-professional consultation and is intended to be compatible with more profession-specific or localised sets of competencies, where these exist, or to fill a gap where they do not.

The Australian College of Health Informatics published a three-level Australian Health Informatics Educational Framework in 2006 [2]. For clinical professionals, who are considered to be at the "users" level of ICT and knowledge resources in health care, it recommends at least basic knowledge and skill in the areas of:

- Health information systems (general characteristics)
- Health information systems (architecture)
- Management of health information systems
- Health data management
- Information management
- Knowledge management
- Bioinformatics
- Epidemiology
- Biometry
- Outcome measurement
- Practice evaluation
- Health care organisation & administration
- Electronic patient records
- Electronic health records

- Health concept representation
- E-health
- Telehealth
- Telemedicine
- Coding & classification
- Health informatics standards
- Decision support systems
- Knowledge based systems
- Expert systems
- Artificial intelligence in medicine
- Organ imaging informatics
- Medical signal processing
- Technology of measurement
- Technology of electrical engineering
- Mathematical models in medicine
- Biomedical modelling
- Medical robotics

The American Medical Informatics Association (AMIA) "10x10" program aims to have 10,000 healthcare professionals in the United States workforce trained, by the year 2010, in three domains of informatics – clinical / health care, public health and translational bioinformatics [3]. Its current base-level training aims to build the following competencies:

- The value proposition of health information technology and how medical informatics and other fields contribute to it.
- The role of various individuals in the health information technology workforce.
- The basic tenets of biomedical computing to enable optimal selection of hardware, software, and network connections for a given setting.
- The essential functions of the electronic health record (EHR) and the barriers to its use.
- The principles of implementing EHRs in ambulatory, hospital, and other settings.
- The role of clinical decision support in health care settings and within the EHR.
- Computerised provider order entry and how it enhances clinical decision support.
- The basic principles of health care quality assessment, including pay for performance programs, and how the EHR enables them.
- The role of health information exchange and Regional Health Information Organisations.
- The personal health record, its interface with the EHR and its value in promoting personal health.
- The importance of standards and interoperability of clinical data and the major initiatives underway.
- Maintaining privacy, confidentiality and security.
- The core principles of evidence-based medicine and their application in clinical practice.
- Accessing medical knowledge resources and linking them to clinical practice.
- People and organisational issues in the use of health information technology.
- The unique aspects of nursing information and practice in relation to clinical information systems.
- The growing impact of genomics on medicine and its implications for health information systems.
- The management of images in clinical settings, including the use of PACS systems.
- The role of telemedicine and barriers to its use.
- The function of public health information systems and their interaction with clinical systems.

- The key issues in organisational, project, and business management in informatics projects and the notion that informatics projects require more than an understanding of technology.

From a comparison of these two base-level competency sets, as shown in Table 1, it can be seen that there are common elements and differences. Both emphasise the dichotomy of electronic health records for personal and clinical use, and the need for interoperability standards. Both emphasise public health and health services informatics, although ACHI may place a greater emphasis on evaluation. ACHI has a specific focus on coding and classification, health concept representation, knowledge management and mathematical modelling, and it has more specific translational bioinformatics competency requirements. AMIA has a specific focus on nursing informatics, and it has a more functional approach to decision support. There are terminology differences between ACHI and AMIA regarding e-health and telehealth; these are possibly related to how the inter-professional health team is organised and governed in different national systems. The table is presented in four sections, 1) basics and common competencies, 2) clinical informatics 3) public health and health services informatics and 4) translational informatics.

Table 1. Comparison of ACHI and AMIA Competencies

ACHI (based on IMIA)	AMIA
*1) **Basics and common competencies***	
• Health information systems (general characteristics)	• The value proposition of health information technology and how medical informatics and other fields contribute to it
• Electronic patient records	• The personal health record (PHR), its interface with the EHR, and its value in promoting personal health
• Electronic health records	• The essential functions of the electronic health record (EHR) and the barriers to its use • The principles of implementing EHRs in ambulatory, hospital, and other settings
• Management of health information systems	• The basic tenets of biomedical computing to enable optimal selection of hardware, software, and network connections for a given setting
• Health informatics standards	• The importance of standards and interoperability of clinical data and the major initiatives underway • The role of health information exchange and Regional Health Information Organisations
• Coding and classification	[no equivalent]
• Health information systems (architecture)	[no equivalent]
• Health data management (*assuming that this includes privacy*)	• Maintaining privacy, confidentiality, and security
• Information management	[no equivalent]
• Knowledge management	[no equivalent]
• Health concept representation	[no equivalent]
• Mathematical models in medicine	[no equivalent]

ACHI (based on IMIA)	AMIA
2) Clinical informatics	
• E-health	[no equivalent]
• Telehealth	[no equivalent]
• Telemedicine	• The role of telemedicine and barriers to its use
• Organ imaging informatics	• The management of images in clinical settings, including the use of PACS systems
[no equivalent]	• The unique aspects of nursing information and practice in relation to clinical information systems.
• Decision support systems	• The role of clinical decision support in health care settings and within the EHR • Computerised provider order entry and how it enhances clinical decision support
• Knowledge based systems	• Accessing medical knowledge resources and linking them to clinical practice
• Expert systems	[no equivalent]

3) Public health and health services informatics	
• Epidemiology	• The core principles of evidence-based medicine and their application in clinical practice • The function of public health information systems and their interaction with clinical systems
• Outcome measurement	• The basic principles of health care quality assessment, including pay for performance programs, and how the EHR enables them
• Practice evaluation	[no equivalent]
• Health care organisation and administration	• The role of various individuals in the health information technology workforce. • People and organisational issues in the use of health information technology • The key issues in organisational, project, and business management in informatics projects and the notion that informatics projects require more than an understanding of technology

4) Translational bioinformatics	
• Bioinformatics	• The growing impact of genomics on medicine and its implications for health information systems
• Biometry	[no equivalent]
• Artificial intelligence in medicine	[no equivalent]
• Medical signal processing	[no equivalent]
• Technology of measurement	[no equivalent]
• Technology of electrical engineering	[no equivalent]
• Biomedical modelling	[no equivalent]
• Medical robotics	[no equivalent]

Developing a full set of competencies for a specific professional context entails deciding which ones are core and which ones are more specialised, and for each one describing an acceptable level of performance, the skill needed to perform in a specific situation, and different levels of proficiency – as well as establishing a formal process for endorsement and regular review by an authoritative advisory group [4].

The focus of health informatics competencies for clinical professions is also determined by the large-scale, long-term requirements of national and regional health and medical systems, as the case of Australia illustrates. The Australian health care system is underpinned by universal basic health insurance and subsidised prescription medications, with a mix of State government, national government and private operators providing hospital care and primary care. The 2008 National Health and Hospitals Reform Commission (www.nhhrc.org.au) placed major emphasis on integrated and coordinated care across all aspects of the health sector and between primary care and hospital services, acute and aged care services and rural and metropolitan health services; a greater focus on prevention, healthy lifestyle and early intervention in chronic illness; improving rural and indigenous health services and outcomes; and a well qualified and sustainable health workforce into the future. The Australian College of Health Informatics (www.achi.org.au) and the Australian Collaboration on eHealth (www.hisa.org.au) have argued for a national e-health strategy that has:

- a solid business case and performance assessment approach,
- a coordinated and standards-based ICT and clinical systems investment plan with credible funding over a realistic timeframe,
- an effort to address capacity building issues to ensure adequately skilled resources are available to support the implementation of a strategy,
- a detailed and open implementation process, accessible for public review and comment,
- appropriate ongoing consultation involving key stakeholders, consumers and clinicians,
- sufficient milestones and review points over the planned timeframe to enable appropriate and timely corrective action or fine tuning of the strategy as required
- a change management and communication strategy,
- a work plan with objectives and key performance indicators, and
- an evaluation research plan to monitor and measure performance outcomes

To implement such a program, which will take at least a decade to complete if sufficiently funded and resourced, requires not only an adequate ICT infrastructure (including broadband, equipment and a national electronic health record system and specialised health informaticians) but critically, a clinical workforce well equipped with a relevant set of competencies to be able to operationalise it in practice. In the State of Victoria in 2008 an integrated ICT initiative for publicly funded healthcare providers (www.health.vic.gov.au/healthsmart) is two years behind schedule, with little to show in terms of informatics capacity-building programs or a skilled workforce to optimise program outcomes; and the situation is similar in other Australian States.

In this case, a quantum leap is needed to move from the current fragmented approaches – profession-by-profession, provider-by-provider and jurisdiction-by-jurisdiction – to a nationally coordinated health informatics capacity-building program. The Australian case is a microcosm of the issues involved in trying to specify a global set of clinical health informatics competencies.

2. Formal Education for Clinical Competence in Health Informatics

Around the world, there is generally poor provision of health informatics learning in entry-level education for clinical healthcare professionals, and very little progress has been made in over a decade [5]. Sometimes pre-clinical learners have access to a required or elective unit of study, but rarely is a set of learning objectives taught across units or years. Prime among the reasons for this is an academic workforce unfamiliar with health informatics competencies and thus unable to lead this aspect of educational reform within their professions [6][7].

Accordingly, this section profiles selected providers of graduate-level education for clinical healthcare professionals, with a focus on established English-language programs that are accessible to international participants who have at least undergraduate qualifications in their clinical field. It also highlights some more localised models of good practice.

The Royal College of Surgeons of Edinburgh in partnership with the University of Edinburgh (previously with the University of Bath) in the UK offers web-based learning, in short courses on topics such as clinical governance, clinical terminology, imaging, information searching, critical appraisal, standards and statistics, as well as in postgraduate programs [8].

The Centre for Health Informatics and Multiprofessional Education at University College London in the UK similarly provides short course and graduate degree options, targeting hospital-based clinical healthcare professionals along with primary and secondary care ICT professionals and librarians, community-based health and social care professionals, healthcare service managers and staff of not-for-profit healthcare foundations [9].

An online Master of Science jointly developed by four Canadian universities (Victoria, Alberta, Calgary and British Columbia) caters for working clinical health professionals such as physicians, nurses, therapists and laboratory technologists, as well as ICT professionals working in the health sector, with the aim of producing champions to lead the implementation of advances in clinical informatics [10].

A range of training options offered at institutions across the United States – the American Colleges of Physicians and Emergency Physicians, the California Healthcare Foundation, the Oregon Health & Science University, the Scottsdale Institute, the Society of Technology in Anaesthesia, Stanford University School of Medicine, the University of Alabama at Birmingham, and the University of Illinois at Chicago – are accredited elements of the AMIA "10x10" program [3]. The AMIA program has promoted existing health informatics education providers in the USA and assisted in boosting their student numbers; however, even though these providers emphasise online delivery and support, many have residential requirements. AMIA has plans to globalise its "10x10" program in the USA, so that it becomes an international collaborative "20x20" program to educate 20,000 healthcare informaticians internationally by 2020.

Another American curriculum model of note is found in the School of Nursing at the University of Washington, which offers an interdisciplinary Master of Science in Clinical Informatics and Patient Centered Technologies, with elements of biomedical and health informatics, health information management, health administration, computer science, and engineering [11].

The provision of formal education and training in health informatics for clinical competence is characterised by study programs with short lifecycles and by rapid turnover among provider organisations and partnerships, making it difficult for a prospective student or a potential training provider to compare options or to make judgements about the quality of a course of study. Because learning and competencies may be recorded and valued differently in different professional and national contexts, before reaching a decision about participating in any formal educational program it is wise to look into key aspects [12]:

- Reputation and history of provider organisation
- Expertise and availability of staff
- Nature of recognition accorded by other relevant professional bodies
- Articulation of credentials and transfer of credit toward further study
- Currency and customisability of content and methods
- Experiences of previous and current participants

3.   Implementing Health Informatics Training Programs in Clinical Work Settings

Given not only the paucity of formal health informatics education in entrants to the clinical workforce, but also the need to build the skills of most existing clinicians, many healthcare organisations and agencies implement work-based health informatics training programs. A training manager needs to consider several options for initiating such a program, and several factors for making it effective.

One model for providing such a program is to adopt or adapt existing training resources. One example is those developed for the Essential IT Skills program of the UK National Health Service, for "anyone who uses a health or care information system in their workplace, whatever their role" [13].

Another model of provision is to develop a package of learning and training activities that staff can undertake while they work, in partnership with vendors of a proprietary technologies, sponsors of industry conference series and industry associations – as listed for example in the European eHealth Directory (www.ehealthnews.eu), CHITTA (www.chitta.ca/membership/members.lasso) and CHIK (www.health-e-directory.com.au). This kind of training package may include approaches such as scheduled individual or group sessions; coaching, mentoring and supervision; action learning projects; or self-paced independent study related to the continuing education requirements of a particular profession.

Any work-based education program needs to be underpinned by a cost-benefit analysis, as well as fundamental principles of workplace learning, adult learning and learning for organisational change:

- Workplace learning by professionals is strongly influenced by factors that include the allocation, structuring, challenge and value of the work, as well as the encounters, relationships, feedback and support involved in the learning experience [14].
- Adult learners are known to be autonomous, experienced and goal-oriented and to require relevance and respect from their education provider [15].
- Learning for organisational change must be part of a framework that also includes visionary leadership, the involvement of staff work teams, enhanced communication strategies, incremental introduction of changes, emphasis on

assimilation of new technologies into routine practice and making performance improvement a priority in workplace culture [16].

4. Using e-Learning Methods to Meet Health Informatics Learning Objectives

When applied to learning and teaching in health professions, e-learning (the use of information and communication technologies in education) is sometimes regarded as a subset of the health informatics knowledge domain. Understood in this way, the ability to use educational technologies effectively is often assumed to be one aspect of clinical health informatics competence. There is a range of levels of such competence:

- Basic: being able to learn by using a web-based training package (for example [17];
- Intermediate: being able to design and deliver training using a course management system (for example [18];
- Advanced: being able to facilitate access to health informatics competencies and e-learning content by using e-learning standards to store and retrieve content-competency associations (for example, [19].

From some perspectives on clinical competence in information management and evidence-based practice, there are areas of overlap between educational technologies and health informatics. Thus health sciences librarians or information technology managers may regard as aspects of clinical health informatics competence the ability to use the electronic database searching and full-text retrieval facilities of health research establishments, and the ability to evaluate the quality of web-based health information [20] [21] for example).

At other times e-learning is treated as a means to the end of developing health informatics knowledge and skills. E-learning can be particularly suitable, for example, to provide an experience with situations which rarely occur in real life, or which are too expensive or dangerous to include in hands-on training. However, most current approaches to learning and teaching with technology contribute very little to building the health informatics competencies required for professional practice. Uses of mainstream course management systems and other e-learning tools are based on generic educational and institutional considerations more often than on authentic informatics applications in clinical workplaces.

Promising new developments in aligning educational technologies with clinical informatics competencies are emerging through the use of some forms of social software [22] and some simulated learning environments (for example, [23] [24]. The use of so-called web 2.0 tools and services for learning, including blogs, social networks, virtual worlds and wikis, brings with it the need to teach new kinds of information literacy and professional communication (as described in [25] [26] for example).

5.   Conclusion: Good Practice in the Provision of Clinical Health Informatics Education

Developing a set of competencies is only one part of a larger educational planning process that is required to produce a competent clinician and a capable clinical workforce. Other critical parts of the process are:

- Curriculum design – mapping the desired competencies across various levels of clinical curriculum in the relevant discipline; aligning the desired competencies with planned learning activities and assessment tasks.
- Teaching / training – offering optimal delivery modes (which may range from scheduled classes through to independent self-paced learning), choosing relevant methods and resources, using an appropriate mix of staff and peer support, and providing timely feedback on learning.
- Assessment – assigning written work, observing performance or reviewing a portfolio of evidence of clinicians' learning in each competency, and granting externally validated (wherever possible) certification of learning achievements at predetermined levels of attainment.
- Evaluation – seeking feedback from learners, teachers / trainers and accreditation bodies, reviewing learning outcomes, teaching performance and curriculum relevance, and making regular improvements to educational quality as indicated.

A number of factors, which are equally important to undergraduate and postgraduate coursework and to continuing professional education programs and just-in-time workplace training programs, will determine the quality of clinical health informatics education offerings (adapted from [27]):

- Relevant, appropriate content and resources: The content and resources should be meaningful to learners and practitioners in their professional context.
- Learner engagement: This is achieved through a meaningful, enjoyable and interactive program, with regular and timely feedback from teachers and other learners. This is a particular challenge for programs offered to independent self-paced learners.
- Effective learning: This is facilitated by catering for the diversity of ways in which learners work at their own pace, study in their own time, and pursue their own path through the material. The most effective programs offer alternative learning pathways which cater for a range of learning styles and preferences.
- Ease of learning: This involves designing, chunking and sequencing learning activities so that they do not make unnecessary cognitive demands on the learner. An e-learning program should be intuitive, requiring a minimum of technical training before use.
- Inclusive practice: Inclusive practice underpins good pedagogy by seeking to develop programs that cater for learners of different age, gender, ethnicity, physical and intellectual ability. E-learning programs must also cater for different levels of access to technology and different ICT skill levels.
- Fitness for purpose: The choice among educational methods or modes of learning including e-learning will be determined as a balance of those which are most authentic in comparison with professional practices and those which are most efficient in the circumstances of the program provider.

In an ideal world, national peak bodies in each clinical healthcare profession would specify types of competence with relevant information and communication technologies that would be standard for members of that profession. These specifications would be based on international benchmarking within professions, and would also represent strong collaboration across healthcare professions. They would underpin the development and accreditation of curricula in which health informatics learning was thoroughly integrated and embedded. These curricula would be the norm at all levels of professional training from entry-level to the level of clinical specialisations, and would be delivered in tertiary education institutions and major clinical education sites, by expert teachers with advanced qualifications, informed by current research in the field and with the aid of authentic educational technologies. The clinical workforce thus educated would be able, indeed would expect, to use state-of-the-art healthcare technologies and to work with professional health informaticians throughout their professional careers – to improve their personal performance, the performance of their clinical teams and the performance of the healthcare systems in which they worked. There is much progress still to be made to achieve such an ideal, especially to build a workforce of well-trained health informatics educators and researchers to teach and support the health workforce in the 21st century world.

References

[1] IMIA International Medical Informatics Association Working Group 1: *Health and Medical Informatics Education. (2000).* Recommendations of the International Medical Informatics Association (IMIA) on education in health and medical informatics. Available from http://www.imia.org/pubdocs/rec_english.pdf

[2] Garde, S., & Hovenga, E. (2006). *Australian Health Informatics Educational Framework.* Australian College of Health Informatics. Available from http://www.achi.org.au/documents/publications/Health_Informatics_Educational_Framework_2006032 6.pdf

[3] AMIA American Medical Informatics Association. (2008). *2008 spring offering.* Available from http://www.amia.org/10x10/partners/ohsu/description.asp

[4] Competency-to-curriculum: Developing curricula for public health workers. (2004). *Centre for Health Policy, Columbia University School of Nursing / Association of Teachers of Preventative Medicine.* Available from http://www.nursing.columbia.edu/chphsr/pdf/toolkit.pdf

[5] Ramasamy, P., & Murphy, J. (2007). *Health informatics education for medical students - International Delphi study.* Web page. Available from http://www.chime.ucl.ac.uk/research/hiems/

[6] Buckeridge, D., & Goel, V. (2002). Medical informatics in an undergraduate curriculum: A qualitative study. *BMC Medical Informatics and Decision Making, 2, 6-16.* Available from http://www.biomedcentral.com/1472-6947/2/6

[7] Nagle, L. (2007). Everything I know about informatics, I didn't learn in nursing school. *Nursing Leadership (CJNL), 20(3), 22-25.* Available from http://www.longwoods.com/product.php?productid=19285

[8] FHI Faculty of Health Informatics of the Royal College of Surgeons of Edinburgh. (2008). Web page. Available from http://www.health-informatics.info/

[9] CHIME Centre for Health Informatics and Multiprofessional Education, University College London. (2008). *Opportunities for Study at CHIME. Web page.* Available from http://www.chime.ucl.ac.uk/study/

[10] UVIC University of Victoria. (2007). Master of Science in Health Informatics Distributed Stream (online) *Handbook for Prospective Students 2007-2008.* Available from http://hinf.uvic.ca/programs/gradprog/DSMc.pdf

[11] SON-UOW School of Nursing at the University of Washington. (2008).*Clinical Informatics and Patient Centered Technologies.Webpage.* Available from http://www.son.washington.edu/eo/cipct/default.asp

[12] Freeth, D., Reeves, S., Koppel, I., Hammick, M., & Barr, H. (2005). *Evaluating interprofessional education: A self-help guide.* Health Sciences and Practice Network, Higher Education Academy (UK). Available from http://www.health.heacademy.ac.uk/publications/occasionalpaper/occp5

[13] NHS National Health Service (UK). (2008) *Essential IT Skills (EITS). Web page.* Available from http://www.connectingforhealth.nhs.uk/systemsandservices/etd/eits/

14] Eraut, M. (2007). Learning the complexity of professional practice. Keynote presentation to Learning in a Complex World: *Facilitating Enquiry Conference, 25-27 June 2007, Guildford, UK.* Available from http://complexworld.pbwiki.com/f/MICHAEL+ERAUT+HANDOUT+FINAL.doc

[15] Russell, S. (2006). An overview of adult learning processes. Originally published in *Urologic Nursing, 26(5), 349-352, 370.* Available from http://www.medscape.com/viewarticle/547417

[16] Nemeth, L., Feifer, C., Stuart, G., & Ornstein, S., (2008). Implementing change in primary care practices using electronic medical records: a conceptual framework. *Implementation Science, 3(3). [11pp.]* Available from http://www.pubmedcentral.nih.gov/articlerender.fcgi?artid=2254645

[17] Lockyer, L., Moule, P., & McGuigan, D. (2007). Web-based learning in practice settings: Nurses' experiences and perceptions of impact on patient care. *Electronic Journal of e-Learning, 5(4), 279-286.* Available from http://www.ejel.org/Volume-5/v5-i4/Lockyer_et_al.pdf

[18] Reeves, P., & Reeves, T. (2008). Design considerations for online learning in health and social work education. *Learning in Health and Social Care, 7(1), 46-58.* Available from http://www.blackwell-synergy.com/action/showPdf?submitPDF=Full+Text+PDF+%28224+KB%29&doi=10.1111%2Fj.1473-6861.2008.00170.x

[19] Hersh, W., Bhupatiraju, R., Greene, P., Smothers, B., & Cohen, C. (2006). Adopting e-learning standards in health care: Competency-based learning in the medical informatics domain. *AMIA Symposium Proceedings, pp. 334-338.* Available from http://www.pubmedcentral.nih.gov/picrender.fcgi?artid=1839696&blobtype=pdf

[20] Intute: Health and Life Sciences. (2008). *Web page. UK: JISC / University of Nottingham / Welcome trust.* Available from http://www.intute.ac.uk/healthandlifesciences/

[21] Tse, J., & McAvoy, B. (2006) Information mastery and the 21st century doctor: Change management for general practitioners. *Medical Journal of Australia, 185(2), 92-93.* Available from http://www.mja.com.au/public/issues/185_02_170706/tse10274_fm.pdf

[22] Boulos, M.N.K., Maramba, I. & Wheeler, S. (2006). *Wikis, blogs and podcasts: A new generation of web based tools for virtual collaborative clinical practice and education.* BMC Medical Education, 6(41). Available from http://www.biomedcentral.com/1472-6920/6/41

[23] Canyon, D., & Podger, D. (2002). Towards a new generation of simulation models in public health education. *Australian Journal of Educational Technology, 18(1), 71-88.* Available from http://www.ascilite.org.au/ajet/ajet18/canyon.html

[24] Cerner Corporation. (2008). *Academic Education Solution.* Web page. Available from http://www.cerner.com/public/Cerner_3.asp?id29911

[25] Skiba, D., & Barton, A., (2006). Adapting your teaching to accommodate the net generation of learners. *Online Journal of Issues in Nursing, 11(2), Manuscript 4.* Available from www.nursingworld.org/ojin

[26] Gray, K., Kennedy, G., & Judd, T. (2006). Teaching health informatics to the Net Generation: A new baseline for building capability? In *Proceedings of Mednet 2006: 11th World Congress on the Internet in Medicine.* Available from http://www.mednetcongress.org/fullpapers/MEDNET-121_GrayKathleenA_e.pdf

[27] Whetton, S., Larson, A., & Liaw, S.T. (2008). Chapter 14. eHealth, eLearning and eResearch for rural health practice. In S.T. Liaw & S. Kilpatrick (Eds.). *A Textbook of Australian Rural Health* (pp. 198-199). Canberra: Australian Rural Health Education Network.

Review Questions

- Find and list a set of health informatics competencies for clinicians in an area of specialisation that is relevant to you, and assess your own level of competence. This could be for a specialisation in medicine or nursing (such as palliative care, paediatrics, psychiatry, etc.), or an allied health profession (such as pharmacy, pathology, physiotherapy, etc.).

- Identify one formal health informatics training program accessible to clinicians in your region and your field of expertise. List the units of study that the program comprises, and nominate the unit/s that would be most beneficial for you.

- Choose a case – from the literature or from your own experience – where a clinical teaching or training body ran / runs a health informatics education program for its clientele (e.g. staff, students, members, trainees). In this case, discuss how major educational considerations were addressed in implementing and evaluating the program.
- For each of the following levels of education – preclinical education, initial clinical training, specialist training and continuing professional development – give an example of an educational technology suited for use at this level. Explain how each of the example technologies you have named may be used effectively to facilitate health informatics learning at this level.

Health Informatics
E.J.S. Hovenga et al. (Eds.)
IOS Press, 2010
© *2010 The authors and IOS Press. All rights reserved.*
doi:10.3233/978-1-60750-476-4-492

35. The Health Informatics Workforce: Unanswered Questions, Needed Answers

William HERSH[1], MD FACP, FACMI

Professor and Chair, Department of Medical Informatics & Clinical Epidemiology, School of Medicine, Oregon Health & Science University, Portland, Oregon 97239, United States of America

Abstract. This chapter gives an educational overview of:
- The value of health information technology in the health industry and the need for well-trained HIT professionals
- The current HI workforce characteristics, occupational status and educational opportunities
- Health informaticians roles and functions

Keywords. Medical Informatics, Credentialing, Computer Literacy, Evidence Based Practice, Workforce

Introduction

There is growing evidence for the value of health information technology (HIT) in improving health, health care, public health, and biomedical research. A number of recent systematic reviews have documented the evidence for information technology (IT) interventions [1], clinical decision support[2], and telemedicine [3]. This has led to programs for widespread adoption around the world [4]. There are also opportunities in other areas of biomedical informatics, such as clinical research informatics [5] [6] and bioinformatics [7], although there is less research explicitly documenting its value.

There are, however, many barriers to wider use of HIT in clinical settings, such as mismatch of return on investment between those who pay and those who benefit, challenges to workflow in clinical settings, lack of standards and interoperability, and concerns about privacy and confidentiality 8] [9]. Another barrier, lesser studied and quantified but increasingly recognized, is the lack of characterization of the workforce and its training needed to most effectively implement HIT systems 10] [11] [12]. We know very little about how the HIT workforce is organized in different health care or biomedical research settings. We know even less about the proper role for individuals who are trained in health informatics, including what jobs need knowledge of health informatics or how much the non-informatics workforce needs to know about health informatics.

The value of a competent workforce can be demonstrated by a "case report" of one study reporting negative findings with computerized provider order entry (CPOE). In late 2005, a paper was published that reported an increased mortality rate after

---

[1] Corresponding Author: hersh@oshu.edu

implementation of CPOE in the pediatric intensive care unit (ICU) of Children's Hospital of Pittsburgh [13]. While the study had some methodological problems, further investigation of their approach demonstrated that their CPOE implementation failed to adhere to known best practices [14] [15]. In particular, centralization of the pharmacy, installing the system without adequate network and computational resources, and not allowing order entry prior to the patient arriving at the ICU were mistakes that those familiar with known best practices would avoid. Indeed, several other pediatric hospitals looked at their own data and failed to find increased mortality after CPOE was implemented [16] [17] [18] [19].

1. Statement of the Problem

There is a growing recognition that the well-trained HIT professional should have knowledge not only of information technology, but also health care, business and management, and other disciplines. A survey of 91 health care chief information officers (CIOs) found 88% in agreement that understanding of health care environment is essential to IT practice in health care settings [20]. Sable et al. [21] surveyed health system managers and found a preference for those with clinical experience, understanding of health care, strong communication skills, and ability to work across boundaries within organizations.

   Another aspect of the problem is that we have little data that characterizes the HIT workforce and, in particular, how it is best trained and deployed for optimal use of the technology. It is traditional in most hospitals and other health care settings to think separately of IT professionals, whom are mostly viewed as technologists, and health information management (HIM) professionals, who are mostly viewed as maintaining the (usually paper) medical record. This view not only creates artificial distinctions, but also ignores the role that others play in HIT, in particular clinicians who gravitate into such roles.

   An additional challenge is that there is no succinct definition of the field of health informatics. Furthermore, the field has difficulty agreeing on the adjective in front of the word informatics (i.e., health vs. medical vs. biomedical) as well as whether a practitioner should be called an informaticist or informatician (this chapter uses the latter). We also do not know where pure IT ends and informatics begins [11]. For example, the individual who installs applications on a desktop computer in a hospital probably does not need formal training in informatics, although the CIO and his or her project leads certainly do. There is also lack of knowledge of the profession by those who advise undergraduates in areas such as biology, in that career opportunities in the field are scarcely mentioned [22]. This has led to calls for health informatics to become a professional discipline [23] and for it to acquire the attributes of a profession, such as a well-defined set of competencies, certification of fitness to practice, shared professional identify, life-long commitment, and a code of ethics [24].

   Also a part of the problem is that informatics is not represented in standard occupational classifications, which results in the field not being represented in some types of workforce analyses. In the US, the Standard Occupational Classification (SOC) has codes for Health Diagnosing and Treating Practitioners (29-1000), Medical Records and Health Information Technicians (29-2070), and Computer Specialists (15-1000), but nothing that combines these elements of what informaticians do into a single code [25]. These codes are updated each decade, and it will be imperative for informatics to have such a code in the next revision of the SOC [26]. The same holds for the International Standard Classification of Occupations (ISCO, http://www.ilo.org/public/english/bureau/stat/isco/), which also has no codes for informatics [27].

2.   What We Know About the HIT Workforce

Although there is some data about the HIT workforce emerging worldwide, most is confined to studies from England and the US. One of the most comprehensive assessments of the HIT workforce was carried out in the English National Health Service (NHS) [28]. An assessment of the English HIT workforce estimated the employment of 25,000 full-time equivalents (FTEs) out of 1.3 million workers in English NHS. This equated to the employment of about one information technology (IT) staff per 52 non-IT workers. The workers were found to be distributed among information and communication technology staff (37%), health records staff (26%), information management staff (18%), knowledge management staff (9%), senior managers (7%), and clinical informatics staff (3%).

Most studies done in the US have focused on one group in the workforce, such as IT or HIM professionals. To our knowledge, no studies have quantified numbers of biomedical informatics (BMI) professionals, although some studies have qualitatively assessed certain types, such as the Chief Medical Information Officer (CMIO) [29] [30]. The value of BMI professionals is also hinted at in the context of studies showing flawed implementations of HIT leading to adverse clinical outcomes [13], which may have been preventable with application of known best practices from informatics [15], and other analyses showing that most of the benefits from HIT have been limited to small numbers of institutions with highly advanced informatics programs [1]. Others have documented the importance of "special people" in successful HIT implementations [31].

There is some US data regarding IT professionals in the clinical setting. Gartner Research assessed IT staff in integrated delivery systems of varying size [32]. Among 85 such organizations studied, there was a consistent finding of about one IT staff per 56 non-IT employees, which was similar to the ratio noted above in England. The major roles for IT staff were listed as programmer/analyst (51%), support (28%), telecommunications (16%).

Another recent assessment of the IT workforce in US health care used the HIMSS Analytics Database (derived from the Dorenfest IDHS+ Database™, http://www.himssanalytics.com) [33]. This database contains self-reported data from about 5,000 US hospitals, including elements such as number of beds, total staff FTE, total IT FTE (as well as broken down by major IT job categories), applications, and the vendors used for those applications. Another component of the HIMSS Analytics Database is the EMR Adoption Model™, which scores hospitals on eight stages to creating a paperless record environment [34] (see Figure 1). "Advanced" HIT is generally assumed to be Stage 4, which includes computerized physician order entry (CPOE) and other forms of clinical decision support that have been shown to be associated with improvements in the quality and safety of health care [1].

Stage 7	Medical record fully electronic; CDO able to contribute to EHR as byproduct of EMR
Stage 6	Physician documentation (structured templates), full CDSS (variance & compliance), full R-PACS
Stage 5	Closed loop medication administration
Stage 4	CPOE, CDSS (clinical protocols)
Stage 3	Clinical documentation (flow sheets), CDSS (error checking), PACS available outside Radiology
Stage 2	CDR, CMV, CDSS inference engine, may have Document Imaging
Stage 1	Ancillaries – Lab, Rad, Pharmacy – All Installed
Stage 0	All Three Ancillaries Not Installed

Figure 1 – Description of Stages for the EMR Adoption Model [34].

This study found the overall IT staffing ratio to be 0.142 IT FTE per hospital bed. Extrapolating to all hospitals beds in the US, this suggested a total current hospital IT workforce size of 108,390 FTE. It also found an IT to total staff ratio of 60.7, which was similar to the Gartner and English numbers described above. Average IT staffing ratios varied based on EMR Adoption Model score. Figure 2 shows a graph of the average staffing ratio for each of the stages (there are currently no hospitals in the US at adoption Stage 7). Average staffing ratios generally increased with adoption score, but hospitals at Stage 4 had a higher average staffing ratio than hospitals at Stages 5 or 6. If all hospitals were operating at the same staffing ratios as Stage 6 hospitals (0.196 IT FTE per bed), a total of 149,174 IT FTE would be needed to provide coverage, an increase of 40,784 FTE.

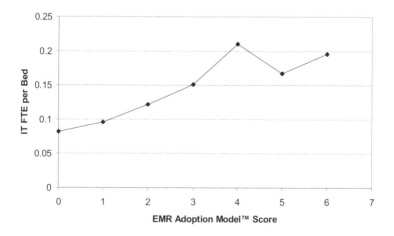

Figure 2 – IT FTE per Bed vs. EMR Adoption.

Also assessed in the US have been HIM professionals, finding that the primary work setting for these individuals was hospital inpatient (53.4%), hospital outpatient (7.8%), physician office/clinic (7.2%), and consulting firm (4.2%) [35]. For those involved in electronic health record (EHR) implementation, two-thirds were on the planning team and half were on implementation team. Study respondents indicated that the largest need for more education was in areas of IT, legal and regulatory issues, reimbursement methodologies, and healthcare information systems.

One additional workforce study has focused on a specific HIT application, estimating the workforce necessary to deploy a Nationwide Health Information Network (NHIN) in the US [36]. For a five-year implementation time frame, there would be an estimated need for 7,600 FTE for installation of EHRs for 400,000 practicing physicians who do not currently have them, 28,600 FTE for the 4,000 hospitals that do not have EHRs, and 420 FTE to implement the infrastructure to connect the network.

There is also data from the US showing that HIT provides well-paying jobs. The 2006 HIMSS Compensation Survey is another self-reported survey [37]. The most recent report of this survey of 1,347 HIMSS members from the US found that the average and median annual salaries were $102,841 and $90,000 respectively. Salaries were highest in consulting firms, vendor firms, health insurance firms, and larger health care delivery systems. Another assessment of US HIT salaries done in 2007 reported on 417 individuals in a variety of health care delivery organizations (hospital and non-hospital), health plans, and IT companies [38]. Median salaries for "C"-level positions (e.g., CIO, CMIO, COO, etc.) were around $100,000 annually. Median salaries for non-"C"-level positions varied by hospital size, clinical background, and level of authority, but were above $100,000 annually for many.

The American Health Information Management Association (AHIMA) also tracks salary data for HIM professionals [39]. Although the salaries are not as high as for IT staff, with a national average of $55,676 annually, there is a large range of salary levels based on job responsibilities, geographical location, and other factors. This economic outlook is not limited to the US. In an assessment of the first 1024 graduates in medical informatics from the University of Heidelberg and Heilbronn (before March, 2001), it was found that 57% had an annual salary above €50,000 [40].

3. What Do We Know About Informaticians?

We know even less about those who are called informaticians. These individuals do have a highly diverse array of job backgrounds, titles, and descriptions [41]. Some have backgrounds as health care professionals, while others bring backgrounds in computer science, other life sciences, and many other disciplines. Indeed, on its Web site, the American Medical Informatics Association (AMIA, www.amia.org) notes that its members consist of physicians, nurses, dentists, pharmacists, and other clinicians; HIT professionals; computer and information scientists; biomedical engineers; consultants and industry representatives; medical librarians; and academic researchers and educators.

Hoffman and Ash [42] surveyed potential employers of informatics graduates, asking them to rate most important skills they desired in graduates. They found that the most important skills desired went well beyond technology and included knowledge of clinical information, interpersonal skills, change management, relational databases, and project management.

Likewise, the Knaup et al. [39] survey of University of Heidelberg and Heilbronn graduates found that graduates were employed in many types of organizations, such as: hardware/software company (33%), other company in industry (19%), academic medical center (13%), self-employed (6%), and non-academic hospital (5%). These graduates reported that the most important topics for their work from their studies included database and information systems, software development/engineering, informatics, economics, and information systems in the health care environment.

Another survey of informatics graduates assessed the biomedical informatics program at the University of Utah [42]. This survey of 209 graduates from the first 35 years of the program found that the most common types of jobs held included operational informatics (67%), academic (18%), medical practice (16%), management (14%), and research (12%). These graduates were most likely to be employed in industry (37%), integrated health care delivery systems (27%), and educational institutions (23%).

How many informaticians do we need? There is no research to quantify this, although a variety of leaders have called for certain numbers of them. In the US, AMIA leaders Drs. Charles Safran and Don Detmer have advocated that there should be at least one physician and one nurse trained in medical informatics in each of the 6,000 hospitals in the US [43]. Likewise, Dr. Charles Friedman, Deputy Director of the Office of the National Coordinator for Health IT has called for 1,000 public health informaticians to be trained based on estimates needed in federal, state, and local public health organizations [44](Keynote Address, Public Health Information Network, August 26, 2007).

Even if we do not have a quantitative handle on the medical informatics workforce, we can define a framework of informatics practice. Table 1 shows an adaptation of a framework originally developed by Covvey et al. [40] used to define job and role competencies. Their original categories included academic/research and applied/professional practitioners (along with the clinical and biomedical research practitioners, whom we omit from this discussion that is focused on the HIT workforce). An additional category of practice added to the framework, seen increasingly in clinical settings, is the local liaison who provides a bridge between the IT staff and clinical users and who represents the user community.

Table 1 - Categories of Informatics Practice, adapted from Covvey et al [40].

Level of Practice	Type of Work	Example Job Titles
Academic	Individual who does research and/or teaching in an academic center	- Professor - Scientist or Researcher
Applied	Individual who works in an operational informatics setting for a majority of his or her working time	- Chief Information Officer - Chief Medical or Nursing Information Officer - Project Manager - Developer - Trainer
Liaison	Individual who spends part of his or her working time as a local expert and interface with informatics or information technology professionals	- Chief Medical or Nursing Information Officer - Clinical IT Liaison

4. What Do We Know About Informatics Leaders?

We know even less about those who are informatics leaders. One survey of member of the Association of Medical Directors of Information Systems (AMDIS) in the US found that of the 82 members who replied, few had formal training in informatics and nearly all of them valued of managerial and clinical over technical skills (Conn 2003). Another analysis looked in depth at five CMIOs [29], finding that the skills they reported to be most important in carrying out their jobs were leadership, communication, and consensus-building. They all expressed a desire to be part of senior physician executive team and did not want to be see as just "techie" doctors.

Another survey of CMIOs was carried out by Gartner and AMDIS [45]. Of the 47 respondents, 70% were employed in integrated delivery organizations. About 38% worked as CMIO full-time, another 25% at >75% time, and the remainder for less. The majority of CMIOs reported to CIO and 60% had no one reporting to them. Three-quarters of them still saw patients part-time and believed it was important for CMIOs to do so. Their top priority was to gain value from investment in clinical information systems. Among the factors they reported as being required for their success were executive-level support and strategic commitment of the organization to IT. The most significant obstacles they reported in their jobs were organizational inertia and physician resistance.

Clearly we need to learn more about informatics professionals and leaders. In many organizations, their role is not well-defined [46]. Of note in the Gartner and AMDIS report[45] is that CMIOs tend not to have reporting relationships to leaders at the highest levels of their organizations, and that they often have no one reporting to them, questioning how much authority they wield in the organizations.

5. What is the Optimal Education of the HIT Workforce?

Just as workforce is one barrier to optimal use of HIT, there are also barriers to educating that workforce. In addition to the problems of unknown needs cited above, their evolving professional status, and a lack of known best practices for their optimal deployment, we also do not have a clear view of the ideal levels of education and most important competencies to teach such individuals. In recognition of the need to promote awareness of the workforce challenges and increase visibility needed, AMIA and AHIMA held a summit in late 2005 that was followed by a report (Anonymous 2006). The report noted the benefits of HIT would not accrue to the US on a wide scale without a well-trained workforce to implement systems. The report advocated:

- Adopting the Institute of Medicine (IOM) "Quality Chasm" [47] vision
- Creating incentives to adopt "systems" that promote quality through use of HIT
- Establishing industry-wide advocacy for workforce training and development
- Building awareness of the need for workforce development
- Utilizing innovative learning environments to train the workforce
- Developing formal educational programs and promoting their value
- Disseminating tools and best practices for these new professionals to succeed

The IOM, which is a high-profile advocate for improving health care in the US, also sees an important role for informatics, designating it as one of three core competencies required for patient-centered care, along with employing evidence-based practice and applying quality improvement [48]. The competences of individual informatics educational programs are less well developed, but were recently analyzed and determined to be quite diverse [49]. Of course, this will likely change as the workforce and the discipline are better characterized.

The optimal education of the HIT workforce is another gap in our knowledge. Not only do we lack good characterization of the workforce as described above, but we cannot even begin to understand its ideal educational criteria. Despite that, informatics educational programs are growing in size and stature. There are comprehensive Web sites that list and link to such programs internationally (http://www.hiww.org/) and in the US (http://www.amia.org/informatics/acad&training/).

These sites demonstrate that there are many models for such training. For example, training in the US, UK, and Canada tends to focus at the graduate level (with some notable exceptions), whereas there are many baccalaureate programs in Germany. Likewise, there is a growing use of distance learning in many programs. Many national medical informatics societies address educational issues for their members and students, and the International Medical Informatics Association (IMIA) has a Working Group on Education devoted to worldwide issues (http://imiawged.pbwiki.com/FrontPage).

Based on the needs in the US advocated by Safran and Detmer [44] quoted above, AMIA launched the 10x10 program, which aims to train 10,000 health care professionals (clinicians and others) in biomedical informatics by the year 2010 [50]. As of mid-2008, the program had provided an in-depth introductory course in biomedical informatics to about 500 individuals. Of course, a single course is not enough to educate a full-scope professional in informatics, but about 15% of those completing the 10x10 program have gone on for further study (unpublished data, Oregon Health & Science University).

There is no dearth of published competencies in health informatics, both for informatics professionals as well as health care professionals. Table 2 provides a list of these competencies, including their year published and targeted professional group.

Table 2 - Inventory of Competencies in Health and Biomedical Informatics.

Organization (Reference)	Year	Discipline
Association for Computing Machinery [51]	1978	Computer science
German Association for Medical Informatics, Biometry and Epidemiology [52]	1992	Informatics
Association of American Medical Colleges [53]	1999	Medical students
University of Pittsburgh Center for Dental Informatics [54]	1999	Dentistry
International Medical Informatics Association [55]	2000	Informatics
UK National Health Service [56]	2001	Informatics
American Nurses Association [57]	2001	Nursing
University of Waterloo, Canada [41]	2001	Informatics
Northwest Center for Public Health Practice [58]	2002	Public health professionals
American Association of Critical-Care Nurses [59]	2003	Nurse Practitioners
American College of Medical Informatics [60]	2004	Bioinformatics
Commission on Accreditation for Health Informatics and Information Management Education [61]	2005	Health Information Management
Commission on Accreditation for Health Informatics and Information Management Education [62]	2005	Health Information Management
Australian College of Health Informatics [63]	2006	Informatics
Journal of Internet Research [64]	2006	"Information age" students
Medical Library Association [65]	2007	Health Science Librarians
University of Washington Center for Public Health Informatics [66]	2007	Public Health Informatics
Methods of Information in Medicine [67]	2007	Informatics
AMIA 10x10 [68]	2008	Informatics

6.   Conclusions

There is growing evidence of the importance of a competent workforce for successful HIT implementation. There are also substantial opportunities in the three major types of professional in IT, HIM, and BMI. These jobs tend to pay well and offer opportunity for career advancement and satisfaction. Indeed, one US newsmagazine recently listed informatics among ten "ahead of the curve" careers [69]. However, both health care leaders and informatics leaders need more information upon which to base implementation of systems, optimal deployment of the workforce, and the best educational options for the workforce.

There is a need for more research to better characterize the workforce of those who develop, implement, and evaluate HIT systems. This will then better inform the development of optimal competencies and curricula for their most effective education and training. Workforce research must go beyond the narrow focus of single groups (e.g., IT staff, HIM professionals, or clinicians) or applications (e.g., EHRs or health information exchanges). Instead, it must focus on the larger picture of all involved in supporting the use of information to improve human health. More effort should also be devoted to establishing occupational coding classifications for informatics jobs and promoting the profession to attract those with passion and competence for it. Additional work must focus on other areas of health and biomedical informatics (such as clinical research informatics, public health informatics, and bioinformatics) as well as other areas of the world (especially outside the US and Europe).

References

[1]   Chaudhry B, et al., *Systematic review: impact of health information technology on quality, efficiency, and costs of medical care.* Annals of Internal Medicine, 2006. 144: 742-752.
[2]   Garg AX, et al., *Effects of computerized clinical decision support systems on practitioner performance and patient outcomes: a systematic review.* Journal of the American Medical Association, 2005. 293: 1223-1238.
[3]   Hersh WR, et al., *Diagnosis, access, and outcomes: update of a systematic review on telemedicine services.* Journal of Telemedicine & Telecare, 2006. 12(Supp 2): 3-31.
[4]   Lorenzi NM, *E-Health Strategies Worldwide*, in *Yearbook of Medical Informatics 2005*, Haux R and Kulikowski C, Editors. 2005, Schattauer: Stuttgart, Germany. 157-164.
[5]   Payne PR, et al., *Breaking the translational barriers: the value of integrating biomedical informatics and translational research.* Journal of Investigative Medicine, 2005. 53: 192-200.
[6]   Zerhouni EA, *Translational research: moving discovery to practice.* Clinical Pharmacology and Therapeutics, 2007. 81: 126-128.
[7]   Baxevanis AD and Ouellette BFF, *Bioinformatics: A Practical Guide to the Analysis of Genes and Proteins, Third Edition.* 2005, Hoboken, NJ: Wiley-Interscience.
[8]   Hersh W, *Health care information technology: progress and barriers.* Journal of the American Medical Association, 2004. 292: 2273-2274.
[9]   Poon EG, et al., *Overcoming barriers to adopting and implementing computerized physician order entry systems in U.S. hospitals.* Health Affairs, 2004. 23: 184-190.
[10] Anonymous, *Building the Work Force for Health Information Transformation.* 2006, American Health Information Management Association and American Medical Informatics Association: Chicago, IL and Bethesda, MD, http://www.ahima.org/emerging_issues/Workforce_web.pdf.
[11] Hersh WR, *Who are the informaticians? What we know and should know.* Journal of the American Medical Informatics Association, 2006. 13: 166-170.
[12] Perlin JB and Gelinas LS, *Electronic Health Records Workgroup Recommendations.* 2008, American Health Information Community: Washington, DC, http://www.hhs.gov/healthit/documents/m20080115/09-ehr_recs_ltr.html.

[13] Han YY, et al., *Unexpected increased mortality after implementation of a commercially sold computerized physician order entry system.* Pediatrics, 2005. 116: 1506-1512.

[14] Phibbs CS, et al., *No proven link between CPOE and mortality.* Pediatrics, 2005. http://pediatrics.aappublications.org/cgi/eletters/116/6/1506.

[15] Sittig DF, et al., *Lessons from "unexpected increased mortality after implementation of a commercially sold computerized physician order entry system".* Pediatrics, 2006. 118: 797-801.

[16] DelBeccaro MA, et al., *Computerized provider order entry implementation: no association with increased mortality rates in an intensive care unit.* Pediatrics, 2006. 118: 290-295.

[17] Longhurst C, et al., *Perceived increase in mortality after process and policy changes implemented with computerized physician order entry.* Pediatrics, 2006. 117: 1450-1451.

[18] Jacobs BR, Brilli RJ, and Hart KW, *Perceived increase in mortality after process and policy changes implemented with computerized physician order entry.* Pediatrics, 2006. 117: 1451-1452.

[19] Rosenbloom ST, et al., *Perceived increase in mortality after process and policy changes implemented with computerized physician order entry.* Pediatrics, 2006. 117: 1452-1455.

[20] Monegain B, *Healthcare IT: is it a breed apart?*, Healthcare IT News. September, 2004. 4. http://www.healthcareitnews.com/story.cms?id=1522.

[21] Sable JH, Hales JW, and Bopp KD. *Medical informatics in healthcare organizations: a survey of healthcare information managers.* Proceedings of the AMIA 2000 Annual Symposium. 2000. Los Angeles, CA: Hanley & Belfus. 745-748.

[22] Eyster KM, *Career counseling: 101+ things you can do with a degree in biology.* Advances in Physiology Education, 2007. 31: 323-328.

[23] Roberts J, *Developing health informatics as a recognised professional domain supporting clinical and health management activity.* World Hospitals and Health Services, 2006. 42(4): 38-40.

[24] Joyub R, *The Professionalisation of Health Informatics in the United Kingdom,* UK Health Informatics Today. Spring, 2004. 42: 1-2, 4. http://www.bmis.org/ebmit/2004_42_spring.pdf.

[25]. Anonymous, *Standard Occupational Classification (SOC) User Guide.* 2004, US Department of Labor - Bureau of Labor Statistics: Washington, DC, http://www.bls.gov/soc/socguide.htm.

[26] Arbuckle DR, *Standard Occupational Classification - Revision for 2010; Notice.* 2006, Federal Register: Washington, DC. 28536-28538, http://www.bls.gov/soc/soc_may06.pdf.

[27] DalPoz MR, et al., *Counting health workers: definitions, data, methods and global results,* in *Background Paper for the World Health Report 2006.* 2006, World Health Organization: Geneva, Switzerland, http://www.who.int/hrh/documents/counting_health_workers.pdf.

[28] Eardley T, *NHS Informatics Workforce Survey.* 2006, ASSIST: London, England, http://www.bcs.org/upload/pdf/finalreport_20061120102537.pdf.

[29] Leviss J, Kremsdorf R, and Mohaideen MF, *The CMIO - a new leader for health systems.* journal of the American Medical Informatics Association, 2006. 13: 573-578.

[30] Shaffer V and Lovelock J, *Results of the 2006 Gartner-AMDIS Survey of CMIOs: Bridging Healthcare's Transforming Waters.* 2007, Gartner: Stamford, CT, http://www.gartner.com/DisplayDocument?ref=g_search&id=504632.

[31] Ash JS, et al., *Implementing computerized physician order entry: the importance of special people.* International Journal of Medical Informatics, 2003. 69: 235-250.

[32] Gabler J, *2003 Integrated Delivery System IT Budget and Staffing Study Results.* 2003, Gartner Corp.: Stamford, CT.

[33] Hersh WR and Wright A, *Characterizing the Health Information Technology Workforce: Analysis from the HIMSS Analytics™ Database.* 2008, Oregon Health & Science University: Portland, OR, http://www.billhersh.info/hit-workforce-hersh.pdf.

[34] Anonymous, *The EHR Adoption Model.* 2007, Healthcare Information Management and Systems Society: Chicago, IL, http://www.himssanalytics.org/docs/EMRAM_att_corrected.pdf.

[35] Wing P, et al., *Data for Decisions: the HIM Workforce and Workplace - 2002 Member Survey.* 2003, American Health Information Management Association: Chicago, IL, http://library.ahima.org/xpedio/groups/public/documents/ahima/bok1_018947.pdf.

[36] Anonymous, *Nationwide Health Information Network (NHIN) Workforce Study.* 2007, Altarum Institute: Ann Arbor, MI, http://aspe.hhs.gov/sp/reports/2007/NHIN/NHINReport.pdf.

[37] Anonymous, *2006 HIMSS Compensation Survey.* 2007, Healthcare Information Management Systems Society: Chicago, IL, http://www.himss.org/surveys/compensation/docs/CompensationSurvey2006.pdf.

[38] Marietti C, Kirby J, and Bennet S, *What Are Healthcare IT Professionals Worth? A Look at Healthcare IT Salaries.* 2007, Healthcare Informatics: New York, NY.

[39] Anonymous, *2006 Salary Study.* 2006, American Health Information Management Association: Chicago, IL, http://www.ahima.org/membership/member_profile_data.asp.

[40] Knaup P, et al., *Medical informatics specialists: what are their job profiles? Results of a study on the first 1024 medical informatics graduates of the Universities of Heidelberg and Heilbronn.* Methods of Information in Medicine, 2003. 42: 578-587.

[41] Covvey HD, Zitner D, and Bernstein R, *Pointing the Way: Competencies and Curricula in Health Informatics.* 2001, University of Waterloo: Waterloo, Ontario, Canada, http://www.cs.uwaterloo.ca/health_info/health_docs/CurriculaMASTERDocumentVersion1Final.zip.

[42] Hoffmann S and Ash J. *A survey of academic and industry professionals regarding the preferred skillset of graduates of medical informatics programs.* MEDINFO 2001 - Proceedings of the Tenth World Congress on Medical Informatics. 2001. London, England: IOS Press. 1028-1032.

[43] Patton GA and Gardner RM, *Medical informatics education: the University of Utah experience.* Journal of the American Medical Informatics Association, 1999. 6: 457-465.

[44] Safran C and Detmer DE, *Computerized physician order entry systems and medication errors.* Journal of the American Medical Association, 2005. 294: 179.

[45] Conn J, *In IT, it pays to think big - survey puts metrics to medical informatics*, Modern Physician. 7: 18-19 2007.

[46] Hersher B, *The essential skills for the Chief Medical Information Officer.* Journal of Healthcare Information Management, 2003. 17(1): 10-11.

[47] Anonymous, *Crossing the Quality Chasm: A New Health System for the 21st Century.* 2001, Washington, DC: National Academy Press.

[48] Greiner AC and Knebel E, eds. *Health Professions Education: A Bridge to Quality.* 2003, National Academy Press: Washington, DC.

[49] Huang QR, *Competencies for graduate curricula in health, medical and biomedical informatics: a framework.* Health Informatics Journal, 2007. 13: 89-103.

[50] Hersh W and Williamson J, *Educating 10,000 informaticians by 2010: the AMIA 10×10 program.* International Journal of Medical Informatics, 2007. 76: 377-382.

[51] Duncan KA, et al. *Health Computing: Curriculum for an emerging profession - report of the ACM curriculum committee on health computing education. Proceedings of the 1978 ACM Annual Conference/Annual Meeting.* 1978. Washington, DC: ACM Press. 277-285. http://portal.acm.org/ft_gateway.cfm?id=804112&type=pdf&coll=GUIDE&dl=GUIDE&CFID=47975758&CFTOKEN=19987037.

[52] Haux R, et al., *Recommendations of the German Association for Medical Informatics, Biometry and Epidemiology for education and training in medical informatics.* Methods of Information in Medicine, 1992. 31: 60-70.

[53] Anonymous, *Medical School Objectives Project: Medical Informatics Objectives.* 1999, Association of American Medical Colleges: Washington, DC, http://www.aamc.org/meded/msop/start.htm.

[54] Schleyer T, *Competencies for Dental Informatics V 1.0.* 1999, University of Pittsburgh Center for Dental Informatics: Pittsburgh, PA, http://www.dental.pitt.edu/informatics/competencies.php.

[55] Anonymous, *Recommendations of the International Medical Informatics Association (IMIA) on education in health and medical informatics.* Methods of Information in Medicine, 2000. 39: 267-277. http://www.imia.org/pubdocs/rec_english.pdf.

[56] Anonymous, *Health Informatics Competency Profiles for the NHS.* 2001, National Health Service Information Authority: London, England, http://www.nhsia.nhs.uk/nhid/pages/resource_informatics/hi_competencyprofiles.pdf.

[57] Staggers N, Gassert CA, and Curran C, *A Delphi study to determine informatics competencies at four levels of practice.* Nursing Research, 2002. 51: 383-390.

[58] O'Carroll PW, *Informatics Competencies for Public Health Professionals.* 2002, Northwest Center for Public Health Practice: Seattle, WA, http://healthlinks.washington.edu/nwcphp/phi/comps/phi_print.pdf.

[59] Curran CR, *Informatics competencies for nurse practitioners.* AACN Clinical Issues, 2003. 14: 320-330.

[60] Friedman CP, et al., *Training the next generation of informaticians: the impact of 'BISTI' and bioinformatics; a report from the American College of Medical Informatics.* Journal of the American Medical Informatics Association, 2004. 11: 167-172.

[61] Anonymous, *Standards for Health Information Management Education - Baccalaureate Degree Program Standards.* 2005, Commission on Accreditation for Health Informatics and Information Management Education (CAHIIM): Chicago, IL, http://library.ahima.org/xpedio/groups/public/documents/accreditation/bok1_026307.pdf.

[62] Anonymous, *Standards for Health Information Management Education - Associate Degree Program Standards.* 2005, Commission on Accreditation for Health Informatics and Information Management Education (CAHIIM): Chicago, IL, http://library.ahima.org/xpedio/groups/public/documents/accreditation/bok1_026306.pdf.

[63] Garde S and Hovenga E, *Australian Health Informatics Educational Framework*. 2006, Australian College of Health Informatics: Brunswick East, Australia, http://www.achi.org.au/documents/publications/Health_Informatics_Educational_Framework_200603 26.pdf.

[64] Ivanitskaya L, O'Boyle I, and Casey AM, *Health information literacy and competencies of information age students: results from the interactive online Research Readiness Self-Assessment (RRSA).* Journal of Medical Internet Research, 2006. 8(2): e6. http://www.jmir.org/2006/2/e6/.

[65] Anonymous, *Health Information Science Knowledge and Skills*. 2007, Medical Library Association: Chicago, IL, http://www.mlanet.org/education/platform/skills.html.

[66] Karras B, *Public Health Informatics Competencies*. 2007, Center for Public Health Informatics: Seattle, WA, http://cphi.washington.edu/competencies.

[67] Pigott K, et al., *An informatics benchmarking statement.* Methods of Information in Medicine, 2007. 46: 394-398.

[68] Hersh W, *Course Description - AMIA-OHSU 10x10 Course*. 2008, American Medical Informatics Association: Bethesda, MD, http://www.amia.org/10x10/partners/ohsu/description.asp.

[69] Nemko M, *Ahead-of-the-Curve Careers*, US News & World Report. December 19, 2007. http://www.usnews.com/articles/business/best-careers/2007/12/19/ahead-of-the-curve-careers.html.

Review Questions

1. What is the value health information technology and why do we need well-trained HIT professionals?

2. What are typical roles of Health Informaticians and how should their education look like?

3. What are the characteristics of the current HI workforce?

Health Informatics
E.J.S. Hovenga et al. (Eds.)
IOS Press, 2010

Subject Index

Author Index